The Social Science of the
COVID-19 Pandemic

The Social Science of the COVID-19 Pandemic

A Call to Action for Researchers

EDITED BY **MONICA K. MILLER**

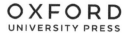

OXFORD
UNIVERSITY PRESS

Oxford University Press is a department of the University of Oxford. It furthers
the University's objective of excellence in research, scholarship, and education
by publishing worldwide. Oxford is a registered trade mark of Oxford University
Press in the UK and certain other countries.

Published in the United States of America by Oxford University Press
198 Madison Avenue, New York, NY 10016, United States of America.

Library of Congress Cataloging-in-Publication Data
Names: Miller, Monica K., editor.
Title: The social science of the COVID-19 Pandemic : a call to action for researchers /
edited by Monica K. Miller.
Description: New York, NY : Oxford University Press, [2024] |
Includes bibliographical references. |
Identifiers: LCCN 2023032667 (print) | LCCN 2023032668 (ebook) |
ISBN 9780197615133 (hardback) | ISBN 9780197615157 (epub) | ISBN 9780197615164 |
Subjects: LCSH: COVID-19 Pandemic, 2020—Social aspects. |
COVID-19 Pandemic, 2020—Research.
Classification: LCC RA644.C67 S62295 2024 (print) |
LCC RA644.C67 (ebook) | DDC 362.1962/4144–dc23/eng/20230921
LC record available at https://lccn.loc.gov/2023032667
LC ebook record available at https://lccn.loc.gov/2023032668

DOI: 10.1093/oso/9780197615133.001.0001

Printed by Sheridan Books, Inc., United States of America

This book is dedicated to those most affected by COVID-19. Although there is likely not a single person on Earth who was not affected by the pandemic, several groups bore the brunt of the pandemic. First, this book is dedicated to the memory of the millions of victims of COVID-19. Second, the book honors those on the front line: medical personnel and researchers and others who worked tirelessly to fight the good fight against COVID-19. Finally, to those who suffered mental health challenges—and it is hoped rose above them—due to the pandemic. May the trials of the pandemic make us all stronger, as individuals and as a society.

CONTENTS

Section Three: Experiences During the Pandemic

Section Four: Outcomes After the Pandemic

Section Five: Conducting COVID-19 Pandemic Research

PREFACE

The idea for this book arose when I was at home during lockdown in the early days of the pandemic. As experts made dire predictions about the loss of life and the lengthy battle that lay ahead, it became clear that COVID-19 was going to be a fierce adversary. The effects of the pandemic were immediate and wide-reaching, touching the lives of every human on Earth. As I started brainstorming the ways that social science and the pandemic interacted, the book began to take shape. It was immediately clear that "The Social Science of the Pandemic" was a broad and multifaceted topic to tackle. But, the team was up to the challenge. Authors from at least 20 different countries came together to create this book. Their perspectives were all unique, drawing on their own background, expertise, and sometimes their own pandemic research. Through countless conversations with dozens of researchers, this book proposal came to life.

Writing a book chapter, editing a book, and publishing a book are big undertakings in general. Doing so during a pandemic—while learning to juggle one's other duties (teaching, administration) online and at home, and while personally experiencing COVID and/or caring for those experiencing COVID—is even more impressive. Our team tackled countless societal and personal challenges over 2 years to make this book a reality.

There are many people I need to thank because, without them, this book would not exist. First, thanks to the chapter authors who provided ideas that shaped the book, wrote these intriguing chapters, and made changes without complaint. Additionally, I'd like to thank Sarah Harrington at Oxford University Press who helped polish up the proposal and offered helpful advice at every phase. Her patience and dedication to this project are remarkable. Thanks also to all the reviewers who made helpful suggestions that certainly improved the book. Finally, thanks to the publishing and production team at Oxford University Press who helped make the book a beautiful reality that arose out of an ugly pandemic.

I'm proud of this team of hard-working professionals. We hope readers find our perspectives on the pandemic interesting and useful. May future researchers use this book as a starting point to challenge and expand the ideas it contains.

LIST OF FIGURES

LIST OF TABLES

CONTRIBUTORS LIST

Maria Babińska, MA, Faculty of Psychology, University of Warsaw, Poland

Ella Selak Bagarić, MA, Clinical psychologist, Zagreb Child and Youth Protection Center, Zagreb, Croatia

Andrea Bayer, JD, PhD, Department of Human Development and Family Science, University of Nevada, Reno, Nevada, USA

Emily R. Berthelot, PhD, Associate Professor, Department of Criminal Justice and Interdisciplinary Social Psychology PhD Program, University of Nevada, Reno, Nevada, USA

Michał Bilewicz, PhD, Faculty of Psychology, University of Warsaw, Poland

Hartmut Blank, Department of Psychology, University of Portsmouth, United Kingdom

Paulo S. Boggio, Mackenzie Presbyterian University, São Paulo, Brazil

Robert Böhm, Department of Psychology and Department of Economics, University of Copenhagen, Denmark; Copenhagen Center for Social Data Science (SODAS), University of Copenhagen, Denmark

Breanna Boppre, PhD, Assistant Professor, Department of Victim Studies, Sam Houston State University, Huntsville, Texas, USA

Rosita Borlimi, PhD, PsyD, Full Professor, Department of Psychology, Sigmund Freud University, Milan, Italy

Brian H. Bornstein, PhD, Research Professor, Arizona State University, Tempe, Arizona, USA; Professor Emeritus, University of Nebraska–Lincoln, Nebraska, USA

Susan G. Bornstein, MD, MPH, Assistant Professor, Health Promotion and Behavioral Sciences, University of Louisville School of Public Health and Information Sciences, Louisville, Kentucky, USA

Tea Brezinšćak, MA, Head of Diagnostics and Treatment Department, Zagreb Child and Youth Protection Center, Zagreb, Croatia

Gianni Brighetti, Full Professor, Department of Psychology, Sigmund Freud University, Milan, Italy

Melissa M. Burnham, PhD, Professor, Human Development, Family Science, College of Education and Human Development, University of Nevada, Reno, Nevada, USA

Jean J. Cabell, MA, PhD candidate, Interdisciplinary Social Psychology PhD Program, University of Nevada, Reno, Nevada, USA

Rachel Calogero, PhD, Professor, Department of Psychology, Western University, London, Ontario, Canada

Valerio Capraro, Economics Department, Middlesex University, London, United Kingdom

Ricky Y. K. Chan, PhD, Department of Marketing, Auckland University of Technology, Auckland, New Zealand

Becky Choma, PhD, Associate Professor, Department of Psychology, Ryerson University, Toronto, Ontario, Canada

Chris Cocking, PhD, School of Humanities and Applied Social Sciences, University of Brighton, Brighton, United Kingdom

Marzena Cypryańska, PhD, Assistant Professor, Center for Climate Action and Social Transformations, SWPS University of Social Sciences and Humanities, Warsaw, Poland

Lydia DeFlorio, PhD, Associate Professor in Human Development and Family Science, College of Education and Human Development, University of Nevada, Reno, Nevada, USA

Paul G. Devereux, PhD, MPH, Professor, School of Public Health and Interdisciplinary Social Psychology PhD Program, University of Nevada, Reno, Nevada, USA

James N. Druckman, Professor of Political Science, Department of Political Science, Northwestern University, Evanston, Illinois, USA

Megan Earle, MA, PhD candidate, Department of Psychology, Brock University, St. Catharines, Ontario, Canada

Samuel E. Ehrenreich, PhD, Assistant Professor, Department of Human Development and Family Science, University of Nevada, Reno, Nevada, USA

A. Christine Emler, MD, MHCM, Deputy Chief of Staff, Durham VA Medical Center, Assistant Professor, Department of Medicine, Duke University School of Medicine, Durham, North Carolina, USA

Kayley D. Estes, MA, PhD student, Department of Psychological Science, University of California, Irvine, California, USA

Victoria Estrada-Reynolds, PhD, Assistant Professor, Department of Psychology, King's College, Wilkes-Barre, Pennsylvania, USA

Pamela M. Everett, JD, Teaching Associate Professor, Department of Criminal Justice, University of Nevada, Reno, Nevada, USA

Gordana Buljan Flander, PhD, Clinical Psychologist, Zagreb Child and Youth Protection Center, Zagreb, Croatia

Kayla Furlano, BA, Interdisciplinary Social Psychology PhD Program, University of Nevada, Reno, Nevada, USA

Dana Rose Garfin, PhD, Assistant Adjunct Professor, Sue and Bill Gross School of Nursing, Program in Public Health, University of California, Irvine, California, USA

Michele J. Gelfand, Stanford Graduate School of Business, Stanford University, Stanford, California, USA

Biljana Gjoneska, MD, PhD, Research Associate, Macedonian Academy of Science and Arts, Skopje, North Macedonia

Jeff Greenberg, PhD, Regents Professor, Department of Psychology, University of Arizona, Tucson, Arizona, USA

Molly M. Hagen, MS, Doctoral student in Epidemiology, School of Public Health, University of Nevada, Reno, Nevada, USA

Sarah Y. T. Hartzell, MA, Doctoral student in Social and Behavioral Health, School of Public Health, University of Nevada, Reno, Nevada, USA

Dylan E. Horner, PhD, Assistant Professor of Psychology, Department of Addiction Studies, Psychology, and Social Work, Minot State University, Minot, North Dakota, USA

Samantha Hughes, MSc, PhD candidate, Department of Psychological Sciences, HERA Lab, University of Gloucestershire, Gloucestershire, United Kingdom

Alma Jeftić, PhD, Postdoc, Department of Cross-cultural and Regional Studies, University of Copenhagen, Denmark; Research Fellow, Peace Research Institute, International Christian University, Tokyo, Japan

Vjekoslav Jeleč, MD, PhD, Neurosurgeon, Department of Neurosurgery, Dubrava University Hospital, Zagreb, Croatia

Eva Jonas, PhD, Full Professor, Department of Psychology, University of Salzburg, Salzburg, Austria

Chiara A. Jutzi, MSc, PhD candidate, Department of Psychology, University of Salzburg, Salzburg, Austria

Jungkeun Kim, PhD, Department of Marketing, Auckland University of Technology, Auckland, New Zealand

Elaine Kinsella, MSc, PhD, Department of Psychology, University of Limerick, Republic of Ireland

Shinobu Kitayama, PhD, Department of Psychology, University of Michigan, Ann Arbor, Michigan, USA

Alex Landry, Stanford Graduate School of Business, Stanford University, Stanford, California, USA

Justin F. Landy, PhD, Assistant Professor, Department of Psychology and Neuroscience, Nova Southeastern University, Fort Lauderdale–Davie, Florida, USA

Jennifer L. Lanterman, PhD, University of Nevada, Reno, Nevada, USA

Sarah Lemon, MSc, PhD candidate, Department of Psychological Sciences, HERA Lab, University of Gloucestershire, Gloucestershire, United Kingdom

Jennifer Lin, PhD student, Department of Political Science, Northwestern University, Evanston, Illinois, USA

Andrew Luttrell, PhD, Assistant Professor, Department of Psychology, Ball State University, Muncie, Indiana, USA

Katarzyna Luzynska, MSc, School of Psychology and Life Sciences, Canterbury Christ Church University, Canterbury, United Kingdom

Roger Marshall, PhD, Department of Marketing, Auckland University of Technology, Auckland, New Zealand

Igor Mikloušić, PhD, Research Associate, Institute of Social Sciences Ivo Pilar, Zagreb, Croatia

Monica K. Miller, JD, PhD, Foundation Professor, Interdisciplinary Social Psychology PhD Program and Department of Criminal Justice, University of Nevada, Reno, Nevada, USA

Jennifer A. Mortensen, PhD, CFLE, Assistant Professor in Human Development and Family Science, College of Education and Human Development, University of Nevada, Reno, Nevada, USA

Steven Mueller, MA, Department of Management, University of Nevada, Reno, Nevada, USA

Evan Murphy, MA, PhD candidate, Interdisciplinary Social Psychology PhD Program, University of Nevada, Reno, Nevada, USA

Mattia Nese, PhD, Postdoctoral Fellow, Department of Psychology, Sigmund Freud University, Milan, Italy

Evangelos Ntontis, PhD, School of Psychology and Counselling, The Open University, Milton Keynes, United Kingdom

Nickola C. Overall, PhD, Professor, School of Psychology, University of Auckland, Auckland, New Zealand

Xinyue Pan, Department of Psychology, University of Maryland, College Park, Maryland, USA

Jooyoung Park, PhD, Department of Management, Peking University HSBC Business School, Shenzhen, China

Clayton D. Peoples, PhD, Interdisciplinary Social Psychology PhD Program, University of Nevada, Reno, Nevada, USA; Department of Sociology, University of Nevada, Reno, Nevada, USA

Matjaž Perc, Faculty of Natural Sciences and Mathematics, University of Maribor, Maribor, Slovenia; Complexity Science Hub Vienna, Vienna, Austria; Department of Medical Research, China Medical University Hospital, China Medical University, Taichung, Taiwan; Alma Mater Europaea, Maribor, Slovenia

Alexander D. Perry, BA, MS candidate in Experimental Psychology, Department of Psychology and Neuroscience, Nova Southeastern University, Fort Lauderdale–Davie, Florida, USA

Richard E. Petty, PhD, Distinguished University Professor, Department of Psychology, Ohio State University, Columbus, Ohio, USA

Paula R. Pietromonaco, PhD, Professor Emerita, Department of Psychological and Brain Sciences, University of Massachusetts, Amherst, Massachusetts, USA

Elvira Prusaczyk, MA, Assistant Professor of Psychology, St. Francis Xavier University, Antigonish, Nova Scotia, Canada

Theron Pummer, PhD, Senior Lecturer, School of Philosophical, Anthropological, and Film Studies, University of St. Andrews, St. Andrews, United Kingdom

Tom Pyszczynski, PhD, Distinguished Professor, Department of Psychology, University of Colorado at Colorado Springs, Colorado Springs, Colorado, USA

Antti Revonsuo, PhD, Professor, Department of Psychology and Speech-Language Pathology, University of Turku, Turku, Finland; Department of Cognitive Neuroscience and Philosophy, University of Skövde, Skövde, Sweden

Greta Riboli, MSc, PhD candidate, Sigmund Freud Privat Universitat, Vienna, Austria

Jon Roozenbeek, PhD, Research Associate, Department of Psychology, University of Cambridge, Cambridge, United Kingdom

Toshiaki Sasao, PhD, Professor, Department of Education and Language Education, International Christian University, Tokyo, Japan

Valentina Sassi, MSc, Trainee psychologist, Department of Psychology, Sigmund Freud University, Milan, Italy

Petra C. Schmid, PhD, Assistant Professor, Department of Management, Technology, and Economics, Swiss Federal Institute of Technology (ETH Zurich), Zurich, Switzerland

Philipp Schoenegger, PhD, Post-Doc, London School of Economics and Political Science, Department of Management, United Kingdom

Sam Scott, PhD, Senior Lecturer in Human Geography, Department of Natural and Social Sciences, University of Gloucestershire, Gloucestershire, United Kingdom

Constantine Sedikides, PhD, Professor of Social and Personality Psychology, Centre for Research on Self and Identity, School of Psychology, University of Southampton, Southampton, United Kingdom

Hugh Shapiro, PhD, Department of History, University of Nevada, Reno, Nevada, USA

Alex Sielaff, BA, PhD student, Department of Psychology, University of Arizona, Tucson, Arizona, USA

Joseph J. Siev, MA, PhD candidate, Department of Psychology, Ohio State University, Columbus, Ohio, USA

Hallgeir Sjåstad, Department of Strategy and Management, Norwegian School of Economics, Bergen, Norway

Angela Spires, MFA, MA, Instructor of English, College of Southern Nevada, Las Vegas, Nevada, USA

Yvonne Stedham, PhD, Interdisciplinary Social Psychology PhD Program, University of Nevada, Reno, Nevada, USA; Department of Management, University of Nevada, Reno, Nevada, USA

Natasha Stonebridge, MSc, PhD candidate, Department of Psychological Sciences, HERA Lab, University of Gloucestershire, Gloucestershire, United Kingdom

Rachel Sumner, MSc, PhD, Health and Human Performance Global Academy, Cardiff Metropolitan University, Cardiff, United Kingdom

Jarno Tuominen, MA, Senior Researcher, Department of Psychology and Speech-Language Pathology, University of Turku, Finland

Michael Tyrala, PhD, Postdoctoral Fellow, Institute for Emerging Market Studies, The Hong Kong University of Science and Technology, Hong Kong

Mete Sefa Uysal, MSc, Independent Researcher, Turkey

Emir Üzümçeker, MSc, Psychology Department, Dokuz Eylül University, Izmir, Turkey

Katja Valli, PhD, Associate Professor, Department of Psychology and Speech-Language Pathology, University of Turku, Turku, Finland; Department of Cognitive Neuroscience and Philosophy, University of Skövde, Skövde, Sweden

Sander van der Linden, PhD, Professor of Social Psychology in Society, Department of Psychology, University of Cambridge, Cambridge, United Kingdom

Bryce Van Vleet, BA, Department of Human Development and Family Science, North Dakota State University, Fargo, North Dakota, USA

Sara Vestergren, PhD, Psychology Department, Keele University, Newcastle, United Kingdom

Matthew P. West, PhD, Assistant Professor, School of Justice and Public Safety, Southern Illinois University Carbondale, Carbondale, Illinois, USA

Sara V. White, BA, PhD candidate, Department of Clinical Psychology, State University of New York, Albany, New York, USA

Tim Wildschut, PhD, Professor of Social and Personality Psychology, Centre for Research on Self and Identity, School of Psychology, University of Southampton, Southampton, United Kingdom

Robin Willardt, MSc, PhD candidate, Department of Management, Technology, and Economics, Swiss Federal Institute of Technology (ETH Zurich), Zurich, Switzerland

Cynthia Willis-Esqueda, PhD, Associate Professor, Department of Psychology, University of Nebraska-Lincoln, Lincoln, Nebraska, USA

Adrian D. Wójcik, PhD, Assistant Professor, Faculty of Philosophy and Social Sciences, Nicolaus Copernicus University, Toruń, Poland

Mengran Xu, PhD, Assistant Professor, School of Management, Fudan University, Shanghai, China

Logan A. Yelderman, PhD, Assistant Professor, Department of Psychology, Prairie View A&M University, Prairie View, Texas, USA

Ethan Zell, PhD, Associate Professor, Department of Psychology, University of North Carolina at Greensboro, Greensboro, North Carolina, USA

The Reciprocal Relationship Between Disease and Society

Historical and Modern Perspectives

MONICA K. MILLER, BRYCE VAN VLEET,
AND HUGH SHAPIRO ■

Disease and society have historically had an uneasy relationship. Society's developments (e.g., global travel, crowded cities, concerts and events with large attendance) shape whether a virus can take hold and spread. And, a virus can bring society to a halt, as it did in the early days of the COVID-19 (coronavirus disease 2019) pandemic. This reciprocal relationship between disease and society prompted the call to action that underlies this book. This introductory chapter outlines both the importance of studying the pandemic from a social science perspective and the challenges that await social scientists who have and will study how society and the pandemic influence each other.

A new virus emerged quietly in the city of Wuhan in China in late 2019, perhaps transmitted from a bat to a human. It soon spread throughout China, forcing the government to take drastic measures, such as compelling inhabitants to stay indoors except for very limited travel—and to wear masks when they did go out. Law enforcement and drones monitored the situation, achieving broad compliance. Makeshift hospitals were built almost overnight to care for those infected. Soon, the virus made its way out of the country in the bodies of unknowing travelers. The first case made its way into the United States in early 2020, at first not garnering much attention from society in general. In early March 2020, Washington State made news after a handful of deaths—most being vulnerable nursing home residents. By then, the United States—and indeed the world—was taking notice.

On February 11, 2020, the World Health Organization named the disease COVID-19. It was named corona because its shape resembles a corona, or crown.

Monica K. Miller, Bryce Van Vleet, and Hugh Shapiro, *The Reciprocal Relationship Between Disease and Society* In: *The Social Science of the COVID-19 Pandemic*. Edited by: Monica K. Miller, Oxford University Press. © Oxford University Press 2024. DOI: 10.1093/oso/9780197615133.003.0001

The underlying virus was called severe acute respiratory syndrome coronavirus 2 (SARS-CoV-2). It thus shares a name with SARS, a virus that swept the globe in 2003, because of their genetic similarities. COVID-19 is often called a "novel coronavirus" because it is just that—something so novel that no one had ever seen it before. Those infected could have symptoms so light that they did not know they were infected; others would die from their infection. Unlike the regular flu virus, COVID-19 could be transmitted for many days before the carrier even knew they were infected; it could live for long periods of time on surfaces; and its R0 (loosely defined as a "transmission rate") was dramatically higher than that of the flu. The World Health Organization first officially called the COVID-19 a pandemic on March 11, 2020. This term is not used lightly: It has been used only a handful times in the last 110 years.

The world has experienced many *epidemics* (i.e., problems that are not as severe as a *pandemic*), including Ebola (2014–2016), SARS (2003), H1N1 influenza (2009–2010) and Zika (2015). Each had a substantial impact on society but was eventually brought under control, and life resumed essentially as it was before. The historical pandemic that arguably affected the United States the most was the 1918 influenza pandemic, which affected nearly a third of the world's population and killed 50 million people. Approximately 675,000 Americans died. However, modern society had never experienced anything like this pandemic until early 2020, when COVID-19 emerged on a global scale.

COVID-19 is remarkable among this list of historical epidemics and pandemics for many reasons: It spread easily due to modern world travel; it spared few areas of the world; it resulted in unprecedented, massive long-term economic consequences; and it was intertwined with politics, as was rarely seen in previous pandemics. What all pandemics and epidemics have in common, however, is that all shaped—and were shaped by—human behavior and other psychosocial factors. COVID-19 has dramatically changed society throughout the world; for example, lockdowns limited travel, and supply shortages caused massive hoarding (see Chapter 2 for detailed descriptions of how society was affected by the pandemic). People's psychological processes shaped the course of the pandemic, as conspiracy beliefs were abundant and antivaxxers and antimaskers caused the pandemic to linger. These are just a few of the examples of the reciprocal relationship between society and the pandemic discussed in this book. By providing a history of the COVID-19 pandemic—and pandemics of the past—it is possible to get a broader understanding of this reciprocal relationship.

The first part of this chapter provides a historical perspective on how past pandemics shaped society/culture, behavior, and way of life. This section is a case study of how the SARS epidemic of 2003 changed the way of life in China—specifically how it gave rise to the habitual use and importance of the Internet. The second part delves into the timeline of the COVID-19 pandemic specifically. This includes many examples of how society was affected by the pandemic. This section documents the pandemic's timeline, which provides a foundation for the rest of the book. The final part of the chapter overviews the contents of the book. These three sections together highlight the importance of the book's purpose—to offer a call to action for researchers to study the relationship between disease, the pandemic, and society.

THE RELATIONSHIP BETWEEN DISEASE AND SOCIETY: A CASE STUDY

A historical perspective on the relationship between disease and society can highlight the magnitude of changes society experiences due to disease—and perhaps help anticipate some of the long-term effects of COVID-19. This part of the chapter provides a foundational and historical perspective on how a past epidemic (SARS) of 2003 shaped one society (China) in one profound way (rise of the Internet). This case study suggests how the current COVID-19 pandemic might have major, lasting effects similar to previous pandemics and epidemics—and provides some context about the importance of studying the social science of a pandemic.

In 2003, as the SARS epidemic broke out, the growth of Internet use in China went from linear to exponential.[1] Today, nearly two decades later, the Internet plays a key role in China's ongoing transformations.[2] Cyberspace is its own ecosystem, impinging on nearly every dimension of daily life. To understand life in 21st-century China, one must understand the role of the internet as a transformative force. This section examines how the rise of the Internet was accelerated by the country's encounter with SARS, and in turn how the how the nature of the Internet in China explains the country's response to COVID-19.

In November 2002, SARS broke out in China's deep south city of Foshan (Guangdong Province), about 80 miles northwest of Hong Kong. Initial investigations were conducted by conscientious local physicians, soon joined by provincial and central government health authorities. These studies were later classified as secret by national authorities, leaving them out of reach of healthcare providers and policymakers, let alone the general public.[3] Naturally, news of the infections spread by informal routes.[4] With the government suppressing news of the outbreak, citizens started going online to find out what was going on.[5] It was in that stressed environment, with large numbers of educated people seeking reliable information on the epidemic and its possible mitigation, that a much less patrolled Internet emerged as a powerful tool for discovering information.

SARS had a second major impact on the Internet in China's daily life: the advent of e-commerce, resulting from the public's desire to stay at home to avoid contact with potentially infected strangers. Thus, the virus created a paradigm shift that can only be described as China's online shopping revolution. The boom in online commerce, or *dianzi shangwu*, began with purchases of food and daily necessities and quickly came to encompass nearly all goods and services. This constituted a major turning point for the Internet in China.[6] Such e-commerce startups as Alibaba grew into some of the world's largest companies. New delivery companies such as Jingdong were developed to service this e-commerce boom. New delivery companies combined sophisticated logistics software and mechanized sorting with a huge fleet of scooters (and later drones) to shorten delivery times from same day to 3 hours—and to 30 minutes for many products.[7]

Not surprisingly, the pervasiveness of the Internet in China's daily life is strongly reflected in the way the government implements its core policy of maintaining social stability, or "stability maintenance" (*weiwen*).[8] The budget for the People's Armed Police (PAP, *wujing*) is larger even than the budget for the nation's armed forces, the People's Liberation Army (PLA).[9] The PLA is oriented outward, internationally, for national defense. In contrast, the PAP is oriented inward, domestically, charged with maintaining order and stability inside China. Within the domestic policing bureaucracy, there exists the Cyberspace Administration of China (CAC), which regulates the Internet.

Nearly 20 years after SARS, the way the COVID-19 pandemic has played out in China illustrates many aspects of the country's relationship with the Internet. When COVID-19 first broke out in China, in early 2020, there were large-scale, short-lived, cell phone-based anonymous collaborations—sort of flash mobs of mass expression. And midnight on one day in January 2020, for instance, a cluster of high-rise apartments coordinated a 1-minute long chant of *Wuhan jiayou*, which is an upbeat, positive phrase roughly translated as "hang tough, Wuhan" or "You're doing great, Wuhan." This flash mob was an expression of support for the 11-million-person city identified as the epicenter of the pandemic.

Not all cell phone-driven flash mobs in early COVID-19 China were so optimistic. In February 2020, another midnight mass expression organized online mourned the death of Dr. Li Wenliang, the Wuhan-based ophthalmologist who warned people of the new virus in late 2019, when few knew of its existence. When Dr. Li first alerted people about the new virus, he was harassed by local police for fomenting rumors. He died of COVID-19 in early February 2020, and his courage and clinical insight are still widely admired. The mass cybermourning of Dr. Li Wenliang was poignant. Organized via cell phone, people stayed at home and remained anonymous. This home-based mass demonstration was first organized via offshore shortwave radio broadcasts in Chile and Uruguay in the early 1980s, in the "breaking-the-silence" protests. Huge numbers of people simultaneously turned out their lights, opened windows, and banged on pots and pans, creating a terrible cacophony.[10]

However, the type of cyberorganized midnight flash mob mourning Dr. Li was uncommon. Very quickly, the authorities won control of the Internet narrative on COVID-19. Internet authorities accomplished this through censorship and by drowning out contrary opinions with a flood of government-endorsed positions, many of which highlighted COVID-19 struggles in other countries, especially the United States.[11] The authorities also silenced specific figures, such as the Wuhan writer, Fang (b. 1955). Fang, already a widely read and respected writer before the pandemic, began a daily blog on January 23, 2020, when Wuhan went into full lockdown. The blog documented both the official response and her personal perceptions. Published daily online, then as a book, Fang Fang's writing led to her being pilloried, censored, and finally denounced as a traitor by anonymous trolls when her *Wuhan Diary: Dispatches From a Quarantined City* was published in translation in the United States in May 2020.

Yet, the story of the Internet and China's battle with COVID-19 is not all dystopic. To the contrary, China's mitigation efforts in handling COVID-19 are extremely successful, and part of that success lies with the imaginative harnessing of the Internet.[12] China was an early adopter of the use of QR codes on cell phones to track COVID-19 status. People must display these QR codes before entering public buildings or spaces such as the subway. For air travel, China implemented dynamic QR codes, embedded with a clock that counts down, showing how much time remains before the negative test no longer allows the person to board a plane. Reverse and contact tracing, telemedicine, and forms of biosurveillance have also been effectively enacted.[13] For sure, mitigation efforts in China also benefit from the state's ability, and willingness, to sustain a strict quarantine policy and to mobilize armies of people to monitor vaccination status and compliance with safety measures. Together with the sophisticated deployment of cybertools, China maintains a robust "ground game."

The profound transformations set in motion by China's embrace of the Internet began with its encounter with SARS in early 2003. Since then, cyberspace has come to impinge on nearly every aspect of life in China. The pivotal role of the Internet in China's daily life is hard to emphasize enough, in not only online, so-cial, and cultural life, but also the public opinion seen in citizen pushback against government policy.

In sum, the SARS epidemic of 2003 transformed society in China in almost unimaginable, enduring ways. This case study is but one example of how a disease can fundamentally alter a country's trajectory. This particular historical perspec-tive suggests that COVID-19 could also shape the society, culture, behavior, and way of life in countries across the globe. Some such long-term social changes are discussed in many chapters throughout the book and in the concluding chapter of this book. This case study of China's experience with SARS emphasizes the im-portance of this book's call to action for researchers to study the social science of the pandemic.

TIMELINE OF THE PANDEMIC

The case study above that detailed how the SARS epidemic of 2003 shaped society in China is one example of the relationship between disease and society. Similarly, COVID-19 is already prompting major societal shifts. This section offers a de-tailed timeline of the major events of the pandemic, up to fall 2021—lest the world forget. The timeline highlights some of the ways the COVID-19 pandemic affected society (this is detailed more specifically in Chapter 2). Whether these changes will be long term is yet to be seen—a topic reserved for the concluding chapter of this volume.

On January 12, 2020, an unknown disease originating from Wuhan, China, was sequenced. The virus was originally named SARS-CoV-2.[14] The first documented case in the United States was on January 20, 2020, in Washington State.[15] Around March 10, the United States began shutting down, 1 day after Italy issued a national lockdown. Music festivals and sport seasons began being cancelled or delayed. U.S. President Donald Trump issued a travel ban for visitors from Europe and assembled a coronavirus task force.[16]

Around March 12, grocery stores around the United States announced shortages of common supplies like toilet paper, hand sanitizer, and disinfectant. Schools started closing down, often for only a couple of weeks and often in conjunction with existing spring breaks. Likewise, businesses advised or required employees to work from home. President Trump and the coronavirus task force advised that Americans avoid gathering in groups of over 10 people. On March 17, seven counties in California's Bay Area issued 3-week stay-at-home orders.[17] Two days later, the entire state of California closed for an unspecified amount of time,[18] and the U.S. State Department issued the highest level warning against global travel.

The situation in America turned dire around March 20. New York City predicted they would run out of medical supplies within 2 weeks, and various states requested military support to house and treat the ill.[19] On March 24, the Summer Olympics were postponed.[20] By April 2, at least 50,000 people globally had died from the coronavirus, with over 1 million confirmed cases globally.[21]

On April 5, U.K. Prime Minister Boris Jonson was admitted to the hospital with a case of COVID-19.[22] By April 12, all 50 U.S. states were under a disaster declaration for the first time in history.[23] Over 2 million people had been diagnosed with COVID-19 globally, with over 119,000 deaths on April 15.[24] On April 20, the price of oil dropped below zero dollars for the first time in history.[25] By April 24, the United States had recorded 50,000 virus-related deaths.

At the end of April, the world had recorded 3 million cases, 1 million of which were in the United States. By May 9, only 9 days later, the global case count had risen to 4 million. Over 300,000 people around the world had died as a result of the virus by May 14. Citing concerns over ties with China, U.S. President Donald Trump withdrew from the World Health Organization, at a time when the United States had 100,000 U.S. deaths and 1.5 million reported COVID-19 cases.[26]

By June 2020, the coronavirus had replicated itself in human beings for at least 9 months and, around June 7, had killed over 400,000 people globally. In Pakistan, hospitals stopped receiving patients due to overcapacity around June 9.[27] On June 24, 36,000 new cases were reported in the United States after some states had reopened. That same day, a report from the International Monetary Fund predicted a 4.9% shrinkage of the global economy.[28] Around June 25, the global death count hit 489,000 deaths from 4.9 million cases. On June 30, Goldman Sachs reported that a federal requirement to wear masks could save the U.S. economy from a 5% gross domestic product loss.[29]

On July 6, the U.S. Immigration and Customs Enforcement announced that international college students would be required to leave the country if schools did not have face-to-face classes. The U.S. Secretary of Education Betsy DeVos told state governors on July 7 that they must open for in-person classes in the fall.[30] The next day, the United States recorded over 3 million cases. On July 17, the United States recorded a new single-day case record of 77,000 and, by July 23, had recorded over 4 million cases, including over 100,000 in children. On July 30, 150,000 Americans had died from the virus.

On August 7, 2020, the Sturgis motorcycle rally began in South Dakota, becoming the first large-scale event to be held in the United States since the start of the pandemic.[31] The following day, the United States reported over 5 million cases. On August 9, Manila, Philippines, reentered a lockdown after an outbreak of the virus. On August 11, New Zealand experienced four new cases of COVID after 100 days of being COVID free. By this point, the world had reported 739,000 deaths from over 20 million cases. Around August 11, Russia announced they had developed a COVID-19 vaccine without the rigorous testing required by global standards.[32] On August 17, the University of North Carolina at Chapel Hill became the first large American university to cancel in-person classes; they were only 1 week into the fall semester.[33] By August 31, the United States had recorded 6 million cases.

On September 16, the Great Synagogue announced it would be closed during the Jewish holidays for the first time in its history.[34] The following day, India had logged a total of 5 million cases within the country. In America, 200,000 Americans had died from the virus by September 20. Eight days later, 1 million people around the world had died from the virus. On October 1, President Donald Trump and his wife tested positive.[35] He had previously promoted the malaria drug hydroxychloroquine to prevent the virus despite fervent governmental warnings about the dangers and ineffectiveness of the drug.[36] He was hospitalized and received the best care available at the time (see Chapter 3 for more details).

On October 23, the United States recorded a new single-day record total of 83,000 new COVID cases. On October 29, the new single-day total rose to 90,000. The next day, France shut down for the second time. During October, U.S. hospitalizations rose by 49%, but hospital stays tended to be shorter.[37]

On November 4, the United States recorded a new single-day total of 100,000 new COVID cases. The next day, the record was broken again with 105,000 new cases. Seventeen states in the country recorded their highest number of daily COVID cases. On November 9, Pfizer announced their vaccine was 90% effective against the virus.[38] The following day, U.S. hospitalizations reached a new record of 61,964. On November 11, Texas became the first state in the United States to surpass 1 million cases, and the country recorded a new single-day total of 140,000 new cases. On November 17, Switzerland announced that every intensive care unit (ICU) bed in the nation was full. The same day, New York City public schools closed down all in-person learning.[39]

December 2, 2020, marked a new record of COVID-19 hospitalizations in the United States, with 100,000 people hospitalized as a result of the virus, as well as a new single-day death record of 2,885. By December 3, over 14 million Americans had been diagnosed with COVID, and hospitalizations rose to 100,667. California announced stay-at-home orders for counties with ICU beds at 85% capacity, and the Centers for Disease Control and Prevention (CDC) officially recommended mask wearing anytime one left their house.[40] On December 8, Margaret Keenan became the first patient in Britain to receive the Pfizer vaccine.[41] The following day, Canada approved the vaccine for use. Mark Meadows, the U.S. presidential chief of staff, threatened to fire the Food and Drug Administration (FDA) commissioner for not approving a vaccine more quickly on December 11. The same day, the vaccine was approved for use in America. Meanwhile, the Australian government canceled $750 million worth of vaccines after volunteers received a false positive for HIV following the vaccine injection.[42]

On December 15, the Supreme Court ordered the states of New Jersey and Colorado to reconsider limits on indoor religious services.[43] On December 16, Germany and the Netherlands announced lockdowns over the Christmas holiday. The Swedish king denounced the country's COVID strategy, and Prime Minister Emmanuel Macron of France tested positive for the virus.[44] On December 18, the FDA approved the Moderna vaccine for use as the United States surpassed 17 million known cases. Vice President Mike Pence and speakers from the houses of congress were vaccinated on national television to bolster confidence in the vaccine. South Africa announced they discovered a new variant of the virus.[45] Global COVID cases reached 76 million, and the United Kingdom announced they had identified a new and more contagious variant of the virus on December 20.[46] The next day, the second economic stimulus package passed in the U.S. Congress.[47] On December 23, Canada approved Moderna's vaccine, which was easier to store and ship than the Pfizer one.[48]

In early January 2021, several U.S. states identified cases of the more dangerous COVID variants. On January 7, the United States reported a new single-day death record of 3,963. Several members of Congress tested positive for the virus after the January 6 capitol riots stemming from the results of the U.S. election. In Japan, Prime Minister Yoshihide Suga declared a state of emergency after the number of cases sharply rose. Israel issued new lockdowns due to rising cases after initially being seen as a model for vaccine distribution.[49] On January 8, the United States reported a new single-day death record of 4,111 deaths.[50] On January 14, Lebanon began its strictest lockdown since the beginning of the pandemic, which was set to last 11 days.[51] By January 15, over 2 million people around the world had died of COVID.[52] On January 20, newly inaugurated President Joe Biden allowed the United States to rejoin the World Health Organization. In Europe, stricter lockdowns and mask requirements were issued to combat the more contagious strains.[53] In late January, drug manufacturers began development of booster vaccines to better combat current and future COVID mutations. Around January 26, over 100 million known cases of the virus had been recorded globally.[54] Around January 29th, forty-eight states reported steady declines in new infections, and Johnson & Johnson announced their single-dose COVID vaccine was effective, although at much lower rates than previously announced vaccines.[55]

By the start of February, at least 90 million people globally had been vaccinated, although vaccination rates were disproportionate between countries and communities. The Sputnik V vaccine released in Russia in August was found to be highly effective against COVID. Covax, an international program aimed at combating vaccine inequality around the world, announced plans to distribute over 300 million doses to lower economic status countries by June 30.[56] On February 7, South Africa stopped its vaccine rollout over concerns the vaccine was ineffective against the dominant strain in the nation.[57] On February 16, the nation gave its vaccines to the African Union after being unable to use them.[58] On February 9, representatives from the World Health Organization traveled to China to investigate the COVID-19 situation; they praised China's response to the virus and denounced ideas that the virus was manufactured in a lab. In mid-February, the number of new cases continued to decline across the world. Globally, countries with strict lockdowns began opening back up, most often by opening schools. On February 26, Canada authorized the AstraZeneca vaccine for use.[59]

On March 2, President Biden announced that the nation would have enough vaccine doses for all adults by the end of May, and the Texas governor announced the state could reopen fully.[60] By March 4, roughly 2 million vaccine doses were being administered daily in the United States.[61] On March 8, the Syrian President Bashar al-Assad tested positive for COVID and British schools reopened.[62] President Biden signed the third stimulus bill into law on March 11. The same day, it was announced that all American adults would be eligible for the vaccine beginning May 1.[63] On March 24, Pfizer began testing its vaccine on children under the age of 12, and on March 31, the company announced vaccines were effective in teens.[64]

About 1 in every 5 American adults was vaccinated by April 9. The same day, India reported a new daily record of 131,968 new cases.[65] On April 12, the United Kingdom began reopening.[66] The following day, the FDA paused Johnson and Johnson vaccines due to blood clot concerns, and India began fast-tracking vaccine approvals for vaccines approved in other countries.[67] On April 22, India broke the world record for the number of single-day new cases with 312,731. The previous record was set on January 8 in the United States at 300,669.[68] The Johnson and Johnson vaccine began being administered again on April 24. India set a new single-day record on the same day, with just under 350,000 new cases.[69]

On May 2, 2021, the New Delhi High Court announced plans to punish government officials due to the nation's lack of oxygen supply.[70] On May 10, the FDA approved the Pfizer vaccine to be used in children between the ages of 12 and 15.[71] On May 13, the CDC dropped mask recommendations for all vaccinated Americans.[72] On May 17, President Biden announced that the United States would donate 20 million vaccine doses to countries in need.[73] India recorded the new highest single-day death total on May 18, with 4,529 deaths.[74] On May 19, New York City reopened.[75] On May 21, the World Health Organization announced that global deaths were likely two or three times higher than official counts.[76] India reached 303,720 total deaths on May 24.[77] On May 25, Moderna announced that its vaccine was safe for children between the ages of 12 and 17.[78] On May 26, Biden ordered U.S. intelligence agencies to investigate the origin of COVID-19.[79] The European Union approved the Pfizer vaccine for use in 12- to 17-year-olds on May 28.[80]

Five percent of the lawmakers in parliament in Congo had died of COVID-19 by June 1, 2021.[81] On June 5, the Indian federal government announced plans to overtake vaccine distribution responsibility from states.[82] On June 8, Pfizer and Moderna announced plans to have COVID vaccines for children as young as 6 months in September 2021.[83] On June 11, leaders in the European Union echoed U.S. and World Health Organization directives to investigate the origins of the COVID-19 virus.[84] A highly transmissible variant dubbed the Delta variant pushed the reopening of Britain back another month[85] around June 14. One day later, the CDC designated the Delta variant as a significant cause for concern due to potential diminished vaccine effectiveness and a higher rate of transmission; government officials pled with the public to get vaccinated.[86] On June 22, the White House acknowledged President Biden would not meet his goal of 70% of U.S. adults being vaccinated, partially due to Americans aged 26 and younger and service members[87] being hesitant to get vaccinated.[88] At the end of June, the Delta variant wreaked havoc on many countries as governments reinstituted safety measures and lockdowns. Deaths increased worldwide, and by July 7, the Delta variant had become the dominant strain the United States.[89]

On July 15, the nation of Haiti began vaccine efforts. On July 23, the CDC specifically targeted "antivaxxers" by decrying the pandemic a "pandemic of the unvaccinated."[90] In France, 100,000 antivax protestors begin weeks-long demonstrations against President Macron's unvaccinated bans.[91] In middle and late July, governors and school leaders hastened the political battle of what the next school year should and would look like. On July 23, the Summer Olympics began in Tokyo after a year delay. COVID-19 had caused over 200 million infections globally by August 4.

In early August, an increase in cases spurred local and federal vaccine and mask mandates.[92] By August 9, U.S. daily cases were averaging over 100,000 per day, and the U.S./Canada border reopened.[93] Common misinformation strategies to discourage vaccinations became a serious problem. Antivaxxers claimed that the vaccines were ineffective, that there was a natural immunity to the virus, and that vaccines contained microchips to track and monitor people who were vaccinated—these tactics delayed the slow of the virus spread.[94] On August 15, the Texas Supreme Court upheld Governor Greg Abbott's mask mandates ban as school districts and governors continued their wars on back-to-school policies.[95] By August 17, a fifth of U.S. ICU beds were at or nearing capacity.[96] On August 21, the U.S. FDA issued a stern warning to Americans to avoid consumption of the unauthorized livestock antiparasitic drug Ivermectin to prevent COVID-19.[97] The drug averaged just under 90,000 prescriptions in mid-August despite a lack of evidence of its effectiveness against COVID-19.[98]

The U.S. Army mandated vaccines for service members on September 15, 2021.[99] In mid-September, China announced that 1 billion of its citizens had been vaccinated. On September 29, YouTube announced a ban on vaccine misinformation in a bid to combat antivaccine content on the platform.[100]

On October 4, New Zealand ended its COVID elimination strategy and eased lockdowns,[101] and in mid- and late October, first responders in Los Angeles and

New York City protested their cities' vaccine mandates. On October 11, Sydney, Australia, ended its 100-day lockdown.[102] In late October, Europe produced more than half of the world's population of COVID cases.[103]

In November 2021, a new variant called Omicron was first identified by scientists in South Africa. At the time of this writing, December 2021, this variant was wreaking havoc globally. The United Kingdom experienced 122,186 new Covid-19 cases, France recorded 94,124 new cases, and Italy reported 50,599 new cases on December 23—a pandemic record for each country.[104] That same day, New York State had 44,431 new cases—also a record.[105] Over 2,000 Christmas Eve flights were cancelled due to staff shortages related to Omicron.[106] Broadway plays, sporting games (National Hockey League, National Basketball Association, and both pro and college football), and Boxing Day matches were postponed due to surges.[107] A host of cities cancelled their New Year's Eve celebrations.[108] On December 23, 2021, the CDC reported that 815,423 people in America had died of COVID-19.

Early studies suggested that this Omicron variant was the most transmissible variant yet; even more disturbing are early findings that some vaccines do not protect against this variant as well as previous variants.[109] Experts have warned that the cloth masks that were typically used during the first 20 months of the pandemic were not effective against Omicron.[110] There is debate about whether a fourth dose of the vaccine is needed or would even be effective.[111] It is clear that the pandemic is far from over.

This brief timeline of the pandemic is woefully inadequate to capture every important event, especially from a global context. However, it does highlight how the pandemic rapidly and exponentially changed society. It also highlights how society's choices (e.g., whether to vaccinate, whether to mandate masks, whether to cancel events) shortened or prolonged the pandemic. This reciprocal relationship between society and the pandemic is the focus of this book.

OVERVIEW OF THE BOOK

Section One of this book contains four chapters that provide the foundation for the remainder of the book. The first chapter offers a glimpse into the experiences of various groups during the pandemic. Through news articles and anecdotes, the chapter describes what it was like to be a policymaker, parent, medical worker, and businessperson, among others. It details pandemic-related changes to education, healthcare, and religion. The second chapter in this section reviews a variety of public health responses to the pandemic. The third discusses some ethical dilemmas that arose from the pandemic, such as medical professionals who struggled with deciding who will get ventilators if there were not enough and policymakers who struggled with how to preserve the economy while saving lives. The last chapter in this section reviews a variety of laws and legal disputes that arose because of the pandemic. These four chapters set the foundation for the rest of the book by providing history and context for the science-based explanations and predictions that follow in Sections Two through Four.

Section Two contains 14 chapters explaining or predicting pandemic-related *behaviors* that shaped the pandemic. Some people behave very rationally, while others panic. This could be due in part to cognitive factors such as one's need for cognition, faith in intuition, and belief in a higher power's control—or individual differences (e.g., introversion, authoritarianism, individualism, narcissism)—or other beliefs (belief in conspiracies, belief in destiny). Additionally, people behaved in both productive and counterproductive ways. They helped their neighbors, hoarded goods, spread misinformation, and chose whether to comply with mandates. Social science can explain many of these behaviors.

As predicted by social contagion, people's behaviors were likely shaped by the behavior of those around them: whether others are panicking; whether others are relying on emotion or science; and whether their culture is "tight" or "loose," for example. Behavior is also shaped by the information one has and seeks. People exhibited behavior such as searching for pandemic-related information—typically from sources with similar views as the self. They chose whether to trust the medical experts, scientists, conspiracy theorists, and politicians. Trying to shape behaviors was a daily challenge for leaders: They had to find ways to encourage people to do behaviors that were seemingly against their own best interest (e.g., shutting their business, avoiding friends and family) for the good of society.

Section Three contains 12 chapters explaining or predicting the *experiences* of individual people during the pandemic. People's experiences of the pandemic (much like any major life event) are shaped by many factors, including internal factors (e.g., coping skills and emotional regulation); external factors (e.g., social support and religious beliefs/participation); individual differences (e.g., age, health condition, socioeconomic status); life situation (e.g., living in an assisted living facility, being imprisoned, being homeless); and family situation (e.g., multigenerational homes, marital strain). Some experiences are shaped by racism or xenophobia. University of California–Berkeley raised controversy by suggesting that xenophobia is a common reaction to a threat posed by a virus from a foreign country.[112] Such prejudices might affect a host of pandemic-related experiences (e.g., a patient refusing medical care from an Asian doctor).

Perhaps the strongest predictor of pandemic experiences is a person's ability to cope with the many new challenges posed by the pandemic. Coping takes many forms, often dictated by culture or technology of the times. For instance, in the Ebola epidemic, African tribes developed songs about the virus; during COVID-19, the Internet was filled with COVID-19 memes. Almost everyone learned how to communicate through Zoom or a similar technology. Some people protested; others organized drive-by graduation or birthday parades. These examples indicate that social, cultural, and personal factors play a role in a person's ability to cope. Such factors could explain individual differences in people's pandemic-related well-being and subjective experience of the pandemic. Because a pandemic creates a type of loss and grief that is different from most losses (e.g., of a loved one, being victimized), typical models and responses to grief might not be applicable. While some will emerge from the pandemic virtually unscathed, others will struggle with the aftermath of the experience (e.g., healthcare providers experiencing many deaths) for the rest of their lives. Such variation is a result of the combination of psychological and sociological influences.

Section Four contains nine chapters explaining or predicting the individual and societal *outcomes* of the pandemic. This includes societal outcomes (e.g., economy, health systems) and personal outcomes (e.g., who gets the accolades or blame) resulting from the pandemic. For instance, theories predict that exposure to illness and other environmental risks lead societies—and the individual people within them—to hold more conservative beliefs and to be less open to outgroup members. This conservatism, in turn, relates to more punitive responses to wrongdoers, including supporting the death penalty. This might suggest that societies might become more punitive postpandemic. Several chapters in this book offer insights to how the pandemic might shape the very moral fabric of society.

Other outcomes are more individual and personal, as they deal with personal interactions with others. Social distancing is likely to have major effects on social communications (e.g., hugging) and behaviors (e.g., public gatherings). If distancing orders are in place for a long period of time, it will fundamentally affect children who will spend months or years having little contact with nonfamily, few opportunities to play with other children, and being schooled in unique ways. Stay-home orders could also shift parenting responsibilities, as fathers who are forced to stay home share the parenting responsibility. The virus could also lead to stigmatization: Those who were infected could be stigmatized because they "didn't stay at home" as ordered. On the other hand, those who recovered from the virus could become more valued members of society as they could go back to work and earn money for their families. In sum, this section discusses social science factors that can play a role in the many outcomes of the pandemic.

Section Five contains seven chapters about best practices in research and practice during and after the pandemic. Because the focus of this book is to highlight how theory can inform COVID-19 pandemic research (and make suggestions for future research), these authors offer chapters that offer best practices for conducting that research. While the other sections suggest theory-based *topics* for study, this section addresses how to *conduct* that research about the pandemic or during the pandemic. One chapter addresses ethical challenges related to COVID-19 research. Three chapters, with authors who have conducted COVID-19-related research, offer best practices for using a variety of theories, research methodologies, and participant samples. Another chapter discusses the importance of self-care for researchers who are studying an emotional topic during an emotional time—a psychological construct called emotional labor. Another chapter offers best practices and lessons learned from authors delivering services and conducting research in the field (with Zagreb Child and Youth Protection Center in Croatia). This will be valuable for researchers working in applied settings. A final chapter discusses the importance of using sophisticated methods and statistics (e.g., modeling) to study such complicated phenomena; this will be valuable for researchers in academic settings who are developing more theoretical aspects of the pandemic. This book is intended to be an essential resource for researchers who heed our "call to action" and begin doing COVID-19-related research.

The final chapter begins with a speculative look at the future. What will the post-COVID-19 world look like? Will people have to carry a "vaccine passport" to enter public places? What changes will lawmakers, medical personnel, educational institutions, and businesses make as a result? How might relationships and personal behavior (e.g., handshakes) change? Will the virus become part of "normal" life, like the flu? Or will restrictions and mandates become the new normal? Will our relationship with China—and the rest of the world—be affected? Will there be serious long-term economic and social effects?

After this speculation of what the post-COVID-19 world will look like, the concluding chapter links common threads from the chapters and synthesizes the "lessons learned" and future research directions for scholars who have found professional inspiration in a new pandemic-related line of research. The concluding chapter ends with an overall take-home message related to how social science did and can shape pandemics.

CONCLUSION

This introductory chapter has offered both a case study of how a historical epidemic shaped society as well as an evolving summary of how COVID-19 was shaping society up until this writing in December 2021. As illustrated, this reciprocal relationship between disease and society is a powerful one. Societies adapt—for good and for bad—to disease and pandemics. On the other hand, viruses and disease are shaped by human decision-making. Decisions about masks, vaccines, travel, and socializing have consequences about to whether the virus can find new hosts in which to replicate and mutate. As such, humans control the pandemic and their own destiny. This book illustrates that pandemic-related human behavior is incredibly complex, however. The pandemic has created a novel context by which to study human behavior using social science theory and methods. The hope is that the book will prompt scientific thought about the social science aspects of pandemics and ultimately help prepare for and reduce the negative impacts of future pandemics and other disasters.

NOTES

1. See https://www.gapminder.org.
2. Yang, G. (2009). *The power of the Internet in China: Citizen activism online.* Columbia University Press; De Lisle, J., Goldstein, A., & Yang, G. (Eds.). (2016). *The Internet, social media, and a changing China.* University of Pennsylvania Press.
3. Huang, Y. (2004). The SARS epidemic and its aftermath in China: A political perspective. In S. Knobler, A. Mahmoud, S. Lemon, A. Mack, L. Sivitz, & K. Oberholtzer (Eds.), *Learning from SARS: Preparing for the next disease outbreak: Workshop*

summary (pp. 116–136). National Academies Press. https://www.ncbi.nlm.nih. gov/books/NBK92479/

4. Tai, Z., & Sun, T. (2011). The rumouring of SARS during the 2003 epidemic in China. *Sociology of Health and Illness, 33*(5), 677–693. https://doi.org/10.1111/ j.1467-9566.2011.01329.x

5. Yu, H. (2007). Talking, linking, clicking: The politics of AIDS and SARS in urban China. *positions: east asia cultures critique, 15*(1), 35–63. https://muse.jhu.edu/arti cle/214311/pdf

6. Ghosh, B. (2016, April 14). *China's Internet got a strange and lasting boost from the SARS epidemic.* Quartz. https://qz.com/662110/chinas-internet-got-a-strange-and-lasting-boost-from-the-sars-epidemic/; Zheng, K. (2020, February 5). How SARS contributed to the birth of China ecommerce. Digital Commerce 360. https:// www.digitalcommerce360.com/2020/02/05/how-sars-contributed-to-the-birth-of-china-ecommerce/; Katz, R., Jung, J., & Callorda, F. (2020). Can digitization mitigate the economic damage of a pandemic? Evidence from SARS. *Telecommunications Policy, 44*(10), 102044. https://doi.org/10.1016/j.telpol.2020.102044

7. Jim Harkness (2022). personal communication.

8. Yang, G. (2017). Demobilizing the emotions of online activism in China: A civilizing process. *International Journal of Communication, 11*, 1945–1965. https:// ijoc.org/index.php/ijoc/article/viewFile/5313/2341

9. Wuthnow, J. (2019). *China's other army: The people's armed police in an era of reform.* National Defense University Press.

10. Kevin Hartigan, personal communication; Uruguayans bang pots to protest army rule. (1983, August 26). The New York Times. https://www.nytimes.com/1983/ 08/26/world/around-the-world-uruguayans-bang-pots-to-protest-army-rule. html; protesters in Iceland in 2009 and in Italy in 2020 emulated the pots and pans protests, in noisy street displays, in public, minus the anonymity.

11. Han, R. (2015). Defending the authoritarian regime online: China's "Voluntary fifty-cent army." *The China Quarterly, 224*, 1006–1025. https://doi.org/10.1017/ S0305741015001216

12. Lin, B., & Wu, S. (2020). COVID-19 (coronavirus disease 2019): Opportunities and challenges for digital health and the internet of medical things in China. *OMICS: A Journal of Integrative Biology, 24*(5), 231–232. https://doi.org/10.1089/ omi.2020.0047

13. Gong, M., Liu, L., Sun, X., Yang, Y., Wang, S., & Zhu, H. (2020). Cloud-based system for effective surveillance and control of COVID-19: Useful experiences from Hubei, China. *Journal of Medical Internet Research, 22*(4), e18948. https:// dx.doi.org/10.2196%2F18948; Ye, Q., Zhou, J., & Wu, H. (2020). Using information technology to manage the COVID-19 pandemic: Development of a technical framework based on practical experience in China. *JMIR Medical Informatics, 8*(6), e19515. https://dx.doi.org/10.2196%2F19515

14. https://www.ncbi.nlm.nih.gov/pmc/articles/PMC7068164/#:~:text=A%20clus ter%20of%20pneumonia%20of,from%20some%20clustered%20cases

15. https://wwwnc.cdc.gov/eid/article/26/6/20-0516_article#:~:text=A%20pati ent%20in%20the%20United,January%202020%2C%202020

16. https://www.nytimes.com/2020/03/11/world/coronavirus-news.html

17. https://www.mercurynews.com/2020/03/16/coronavirus-six-bay-area-counties-to-shelter-in-place/

18. https://paloaltoonline.com/news/2020/03/19/governor-newsom-declares-statewide-shutdown

19. https://www.nytimes.com/2020/03/19/health/coronavirus-masks-shortage.html

20. https://www.nytimes.com/2020/03/24/sports/olympics/coronavirus-summer-olympics-postponed.html

21. https://www.bbc.com/news/world-52144390

22. https://www.nytimes.com/2020/04/05/world/europe/coronavirus-queen-elizabeth-speech.html

23. https://www.nytimes.com/2020/04/11/us/coronavirus-live-updates.html

24. https://www.nytimes.com/2020/04/15/world/coronavirus-cases-world.html

25. https://www.nytimes.com/2020/04/20/business/stock-market-live-trading-coronavirus.html

26. https://www.nytimes.com/2020/05/29/health/virus-who.html

27. https://www.nytimes.com/2020/06/15/world/asia/pakistan-coronavirus-hospitals.html

28. https://www.nytimes.com/2020/06/24/business/imf-world-economic-outlook.html

29. https://www.forbes.com/sites/sarahhansen/2020/06/30/a-national-mask-mandate-could-save-the-us-economy-1-trillion-goldman-sachs-says/?sh=1e19d35f56f1

30. https://www.nytimes.com/2020/07/14/us/coronavirus-international-foreign-student-visas.html

31. https://www.nytimes.com/2020/08/07/us/sturgis-motorcyle-rally.html

32. https://www.nytimes.com/2020/08/11/world/coronavirus-covid-19.html

33. https://www.nytimes.com/2020/08/17/us/unc-chapel-hill-covid.html

34. https://www.nytimes.com/2020/09/18/world/middleeast/israel-lockdown-high-holidays.html

35. https://www.nytimes.com/2020/10/02/us/politics/trump-positive-coronavirus-test.html

36. https://www.nytimes.com/article/hydroxychloroquine-coronavirus.html

37. https://www.nytimes.com/live/2020/10/28/world/covid-19-coronavirus-updates

38. https://www.nytimes.com/2020/11/09/health/covid-vaccine-pfizer.html

39. https://www.nytimes.com/2020/11/17/us/coronavirus-today.html

40. https://www.nytimes.com/2020/12/03/us/coronavirus-today.html

41. https://www.nytimes.com/2020/12/08/us/coronavirus-today.html

42. https://www.nytimes.com/2020/12/11/us/coronavirus-briefing-what-happened-today.html

43. https://www.nytimes.com/2020/12/15/us/coronavirus-today.html

44. https://www.nytimes.com/2020/12/16/us/coronavirus-today.html

45. https://www.nytimes.com/2020/12/18/us/coronavirus-briefing-what-happened-today.html

46. https://www.nytimes.com/2020/12/20/briefing/virus-mutation-uk-china-censorship-muppets.html

47. https://www.nytimes.com/2020/12/21/us/coronavirus-briefing-what-happened-today.html

48. https://www.nytimes.com/2020/12/23/us/coronavirus-briefing-what-happened-today.html

49. https://www.nytimes.com/2021/01/07/us/coronavirus-today.html

50. https://www.nytimes.com/2021/01/08/us/coronavirus-briefing-what-happened-today.html
51. https://www.nytimes.com/2021/01/14/us/coronavirus-today.html
52. https://www.nytimes.com/2021/01/15/us/coronavirus-today.html
53. https://www.nytimes.com/2021/01/20/us/coronavirus-today.html
54. https://www.nytimes.com/2021/01/26/us/coronavirus-today.html
55. https://www.nytimes.com/2021/01/29/us/coronavirus-briefing-what-happened-today.html
56. https://www.nytimes.com/2021/02/01/us/coronavirus-today.html
57. https://www.nytimes.com/2021/02/07/briefing/your-monday-briefing.html
58. https://www.nytimes.com/2021/02/16/us/coronavirus-today.html
59. https://www.nytimes.com/2021/02/26/us/coronavirus-today.html
60. https://www.nytimes.com/2021/03/02/us/coronavirus-today.html
61. https://www.nytimes.com/2021/03/04/us/coronavirus-today.html
62. https://www.nytimes.com/2021/03/08/us/coronavirus-briefing-what-happened-today.html
63. https://www.nytimes.com/2021/03/11/us/coronavirus-briefing-what-happened-today.html
64. https://www.nytimes.com/2021/03/24/us/coronavirus-today.html   https://www.nytimes.com/2021/03/31/us/coronavirus-today.html
65. https://www.nytimes.com/2021/04/09/us/coronavirus-today.html
66. https://www.nytimes.com/2021/04/12/us/coronavirus-today-vaccines.html
67. https://www.nytimes.com/2021/04/13/us/coronavirus-today-vaccines.html
68. https://www.nytimes.com/2021/04/22/us/coronavirus-today.html
69. https://www.nytimes.com/2021/04/23/briefing/johnson-johnson-india-oscars.html
70. https://www.nytimes.com/2021/05/02/world/with-india-drowning-in-crisis-modis-party-loses-big-in-a-key-election.html
71. https://www.nytimes.com/2021/05/10/us/coronavirus-today-vaccines.html
72. https://www.nytimes.com/2021/05/13/us/coronavirus-briefing-what-happened-today.html
73. https://www.nytimes.com/2021/05/17/us/coronavirus-masks-cdc-covid-pandemic.html
74. https://www.nytimes.com/2021/05/18/us/coronavirus-today-masks.html
75. https://www.nytimes.com/2021/05/19/us/coronavirus-today-new-york-city.html
76. https://www.nytimes.com/2021/05/21/us/coronavirus-today.html
77. https://www.nytimes.com/2021/05/24/us/coronavirus-briefing-what-happened-today.html
78. https://www.nytimes.com/2021/05/25/us/coronavirus-today-vaccines.html
79. https://www.nytimes.com/2021/05/26/us/coronavirus-today-vaccines-immunity.html
80. https://www.nytimes.com/2021/05/28/us/coronavirus-today-summer.html
81. https://www.nytimes.com/2021/06/01/us/coronavirus-today-vaccines-work-office.html
82. https://www.nytimes.com/2021/06/07/us/coronavirus-today-vaccines.html
83. https://www.nytimes.com/2021/06/08/us/coronavirus-briefing-what-happened-today.html

84. https://www.nytimes.com/live/2021/06/10/world/covid-vaccine-coronavi
rus-mask#lab-leak

85. https://www.nytimes.com/2021/06/14/us/coronavirus-today.html

86. https://www.nytimes.com/live/2021/06/15/world/covid-vaccine-coronavirus-
mask#the-cdc-designates-the-delta-version-of-the-virus-a-variant-of-concern

87. https://www.nytimes.com/live/2021/07/02/world/covid-19-vaccine-coronavirus-
updates#the-us-military-and-va-hospitals-struggle-to-increase-their-vaccinat
ion-rates

88. https://www.nytimes.com/live/2021/06/22/world/covid-vaccine-coronavirus-
mask#biden-covid-vaccine-july-4

89. https://www.nytimes.com/2021/07/07/us/coronavirus-briefing-what-happened-
today.html

90. https://www.nytimes.com/live/2021/07/16/world/covid-variant-vaccine-upda
tes#cdc-covid-vaccine-delta-variant

91. https://www.nytimes.com/2021/07/19/world/france-covid-vaccine-pass-prote
sts.html

92. https://www.nytimes.com/2021/08/10/us/coronavirus-today-misinformation-
delta.html

93. https://www.nytimes.com/2021/08/09/us/coronavirus-today-children-delta-milit
ary-vaccine-mandate.html

94. https://www.nytimes.com/2021/08/10/us/coronavirus-today-misinformation-
delta.html

95. https://www.nytimes.com/2021/08/15/us/texas-covid-masks-ban-abbott.html

96. https://www.nytimes.com/2021/08/17/us/coronavirus-briefing-what-happened-
today.html

97. https://www.nytimes.com/2021/08/21/world/ivermectin-fda-covid-19-treatm
ent.html

98. https://www.nytimes.com/live/2021/08/30/world/covid-delta-vari
ant-vaccine#demand-surges-for-a-deworming-drug-despite-no-evide
nce-it-can-treat-covid

99. https://www.nytimes.com/2021/09/15/us/coronavirus-today-us-future.html

100. https://www.nytimes.com/2021/09/29/us/coronavirus-today-california-vaccine-
mandates.html

101. https://www.nytimes.com/2021/10/04/us/coronavirus-briefing-what-happened-
today.html

102. https://www.nytimes.com/2021/10/11/us/coronavirus-briefing-what-happened-
today.html

103. https://www.nytimes.com/2021/10/29/us/coronavirus-briefing-what-happened-
today.html

104. https://www.reuters.com/world/uk/uk-reports-new-record-122186-covid-cases-
2021-12-24/; https://www.bloomberg.com/news/articles/2021-12-24/france-new-
covid-19-infections-reach-record-for-second-day; https://www.reuters.com/arti
cle/us-health-coronavirus-italy-tally/italy-reports-record-50599-coronavirus-
cases-on-friday-141-deaths-idUSKBN2J30YT?feedType=RSS&feedName=hea
lthNews

105. https://abcnews.go.com/Health/live-updates/coronavirus/?id=81852482

106. https://www.cnn.com/2021/12/23/business/united-delta-cancellations-christmas-eve/index.html
107. https://www.cnn.com/2021/12/23/entertainment/broadway-shows-coronavirus-cancellations/index.html; https://www.cnn.com/2021/12/20/sport/nhl-nfl-nba-ncaa-games-postponed-coronavirus-spt/index.html; https://www.foxsports.com.au/football/premier-league/football-news-2021-premier-league-fixture-boxing-day-games-cancelled-postponed-liverpool-vs-leeds-watford-vs-wolves-everton-forced-to-play/news-story/089f4d36a4ddc6f4e313ef5ca8bd188d
108. https://www.cnn.com/travel/article/new-years-eve-2021-celebrations-cancellations-pandemic/index.html
109. https://www.bloomberg.com/news/articles/2021-12-09/omicron-four-times-more-transmissible-than-delta-in-japan-study
110. https://www.cnn.com/2021/12/24/health/cloth-mask-omicron-variant-wellness/index.html
111. https://www.cnn.com/2021/12/24/health/fourth-dose-covid-19-vaccine-us/index.html
112. https://www.cnn.com/2020/02/01/us/uc-berkeley-coronavirus-xenophobia-trnd/index.html

FURTHER READING

Fang, F. (2020). *Wuhan Diary: Dispatches From a Quarantined City*. HarperVia.
Spinney, L. (2017). *Pale Rider: The Spanish Flu of 1918 and How It Changed the World*. Public Affairs.
Tooze, A. (2021). *Shutdown: How Covid Shook the World's Economy*. Viking.

Foundation of the COVID-19 Pandemic

2

How the Pandemic Changed People, Experiences, and the World

ANGELA SPIRES AND MONICA K. MILLER ■

INTRODUCTION

In February 2020, passengers boarded the *Diamond Princess* expecting an exciting cruise but got more than they bargained for when one or more passengers unknowingly brought on board a virus that ultimately infected 700 people—and quarantined 3,600 passengers.[1] This news story was how many Americans learned about the coronavirus—the cause of COVID-19. The virus affected everyone, whether through changed routines, school, employment, religion, entertainment, or mask mandates. Couples canceled weddings; skeptics organized antimask protests; families kept their children indoors; entire states went into lockdown. Politicians struggled to save businesses and the economy while calculating risk factors and virus spread. COVID-19 created enemies of friends but also brought people together for a common cause. Societies were transformed by this unique enemy—leaving all to wonder when things would return to normal or what postpandemic "normal" would even look like. This chapter details the ways the pandemic changed nearly all aspects of life.

DAILY LIFE

The COVID-19 pandemic dramatically altered daily life. Of note are changes to travel, personal care, entertainment, hobbies, and the experience of loss; these are discussed below.

Angela Spires and Monica K. Miller, *How the Pandemic Changed People, Experiences, and the World* In: *The Social Science of the COVID-19 Pandemic*. Edited by: Monica K. Miller, Oxford University Press. © Oxford University Press 2024.
DOI: 10.1093/oso/9780197615133.003.0002

Travel

At the start of the pandemic, travel restrictions reducing passenger numbers by up to 80%—or prohibiting passenger entrance altogether—began in East Asia and soon spread worldwide. Thousands of tourists were stranded abroad; some lost jobs, ran out of money, or had difficulty acquiring medications. Some like Jonatan Lopez lived in empty houses or shared motel rooms with strangers.[2] By April, air traffic was down by 30%. Airlines filled flights with only 20%–30% capacity by not filling middle seats. In the United States, 750,000 airline workers were furloughed or fired.[3] Even when airlines opened back up with mask requirements, social media "travel-shamed" travelers like Matt Long.[4] Others traveled in secret due to the stigma and backlash.

Personal Care

During shutdowns, people lost access to personal care in salons, spas, and gyms, and other nonessential treatments ceased. Those who managed to get treatments, including Congresswoman Nancy Pelosi, faced backlash.[5] People were not able to get massages, facials, or even work out on their regular schedules. Many of these activities typically lower stress, forcing people to find new ways to manage their personal care and stress release. People turned to social media for DIY (do-it-yourself) haircuts, home hair dying, and exercise. Actor Chris Hemsworth gave free access to his workout app during the pandemic.[6] Despite increased access to online health resources, the media was rife with reports of people struggling with weight problems spanning the spectrum from obesity to anorexia.[7]

Entertainment

As states went into lockdown, the entertainment industry came to a halt. Movie theaters, bars, casinos, and concerts were closed, canceled, or limited. This restricted entertainment both inside and outside the home. College basketball's March Madness was canceled for the first time since 1939,[8] and other college and professional sports followed; sports channels showed reruns. Movie and television production ceased; for instance, *Supernatural*, in its final (15th) season could not film its two final episodes.[9] Viewers looked to streaming networks for new shows or reruns. Some people created "bubbles" of friends with whom they would socialize in person, while others fully isolated themselves, choosing only online interaction. Even when restaurants were allowed to reopen, many could only open at limited capacity with reservations.

Hobbies

Some hobbies were strongly discouraged during the pandemic. Parks taped off playgrounds and removed basketball nets. One Swedish city used manure spread all over the park to deter visitors.[10] With conventions (e.g., comic cons) canceled, vendors and artists took to social media to sell their products. Collectors visited online auction houses, organized online gameplay, or developed other virtual ways to maintain their hobbies. With people's normal hobbies put on hold, many took up new hobbies, like golf, camping, and home-based hobbies like baking, puzzles, gardening, and learning to raise farm animals. Those who wanted to avoid being homebound purchased campers.[11] Illegal camping and fires contributed to record high California wildfires. Controversy arose when some events were not canceled, such as political rallies or the Sturgis, North Dakota, motorcycle rally that attracted 365,000 people.

Losses in Daily Life

COVID-19 brought many types of losses to daily life. People experienced loved ones' deaths, were not allowed hospital visits with COVID-19 patients, and often were unable to attend funerals due to the gathering regulations. Nursing homes forbid visitations, leaving loved ones to visit through windows or, like M. J. Ryan, take a job at the nursing home.[12]

Students lost the chance to attend proms and graduations, although some schools held graduations virtually or invented new ways to hold events. A Florida school held a jet ski graduation,[13] a Texas university held a drive-through graduation,[14] and a town in Oklahoma put on a "prom parade."[15]

Worry and loss varied by generation. Baby boomers were more at risk for death but worried less about financial loss. Generation Xers worried about not only losing older relatives, but also their children's health and their finances. Millennials worried about financial losses and medical care, as many lacked insurance. Young workers of Generation Z were often hardest hit by job loss and furlough.[16]

EDUCATION

Both K–12 and college systems were changed dramatically by the pandemic. There was great variation among states—and even among schools within the same state—in pandemic responses. Even so, few schools, students, and employees were untouched by the pandemic.

K–12

In March of 2020, K–12 schools across the United States went online. Andreas Ortner, a single mother, homeschooled her students while also working from home. She had to relearn math and accept that her children would interrupt her work video calls—like when her youngest child said "what you are talking about is boring" after unmuting her computer. Ortner also said she learned how to "slow down properly," and that homeschooling was also about being a pupil again.[17]

As teachers were not prepared to teach online, many parents complained that their children were not learning or receiving proper instruction. Some schools printed out work that parents had to pick up, and some schools required students do all assignments online. Subscriptions to services like Zoom soared as teachers tried to find a way to connect with students. However, going online further increased the learning gap between low-income and higher income households, as many low-income households did not have computers or access to reliable Internet service (see Chapter 24 for more about inequities during the pandemic). Even when tablets were offered, parents were often afraid to borrow them because they could not afford to replace them if they were broken. A 10th grader in New Jersey explained that his phone was the only tool he had to keep up with his seven high school classes, and he had no help at home as neither of his parents spoke much English. He was one of the millions of students who lacked the resources needed to complete assignments.[18]

In addition to students lacking the resources, many parents tried to home-school their children. Students in grades as early as kindergarten had five or more apps required for homework, requiring parent support. Students in high school could have as many as seven different classes, all with different requirements and methods, some that parents struggled to understand.[19] Parents had to play the role of teacher's aide while working full time or searching for jobs. Math test results dropped dramatically in Grades 3 through 8, as parents had to relearn skills they had not used in years, or the "new" way math was taught.[20] When parents were unable to assist their children, the children's performance suffered. Student Christopher Lamar, a senior at Lake Nona High School, in Orlando, Florida was excelling at school until he had to take care of his younger siblings, cook for the family, and help manage the household. He soon fell behind at school. Eventually, he realized he was failing, and his dream of being a firefighter could be over.[21]

In fall 2020, parents and schools debated whether to bring students back. The Orange County California board of education approved students' return to school with no requirements of social distancing or wearing masks, but schools and parents protested. School administrators said they would not return students to school without masks or social distancing in place.[22] Some school districts offered the option of in-person or online learning, while other schools only offered online education. Schools reopened, and many took precautions: (1) mask and distancing requirements, (2) splitting classes in half and meeting on alternate days, (3) closing one day midweek for sanitizing, (4) temperature checks, and (5) distributing hand sanitizer (see Chapter 29 for more on school health policies).

College

Most colleges went online in mid-March 2020, even though many college instructors had never taught online. Professors struggled to learn how to use Zoom and other video applications and adapt a class in real time. Most study abroad programs were canceled, but some innovative people like the founders and directors of the Study Abroad Association, Christian Alyea and Leonardo Gubinelli, worked with professionals in other countries to provide virtual learning sessions, beginning with Mayan hieroglyphs and Italian cooking.[23] Colleges had to weigh the risk of reopening in the fall, taking into consideration the money made from on-campus living, food, and parking, as well as the exposure rate to students living in the dorms. Other colleges brought students back in person, but then went online after Thanksgiving when holiday travel contributed to increasing virus infections across the United States.

Many colleges and universities struggled with enforcing COVID-19 restrictions. For instance, Syracuse University suspended students for violating restrictions on gatherings by having a party. Such punishments were met by legal challenges.[24]

The virus also affected many college athletes, as athletics were shut down because cases of the virus were higher in college athletic programs. Some sports continued, albeit on shortened seasons with many restrictions.

RELATIONSHIPS AND FAMILY

Relationships were taxed greatly during the pandemic. Families experienced stress due to the lockdown, parents adjusted to new roles, and people experienced challenges to their social and love lives.

Household Stress

Being confined to home caused a variety of stressors. Many employees worked from home, creating crowded households with children online and parents working. Finding space and sharing computers and Internet was an issue for many.

Children struggled with missing friends and family. As extracurricular activities closed down, many parents tried to find ways to keep children active. Newspapers, social media, and the Centers for Disease Control and Prevention (CDC) offered ideas to help parents keep children fit, including having the child create their own exercise videos. Some extroverted children were able to connect virtually with friends, but not all had the means to do so.

Crowded households also caused domestic abuse to become more common and sometimes more brutal.[25] With schools closed down, the number one reporter of child abuse was no longer available, and many children suffered.

New Roles

In addition to struggling with disruptions in daily routines, people were also struggling in new roles. Gender roles of parents sometimes changed; for instance, emergency room nurse Katherine Cargill quarantined away from her family, moving her husband from "helper" to full-time parent of their three children.

He took leave from work and expressed how tired he was all the time.[26] Because women made up 76% of healthcare workers, this became a new norm for many. This was also complicated when parents had different viewpoints or parenting styles and thus had to find compromises.

Love Life

People grappled with dating during the pandemic, meeting new people virtually. Allison Stevenson wanted someone to connect with; after a month of discussion with a friend, they agreed to conditions for their meeting, including a negative COVID-19 test, masks, and exclusiveness.[27] Many others tried dating apps, like Sara Estan, who met someone online during the pandemic. They texted, used Snapchat, played online games, and streamed television shows together.[28]

Some older couples were separated due to residential housing restrictions. Dick and Susan Williams were apart for 8 months due to her nursing home regulations but were finally reunited in person after being vaccinated.[29] Other couples were not as lucky. Sam and Joanne Reck were separated in their retirement facility, but she would sit in her wheelchair and talk to him as he sat in his balcony above—leading them to be dubbed "Romeo and Juliet." The nursing home allowed the pair to reunite briefly before she passed from COVID-19.[30]

EMPLOYMENT AND THE ECONOMY

By April 2020, unemployment skyrocketed to 14.8%, then leveled to an elevated 6.7% in December.[31] Congress took action in March 2020, passing the first stimulus package designed to help schools, small businesses, and both employed and unemployed people. The airline industry lost over $100 billion in 2020 and projected the losses to continue into 2021. With people and businesses still struggling, a second package was approved at the end of 2020, followed by a third package, totaling $1.9 trillion, on March 11, 2021. The third package extended unemployment benefits and cut larger stimulus checks to Americans in an attempt to boost the economy.

The Vegas strip went dark, and slot machines grew silent; casino profits plummeted 40%,[32] and unemployment topped at 30% in Nevada. A casino pit boss on the strip reported being nauseous every shift as managers turned a blind eye to maskless patrons when casinos opened at 50% capacity.[33] Convention centers sat empty; cruise lines were closed into the beginning of 2021. Even Disneyland closed its doors.

Supply chains were broken during the pandemic, causing food and supply shortages. Shelves of discount and supply stores were bare, and sales of many items were limited to one per person when they restocked. With supply chains broken, some farmers and ranchers had to deal with excess of vegetables or milk that could not be distributed. This caused farmers to have to dump stock and euthanize some livestock.[34] This affected other businesses as well, including restaurants.

However, many restaurants had to shut down immediately and then were allowed to reopen for delivery and take-out only or with very limited seating inside.

Communication was also an employment-related issue during the pandemic, as many people who were allowed to work from home lacked the equipment or Internet service to do so. Workers in rural areas often did not have strong enough Internet service to successfully work from home.

Not all businesses suffered, however. Delivery businesses boomed during the pandemic. Business boomed for food delivery (e.g., Uber Eats, Grubhub) and product delivery companies (e.g., Instacart and Amazon).

RELIGION

The first major holiday during the pandemic was Easter; many services were canceled, held over the Internet, or moved outdoors, where worshipers could social distance. With limitations on gatherings, many churches were forbidden from holding large services. Churches in California, Minnesota, and Oregon (to name a few) sued their governors, claiming that size restrictions on their gatherings violated their religious rights.

At some Muslim churches, people were required to bring their own prayer rugs, have temperature checks, and wear masks. Young Jewish couples prepared to have their first seders had to meet virtually. Jews used the platform OneTable for Seder-in-Place and virtual Pandemic Passover.[35] Some people even embraced the pandemic with humor; after one baptism, a family took staged photos of the priest holding a squirt gun as a way to reach the child from six feet away.[36]

POLITICS

Because 2020 was an election year, pandemic-related problems arose as early as the primaries. With social distancing and gatherings limited, people lined up for multiple blocks to vote. Many people had to decide between virus exposure and not voting. After the primaries, Democratic candidate Joe Biden limited his appearances and wore a mask, while Republican candidate Donald Trump attended rallies and refused to wear a mask. The voting experience of 2020 was dramatically different for many people, as 46% of people voted by absentee or mail-in votes.[37] Others chose to wait in socially distanced lines. The two parties disagreed over mail-in voting, which would protect people from exposure, and President Trump tried to have the election delayed.

The pandemic divided the country dramatically, with conservative states resisting restrictions more than liberal states. Many policies became political hot topics (see Chapter 3 for more on the politics of the pandemic). Republicans in California even pushed to have Democratic Governor Gavin Newsom recalled from office due to his policies of closing businesses and schools to limit COVID exposure.[38] As these examples illustrate, the pandemic affected the political life of many Americans.

COVID-19 VICTIMS AND LOVED ONES

The pandemic most strongly affected those who were infected by—or had loved ones infected by—the virus. Brittany Boccia thought her upset stomach was anxiety, but muscles in her neck and spine began to ache, so she self-quarantined, still not fully considering she might have COVID-19. Soon, her heart rate became elevated, she had trouble breathing, and her temperature spiked to 103°F. She then went to urgent care, where she was tested for COVID-19 and sent home. The test was positive, and the doctor recommended going to the hospital, but Brittany did not want to take beds away from other people, especially because she was considered low risk. She finally called ahead and was admitted to the hospital, where her lungs showed a possible case of pneumonia in both lungs, and she was admitted for a few days.[39] Though COVID-19 symptoms and severity varied from person to person, many people who experienced it said it was the sickest they had ever been. Energy levels were depleted, appetites were gone, and many lost their sense of taste and smell. The recovery for some was 2 weeks or more. But one element that followed was the effect on their mental health, fearing that leaving their house might cause them to get sicker or make someone else sick, even after their symptoms subsided. Some people, called "long haulers," had lingering effects for many months. The long-term effects of the virus are yet undiscovered at the time of this writing.

While many tips were posted by the CDC, Mayo Clinic, and other health organizations, reading the information and living it were two different things. Some people who cared for others with COVID-19 wore masks and frequently washed their hands as advised to try not to catch the virus. Spouses slept in separate rooms and tried to keep children away from the infected member. Often, COVID-19 infected the entire household. Those with less severe symptoms often took care of the others, helping them to follow orders for rest and eating.

The average length of a hospital stay with COVID-19 declined as the pandemic progressed, and doctors and researchers had a better understanding of the disease. In March 2020, the average was 10.5 days but decreased to 4.6 days by September 2020,[40] although there have been some anomalies, like Deanna Hair, who spent 196 days in the hospital.[41] But the hospital stay was just the start, as her rehabilitation (e.g., receiving ventilation at night) continued after she returned home.

In addition to the health effects of the virus, some people had to deal with anger from others and a stigma that maybe they had done something wrong, like not follow mandates. This was especially true in the case of the Goldmans, who were on the *Diamond Princess* cruise ship. They received threats for weeks after recovering and returning home.[42]

ADDRESSING HEALTH AND SAFETY NEEDS

Addressing health and safety was a critical need and a serious challenge during the pandemic. While all businesses were affected, some were particularly so. The medical profession was the most affected by the pandemic, and healthcare itself changed as a result of safety precautions. More broadly, the pandemic resulted in a number of health and safety concerns even for people who were not themselves infected.

COVID-9 Hotspots

As noted above, many businesses shut down, but others deemed "essential" were tasked with the challenge of addressing the health and safety of their employees and customers. Nearly every business constructed Plexiglass windows to separate cashiers from customers; businesses closed early to clean; the number of customers in a store a time was restricted.

Two of the biggest hot spots for COVID spread were nursing homes and meatpacking plants. Meatpacking plants' environments are great breeding ground for virus spread due to their cold, damp nature. Nursing homes were deadly due to the age and underlying conditions of many of the patients. To make things worse, some nursing homes hid deaths and turned in false numbers. One facility in Harlem was actually shipping bodies out of the facility to make their numbers look better[43] (see Chapter 25 for more on the impact of COVID-19 on nursing homes).

Medical Personnel

Early on, medical professionals had to reuse one-use masks and wear only re-usable cloth gowns. Although a photo of nurses wearing trash bags as gowns was circulated, it is believed that they were wearing proper medical attire underneath.[44] Most medical facilities did not allow medical personnel to attend to patients without proper personal protective equipment (PPE). However, supplies were short in some places, and at times equipment had to be reused. The U.S. Food and Drug Administration issued instructions on how two patients could share a ventilator because of the shortage.[45] At the height of the virus, many cities set up makeshift hospitals in event centers or parking garages. Because of the overabundance of patients, some medical care professionals were allowed to perform procedures above their normal role, and some medical students were given privileges to administer care earlier than planned.

These situations took a mental health toll on many healthcare workers. They struggled with the daily exposure to death, being overworked, and fearing infection—which they could pass on to their family. Their efforts were rewarded in many places, with handclapping, horns, and cheers from people showing their appreciation.

Use of Healthcare

The pandemic caused havoc on healthcare in many ways. At the beginning of the pandemic, elective medical procedures were canceled so doctors could focus on

COVID-19 patients. People often feared going to the doctor or dentist because they might catch COVID-19 from the staff or other patients. And with thousands of people out of work, people began applying for Medicaid. Others, who still had income that put them above the Medicaid limit, had to search for insurance because the employer did not pay for it. Insurance—and healthcare itself—could be expensive and hard to find as many doctors were not taking new patients. These examples illustrate some difficulties in obtaining healthcare.

When available, people often used healthcare services differently due to the pandemic. Teledoc services increased, and virtual doctor visits for physical and mental health rose significantly. People began considering in-home health aids in lieu of nursing homes. While people joked that there would be a COVID-19 baby boom, births in late 2020 and early 2021 decreased in the United States and were projected to be 300,000 fewer in 2021, however births actually increased in 2021 by 1%, the first increase since 2014.[46]

COVID-19 Stress and Other Health Issues

People also struggled with medical issues related to the pandemic. Stress increased during COVID-19 due to multiple factors, including fear of catching the virus, financial concerns, learning new technologies, adjusting to new roles, and living in lockdown. Broken heart syndrome spiked during the virus, with the stress of losing someone and additional stresses making the heart muscles weak. In addition, opioid and stimulant use increased during the pandemic, with 13% of Americans starting or increasing use to deal with stress.[47] Suicidal thoughts also increased, but suicide rates did not statistically change in the United States. However, in countries such as Japan, suicide rates increased significantly.[48]

People, now taking on new roles and having new stresses, struggled more with mental illnesses such as depression and anxiety. People had to find new ways of coping with stress, such as breaks from social media and news outlets, as news was a major form of stress. Other ways of coping included getting more sleep, eating healthier, and exercising regularly—but these were sometimes hard to do due to limited finances for healthy food, worries that kept people awake at night, and lack of places to exercise. In addition, Zoom fatigue became a new phenomenon, causing stress, fatigue, and burnout. Contributing factors included auditory and visual issues on-screen that caused mental fatigue, as well as underlying stress from financial situations.[49]

ENVIRONMENT

The pandemic had various effects on the environment. Air quality improved and greenhouse gas emissions lowered in many cities due to the shutdown of some businesses and restrictions on travel. With businesses shut down and supply chains broken, people used fewer products and therefore had less waste. Water destinations such as lakes were cleaner because of fewer visitors to leave trash. Noise pollution from machines and vehicles also lowered. But the use of single-use PPE (e.g., face masks, gloves) and high medical waste had negative impacts on the environment. Biomedical waste increased significantly on a global level. For instance, Wuhan, China, created over 240 metric tons of medical waste each day of the outbreak.[50] The blatant discarding of single-use masks and gloves has littered parking lots, and other places where they were required, adding to land waste.

ANIMALS

Animals have also felt the impact of the pandemic. The virus posed a direct threat mainly to wild animals, especially large cats (e.g., tigers and lions) in captivity, which likely caught the virus from an asymptomatic human carrier. The virus has also been deadly to animals on fur farms, including mink and foxes. Livestock that contracted the virus could easily spread it to the entire farm. In addition to animals catching the virus from humans, many animals were experimented on to find a potential cure or vaccine for the virus, although animal testing was largely ineffective.[51]

In addition, household pets were affected. Pets belonging to people who were hospitalized by or died from COVID-19 were sent to local animal shelters. Though some shelters were able to use mobile units to care for pets of those hospitalized, not all places had this option. Some people, after losing jobs and being under financial strain, abandoned their pets or dropped them off at shelters. On the other hand, many shelters were empty because people decided to adopt a pet to fill their time during the lockdown. Unfortunately, many of these pets ended up in shelters as the pandemic ended and families went back to "normal."

DEVIANT AND FRINGE BEHAVIOR

The pandemic prompted changes in both deviant behavior and the way the government addressed deviant behavior. This included disobedient behavior (e.g., refusing to follow stay-home orders), fringe behavior (e.g., belief in conspiracy theories), and violent behavior.

The pandemic also resulted in dramatic changes to the court and prison systems.

Disobedience

Many people disobeyed stay-home orders or attended large gatherings despite government mandates. In Georgia, many people traveled to Tybee Island beach in part due to confusing government messages from the mayor and the state governor; the beach was eventually closed down. In Florida, 16 friends went to the bars to celebrate a birthday; all 16 got COVID-19.[52] A California church was fined for refusing to comply with a court order to stop holding large church services in which many attendees did not wear masks.[53]

A park ranger in Texas was in the midst of telling a crowd of visitors to practice social distancing. One of the visitors pushed him into a lake.[54] This event was caught on video and the visitor faced charges of assault.

Similar disobedience happened with mask regulations. Many people refused to wear masks even after they were mandated and required to enter stores. Videos of fights over masks continually popped up online. Fights were with security guards, police, employees, or other customers. Some people even devolved to spitting on people who were not wearing a mask or wiping their face on an employee telling them to wear a mask.[55] Some of these altercations ended in major injuries or death.[56]

Conspiracy Beliefs

While most people had at least a basic understanding of the virus that was in line with the "mainstream" messages from experts and country leaders, others had beliefs that were more "fringe." Conspiracy theories during the pandemic led to people believing that COVID-19 was a bioweapon created by China, causing misplaced hatred toward Chinese people and hate crimes against them and their businesses in the United States (see Chapter 36 for more on conspiracies and Chapter 23 for more on prejudice during the pandemic). Others believed the virus was a hoax, was related to 5G phone towers, was a way to eventually inject every person with a device that could track and/or control people's behavior, or was a way to get people to wear masks and poison people with their own carbon dioxide. Mistrust and misinformation (see Chapters 18 and 36, respectively) led to individual or group protests, some of which got unruly or violent.[57] Finally, some believed the pandemic was part of a larger political agenda to allow Democrats to take back political control, a belief that contributed to the capital building being stormed and desecrated on January 6, 2021, when the electoral votes were being counted.

Courts

The court system struggled during the pandemic. Jury trials came to a halt because of fears of virus transmission. But this threatened defendants' right to a speedy trial. Some courts experimented with virtual trials over Zoom, with mixed success. Many defendants chose to plea bargain, perhaps to avoid being imprisoned until a trial could be held or perhaps just to bring resolution to the situation. A survey of defense attorneys found that most (81%) believed that the pandemic changed the plea bargaining process. Attorneys often had problems communicating with their clients (especially those who were detained). Many believed that prosecutors offered more lenient deals during the pandemic, and some reported that they had clients accept plea deals because of COVID-19 conditions—deals they might not have accepted under normal circumstances.[58]

Prisons

Most prisons were unable to allow their prisoners to social distance, so prison officials planned to release some offenders (see Chapter 24 for more on prisons during the pandemic). However, data published in March 2021 showed that the decline in prisoners was due to not taking in as many *new* inmates, not due to the release of *current* offenders. Prisons were still at or above 90% capacity.[59] Not only were many prisons not releasing offenders early, but fewer parolees were approved in 2020. Some states, such as New Jersey, began to release prisoners early, but not until November 2020—and not enough were released to reduce the spread of COVID. Inmates in a Los Angeles correctional facility, in an attempt to get a COVID-19 release, went as far as sharing a mask and drinking from the same cup to try to get infected with the virus; this plan successfully infected 21 prisoners.[60]

PEOPLE HELPING PEOPLE

While the virus brought out the worst in some people, it also brought out the best in others (see Chapter 13 for more about prosocial behavior during the pandemic). In Maryland, 7-year-old Cavanaugh Bell started making and delivering care packages to his elderly neighbors. The idea was born when he realized his grandmother—and others in his neighborhood—were at high risk.[61] Many people brought food and supplies to elderly neighbors or homeless people. Stores set special hours in which only older people could shop. Crafters and sewers across the country made masks and sent them to family, friends, medical professionals, and other organizations. The Girl Scouts started an online program to donate cookies to communities in need.[62] In Pennsylvania, over 40 employees spent 28 days living at the Braskem America plant making polypropylene, the material used to make masks, medical gowns, and other protective gear.[63] Throughout America, many people donated time and money to help those who needed it most during the pandemic.

CONCLUSION

At the time of this writing, June 2021, the pandemic is seemingly at a turning point. While the pandemic created a "new norm" for many people, some people hope that society will go back to the "old norm" of prepandemic times. Postpandemic life may actually fall somewhere in the middle of the "new norm" and "old norm." Whether the changes to life that are discussed above are permanent or temporary, there is no dispute that the pandemic had an impact on virtually every human.

Teachers learned how to use online tools and teach online. Businesses learned to operate with many employees working at home. People lost loved ones, jobs, and a sense of security as things changed throughout the pandemic. But people also joined together, helped one another, and learned some new coping skills to address stress. While the pandemic changed many things about how people live, it also shed light on underlying issues of inequality and the environmental benefits of less travel and business. While the pandemic was difficult in myriad ways, people coped and changed to survive COVID-19. This coping (as discussed in Chapter 21) represents the collective resilience of society and its people to overcome any obstacle.

NOTES

1. https://www.webmd.com/lung/news/20200729/gene-study-shows-how-coronavi rus-swept-through-the-idiamond-princessi#1
2. https://www.nbcnews.com/news/latino/we-are-abandoned-these-tourists-stran ded-u-s-because-coronavirus-n1206386
3. https://www.washingtonpost.com/graphics/2020/business/coronavirus-airline-industry-collapse/
4. https://www.insider.com/travelers-face-backlash-for-posting-photos-and-videos-during-pandemic-2021-1
5. https://www.foxnews.com/politics/pelosi-san-francisco-hair-salon-owner-calls-it-slap-in-the-face
6. https://www.abcactionnews.com/news/region-hillsborough/chris-hemsworth-makes-workout-app-available-for-free
7. http://med.stanford.edu/news/all-news/2021/03/pandemic-worsens-weight-woes-among-young-people.html
8. https://www.cbssports.com/college-basketball/news/2020-ncaa-tournament-canceled-due-to-growing-threat-of-coronavirus-pandemic/#:~:text=In%20a%20h istoric%20move%2C%20the,was%20first%20held%20in%201939.
9. https://ew.com/tv/supernatural-halts-production-final-season/
10. https://www.bbc.com/news/world-europe-52481096
11. https://www.nbcnews.com/health/health-news/live-blog/2020-04-30-coronavi rus-news-n1196031/ncrd1196301#blogHeader
12. https://boston.cbslocal.com/2020/10/22/norton-woman-part-time-laundry-nurs ing-home-visit-mother-coronavirus/
13. https://www.wdrb.com/wdrb-in-the-morning/key-west-high-school-follows-coro navirus-social-distancing-measures-with-jet-ski-graduation/article_773dbe46-a3fc-11ea-a6b1-a3d6f9d87616.html
14. https://dfw.cbslocal.com/2020/12/11/texas-womans-university-hosts-drive-thru-graduation-at-texas-motor-speedway/
15. https://dfw.cbslocal.com/2020/12/11/texas-womans-university-hosts-drive-thru-graduation-at-texas-motor-speedway/
16. https://www.wellmark.com/blue-at-work/healthy-employees/generational-impa cts-from-covid-19
17. https://www.vogue.com/article/working-from-home-kids-pandemic

18. https://www.cnn.com/2020/04/17/us/coronavirus-education-distance-learning-challenges/index.html
19. https://www.nytimes.com/2020/04/27/nyregion/coronavirus-homeschooling-parents.html
20. https://edsource.org/2020/early-data-on-learning-loss-show-big-drop-in-math-but-not-reading-skills/644416.
21. https://www.usatoday.com/story/news/education/2020/12/23/students-failing-grades-online-class-coronavirus/3967886001/
22. https://www.cnn.com/2020/07/14/us/california-orange-county-reopen-school-no-masks-trnd/index.html
23. https://www.nytimes.com/2020/04/23/education/learning/coronavirus-online-learning.html
24. https://www.npr.org/2020/09/17/914046958/students-accused-of-breaking-college-covid-19-rules-fight-their-punishments
25. https://time.com/5928539/domestic-violence-covid-19/
26. https://www.theguardian.com/us-news/2020/jun/17/gender-roles-parenting-housework-coronavirus-pandemic
27. https://www.nytimes.com/2021/01/10/style/coronavirus-sex-hookups-dating.html
28. https://www.nbcboston.com/news/coronavirus/covid-dating-whats-it-like-looking-for-love-in-a-pandemic/2303484/
29. https://local21news.com/news/nation-world/were-happy-elderly-couple-separated-for-8-months-due-to-covid-finally-reunites
30. https://www.usatoday.com/story/news/nation/2020/07/18/elderly-florida-couple-separated-pandemic-meets-one-last-time/5444919002/
31. https://fas.org/sgp/crs/misc/R46554.pdf
32. https://apnews.com/article/us-news-pandemics-las-vegas-coronavirus-pandemic-nevada-3af6106c5dd0134d46783303eb204c93
33. https://www.thedailybeast.com/these-casino-staffers-are-working-in-fear-amid-coronavirus
34. https://www.usda.gov/media/blog/2020/09/24/americas-farmers-resilient-throughout-covid-pandemic
35. https://www.cnn.com/2020/04/08/world/passover-2020-coronavirus-real-plague/index.html
36. https://www.catholicnewsagency.com/news/priest-says-water-gun-baptism-photo-meant-to-be-funny-51057
37. https://www.pewresearch.org/politics/2020/11/20/the-voting-experience-in-2020/
38. https://www.wsj.com/articles/california-governor-faces-recall-effort-amid-anger-over-covid-19-restrictions-11611583254
39. https://www.northwell.edu/infectious-disease/patient-testimonials/i-had-covid19-one-young-womans-coronavirus-story
40. https://www.statnews.com/2020/11/23/hospitalized-covid-19-patients-surviving-at-higher-rates-but-surge-could-roll-back-gains/
41. https://www.nbcnews.com/news/us-news/67-year-old-woman-survives-covid-19-after-196-days-n1243769
42. https://www.cnn.com/2020/04/08/us/coronavirus-stigma-diamond-princess-passengers/index.html

43. https://www.aclu.org/news/disability-rights/how-nursing-homes-got-away-with-hiding-bodies-during-the-covid-19-outbreak/
44. https://www.today.com/health/nyc-hospital-responds-photos-nurses-wearing-trash-bags-t176939
45. https://www.fda.gov/medical-devices/letters-health-care-providers/using-ventilator-splitters-during-covid-19-pandemic-letter-health-care-providers; see also https://www.nytimes.com/2020/03/26/health/coronavirus-ventilator-sharing.html
46. https://www.usatoday.com/story/news/nation/2020/12/16/covid-19-baby-bust-coronavirus-pandemic-lead-birth-decline/6507974002/
47. https://www.apa.org/monitor/2021/03/substance-use-pandemic
48. https://www.nature.com/articles/s41562-020-01042-z
49. https://www.psychiatrictimes.com/view/psychological-exploration-zoom-fatigue
50. https://www.ncbi.nlm.nih.gov/pmc/articles/PMC7498239/#:~:text=Overall%2C%20the%20pandemic%20has%20caused,et%20al.%2C%202020).
51. https://www.news-medical.net/health/COVID-19-and-Animals.aspx
52. https://www.cnn.com/videos/us/2020/06/17/friends-test-positive-coronavirus-after-night-out-florida-bar-warning-cpt-vpx.cnn
53. https://www.nbcnews.com/news/us-news/california-pastor-church-found-contempt-fined-over-covid-rules-n1250481
54. https://www.cnn.com/2020/05/04/us/social-distancing-ranger-pushing-lake-covid-19-trnd/index.html
55. https://www.cnn.com/2020/05/05/us/dollar-tree-wiping-face-trnd/index.html
56. https://people.com/crime/man-charged-in-death-of-80-year-old-man-after-fight-over-wearing-mask-in-bar/#:~:text=A%20New%20York%20man%20has,face%20mask%20inside%20the%20venue; https://www.fox23.com/news/trending/man-shot-killed-by-police-after-fight-over-wearing-mask-reports-say/CE6ORWE6UVBBPGOLCZZTREBRQI/
57. https://en.wikipedia.org/wiki/Protests_over_responses_to_the_COVID-19_pandemic
58. https://doi.org/10.1037/lhb0000442
59. https://www.prisonpolicy.org/virus/virusresponse.html
60. https://www.cnn.com/2020/05/11/us/california-inmates-coronavirus-self-infection/index.html
61. https://www.cnn.com/2020/04/05/us/7-year-old-care-packages-elderly-iyw-trnd/index.html
62. https://www.girlscouts.org/en/girl-scouts-at-home/troop-leaders/national-service-projects.html
63. https://www.washingtonpost.com/nation/2020/04/23/factory-masks-coronavirus-ppe/

3

U.S. Public Health Policy Responses to COVID-19

SUSAN G. BORNSTEIN AND MONICA K. MILLER ■

The first case of what became known as coronavirus SARS-CoV-2 (COVID-19; severe acute respiratory syndrome coronavirus 2) was announced by China on December 31, 2019. The first case detected in the United States presented in a traveler from Wuhan, China, on January 21, 2020.[1] The first residential domestic cases appeared in a nursing home in the Seattle, Washington, area on February 2, 2020 (McMichael et al., 2020), leading to a variety of infection control measures throughout the country. These included mask mandates, stay-home orders, business shutdowns, travel restrictions, and an unparalleled effort to develop and distribute a preventive vaccine.

The World Health Organization (WHO) declared an international health emergency on January 31, 2020, followed by the United States on February 3.[2] However, the global response was hampered by "contradictory and misleading advice," as well as denial and minimization of the risks of asymptomatic spread; these messages were delivered by health officials (including WHO's emergency director) and political leaders.[3] Although WHO offered some global guidance, the United States itself distanced from WHO early in the pandemic and issued a letter of withdrawal in July.[4]

For the first year of the pandemic, the only national-level U.S. response pertained to international travel restrictions. The vast majority of infection control orders were promulgated by leaders at the city, county, and state levels. In addition, these were materially and consequentially influenced by the elected leaders' prevailing political party affiliation. Generally, Democratic mayors and governors were more inclined to implement measures expected to prevent and/or limit the spread of infection than were Republican officials. Discordant actions and messaging among local, state, and national leaders—and between government officials versus physicians, scientists, epidemiologists, and other health experts—influenced

Susan G. Bornstein and Monica K. Miller, *U.S. Public Health Policy Responses to COVID-19* In: *The Social Science of the COVID-19 Pandemic*. Edited by: Monica K. Miller, Oxford University Press. © Oxford University Press 2024.
DOI: 10.1093/oso/9780197615133.003.0003

individual attitudes toward and compliance with recommended control measures, as well as subsequent willingness to receive COVID-19 vaccinations.

The Centers for Disease Control and Prevention (CDC), operating under the
Department of Health and Human Services (HHS), is the primary agency responsible for public health safety and emergency preparedness, including the detection
and prevention of communicable diseases, in the United States.[5] With respect to
COVID-19, the CDC was responsible for assessing the threat of danger to the
U.S. public, developing and/or delivering a test capable of accurately detecting the
infection, synthesizing and publicizing the evolving scientific evidence regarding
transmission, consulting/assisting with community tracking, and promulgating
guidelines designed to prevent further spread of the disease. A White House task
force, led by Vice President Mike Pence and comprising others appointed by then-
President Trump, issued updates daily, then weekly, then less often throughout the
pandemic, essentially ceasing by November 2020.

Meanwhile, most of the strategy decisions aimed at controlling the outbreak
were made at the state level, with considerable local, state, and regional variation. For instance, California was the first to issue stay-home orders instructing
residents not to leave the house except for essential tasks (work, groceries), and
ordered nonessential businesses to close or dramatically alter their operations.
In contrast, states such as Nebraska, Utah, and Arkansas did not issue stay-home
orders.[6]

Cities also enacted policies, at times conflicting with their state leaders to the
point of litigation, creating confusion and sowing mistrust among their citizenry.
For example, Georgia's Republican (R) Governor Kemp sued Democrat (D) Atlanta
Mayor Keisha Lance Bottom over Atlanta's mask mandate.[7] In Kentucky, Attorney
General Daniel Cameron (R) challenged Governor Andy Beshear's (D) ability to
enact emergency executive orders, including a mask mandate.[8] The net result of
these conflicts was reduced compliance with public health measures aimed at reducing the spread of disease.

A review of the global pandemic response, or even the guidelines of every state,
is beyond the scope of this chapter, particularly because they continuously and
frequently changed over time. Such summaries are available elsewhere.[9] This
chapter offers a brief discussion of U.S. policies, mandates, ordinances, and other
government orders enacted to protect public health.[10]

TRAVEL RESTRICTIONS

Following the emergence of the coronavirus in China, one of the first responses
of national governments was to institute travel bans restricting entry of travelers
from other countries experiencing COVID-19 outbreaks. On February 2, 2020,
the United States banned "foreign nationals who had visited China in the last
14 days" from entering the country, excluding U.S. citizens and permanent
residents.[11] However, by that time the virus was already endemic in the United
States and in other countries from which travelers were able to freely enter the

United States. Later in the pandemic, when the United Kingdom was found to have a more virulent variant of the virus, additional bans were instituted.

The CDC guidelines did not specifically prohibit travel, but recommended inquiry into destination infection control policies and procedures and wearing a mask in common areas.[12] It joined with the Department of Homeland Security on a "do not board" list or "lookout" list to prevent people with known COVID-19 infections from boarding planes. This was not entirely successful, with reports of people who knew that they were COVID-19 positive deliberately boarding airline flights.[13] By early 2021, anyone traveling by air into the United States from another country had to show negative coronavirus testing results dating within 3 days of departure or proof of successful recovery from the virus. Quarantine on arrival was not required.[14]

At the state level, there was a mixed assortment of rules and regulations, varying across time and location, ranging from no rules in some places, rules applying only to specified travelers, or rules that applied universally. Furthermore, the rules might apply only to those departing, those arriving, or both. Some states forbade all but nonessential travel. At one point, New York banned incoming travel from 41 states. Multiple states required official notification of intent to travel, and many required quarantining on arrival to the state. Failure to follow quarantine rules could result in penalties (e.g., in Hawaii). In some cases, the rules applied to travel from specifically named states, while other state restrictions were based on the infection or COVID-19 positivity rates in the states from which the traveler departed. Colorado required travelers to certain in-state locations to submit affidavits and to show proof of negative COVID-19 testing.[15] There could be additional entry requirements by cities or counties within a given state. For example, Chicago required visitors from any state with more than 15 average cases/ 100,000 residents to have a negative COVID test no more than 72 hours prior to arrival or to quarantine for 10 days.[16] Kentucky, on the other hand, had general recommendations against travel and for quarantine on return/arrival, but without legal requirements to do so[17]; Florida had no guidelines or requirements whatsoever.[18]

The ramifications of travel restrictions on people's lives and jobs, as well as on the tourism industry, were substantial. As COVID-19 rates surged and fell throughout the United States and across the globe, travel restrictions, and individual concerns about travel, continued to wax and wane throughout the pandemic.

STAY-HOME ORDERS

The first major mandates required people to stay home unless they were engaging in essential tasks, such as school, work, medical visits, or purchasing food. Unlike many other countries, in the United States there were no *national* orders limiting or restricting activity. The first statewide stay-home order was issued in California on March 20, 2020.[19] Throughout the pandemic, stay-home orders varied by state and duration and over time. Between March 1 and May 31, 2020, of 50 U.S. states, the District of Columbia, and the 5 U.S. territories (American Samoa, Guam, Northern Mariana Islands, Puerto Rico, and the U.S. Virgin Islands), 42 issued mandatory stay-home orders, 8 made recommendations or advisories, and 6 took no action (American Samoa, D; Arkansas, R; Connecticut, D; Nebraska, R; North Dakota, R; and Wyoming, R) (Moreland, 2020). As time progressed, states and territories completely reopened, paused, imposed new restrictions, or vacillated between more and less liberal restrictions, depending on levels of infections and perceived risks. On January 25, 2021, California Governor Newsom lifted the last remaining state's stay-home orders.[20]

In the setting of a highly communicable virus, without adequate capacity to diagnose COVID-19 infections, with no vaccine available, and without certain and effective treatments, the only public health strategy available to prevent the spread of disease was to keep people away from one another, most effectively by confining everyone to their own homes. Therefore, this was one of the earliest pandemic policies enacted by state and local governments. As infection rates diminished over the summer of 2020, these policies were relaxed, only to resume with rising infection rates and diminishing hospital beds and intensive care unit (ICU) capacity. With the Food and Drug Administration's approval of two COVID-19 vaccines in December 2020 and mass vaccination programs underway by early 2021, stay-home orders slowly ended.

LIMITING GATHERING SIZE

The term "social distancing" was quickly invented, based on the concept that the majority of expelled respiratory droplets containing viral particles fell to the ground within 6 feet from their source.[21] Thus, the CDC recommended avoidance of large groups, particularly indoors, and staying at least 6 feet away from persons outside of one's household. Mardi Gras, which concluded on February 25, 2020, was ultimately considered a nidus of many infections, hospitalizations, and deaths in New Orleans[22] and may have well been the first "superspreader" event in the United States. Concerts and sporting events were cancelled (see Chapter 2 for more on how COVID-19 changed life). Eventually, home gatherings of as few as 10 people or 2 households were prohibited in some areas, while others prohibited anyone from gathering with anyone else outside their household.

The CDC recommended staying home if ill, staying at least 6 feet away from others, and frequent handwashing or sanitization. However, there were no national limits on crowd size, leaving these decisions to state and local governments.[23] States, including South Dakota, Missouri, and Florida, issued no limits on gatherings, while South Carolina allowed up to 250 people. In South Dakota, not only did Governor Kristi Noem decline to limit gatherings, the state permitted an Independence Day celebration event for President Trump at Mt. Rushmore in early July, attended by a crowd of 3,700[24] and diverted $5 million in federal COVID-19 relief funds to promotion of tourism.[25] A massive motorcycle rally in Sturgis, South Dakota, in August, attended by a crowd of 462,000 people, was identified by some researchers as yet another superspreader event.[26] Meanwhile, other states enacted stricter regulations. Minnesota prohibited gatherings of over 10 people, Texas required approval by local officials for gatherings of more than 10, and Nashville, Tennessee, had a limit of 8 people. Sometimes regulations distinguished between indoor versus outdoor settings; for example, Mississippi allowed groups of 10 indoors, but 20 outdoors. At the opposite end of the spectrum, Vermont prohibited any gatherings of more than one household, and Puerto Rico restricted gatherings of ANY size. Many states had standards that varied by county or city and that changed with prevalence of virus.

Throughout the pandemic, there were varying restrictions on crowd size. However, given the absence of national guidance, these ranged from complete bans on gatherings to no limitations whatsoever. Overall, the restrictions decreased over time. By February 2021, state restrictions varied from no indoor social gatherings in some counties (Washington); limited to three households (California); groups no larger than six people in high-risk regions (Illinois, Oregon); limitations by county and attached to color-coded level of risk (Colorado); limitations varying according to type of venue (e.g., lower caps in private homes compared to dining, social, and cultural activities; Connecticut, Nevada); to no limits on crowd size altogether (Iowa and others).[27]

CLOSING SCHOOLS

In March 2020, schools began shutting down, typically by order of the local school boards or state governors. This included universities, which suspended classes, sports, and campus clubs and recalled study abroad students. While many schools and universities reopened in fall 2020, this proved temporary, and most were closed to on-campus learning again by Thanksgiving as infection rates surged.

The CDC issued guidance concerning ventilation and food service provision in hopes that improving air circulation and distancing would prevent spread of the virus.[28] The CDC also offered schools advice for managing students who were unable to wear masks and students with disabilities or healthcare needs. They suggested strategies for cleaning surfaces and screening students for COVID-19. Other recommendations included the creation of smaller class sizes to limit in-person contact. Specifically, with respect to colleges and universities, the CDC provided guidance for virus testing, treatment, and tracking; quarantining; operating shared housing; and cleaning and ventilating buildings.[29]

Across states and even within jurisdictions, there was wide variation of educational response to the pandemic. While K–12 decisions were largely made by local school boards or local and state governments, most universities were permitted to make decisions independently. K–12 schools converted face-to-face instruction into online ("distance") methods of instruction, thereby reducing potential for viral spread. By fall 2020, many K–12 schools that elected to hold on-site sessions implemented new protections, including outdoor classes, use of Plexiglas barriers, reduced class sizes, and requiring face masks. Some schools adopted staggered or alternate attendance in which, for example, half the students attended Monday and Tuesday, while other half attended Thursday and Friday (with Wednesdays hallmarked for cleaning). Research had indicated that children were less at risk of catching the virus than adults, but by the holidays, most schools had returned to distance learning.

In the spring of 2020, more than 1,300 colleges and universities across the United States closed their campuses.[30] While some continued their usual educational delivery methods, most transitioned to online education, and others ended the semester prematurely.[31] For the start of the fall 2020 classes, schools took myriad steps to inhibit the spread of the virus.[32] Many campuses required students to have a negative COVID-19 test before returning to campus, forbade off-campus parties, substituted carry-out foods for cafeteria dining, restricted both personal and professional travel, and cancelled sports activities entirely. Some even expelled students for violating the rules. Universities cancelled fall breaks and spring breaks out of concern that students would travel and bring the virus back to the classrooms and dormitories. Under similar reasoning, many universities extended the Thanksgiving holiday until after the New Year—ending the semester early. Conversely, some universities and colleges (e.g., Duke, Wagner College, Liberty University) remained open for face-to-face instruction.

In sum, both K–12 and institutions of higher education took many steps aimed at protecting the safety of students and staff. These included converting some or all classes to online platforms, cleaning, testing, and social distancing.

BUSINESS CLOSURES

In order to reduce the risk of viral exposure among employees, between employees and their customers, and among customers patronizing public and private enterprises, orders were issued restricting business operations across the United States. As with other policies related to COVID-19, the extent and duration of business closures varied by time and place.

When they occurred, business closures were typically determined by whether or not they provided "essential services." Although there were no national mandates affecting business operations, the Cybersecurity and Infrastructure Security Agency issued a document, "Guidance on the Essential Critical Infrastructure Workforce: Ensuring Community and National Resilience in COVID-19 Response" on March 23, 2020.[33] This provided information on the types of businesses and operations considered essential, including grocery stores, banks, gas stations, and hardware stores, as well as such activities as healthcare operations, governmental functions, public safety, and food and agriculture.[34] The U.S. Department of Homeland Security defined essential workers.[35] However, states were allowed to adopt their own definitions, and what constituted "essential businesses" could be spurious, such as doggy daycare.

The first business shutdowns occurred on March 15, 2020, in Los Angeles and New York City, affecting restaurants, bars, theaters, and movie houses—closures that New York State subsequently extended to all nonessential businesses.[36] Throughout the pandemic, there was particular attention directed toward bars and restaurants, patronage of which is neither compatible with continual mask wearing nor conducive to social distancing. Restrictions in drinking and dining establishments ranged from complete bans on in-person dining, to indoor capacity limits of 25%–75% of the fire code, to outdoor dining only. Sometimes the restrictions took the form of hours of operation, for example, not allowing patrons between 10 PM and 5 AM. For the most part, carry-out orders were permitted throughout the pandemic. Pennsylvania exemplified the seesawing of regulations experienced by some cities and states. Bars and restaurants were closed for in-person dining March 19, 2020, opened for in-person dining at 25% capacity on June 19, 2020, fully opened on July 16, 2020, reduced to 25% capacity on indoor service November 27, 2020, closed entirely on December 12, 2020, and reopened for bars at 25% of the fire code and restaurants at 75% capacity April 4, 2021.[37]

Beyond bars and restaurants, restrictions were most likely to apply to hair and nail salons, personal care services, movie theaters, tattoo parlors, museums, gyms, amusement parks, and pools. Decisions to reduce or eliminate in-person religious worship and sporting activities were particularly contentious. While Texas had no statewide closures, it reduced capacity at some businesses to 50%–75%, while specifically exempting religious services and recreational sports programs from any occupancy limits.[38] Among the states, only South Dakota refrained from any business closures.[39]

In summary, across the United States, the approach to business closures varied widely. New York, and New York City, which suffered the greatest numbers of infections and deaths in the early part of the pandemic, imposed some of the strictest control measures for the longest duration. Some states opened businesses, then paused their reopenings due to rising COVID-19 cases. Other times, limitations were based on statistics such as ICU bed availability or tiers of COVID-19 testing positivity results. As of this writing, late April 2021, with 133 million Americans vaccinated so far,[40] business restrictions are slowly being relaxed, although the country is not fully reopened.

MASK MANDATES

Perhaps the most politically, although not medically, controversial government orders were mask mandates. Facial covering of the mouth and nose has been shown to reduce the risk of contracting COVID-19.[41] Mask mandates reduce the numbers of infections in counties where mandates are implemented, compared to those where they are not.[42]

For the first year of the pandemic, there were no federal or national orders *requiring* masks in the United States. Initially, the CDC only recommended that people who were sick wear a mask. On February 29, 2020, the U.S. Surgeon General Dr. Jerome Adams tweeted: "Seriously people-STOP BUYING MASKS!"[43] The CDC's position was later attributed to inadequate stores of personal protective equipment (PPE) for healthcare personnel, stigma attached to mask wearing, concern that it would not be accepted by the public, and worry over inciting fear. On April 3, 2020, following debate with the White House and a change in the CDC's position, the United States finally issued a recommendation (not a mandate) for face coverings in public.[44] An April 2020 plan by the U.S. Postal Service to distribute five reusable face masks to all U.S. households was never implemented.[45] The CDC did not encourage universal mask use indoors until December 4, 2020, nearly a year into the pandemic (Honein, 2020).

Regardless, based on theoretical, and ultimately empirical, evidence of the effectiveness of mask wearing in reducing the spread of COVID-19, mask mandates slowly began to emerge within U.S. cities, counties, states, and territories. The first states to issue mandates were Connecticut and New York on April 17, 2020, with Wyoming last, on December 9, 2020 (Harcourt et al., 2020). Ultimately, the majority of states issued mask-wearing mandates applicable to the general public. However, in Georgia and Arizona, masks were only required statewide for certain employees, with local officials allowed to require mask wearing for the general public. Eleven states, all with Republican governors (Alaska, Arizona, Indiana, South Dakota, Nebraska, Oklahoma, Missouri, Tennessee, Georgia, Florida, South Carolina), had no statewide mask mandates.[46]

The absence of statewide mandates produced some interesting responses. For instance, following a Republican caucus postelection dinner celebration, in which masks were not worn and four senators in attendance subsequently tested positive for COVID-19 (one of whom died), the Minnesota state legislature *defeated* a proposal to require mandatory mask usage in public areas of the state capitol (which was exempt from the state mandate).[47] State Republican majority leader Senator Paul Gazelka, one of the legislators who tested positive following the dinner, said: "Our future cannot be prolonged isolation, face coverings, and limited activities."[48] At the opposite end of the spectrum, New York City and Glendale, California, imposed financial penalties for failures to wear masks.[49]

Of note, in an effort to protect their employees and their customers, in July 2020 some of the country's largest retail chains began requiring everyone to wear masks inside their establishments, including Walmart, Amazon, Kroger, Costco, Walgreens, Home Depot, CVS, Target, Apple, and Starbucks.[50]

Beginning with the initial response by the CDC and followed by continued mixed messaging, mask wearing in the United States was a contentious and politically charged subject, to the point of provoking physical conflict between those wishing to assert their individual freedom not to wear a mask and those trying to follow orders or to protect their personal safety. President Biden's inauguration on January 20, 2021, marked a sharp change in the U.S. approach to mask wearing. Within hours of assuming office, he began requiring the wearing of masks on federal property.[51] The next day, he issued an executive order mandating masks for travel on airplanes, trains, and public transportation, as well as in airports.[52]

OTHER TYPE OF ORDERS

There have been a variety of other types of orders related to the COVID pandemic. One of the most critical issues early on was inadequate PPE, needed to reduce the risk of medical personnel and first responders becoming infected themselves. Activation of the Defense Production Act (DPA) was considered as early as February 2020[53] to allow ramped up manufacturing of masks, gowns, ventilators, and other necessary medical and protective supplies. In March through September 2020, approximately $3.9 billion was spent on contracts and agreements executed by governmental agencies under the DPA and included purchases of ventilators, swabs, gloves, and vaccine supplies.[54] The DPA was enacted again on January 21, 2021, to increase supplies for testing.[55]

The CARES Act was signed into federal law on March 27, 2020, providing $2 trillion in aid to healthcare organizations, businesses, and state and local governments. It directed suspension of student loan payments and stopped collections on defaulted loans. The CARES Act also provided for mortgage payment forbearance for an initial term of 180 days, which could be extended for another 180 days on request,[56] and prohibited evictions for 120 days from federally insured or backed multifamily rental housing.[57] The CDC issued an order September 4, 2020, to halt evictions from residential property, which was extended through January 31, 2021. Ten states had protections that were more comprehensive than the CDC, and some states (Arizona, Delaware, Montana, Ohio, Iowa, and New York) allocated funds for rental assistance.[58] Nonetheless, families were evicted despite this ban.[59]

COVID-19 testing, unlike most other healthcare services in United States, was provided without charge to recipients. On January 16, 2020, HHS announced that the COVID-19 vaccine, when available, would also be free of charge to those who could not afford it,[60] and on September 16, 2020, HHS and the Department of Defense released a plan to have the COVID-19 vaccine provided free to all Americans.[61]

Nursing homes, with their predominantly frail and elderly populations, were afflicted by a disproportionate share of COVID-19 illness and deaths. Based on CDC guidance,[62] the Centers for Medicare and Medicaid Services issued a memorandum on March 13, 2020, directing nursing homes to restrict visitors except for compassionate care situations, as well as restricting communal activities.[63] Given the mental toll on residents, this guidance was relaxed in September, and outdoor visitation encouraged.[64] In an effort to protect their vulnerable residents during the pandemic, some facilities completely sequestered staff and residents for weeks; others prohibited visitation, while allowing staff to come and go; some limited the number of visitors; and some required proof of negative testing before family and friends were allowed to see their loved ones.

Innumerable actions and orders arose in response to the extensive repercussions of the COVID-19 pandemic. These occurred at the executive, legislative, and judicial levels, by communities, cities, and states, as well as within individual sectors such as nursing homes. They were influenced by political affiliation, perceived risk, prevalence of disease, economic concerns, individual values, and more.

VACCINE ADMINISTRATION

On December 11, 2020, the U.S. Food and Drug Administration approved the first vaccine for COVID-19. The CDC issued recommendations on administration of the vaccine. However, these were only guidelines, and states could establish their own plans for determining who would receive the vaccine, and in what order. Vaccine quantity was allocated to states based on population, rather than the number of higher risk individuals, such as healthcare workers, the number of elderly persons, or those in long-term care facilities. With vaccines in limited supply, states were forced to make difficult decisions about how to prioritize administration.[65]

The CDC Advisory Committee on Immunization Practices (ACIP) recommended that the first people to receive the vaccine (1a) should be healthcare workers and long-term care residents, such as those living in nursing homes. The second group (1b) to receive the vaccine would be essential workers outside of healthcare and people over the age of 75. The third group (1c) comprised people ages 65–74 and those aged 16–64 with high-risk medical conditions, along with essential workers not in Group 1b.[66]

There was considerable variety in prioritization of the vaccine from state to state.[67] Approximately 45 states followed the ACIP guidelines to initially vaccinate healthcare workers and long-term care residents, although some chose to vaccinate both groups simultaneously, while others vaccinated sequentially as more vaccines became available. Over 20 states (e.g., Alabama) had subcategories for healthcare workers, allowing those at highest risk to get vaccinated before those at lower risk. States such as Maryland and Tennessee deviated by prioritizing people over 65 before nonhealth essential workers. A few states also included law enforcement (e.g., New Hampshire), while others included incarcerated or homeless people (e.g., Massachusetts, Oklahoma) or educators in the early phases of vaccination.

By January 15, 2021, states had begun vaccinating groups beyond Phase 1a, even if vaccinations of the 1a group had not been completed, albeit according to diverse criteria. Interestingly, some states, such as Florida, did not require proof of residency, leading motivated visitors from out of state to travel to Florida to obtain shots that were less readily accessible in their home state, a practice that became known as "vaccine tourism."[68]

On his first day in office, President Joe Biden took steps to improve the national vaccination effort. He created a federal office to coordinate the COVID-19 response and restored the White House National Security Council directorate for global health security and defense, which had been dismantled under the previous administration.[69] President Biden directed the Federal Emergency Management Agency and the National Guard to build clinics across the country to increase administration of the COVID-19 vaccine.[70]

In sum, states varied considerably in their administration of the vaccine. While most generally adhered to CDC guidelines, many deviated—perhaps in response to their residents' community sentiment (vaccinating teachers to get children back in school in Elberton, Georgia),[71] economic needs, or political favoritism (e.g., a pop-up vaccination clinic in a wealthy section of Manatee County, Florida).[72]

SUMMARY

The pandemic brought about near daily orders, policies, and practices—some of which were revoked within days of being issued. Although the quickly changing environment confounded analysis, a preliminary study of multiple countries indicated that the most successful measures were curfews, lockdowns, school and business closures, and restricting size of gatherings, although the degree of success was dependent on infection rates and compliance (Brauner et al., 2021; Haug et al., 2020; Wibbens et al., 2020). Mask mandates were also effective in reducing the risk of COVID-19 infections and death (Guy, 2021).

This overview described many of the government regulations regarding COVID-19 designed to protect public health by limiting or preventing spread of the virus. The chapters that follow discuss many of these regulations in detail, and how social science theories can help explain COVID-related behaviors and experienced outcomes.

NOTES

1. https://www.cdc.gov/media/releases/2020/p0121-novel-coronavirus-travel-case.html
2. https://www.ajmc.com/view/a-timeline-of-covid19-developments-in-2020
3. https://www.nytimes.com/2020/06/27/world/europe/coronavirus-spread-asymptomatic.html
4. https://www.statnews.com/2020/07/07/trump-administration-submits-formal-notice-of-withdrawal-from-who/
5. https://www.cdc.gov/about/history/index.html
6. https://ballotpedia.org/States_that_did_not_issue_stay-at-home_orders_in_response_to_the_coronavirus_(COVID-19)_pandemic,_2020
7. https://www.cnn.com/2020/08/13/politics/brian-kemp-atlanta-mask-lawsuit-withdrawing/index.html
8. https://www.courier-journal.com/story/news/politics/2020/07/10/judges-order-block-beshears-mask-order-going-into-effect/5412862002/
9. https://www.aarp.org/politics-society/government-elections/info-2020/coronavirus-state-restrictions.html
10. Note that these regulations changed regularly, and thus the online sources are updated regularly. The information presented was current at some point, but as regulations changed, so did the restrictions. Thus, the references provided might not currently reflect the information presented here.

11. https://www.washingtonpost.com/outlook/2020/10/01/debate-early-travel-bans-china/
12. https://www.cdc.gov/coronavirus/2019-ncov/travelers/travel-during-covid19.html
13. https://www.washingtonpost.com/travel/2020/12/28/passenger-covid-flight-airlines-positive
14. https://www.nytimes.com/2021/01/14/travel/international-travel-covid-test.html
15. https://www.usatoday.com/story/travel/news/2021/01/11/covid-travel-restrictions-which-states-require-covid-test-quarantine/6566179002/
16. https://www.usatoday.com/story/travel/news/2021/01/11/covid-travel-restrictions-which-states-require-covid-test-quarantine/6566179002/
17. https://www.usatoday.com/story/travel/news/2021/01/11/covid-travel-restrictions-which-states-require-covid-test-quarantine/6566179002/
18. https://floridahealthcovid19.gov/travelers/
19. https://www.reuters.com/article/us-health-coronavirus-timeline-idUSKBN23Z0UW
20. https://apnews.com/article/california-lifts-stay-home-order-virus-1c298c67338a5914f7c3857cd167edcc
21. https://www.cdc.gov/coronavirus/2019-ncov/more/scientific-brief-sars-cov-2.html
22. https://www.nytimes.com/2020/03/26/us/coronavirus-louisiana-new-orleans.html
23. https://www.northstarmeetingsgroup.com/News/Industry/Coronavirus-states-cities-reopening-COVID-19-new-cases
24. https://abcnews.go.com/Politics/trump-mount-rushmore-controversy-fireworks-personal-fascination/story?id=71595321
25. https://www.nytimes.com/2021/01/17/us/covid-deaths-2020.html
26. https://www.webmd.com/lung/news/20200909/sturgis-bike-rally-superspreading-event-or-not
27. http://www.aarp.org/politics-society/government-elections/info-2020/coronavirus-state-restrictions.html
28. https://www.cdc.gov/coronavirus/2019-ncov/community/schools-childcare/schools.html
29. https://www.cdc.gov/coronavirus/2019-ncov/community/colleges-universities/index.html; https://www.cdc.gov/coronavirus/2019-ncov/community/colleges-universities/considerations.html
30. https://www.ncsl.org/research/education/higher-education-responses-to-coronavirus-covid-19.aspx
31. https://www.insidehighered.com/news/2020/03/12/why-are-some-colleges-closing-over-virus-concerns-while-others-stay-open
32. https://www.npr.org/2020/03/06/812462913/6-ways-universities-are-responding-to-coronavirus
33. https://www.hsdl.org/?abstract&did=835403
34. https://content.next.westlaw.com/Document/Id9e2366772d611ea80afece799150095/View/FullText.html?transitionType=Default&contextData=(sc.Default)
35. https://www.ncsl.org/research/labor-and-employment/covid-19-essential-workers-in-the-states.aspx#:~:text=According%20to%20the%20U.,to%20defense%20to%20agriculture

36. https://www.reuters.com/article/us-health-coronavirus-timeline-idUSKB N23Z0UW

37. https://content.next.westlaw.com/Document/Id9e2366772d611ea80afece799150 095/View/FullText.html?transitionType=Default&contextData=(sc.Default)

38. https://content.next.westlaw.com/Document/Id9e2366772d611ea80afece799150 095/View/FullText.html?transitionType=Default&contextData=(sc.Default)

39. https://ballotpedia.org/States_that_did_not_issue_stay-at-home_orders_in_respo nse_to_the_coronavirus_(COVID-19)_pandemic,_2020

40. https://www.nytimes.com/interactive/2020/us/covid-19-vaccine-doses.html

41. https://www.cdc.gov/coronavirus/2019-ncov/more/masking-science-sars-cov2.html

42. https://www.usnews.com/news/best-states/articles/these-are-the-states-with-mask-mandates

43. https://www.nytimes.com/2020/06/27/world/europe/coronavirus-spread-asymp tomatic.html

44. https://www.washingtonpost.com/health/2020/04/03/white-house-cdc-turf-bat tle-over-guidance-broad-use-face-masks-fight-coronavirus/

45. https://www.cnbc.com/2020/09/17/white-house-abandoned-plan-to-deliver-650-million-face-masks-across-us-report-says.html

46. http://www.aarp.org/health/healthy-living/info-2020/states-mask-mandates-coro navirus.html

47. https://www.nytimes.com/2021/01/18/us/politics/relph-covid-minnesota.html

48. https://minnesota.cbslocal.com/2020/11/15/republican-senate-majority-leader-paul-gazelka-tests-positive-for-covid/

49. https://www.marketplace.org/2020/09/16/penalties-behavioral-economics-fine-people-who-refuse-wear-mask/

50. http://www.aarp.org/health/healthy-living/info-2020/retailers-require-face-masks-coronavirus.html

51. https://www.wlky.com/article/bidens-first-act-orders-on-pandemic-climate-immi gration/35265918

52. https://www.wlky.com/article/president-biden-puts-forth-virus-strategy-requi res-mask-usc-to-travel/35275720

53. https://www.usnews.com/news/health-news/articles/2020-03-01/us-announces-more-travel-restrictions-as-first-coronavirus-death-reported

54. https://www.gao.gov/products/GAO-21-108

55. https://www.wlky.com/article/president-biden-puts-forth-virus-strategy-requi res-mask-use-to-travel/35275720

56. https://www.hud.gov/sites/dfiles/SFH/documents/IACOVID19FBFactSheetC onsumer.pdf

57. https://www.hud.gov/coronavirus/renters

58. https://www.cnbc.com/2020/09/08/most-evictions-in-the-us-are-now-ban ned-what-you-need-to-know-.html

59. https://www.npr.org/2020/12/20/947992198/why-the-cdc-eviction-ban-isnt-rea lly-a-ban-i-have-nowhere-to-go

60. https://www.ajmc.com/view/us-releases-more-details-about-covid19-vaccine-process-says-some-doses-will-be-free

61. https://www.ajmc.com/view/a-timeline-of-covid19-developments-in-2020

62. https://www.cdc.gov/coronavirus/2019-ncov/hcp/long-term-care.html
63. https://www.cms.gov/newsroom/press-releases/cms-announces-new-measures-protect-nursing-home-residents-covid-19
64. https://www.cms.gov/newsroom/press-releases/cms-announces-new-guidance-safe-visitation-nursing-homes-during-covid-19-public-health-emergency
65. https://www.kff.org/policy-watch/how-are-states-prioritizing-who-will-get-the-covid-19-vaccine-first/
66. https://www.cdc.gov/coronavirus/2019-ncov/vaccines/recommendations-process.html
67. https://www.kff.org/policy-watch/how-are-states-prioritizing-who-will-get-the-covid-19-vaccine-first/
68. https://www.wsj.com/articles/floridas-covid-19-vaccines-draw-foreigners-snowbirds-11610620200
69. https://www.wlky.com/article/bidens-first-act-orders-on-pandemic-climate-immigration/35265918
70. https://www.wlky.com/article/president-biden-puts-forth-virus-strategy-requires-mask-use-to-travel/35275720
71. https://www.washingtonpost.com/nation/2021/01/29/elberton-georgia-vaccine-teachers-suspended/
72. https://www.cnn.com/2021/02/17/politics/ron-desantis-vaccines/index.html

REFERENCES

Brauner, J. M., Mindermann, S., Sharma, M., Johnston, D., Salvatier, J., Gavenčiak, T., Stephenson, A. B., Leech, G., Altman, G., Mikulik, V., Norman, A. J., Monrad, J. T., Besiroglu, T., Ge, H., Hartwick, M. A., Teh, Y. W., Chindelevitch, L., Gal, Y., & Kulveit, J. (2021). Inferring the effectiveness of government interventions against COVID-19. *Science, 371*(6531). https://doi.org/10.1126/science.abd9338

Guy, G. P. (2021). Association of state-issued mask mandates and allowing on-premises restaurant dining with county-level COVID-19 case and death growth rates—United States, March 1–December 31, 2020. *MMWR. Morbidity and Mortality Weekly Report, 70*, 350–354. https://doi.org/10.15585/mmwr.mm7010e3

Harcourt, J., Tamin, A., Lu, X., Kamili, S., Sakthivel, S. K., Murray, J., Queen, K., Tao, Y., Paden, C. R., Zhang, J., Li, Y., Uehara, A., Wang, H., Goldsmith, C., Bullock, H. A., Wang, L., Whitaker, B., Lynch, B., Gautam, R., . . . Thornburg, N. J. (2020). Severe acute respiratory syndrome coronavirus 2 from patient with coronavirus disease, United States. *Emerging Infectious Diseases, 26*(6), 1266–1273. https://doi.org/10.3201/eid2606.200516

Haug, N., Geyrhofer, L., Londei, A., Dervic, E., Desvars-Larrive, A., Loreto, V., Pinior, B., Thurner, S., & Klimek, P. (2020). Ranking the effectiveness of worldwide COVID-19 government interventions. *Nature Human Behaviour, 4*(12), 1303–1312. https://doi.org/10.1038/s41562-020-01009-0

Honein, M. A. (2020). Summary of guidance for public health strategies to address high levels of community transmission of SARS-CoV-2 and related deaths. *MMWR. Morbidity and Mortality Weekly Report, 69*(49), 1860–1867. https://doi.org/10.15585/mmwr.mm6949e2

McMichael, T. M., et al. (2020). COVID-19 in a long-term care facility—King County, Washington. *MMWR. Morbidity and Mortality Weekly Report, 69*(12), 339–342. https://doi.org/10.15585/mmwr.mm6912e1

Moreland, A. (2020). Timing of state and territorial COVID-19 stay-at-home orders and changes in population movement—United States, March 1–May 31, 2020. *MMWR. Morbidity and Mortality Weekly Report, 69*(35), 1198–1203. https://doi.org/10.15585/mmwr.mm6935a2

Wibbens, P. D., Koo, W. W.-Y., & McGahan, A. M. (2020). Which COVID policies are most effective? A Bayesian analysis of COVID-19 by jurisdiction. *PLoS One, 15*(12), 1–19. https://doi.org/10.1371/journal.pone.0244177

4

The Ethics of the COVID-19 Pandemic

JENNIFER L. LANTERMAN ■

Public health challenges, crises, prevention efforts, and risk mitigation measures are often fraught with ethical issues and dilemmas. The COVID-19 pandemic required individual and organizational decision-making that collectively influenced the trajectory of the pandemic. Macrolevel ethical issues and microlevel ethical dilemmas related to individual behavior, decision-making by medical professionals, leadership, and the economy have all emerged as a result of the COVID-19 pandemic. People make decisions based on a variety of factors, including individual ethical orientations and professional ethics. This chapter introduces ethical issues and dilemmas, initial ethics considerations in the United States context, and areas for research. Ethics scholars and other researchers are encouraged to more thoroughly assess these and other issues to establish a historical record and guidance for ethical conduct in future pandemics.

BRIEF THEORETICAL FRAMEWORK

Deontology, utilitarianism, and Rawls's theory of justice (hereafter, social justice) are three ethics theories that aid in framing the ethical issues and dilemmas observed during the COVID-19 pandemic. Deontology posits that actions are ethical if they are guided by a set of universal rules, motivated by a sense of duty and obligation, rational, and reflect a respect for all people regardless of their qualities or rank (Benn, 1998; Hill, 2000; Kant, 1785/1998). Deontologists are not concerned about the impact or outcomes of their actions for themselves or anyone else. For example, an adherent of deontology would comply with rational, universal rules regardless of outcomes unless there was some overriding harm caused by compliance with the universal rule (Dancy, 1991).

Jennifer L. Lanterman, *The Ethics of the COVID-19 Pandemic* In: *The Social Science of the COVID-19 Pandemic*. Edited by: Monica K. Miller, Oxford University Press. © Oxford University Press 2024. DOI: 10.1093/oso/9780197615133.003.0004

Utilitarianism posits that actions are ethical or unethical based purely on the nature and magnitude of the outcomes they produce (Bentham, 1789; Mill, 1867). Utilitarians assess an action as ethical if it produces the greatest possible benefits for the people who are impacted by the action, regardless of the circumstances associated with how the action was executed (Rachels & Rachels, 2018). Modern utilitarians define benefits as mental state or experience views, preference or desire views, and objective or substantive views (Mulgan, 2014). Utilitarians who define benefits as mental state assess an action as ethical if it produces a positive state of mind for them (Mulgan, 2014). Those who define benefits as preferences assess an action as ethical if it satisfies their preferences, which is consistent with the original utilitarian concept of hedonism (Mulgan, 2014). Finally, utilitarians who define benefits as objective goods assess an action to be ethical if it produces an outcome that would be good for any person, such as good health (Mulgan, 2014).

Rawls's (1999) theory of justice informs contemporary social justice theory. This theory of justice emphasizes individual rights and focuses on the creation of institutions and societies that assign duties and equitably distribute the benefits and burdens of life in societies in ways that support those individual rights (Rawls, 1999). A just society will be governed by two principles (Banks, 2020; Rawls, 1999):

- Every person in the society has the right to the most extensive liberties compatible with equivalent liberties for others, and
- Social and economic inequalities are distributed in ways that are to everyone's advantage and accessible to everyone, regardless of position.

According to this theory, people in just societies use the government as an instrument to express solidarity with other members of the society, and the government regulates people in ways that prevent people with more resources from exploiting the system to their advantage and to the disadvantage of others with fewer resources (Alejandro, 1998; Rawls, 1999). In societies governed by social justice theory, individual and institutional behaviors are assessed as ethical if they support equitable access to resources and exposure to harms.

These three theories can be used to understand ethical issues and dilemmas. Ethical issues are macrolevel or big-picture issues that present ethical or moral problems (e.g., the impact of a lockdown on the economy). Ethical dilemmas are microlevel or specific instances in which a person must apply their ethical standards or morals to make a decision (e.g., deciding whether or not to attend a party during a pandemic).

ETHICS AND PUBLIC HEALTH

Public health is the collective effort of individuals and institutions to ensure the conditions necessary for people to live healthy lives (Institute of Medicine, 2003). It is critical to understand that public health as an outcome is dependent on the efforts of both individual people and organizations. If individual people refuse to engage in behaviors that support public health, particularly if a large enough proportion of the population is noncompliant with prevention or risk mitigation measures, then the public health is compromised, and institutions cannot compensate for the effects of noncompliant health behaviors. Abbasi and colleagues (2018) conducted a systematic review of research on public health ethics frameworks and the values and normative behaviors reflected in public health policy and practice. They found that most contemporary public health frameworks seek to balance the obligations to prevent harm, improve health, and respect individual autonomy (Abbasi et al., 2018). As such, achieving public health as an outcome requires a balance of deontological, utilitarian, and social justice considerations at the individual, community, and societal levels.

ETHICS AND INDIVIDUAL BEHAVIOR

Pandemic-related decision-making started at the individual level. People were required to make numerous choices for themselves and their families. There were numerous microlevel choices people had to make every day with respect to compliance with lockdowns, stay-home orders, mask mandates or recommendations, and physical distancing practices (see Bornstein & Miller, Chapter 3, for more information on public health responses and government mandates). In addition to compliance with public health measures to mitigate disease spread, people had to make decisions about how to procure supplies that might be necessary, but in short supply (e.g., personal protective equipment [PPE], disinfecting supplies, toilet paper). These individual decisions involved, broadly speaking, choices to purchase what people actually needed versus hoarding supplies so they and their families had sufficient resources, but other people might have been unable to access these resources. As of December 2020, people had to make decisions about seeking COVID-19 vaccines as they became eligible under their states' guidelines or electing not to be vaccinated (see Bornstein & Miller, Chapter 3, for more information on vaccine administration).

There are two aspects of utilitarianism that are useful in understanding how people make these individual decisions throughout the pandemic. First, how a person defines benefits impacts how they evaluate options. People who define benefits as mental state or individual preferences are more likely to make choices that benefit them personally, regardless of the consequences of those choices for other people. Conversely, people who define benefits as objective goods are more likely to consider people beyond themselves and their families when they evaluate their options. Second, how people define their groups or communities of interest (i.e., ingroup and outgroup) will influence how they evaluate options. Group identities can be very narrow (e.g., immediate family) or expansive (e.g., state of residence, racial or ethnic group). The scope of individual conceptions of group identity or communities of interest influence decision-making; people tend to make decisions that benefit their ingroup (Roets et al., 2020). People who narrowly define their communities of interest will consider the effects of their decisions on a smaller population of people relative to people who more broadly define the ingroup. More objective good definitions of benefits and expansive definitions of groups or communities of interest also relate to the deontological principle of respect for all persons and the social justice principles of equity and fairness.

Ethics and social psychology scholars should consider these individual assessments in the context of personality differences (see Devereaux, Chapter 46, for more information on personality and individual difference theories) and people residing or having been socialized in individualist or collectivist cultures (Torelli & Shavitt, 2010). Personality and cultural differences influence the values a person espouses. Values influence individual ethical assessments (see also Chapter 37 for more on the related topic of moral foundations).

ETHICS AND DECISION-MAKING BY MEDICAL PROFESSIONALS

The COVID-19 pandemic, by definition, presented myriad ethical issues for medical professionals. First, COVID-19 was a novel virus. The novelty of the disease meant that medical professionals initially knew very little about its cause, method of spread, and most effective treatment. Thus, they had to make decisions about treatment without being able to thoroughly assess the benefits and risks of a course of treatment.

Second, medical professionals must decide how to allocate resources when hospitals or intensive care units reach or exceed capacity,[1] have more patients who require ventilators than are available or have insufficient specialized medical personnel to operate the ventilators,[2] or if hospitals exhaust their oxygen supplies.[3] Their options include providing the best care available to people in the order that they arrive in the hospital and the order in which their deteriorating conditions require additional interventions, or they must decide who receives which limited resources (Kisner, 2020). Savulescu and colleagues (2020) identified some of the criteria that medical professionals could consider in determining who receives what care, including how to maximize care for the largest number of patients, age of patients and life expectancy should they recover, the quality of life a person will have should they recover, and the "social worth" of patients or what they contribute to society (e.g., a respiratory therapist vs. a drug-dependent homeless person). These criteria are fraught with ethical issues and bias. In the United States, medical professionals cannot ignore how race and ethnicity are inextricably linked to the pre-existing health conditions that increase the likelihood of severe COVID-19 illness and prognosis (Lopez et al., 2021; see Berthelot & Bornstein, Chapter 25, for more information on healthcare inequities in the United States).

Third, the COVID-19 pandemic struck during a time of extreme political polarization and racial tension in the United States. (See Chapter 15 by Lin and Druckman for more on political polarization). It is possible that physicians, nurses, and other medical personnel will encounter people who express bigoted views that are offensive to them or diminish them as people. For example, a physician who is an immigrant or the child of immigrants could encounter a patient wearing attire that expresses anti-immigrant sentiment. A Jewish nurse could encounter a patient with a swastika tattoo. An African American respiratory therapist could encounter a patient wearing a T-shirt depicting a confederate flag or who is using racial slurs.

Physicians, nurses, and other medical professionals espouse their own personal ethics. Their work duties are bound by professional ethics, which are enshrined in the Hippocratic Oath, Nightingale Pledge, and other professional codes of ethics. Physicians swear a modern version of the Hippocratic Oath on graduation from medical school (Tyson, 2001). This oath requires that physicians provide the best care they are able to provide to people who present to them with a need for medical care. Similarly, nurses take the Nightingale Pledge on graduation from nursing school (VSUN Communications, 2010). The premise of this pledge is that nurses will act in the best interest of patients and will support physicians in their care of patients. Other medical professionals are also bound by codes of ethics. For example, respiratory therapists are bound by the American Association for Respiratory Care (AARC) Statement of Ethics and Professional Conduct (2015). This code of ethics, like the Hippocratic Oath and the Nightingale Pledge, requires respiratory therapists to provide care to patients without bias of any kind.

In situations where personal ethics and professional ethics are in conflict, medical professionals are expected to abide by their professional ethics. The superordinate role of professional ethics can be understood through deontology. Deontology requires the use of universal rules guided by a motive of duty. According to the oaths, pledges, and codes of ethics that guide medical professionals, medical care can only be ethically provided if universal rules are free from bias and discrimination. This duty requires, for example, a Jewish medical professional to provide the same level of care to an anti-Semitic patient as they would provide to a patient who is not anti-Semitic, regardless of that medical provider's personal values, individual ethical assessment of the situation, or the impact that providing that care under abusive circumstances has on the medical professional.

The prohibition of bias and discrimination in medical care is ideal. However, this goal is particularly challenging in the United States given the pernicious challenge of racial inequities in healthcare in the United States. This persistent inequity complicates the ethical provision of care. This inequity is amplified when personnel and material resources during a pandemic are scarce, and medical professionals may need to make more frequent decisions about who receives care. In this scenario, in the United States, deontological duties, social justice concerns, and utilitarian criteria for resource allocation clash with professional ethics. Medical ethics researchers should use the historic event of the COVID-19 pandemic to explore how medical professionals around the United States made decisions about resource allocation given the stress to many healthcare systems. It would be useful for researchers to inquire if professionals think their decision-making processes have been changed given the intense focus on racial inequity in every aspect of U.S. life in recent years. Furthermore, it would be useful to explore the impact of providing care to patients, in a manner consistent with professional ethics, when those patients clearly do not respect or value medical professionals as people due to their race, gender, or perceived religious beliefs.

ETHICS AND LEADERSHIP

People in positions of leadership were required to make decisions for constituencies of varying size throughout the pandemic. Assessments of many of these performances have varied over time (see Blank, Chapter 38, for more information on hindsight and outcome bias), while other performances have received steady assessments over time (see Stedham & Mueller, Chapter 32, for more information on transformational leadership). The case of U.S. Navy Captain Brett Crozier offers an interesting case of decision-making in the instance of conflicting professional duties in which professional codes of ethics do not offer clear guidance and the way people weigh duties is influenced by their roles.

Captain Crozier was the commanding officer of the *Theodore Roosevelt*, a U.S. Navy aircraft carrier, served by approximately 5,000 sailors. He was frustrated by what he perceived to be the slow response and inadequate efforts to get sailors off of the carrier and into safer conditions on land in Guam. He sent an e-mail about the circumstances on the carrier through unclassified channels and the e-mail was leaked, which was an embarrassment to military leadership senior to him and to then-President Trump.[4] The U.S. Navy classified Captain Crozier's response to the COVID-19 outbreak on the carrier as poor and determined that he violated the chain of command. He was subsequently relieved of his command. He indicated that he knew he was jeopardizing his career with this action, but he was alarmed by the rapidly deteriorating situation on the carrier that ultimately resulted in 1,200 crew testing positive for COVID-19, several being hospitalized, and one crew member dying from COVID-19 complications.[5] He was dismissed by his superiors, but received a hero's send off by his crew who believed he saved their lives.

Captain Crozier's choice to communicate outside of the chain of command to accelerate a response to the COVID-19 outbreak on the *Theodore Roosevelt* can be understood through the interaction of a personal deontological orientation and the Department of the Navy Code of Ethics. People in positions of military leadership have an obligation to execute lawful orders in support of their respective branch's mission and a duty of care to the subordinates under their command while executing those orders. Ideally, these dual obligations are compatible and can be satisfied. However, sometimes these obligations are in conflict, which creates ethical dilemmas for military leaders. The Department of the Navy's (2005) Code of Ethics requires all sailors and Marines to be loyal to the Constitution, the laws, and ethical principles and to protect and conserve federal property while explicitly stating that all sailors and Marines should avoid taking actions that appear to be illegal or unethical. Captain Crozier viewed his obligations to include the faithful execution of lawful orders, good order and maintenance of the *Theodore Roosevelt*, and a duty of care to his crew. His perception of the slow and inadequate response to the COVID-19 outbreak on the carrier created a set of conflicting duties. Consistent with Dancy (1991), Captain Crozier ceased executing orders or abiding by the chain of command when he thought that those orders unnecessarily jeopardized the safety of his crew.

In this case, Captain Crozier chose to violate one set of universal rules to satisfy another duty at great personal expense. Other warship captains communicated with him indicating that they thought he was "doing the right thing."[6] People in other positions have criticized Captain Crozier's actions, including then-Acting Navy Secretary Thomas Modly and Admiral Mike Gilday,[7] retired naval officers,[8] and retired officers from other branches of the military.[9] These different perspectives can be partially explained by different roles, which involve different scopes of responsibility. Captain Crozier and other warship captains occupy operational roles. These roles involve daily operations and care for their crews. The secretary of the Navy, admirals, and retired generals across the branches occupy strategic roles. They are focused on "bigger picture" issues and less focused on daily operations. Leaders in strategic roles might be more inclined to value and expect deference to orders than they are to be concerned with the daily effects of compliance with those orders.

This case raises several issues for military ethicists to consider. First, they should explore how militaries can expect to cultivate ethical leaders when those leaders are punished for pursuing a course of action that can reasonably be considered ethical. If military personnel are expected to follow all lawful orders, regardless of the outcomes of those orders, then the Uniform Code of Military Justice and the codes of ethics guiding each branch of the U.S. military ought to be revised to reflect this change to conduct expectations. Second, military ethicists should consider ways to reduce the occurrence of situations in which military leaders are given orders that are in conflict with fundamental duties and obligations as a leader.

ETHICS AND THE ECONOMY

The COVID-19 pandemic has raised numerous ethical issues in relation to the economy. Lawmakers had to determine who was classified as "essential" staff, which would require those people to continue to work in in-person settings. Some sectors of the economy had to remain operational, including essential and emergency medical care, grocery stores, and gas stations, among others. Women and people of color are less likely to have employment that allows them to work at home, and they are more likely to work in jobs that are high risk (e.g., at grocery stores) during a pandemic (see Willis-Esqueda & Estrada-Reynolds, Chapter 24, for more information on inequality and employment). People who work in these sectors of the economy had to return to the workplace if they wished to retain their jobs, but this return was complicated by the absence of guarantees to adequate access to PPE.[10,11,12,13]

Lawmakers also had to determine whether and how to safely open day-care centers and schools (see Bornstein & Miller, Chapter 3, for more information on school closures). These complicated decisions involved the safety of infants and children, childcare providers, teachers, and school staff. These decisions exerted significant economic and professional impacts on the parents of young children (Igielnik, 2021), particularly the mothers of young children (Barroso & Menasce Horowitz, 2021; see Mortensen et al., Chapter 29, for more information on the effects of the pandemic on the mothers of young children).

These decision points raised ethical issues regarding the safety of individual people and their families, as well as highlighted substantial gender and racial inequities. Some lawmakers struggled to achieve a balance of orders that mitigate harms to the economy while saving lives and taking into consideration the impact of these orders on various groups of people. Other lawmakers either primarily focused on reducing the spread of illness regardless of the economic impacts, and still other lawmakers primarily focused on saving the economy without concern for the loss of life that could result. These approaches can be understood through an understanding of lawmakers' ethical orientations. Lawmakers who sought to craft orders that balanced needs and were conscious of the impacts of the orders on people were adopting both a utilitarian lens that defined benefits as objective goods and a social justice lens. Lawmakers who sought to solely focus on the economy without regard for the loss of life that may result[14,15] were adopting a utilitarian lens that both defined benefits as preference satisfaction and made assessments based on "social worth."

Scholars in the areas of ethics and economics have a wide array of issues to study. First, a cost-effectiveness study of economic management approaches (i.e., balancing orders, people-focused orders, economy-focused orders) would be useful for consideration during the next pandemic. A second useful study would explore the relative health impacts of COVID-19 on essential and nonessential workers. The results of this study would be useful in planning for how to allocate PPE during the next pandemic. Third, a longitudinal study of the economic and professional effects of COVID-19 on mothers of young children is warranted. Finally, the disparate impact of COVID-19 on women, people of color, and people who occupy the lower socioeconomic strata suggest the need for ethical and economic assessments of structural reform that would rectify the inequities highlighted or exacerbated by the pandemic.

CONCLUSION

Ethics can guide or help people understand behavior. The COVID-19 pandemic raised myriad ethical issues and dilemmas. Decisions regarding these issues had to be made at the individual and organizational levels, which were influenced by individual ethical orientations and professional ethics. These individual and organizational choices collectively impacted public health outcomes, such as the rate of new COVID-19 infections and deaths. These decisions also collectively highlighted and exacerbated gender, racial, ethnic, and socioeconomic inequities in the United States. The nature of the choices made by individuals and organizations have created a substantial research agenda for scholars of ethics, public health, psychology, medicine and bioethics, leadership, government, and economics. Scholars would do well to examine these issues to establish a historical record and identify lessons learned for consideration during the next pandemic.

NOTES

1. https://www.cnn.com/2020/12/10/health/us-coronavirus-thursday/index.html
2. https://www.nytimes.com/2020/11/22/health/Covid-ventilators-stockpile.html
3. https://www.usnews.com/news/health-news/articles/2021-01-06/us-covid-hospitalizations-reach-record-high-as-california-hospitals-run-out-of-oxygen
4. https://www.navytimes.com/news/your-navy/2020/09/19/captain-says-he-knowingly-risked-career-with-virus-warning/
5. https://www.navytimes.com/news/your-navy/2020/09/19/captain-says-he-knowingly-risked-career-with-virus-warning/
6. https://www.businessinsider.com/warship-captains-praised-capt-crozier-before-navy-fired-him-emails-2021-3
7. https://www.reuters.com/article/us-usa-navy-coronavirus-carrier-exclusiv/in-reversal-navy-wont-reinstate-captain-of-coronavirus-hit-aircraft-carrier-idUSKBN23Q31H
8. https://www.defenseone.com/ideas/2020/07/13-lessons-crozier-controversy/166751/
9. https://sites.duke.edu/lawfire/2020/04/27/eight-leadership-lessons-from-the-navy-carrier-captains-case/
10. https://www.bmj.com/company/newsroom/we-cant-and-shouldnt-expect-clinicians-without-ppe-to-treat-covid-19-patients/
11. https://www.rgj.com/story/news/2020/11/13/covid-updates-nevada-reno-hospitals-overwhelmed-virus-spread/6271909002/
12. https://www.networkforphl.org/news-insights/workplace-disparities-gaps-in-covid-19-protections-for-grocery-workers/
13. https://www.usatoday.com/story/money/2020/11/23/covid-19-grocery-workers-demand-masks-hazard-pay-amid-virus-surge/6396541002/
14. https://www.cnn.com/2020/04/14/politics/trey-hollingsworth-coronavirus/index.html
15. https://www.rollingstone.com/politics/politics-news/official-ousted-after-endorsing-herd-immunity-killing-elderly-and-homeless-993356/?fbclid=IwAR3R1VIQoU7LcYRkDCYqX33ZBVpwsY0SI0h2qlllisvRIhq-QBHZZpnAWvk

REFERENCES

Abbasi, M., Majdzadeh, R., Zali, A., Karimi, A., & Akrami, F. (2018). The evolution of public health ethics frameworks: Systematic review of moral values and norms in public health policy. *Medicine, Health Care and Philosophy, 21*, 387–402. https://doi.org/10.1007/s11019-017-9813-y

Alejandro, R. (1998). *The limits of Rawlsian justice.* Johns Hopkins University Press.

American Association for Respiratory Care. (2015). AARC statement of ethics and professional conduct. https://www.aarc.org/wp-content/uploads/2017/03/statement-of-ethics.pdf

Banks, C. (2020). *Criminal justice ethics: Theory and practice* (5th ed.). Sage Publications.

Barroso, A., & Menasce Horowitz, J. (2021, March 17). The pandemic has highlighted many challenges for mothers, but they aren't necessarily new. *Pew Research Center.* https://www.pewresearch.org/fact-tank/2021/03/17/the-pandemic-has-highligh ted-many-challenges-for-mothers-but-they-arent-necessarily-new/

Benn, P. (1998). *Ethics: Fundamentals of philosophy.* McGill-Queen's University Press.

Bentham, J. (1789). *An introduction to the principles of morals and legislation.* T. Payne and Son.

Dancy, J. (1991). An ethic of prima facie duties. In P. Singer (Ed.), *A companion to ethics* (pp. 219–229). Blackwell.

Department of the Navy. (2005, November 10). Navy code of ethics. https://www.secnav.navy.mil/Ethics/Pages/codeofethics.aspx

Hill, T. E. (2000). *Respect, pluralism, and justice: Kantian perspectives.* Oxford University Press.

Igielnik, R. (2021, January 26). A rising share of working parents in the U.S. say it's been difficult to handle child care during the pandemic. Pew Research Center. https://www.pewresearch.org/fact-tank/2021/01/26/a-rising-share-of-working-parents-in-the-u-s-say-its-been-difficult-to-handle-child-care-during-the-pandemic/

Institute of Medicine. (2003). *The future of the public's health in the 21st century.* National Academies Press. https://doi.org/10.17226/10548

Kant, I. (1998). *Groundwork of the metaphysics of morals* (M. Gregor, Ed.). Cambridge University Press. (Original work published 1785)

Kisner, J. (2020, December 8). What the chaos in hospitals is doing to doctors. *The Atlantic.* https://www.theatlantic.com/magazine/archive/2021/01/covid-ethics-committee/617261/

Lopez, L., 3rd, Hart, L. H., 3rd, & Katz, M. H. (2021). Racial and ethnic health disparities related to COVID-19. *JAMA, 325*(8), 719–720. https://doi.org/10.1001/jama.2020.26443

Mill, J. S. (1867). *Utilitarianism* (3rd ed.). Longmans, Green, Reader, and Dyer.

Mulgan, T. (2014). *Understanding utilitarianism.* Routledge. http://doi:10.4324/978131 5711928

Rachels, J., & Rachels, S. (2018). *The elements of moral philosophy* (9th ed.). McGraw-Hill Education.

Rawls, J. (1999). *A theory of justice* (Rev. ed.). Harvard University Press.

Roets, A., Bostyn, D. H., De keersmaecker, J., Haesevoets, T., Van Assche, J., & Van Hiel, A. (2020). Utilitarianism in minimal-group decision making is less common than equality-based morality, mostly harm-oriented, and rarely impartial. *Scientific Reports, 10*(6), 13373. https://doi.org/10.1038/s41598-020-70199-4

Savulescu, J., Persson, I., & Wilkinson, D. (2020). Utilitarianism and the pandemic. *Bioethics, 34*, 620–632. https://doi.org/10.1111/bioe.12771

Torelli, C. J., & Shavitt, S. (2010). Culture and concepts of power. *Journal of Personality and Social Psychology, 99* (4), 703–723. https://doi.org/10.1037/a0019973

Tyson, P. (2001, March 26). The Hippocratic Oath today. NOVA. https://www.pbs.org/wgbh/nova/article/hippocratic-oath-today/

VSUN Communications. (2010, November 3). Florence Nightingale Pledge. Vanderbilt School of Nursing. https://nursing.vanderbilt.edu/news/florence-nightingale-pledge/

FURTHER READING

Ciulla, J. B. (2020). *The search for ethics in leadership, business, and beyond.* Springer.

Garran, A. M., & Rasmussen, B. (2019). How should organizations respond to racism against health care workers? *AMA Journal of Ethics, 21*(6), E499–E504.https://doi.org/10.1001/amajethics.2019.499

Rosoff, P. M. (2017). Who should ration? *AMA Journal of Ethics, 19*(2), 164–173.https://doi.org/10.1001/journalofethics.2017.19.2.ecas4-1702

Scheunemann, L. P., & White, D. B. (2011). The ethics and reality of rationing in medicine. *Chest, 140*(6), 1625–1632. https://doi.org/10.1378/chest.11-0622

Triandis, H. C. (1995). *Individualism and collectivism.* Westview Press.

Wight, J. B. (2015). *Ethics in economics: An introduction to moral frameworks.* Stanford Economics and Finance.

5

Legal Actions and Impacts of the COVID-19 Pandemic

PAMELA M. EVERETT ■

After the COVID-19 virus began spreading in the United States, public health advisors at all levels quickly determined that much of American life, except its most essential operations, would have to shut down. The pandemic stopped the flow of people and money with unprecedented speed and breadth. Contracts in a variety of realms were imperiled as payments and obligations could not be performed. Rents went unpaid, while landlords were prevented from evicting tenants and lenders were unable to foreclose on mortgages in default. College students were forced to learn remotely, with no reduction in their tuition and, in some cases, increased student fees. And inmates in the nation's prisons and jails were trapped in conditions proven to cause rapid transmission of the virus. As Americans watched these and other effects impact their freedoms, and their mental, physical, and financial health, many turned to the courts for relief. More than 1,400 pandemic-related class action lawsuits, and hundreds of individual-plaintiff actions, were filed in 2020 alone. This chapter provides a sample of some of the most litigated issues and the opportunities they present for further observation and analysis.

GOVERNMENT RESTRICTIONS

In addition to initial stay-home orders, state and local governments imposed mask requirements, occupancy limits on indoor spaces, bans on in-person religious services, and closure orders for other business environments that posed the greatest risk for disease transmission (see Chapter 3 of this volume for more on Covid-19-related health policies). The restrictions triggered a wide variety of legal actions around the country. California officials issued some of the most restrictive

Pamela M. Everett, *Legal Actions and Impacts of the COVID-19 Pandemic* In: *The Social Science of the COVID-19 Pandemic*. Edited by: Monica K. Miller, Oxford University Press. © Oxford University Press 2024.
DOI: 10.1093/oso/9780197615133.003.0005

orders because of the state's massive population; as a result, many novel legal cases originated there, samples of which are outlined below.

Lockdowns and Stay-Home Orders

In March 2020, California's Governor Newsom issued an executive order instructing Californians to stay home unless going out was necessary to maintain essential infrastructure. One plaintiff challenged the order by arguing that he and all others similarly situated were "unjustly confined" in violation of the Fourteenth Amendment's due process guarantee (*Armstrong v. Newsom*, 2020; U.S. Const. amend. XIV).

Other plaintiffs included a bride who claimed financial and emotional distress resulting from her cancelled wedding, a musician limited to playing his saxophone over Zoom, a high school senior deprived of an in-person graduation, and a yoga instructor aggrieved because he and his clients were suffering from mental health deterioration; all claimed violations of various state and federal constitutional rights.[1] Some cases were quickly dismissed, but others remain pending at this time (May 2021) and offer an opportunity to explore new constitutional challenges to state action.

Churches

Most states limited attendance at church services, but California's restrictions on religious gatherings were the most extreme in the country, banning indoor worship, including singing and chanting, in all but the most sparsely populated areas (Cal. Exec. Order No. N-33-20, 2020). Many religious entities brought legal challenges, but a suit by South Bay United Pentecostal Church in Chula Vista was the first to reach the U.S. Supreme Court, which initially deferred to public health officials in upholding the restrictions (*South Bay United Pentecostal Church v. Newsom*, 2020).

But in a second suit, which Pasadena's Harvest Rock Church joined, the churches challenged the state's later action of lifting restrictions for other businesses, such as nail salons and liquor stores, while maintaining the ban on indoor worship. In this second action, and after a key decision in a similar case against New York's Governor Cuomo,[2] the U.S. Supreme Court justices voted 6–3 in favor of the churches, allowing indoor worship but also allowing California officials to limit occupancy to 25% and to restrict indoor singing and chanting. The justices reasoned California could not treat secular businesses more favorably (*South Bay United Pentecostal Church v. Newsom*, 2021).

K–12 School Closures and Reopenings

The stay-home order forced California's schools to move instruction online for nearly a year. An eventual reopening plan was based primarily on the number of

COVID-19 cases per number of residents (with disparate impacts on different districts), and it required a 4-foot distance between students in classrooms. In February 2021, a group of plaintiffs in San Diego challenged the state's plan, claiming it violated constitutional and statutory guarantees of a quality and equal education, separation of powers, and due process. A superior court judge agreed, staying enforcement of the plan because it was "selective in its applicability, vague in its terms, and arbitrary in its prescriptions" (*A.A. v. Newsom*, 2021). Other challenges are pending as of May 2021, and their outcomes will surely guide government and school officials if they face a fall or winter 2021 resurgence or a future public health emergency of similar scope.

Gun Sales

Shortly after the stay-home order was issued, the National Rifle Association and several firearm advocacy groups filed suit against Governor Newsom and other state officials in federal court. They argued that Californians could buy and transfer guns only through state and federally licensed dealers, and as such, those dealerships were essential for consumers to exercise their constitutionally guaranteed right to keep and bear arms. Newsom left the ultimate decision about gun sales to local officials, which resulted in inconsistent enforcement. The sheriff in Los Angeles County worked to close gun shops, while San Diego's sheriff refused because such shops provided a "valuable public service." Plaintiffs brought similar suits around the country, and officials in 30 states eventually eased restrictions, citing those legal actions and pressure from the Trump administration.[3] But the plaintiffs' arguments that gun shops are essential to the exercise of Second Amendment rights have provided opportunities for further constitutional analysis (U.S. Const. amend. II).

Masks

The majority of state mask requirements were for public places or mandates that businesses require their employees and customers to wear masks. The latter have been the target of the majority of suits, with the Americans With Disabilities Act (ADA) providing the basis for many challenges (ADA, 1990).

For example, a customer who claimed to suffer from severe hearing loss sued Nike under the ADA, alleging discrimination in Nike's San Diego store because their salespeople were wearing masks and preventing her from reading lips and from seeing other cues, which deprived her of "friendly and personalized customer service." The class action suit was settled in January 2021, and Nike agreed to provide its employees with clear face masks and other equipment to accommodate hearing impaired customers (*Bunn v. Nike, Inc.*, 2020).

Similar suits in other states have alleged discrimination against customers with respiratory conditions, nervous system issues, and post-traumatic stress disorder.

And employees have brought actions against business owners alleging failures to ensure a safe work environment by not complying with mask regulations, so employers and their labor attorneys will need to find solutions that work on both sides of customer interactions when these requirements are in effect.

CONTRACTS

The pandemic has tested the law of contracts perhaps more than any other legal construct. When COVID-19 brought the business world to a near standstill, many parties found it impossible or impractical to carry out contractual promises in arenas such as real property transactions, travel, events, and insurance.

Typically, parties to a contract must perform unless the contract provisions or applicable laws excuse such performance. Arguing that performance has become more difficult or expensive is not enough. The law requires proof of a more substantial block to performance under force majeure clauses and/or the common law doctrines of impossibility and frustration of purpose.

Force Majeure

Force majeure refers to unforeseeable circumstances or a "greater force" that parties to a contract cannot control. Historically, courts construed force majeure clauses rather narrowly and focused on "acts of God," such as natural disasters. Today, most courts take a somewhat broader view, and such clauses can encompass a variety of unexpected events, which is why a typical modern force majeure clause will include not only specific events such as labor disputes, terrorism, and civil commotions, but also other causes beyond the parties' reasonable control. And, many state laws require courts to examine the contract language when interpreting these clauses, so the events listed, or omitted, can become critically important.

Of course, most contracts do not include references to a pandemic and its related effects, so the broader provisions that refer to acts of God and causes beyond the parties' reasonable control are the focus of many COVID-19 cases. But some breaching parties have still had to establish a connection between a government order and the party's inability to perform. Establishing that connection can be problematic because, in a suit for nonpayment of rent, for example, the landlord can argue that the tenant could have insured against the peril or could have drawn from its personal funds or a short-term loan to honor its obligations.

Indeed, a federal trial court judge in Florida rejected just such a claim from a commercial tenant. The court noted that the tenant failed to make "factual allegations in the complaint that show the government regulations themselves actually prevented [the defendant] from making rent payments" (*Palm Springs Mile Assoc., Ltd. v. Kirkland's Stores, Inc.*, 2020). And a Massachusetts court rejected a similar argument, noting that the party's obligations to pay preceded the pandemic and the party had even made some payments in late 2020, evidencing their ability to perform during the crisis (*Future St. Ltd. v. Big Belly Solar, LLC,* 2020).

The concepts of foreseeability and "superhuman" force can also frustrate the use of force majeure clauses. While the initial COVID-19 crisis may not have been foreseeable in its duration or scope of damage, it is not the first pandemic in the United States or the world, and the fairly recent Ebola, SARS (severe acute respiratory syndrome), and H1N1 outbreaks would support an argument that the current crisis was foreseeable. The several surges in the United States also make foreseeability a difficult issue if a defendant is trying to use a force majeure argument for nonperformance after the initial outbreak. Further, the disease might be reasonably construed as a superhuman force or an act of God, but the government shutdowns and related effects are, for contract purposes, almost certainly human caused.[4]

And again, courts must consider specific contract language to determine the effect of a force majeure clause, many of which do not excuse monetary payments, such as monthly rent and common area charges, in a commercial lease. So, even if a force majeure clause is construed as applying to the pandemic and its effects, that finding provides no relief to a struggling commercial tenant whose business income stops flowing but whose monetary obligations do not.

Impossibility and Frustration of Purpose

A party may also be excused when its performance is objectively impossible because of an event that could not be addressed at the time of contracting. The event must be genuinely unforeseeable and not simply more expensive or complicated. A classic example of impossibility that became a reality during the pandemic is when a promoter is not able to hold a scheduled event because of a government order prohibiting large gatherings, which then impacts service providers who were contracted for the event. These cases will test and define the future limits of impossibility, particularly when a virtual event option was available as a substitute. But some situations without a virtual alternative are more easily resolved through this doctrine.

The majority of plaintiffs in class actions for travel-related refunds and damages have sued under contract theories, with some arguing that travel vendors/carriers should not have cancelled trips at all and defendants arguing it was impossible for them to fly or cruise. In September 2020, a California court defeated one of these actions, finding that an airline could not be held liable for cancelling a flight when the COVID-19 travel ban rendered its performance impracticable (Daversa-Evdyriadis v. Norwegian Air Shuttle ASA, 2020). This case may provide other defendants guidance and a framework for dismissal in the multitude of pending class action cases against travel providers.

Frustration of purpose is a similar doctrine, addressing an event that interferes with the essential purpose of the contract. For example, a restaurant operator may argue that its lease with a landlord is useless if the restaurant cannot operate because of government closures. But the landlord can argue that the operator should simply pivot, as so many restaurant owners have, to provide curbside service, deliveries, or other alternatives to indoor dining.

Given the geographic and subject matter breadth of COVID-19 contract cases, attorneys are encouraged to research pending cases and ultimate outcomes in cases that have been fully adjudicated and that apply in their cases and jurisdiction. Reviewing these outcomes can assist attorneys to draft future provisions with specificity, including the now more familiar universe of pandemic-related effects and perhaps the future effects of climate change.[5]

EVICTIONS AND FORECLOSURES

The compounding effect of COVID-19's impacts has been especially pronounced in the real estate arena. Suddenly unemployed residential tenants stopped paying rent and landlords had to continue paying their ownership expenses even though their rental income stream had stopped. Some landlords then defaulted on their mortgages and lenders moved to foreclose. Aside from the widespread economic impact, communities braced for an influx of newly homeless people seeking assistance and shelter at a time when isolating at home was critical to containing the pandemic. Evictions would cause people to be on the move, carrying the virus with them.

The federal response came first in September 2020, through the Centers for Disease Control and Prevention (CDC), which issued an order to prohibit residential evictions for certain tenants through the end of December 2020 (later extended through June 30, 2021) (Order Under 42 U.S.C. 264 and 42 C.F.R. 70.2, 85 Fed. Reg. 55,292, 2020).

The order provided protection for tenants who met certain noneconomic criteria, such as showing best efforts to obtain government assistance for housing, being unable to pay rent due to a substantial income loss, making best efforts to timely pay partial rent, and demonstrating they would become homeless or would have to move into a shared living arrangement if evicted. Tenants also had to meet certain economic requirements, including showing they had no or limited income expected for 2020 or receipt of a stimulus check in 2020 or 2021. Tenants were required to sign declarations under penalty of perjury to qualify, and landlords would face criminal charges for violating the order (landlords were allowed to evict tenants who were, e.g., violating criminal laws or health and safety regulations).[6]

State governments were free to enact their own legislation and could provide broader, but not less, protection than the CDC's order. States provided varying levels of temporary and longer term eviction protection and/or more traditional relief, such as housing assistance and restrictions on utility companies' ability to shut off services.[7]

Some states provided protection to landlords as well, preventing lenders from foreclosing on smaller rental properties as long as the owner could demonstrate a COVID-19-related hardship.[8] But with property owners typically still responsible for mortgages, taxes, water, and heating bills, they carried most of the economic burden while staving off foreclosure.

Landlords and realtor groups filed federal court actions in multiple states, with suits based primarily on arguments that the CDC had exceeded its authority (e.g., the moratorium violated the doctrine that limits the extent to which Congress can delegate its legislative authority to the executive branch, and the agency lacked constitutional authority, and that such action illegally intruded into real estate, which is an inherently local domain) (*Brown v. Azar*, 2020; *Chambless Enters., LLC. v. Azar*, 2020; *Terkel v. CDC*, 2021). And landlords in New York challenged that state's act, claiming it violated their constitutional rights to due process and certain First Amendment protections (Chrysafis v. James, 2021; U.S. Const. amend. I). The bases for claims and outcomes were mixed, and the stage was set for a court to rule more definitively.

On May 5, 2021, a federal court struck down the CDC. In a suit by the Alabama Association of Realtors, the judge ruled more broadly that the CDC does not have the authority to impose a nationwide eviction moratorium (Alabama Assoc. of Realtors v. DHS, 2021). The Justice Department then appealed and requested a stay of the court's order, and the ultimate outcome on appeal could guide other courts, and Congress, in defining the limit of government's reach into private contracts during public emergencies.[9]

The pandemic caused severe hardships for commercial tenants as well, and many state and local officials used a variety of methods to temporarily stay these evictions during the crisis (Practical Law Real Estate, 2021). The majority of litigation in the commercial arena has focused on business interruption insurance coverage, which is typically triggered when a business loses income because of physical damages caused by fires or natural disasters. As of May 2021, business owners were arguing that the pandemic was indeed a natural disaster even though the damage was economic rather than physical, while insurers were asking courts to deny coverage by following the specific language in insurance contracts that requires physical damage.[10]

HIGHER EDUCATION

The pandemic impacted higher education on multiple fronts when it closed campuses and imperiled the future of in-person learning. The two primary types of legal challenges have been the result of moving students off campus to learn remotely in early 2020 and bringing them back to campus in the fall of 2021.

Student Contract Claims

When students were forced off campus early in the pandemic, many observed that they had paid for in-person instruction and an on-campus experience, but they would be getting neither, and their attorneys took these complaints to the courts.

Like so many of the pandemic-related legal issues, most of the higher education suits were essentially breach of contract cases and claims for unjust enrich-
ment and conversion, with students alleging that institutions were not delivering
bargained-for services and education. Accordingly, courts were required to look
closely at the specific agreements between institutions and their students and the
facts of each case.

Potentially bolstering the students' argument is the fact that most defendant
institutions charge less for online classes, evidencing that such classes are different
from in-person instruction. With respect to some classes, such as labs or those
involving dance, music, or engineering projects, students have further argued the
contract law principle that the goods and services for which they contracted are
unique and not replaceable through substitution or accommodation. But delivery
of an education is not like any other goods or services, and early results in the
courts reflected the unique nature of these suits.

A student sued Florida Southern College in June 2020, highlighting the many
differences between in-person and online learning, including the learning environment, the lack of face-to-face interactions with faculty, and access to laboratories
and other on-campus learning resources. The federal court judge allowed the case
to move forward, noting the absence of any applicable legal precedent to block it
(*Salerno v. Fla. S. Coll.*, 2020).[11]

In contrast, in October 2020, a federal judge dismissed a class action suit
against Northeastern University for breach of contract and unjust enrich-
ment, finding the university had never promised in-person instruction.
Attorneys for Northeastern invoked the specific language of the institution's
financial agreement with students, with its general provision that tuition is
"in exchange for the opportunity to enroll at Northeastern [and] to receive
educational services." Northeastern's counsel also noted other agreements in
which Northeastern was protected from liability for delay or failure to provide services due to causes beyond the university's reasonable control. The
judge agreed and dismissed all claims except those for reimbursement of a
nominal recreation fee that was tied to use of closed campus facilities (*Chong
v. Northeastern Univ.*, 2020).

Further, in California, several systems faced claims of wrongfully withholding
federal COVID-19 relief funds. Student plaintiffs argued these funds should be
used in part to refund student tuition and fees, but those case outcomes were still
uncertain as of May 2021.[12]

Despite some early defeats for students, many contract-based cases remain
pending around the country, even as institution administrators move forward
with plans for a robust in-person experience in fall of 2021. And again, because
courts issue decisions based on specific contract language and case-by-case facts,
establishing legal precedent for pending and future cases could be difficult unless contracts and facts are substantially similar. Many institutions have proactively refunded significant amounts to students for tuition, room and board, and
student services fees and/or have discounted tuition for upcoming semesters to
promote settlement and to avoid future litigation, but much remains uncertain

for the 2021–2022 academic year, and research into these case outcomes will be critical to providing administrators guidance for the future.

Vaccine Mandates

In late March 2021, Rutgers University officials were the first to announce a COVID-19 vaccine requirement for students returning to campus. Reports released earlier in the pandemic indicated a consensus among administrators to reject the idea because the available vaccines were approved by the Food and Drug Administration (FDA) for emergency use only and because there was no precise legal precedent. But after Rutgers announced its mandate, other institutions followed, and, by late April, officials from nearly 200 campuses adopted similar policies. Predictably, Rutgers was the first target for potential legal action.

Attorneys for the antivaccine advocacy group Informed Consent Action Network demanded that President Jonathan Holloway rescind the mandate, which they claimed was illegal as applied to a vaccine with only emergency approval. In a letter to Holloway, they cited a variety of laws and public policies, arguing: "Rutgers is effectively forcing each student to choose between receiving an education or receiving an experimental medical treatment to which they do not consent," and that informed medical consent is "considered a fundamental, overriding principle of medical ethics." Rutgers officials say they are relying on well-settled law authorizing immunization requirements and defend the move by arguing they are merely adding COVID-19 vaccines to existing requirements.[13]

Indeed, the law is well settled but only with respect to vaccines with full FDA approval. The most recent case involved a suit against the University of California (UC) system for its requirement that students be vaccinated for the 2020–2021 flu season. The UC system prevailed under applicable precedent because the FDA has fully approved the flu vaccine (*Kiel v. Regents of the Univ. of Cal.*, 2020).[14]

Formal suits against universities for the COVID-19 vaccine requirement are anticipated, and attorneys defending those actions could extrapolate from prior cases like *Kiel* or craft new arguments stressing COVID-19's serious medical impacts and death toll as compared to the flu and justifying mandates for vaccines with limited FDA approval because of the extraordinary nature of the COVID-19 public health crisis.

While the outcome of civil suits is uncertain, executive and legislative actions can provide more direct and expedient results, as governors in Texas and Florida have already demonstrated. The governor of Texas issued an executive order in early April 2021 prohibiting state agencies and organizations that receive public funds through any means from requiring vaccine "passports," and Florida's governor issued a similar order that applies more broadly to public and private institutions and any other businesses (Fla. Exec. Order 21-81, 2021; Tex. Executive Order GA 35, 2021). At least one Texas institution, St. Edwards University, has responded by carving out an exemption for any student who declines to provide the university with their COVID-19 vaccine status.

Some institutions have taken yet another approach of providing financial incentives for students who get vaccinated. Rowan University in New Jersey, for example, has offered $500 for tuition and $500 for on-campus housing, while other schools are holding lotteries in which vaccinated students can win similar gifts.[15] No legal challenges to vaccine incentives have yet surfaced, but they trigger ethical and constitutional questions similar to those associated with the immunization mandates.[16]

INMATE LAWSUITS

Legal challenges have also proliferated because of conditions in the nation's jails and prisons. The virus impacted institutions around the country, causing deaths and severe illness, which inmates claim have resulted from prison administrators' negligent or reckless failures to implement reasonable cleaning and other procedures to contain the virus. Inmates have responded with class actions claiming violations of their protections against cruel and unusual punishment and their rights under applicable disability laws (U.S. Const. amends. VIII and XIV).

Most inmates have sought injunctive relief, asking the courts to force prison officials to take appropriate actions like establishing cleaning protocols, providing hand sanitizer and masks, performing virus testing and quarantining, and reducing population densities. Other plaintiffs are seeking transfer to home confinement or even monetary damages.

Results have been mixed. The cases are complex in part because of federal law that requires an inmate to first exhaust actions available through the institution's grievance system before resorting to outside litigation (Prison Litigation Reform Act, 1996). Inmates have argued in response that, given COVID-19's rapid spread and potentially deadly outcomes, they cannot avoid irreparable harm without seeking immediate relief through the courts because internal grievance procedures will take too long and are likely to offer little to no relief. Corrections officials have argued that any failures have not and cannot amount to cruel and unusual punishment.

One involves Texas inmates housed in a prison for older and medically vulnerable prisoners. They allege that prison officials have failed to provide even the most basic COVID-19 safeguards. The trial court ordered the prison to take action, but the Fifth Circuit Court of Appeals stayed that order, and the prisoners appealed to the U.S. Supreme Court for relief while they sought review of the Fifth Circuit Court's decision. The court denied the request but Justice Sotomayor published a statement with the denial in which she detailed the "disturbing" violations and mistreatment, concluding:

It has long been said that a society's worth can be judged by taking stock of its prisons. That is all the truer in this pandemic, where inmates everywhere have been rendered vulnerable and often powerless to protect themselves from harm. May we hope that our country's facilities serve as models rather than cautionary tales (*Valentine v. Collier*, 2020).

The ultimate outcome of these suits will provide opportunities for further constitutional analyses and potential reforms to address future pandemics or similar crises.

CONCLUSION

The pandemic's full effects on American law will continue to be revealed in the coming months and years. But the issues and cases outlined here demonstrate how seemingly long-established legal principles are deeply woven into American life and how quickly they can be challenged when that lifestyle changes so significantly. These cases also illustrate the important judicial tradition of recognizing, as former U.S. Supreme Court Justice Oliver Wendell Holmes did, that "the life of the law has not been logic, it has been experience," and from this experience like no other, the law must evolve as part of the changing world in which it operates, with opportunities for researchers and scholars to help guide the process.

NOTES

1. https://calmatters.org/health/coronavirus/2020/05/california-shutdown-lawsuits-newsom-dhillon-coronavirus-shelter-in-place-executive-orders/
2. https://www.nytimes.com/2020/11/26/us/supreme-court-coronavirus-religion-new-york.html
3. https://www.nbcnews.com/politics/politics-news/buckling-pressure-many-states-deem-gun-stores-essential-allow-them-n1177706
4. https://www.pillsburylaw.com/en/news-and-insights/tour-de-force-evolving-force-majeure-considerations-one-year-into-the-pandemic.html
5. https://www.kirkland.com/publications/article/2020/07/covid19-force-majeure-lessons-climate-planning
6. https://www.cbsnews.com/news/cdc-renter-eviction-moratorium-coronavirus-spread/
7. https://www.nolo.com/evictions-ban
8. https://www.nysenate.gov/newsroom/articles/2021/covid-19-emergency-eviction-and-foreclosure-prevention-act
9. https://www.nytimes.com/2021/05/05/us/politics/eviction-moratorium-biden.html
10. https://www.jdsupra.com/legalnews/covid-business-interruption-coverage-9640892/
11. https://www.theledger.com/story/news/local/2020/07/09/florida-southern-college-student-sues-for-tuition-refund-over-online-classes/41964833/; https://www.sandiegouniontribune.com/news/courts/story/2020-10-18/lawsuits-refunds-coronavirus-universities-san-diego

12. https://www.sandiegouniontribune.com/news/courts/story/2020-10-18/lawsuits-refunds-coronavirus-universities-san-diego
13. https://www.chronicle.com/blogs/live-coronavirus-updates/anti-vaccine-group-challenges-rutgers-u-s-covid-19-vaccination-requirement?cid2=gen_login_refresh&cid=gen_sign_in
14. https://www.crowell.com/NewsEvents/Publications/Articles/Kiel-et-al-v-The-Regents-of-the-University-of-California-et-al-Major-Takeaways-from-a-California-Court-Decision-Upholding-a-Flu-Vaccination-Mandate-and-Implications-for-the-COVID-19-Vaccine
15. https://www.forbes.com/sites/tommybeer/2021/05/06/rowan-university-to-offer-up-to-1000-to-students-who-are-fully-vaccinated/?sh=4ccafccc3b87
16. https://newsroom.uw.edu/news/bioethicist-argues-against-paying-employees-get-vaccinated

REFERENCES

A.A. v. Newsom, No. 37-2021-00007536-CU-WM-NC, Minute Order, p.9 (Cal. Super. Ct. Mar. 15, 2021).
Alabama Assoc. of Realtors v. DHS, No. 1:20-cv-03377 (DC May 5, 2021).
Americans With Disabilities Act of 1990 (ADA). Public Law 101-336. 108th Congress, 2nd session (July 26, 1990).
Armstrong v. Newsom, No. 2:20-cv-03745 (CD Cal. Apr. 23, 2020).
Brown v. Azar, No.1:20-cv-03702, 2020, WL 6364310, at *9–11 (N.D. Ga. Oct. 29, 2020), appeal filed No. 20-14210H (11th Cir. 2020).
Bunn v. Nike, Inc., No. 4:20-cv-07403 (ND Cal. Oct. 22, 2020).
Cal. Exec. Order No. N-33-20 (Mar. 19, 2020).
Chambless Enters., LLC. v. Azar, No. 20-cv-01455, 2020 WL 7588849, at *5–9 (W.D. La. Dec. 22, 2020), appeal filed No. 21-30037 (5th Cir. 2021).
Chrysafis v. James, No. 2:21-cv-00998 (E.D.N.Y. Feb 2021).
Daversa-Evdyriadis v. Norwegian Air Shuttle ASA, No. 5:20 Civ. 00767 (C.D. Cal. Sept. 17. 2020).
Fla. Exec. Order No. 21-81 (Apr. 2, 2021).
Future St. Ltd. v. Big Belly Solar, LLC, No. 20-cv-11020-DJC (D. Mass. Jul. 31, 2020).
Kiel v. Regents of the Univ. of Cal., No. HG20072843 (Cal. Super. Ct. Dec. 4, 2020).
Order Under 42 U.S.C. 264 and 42 C.F.R. 70.2, "Temporary Halt in Residential Evictions to Prevent the Further Spread of COVID-19," 85 *Fed. Reg.* 55,292 (Sept. 4, 2020).
Palm Springs Mile Assoc., Ltd. v. Kirkland's Stores, Inc., No. 20-21724-CIV-RNS (S.D. Fla. 2020).
Practical Law Real Estate (2021, February 12). COVID-19: Commercial mortgage foreclosure and payment relief programs state tracker (US). Thomas Reuters Practical Law. https://content.next.westlaw.com/Document/I58c9c1ba832411ea80afece799150095/View/FullText.html?originationContext=document&transitionType=DocumentItem&contextData=(sc.Default)&firstPage=true
Prison Litigation Reform Act, 42 U.S.C. § 1997e (1996).
Salerno v. Fla. S. Coll., No. 8:20-cv-01494 (M.D. Fla 2020).
South Bay United Pentecostal Church v. Newsom, 590 U.S. _____ (2020).

South Bay United Pentecostal Church v. Newsom, 593 U.S. ____ (2021).

Student "B" v. Howard Cnty. Cmty. Coll., No. SAG-20-1820 (D. Md. 2020).

Terkel v. CDC, No. 6:20-cv-564, 2021 WL 742877, at *1–2, 10–11 (E.D. Tex. Feb. 25, 2021), appeal filed, No. 21-40137 (5th Cir. 2021).

Tex. Exec. Order No. GA 35 (Apr. 5, 2021).

U.S. Const. amends. I, II, VIII and XIV.

Valentine v. Collier, 590 U.S. ____ (2020).

Valentine v. Collier, No. 4:20-cv-01115, 2020 BL 372012 (S.D. Tex. Sep. 30, 2020).

FURTHER READING

Class action litigation related to COVID-19: Filed and anticipated cases in 2020. (2021, March 9). *The National Law Review*, *13*(203). https://www.natlawreview.com/arti cle/class-action-litigation-related-to-covid-19-filed-and-anticipated-cases-2020

Harvard Law Review. (2021, March 15). Covid-19. *Harvard Law Review Blog.* https:// blog.harvardlawreview.org/category/covid-19/

Lawsuits about state actions and policies in response to the coronavirus (COVID-19) pandemic, 2020–2021. (n.d.). Ballotpedia. https://ballotpedia.org/Lawsuits_about_ state_actions_and_policies_in_response_to_the_coronavirus_(COVID-19)_pande mic,_2020-2021

Pandemic-Related Behavior During the Pandemic

6

Confirmation Bias, Cognitive Dissonance, and the COVID-19 Pandemic

MONICA K. MILLER AND JEAN J. CABELL ∎

The global COVID-19 pandemic presented challenges, including stay-home orders and mask mandates. People quickly developed attitudes about the pandemic and the virus that could be challenged by contradictory information, forcing people to decide how to react. The psychological principle of confirmation bias suggests that people intentionally avoid information that challenges their viewpoints while seeking information that supports their viewpoints. When they cannot avoid disconfirming information, they might use biased reasoning to discount or forget this information. People selectively accept, interpret, and remember information to reduce the uncomfortable cognitive dissonance caused by holding inconsistent beliefs (e.g., not wanting to wear a mask but knowing that research says masks will save lives). Simply put, people have preferred conclusions (e.g., opinions) that lead them to seek, evaluate, and remember information in a way that supports their preferred conclusions. These are the three-component confirmation bias, which can be applied to pandemic-related behaviors. For instance, a person who wants to go out with friends despite stay-home orders might consciously or unconsciously avoid sources contradicting his preferences (e.g., expert news sources), seek out and believe sources supporting his preferences (e.g., selecting similar-minded friends on social media), or misremember or forget information contradicting personal preferences (e.g., erroneously forget the stay-home orders). To reduce dissonance, the person might take steps such as discounting experts who say the risk of catching and spreading COVID-19 is high. This chapter discusses how confirmation biases and cognitive dissonance can explain pandemic-related behaviors.

Monica K. Miller and Jean J. Cabell, *Confirmation Bias, Cognitive Dissonance, and the COVID-19 Pandemic* In: *The Social Science of the COVID-19 Pandemic*. Edited by: Monica K. Miller, Oxford University Press. © Oxford University Press 2024. DOI: 10.1093/oso/9780197615133.003.0006

CONFIRMATION BIAS

Confirmation bias refers to the tendency to interpret, search for, and remember information consistent with previously held beliefs (Nickerson, 1998). The following section reviews the three components of confirmation bias (biased interpretation, information search, and memory), citing research most relevant to pandemic-related beliefs and behaviors.

Biased Interpretation and Motivated Reasoning

Motivated reasoning occurs when people hold nonpreferred information to heightened scrutiny and analysis, while easily accepting preferred information (Ditto & Lopez, 1992). Motivated reasoning has been widely found in the social cognition literature, such as in political beliefs and medical behaviors. As the pandemic is both political and health related, we discuss two relevant studies. First, participants were more critical of information that was inconsistent with their previously held beliefs regarding capital punishment (Lord et al., 1979), affirmative action, and gun control policies (Taber & Lodge, 2006). Such studies suggested that people criticize and discount information that contradicts their political beliefs. Second, participants given an unhealthy medical diagnosis took more time to accept the results and replicated the original medical test—paralleling how patients who are unsatisfied with a medical diagnosis might seek a second opinion (Ditto & Lopez, 1992). Participants were also more likely to question the accuracy and generate more alternative explanations of a medical test that indicated an *unhealthy* medical condition than a *healthy* medical condition. These findings suggest that people are likely to be critical of medical results that do not support their preferred conclusion (i.e., about a COVID-19 test result) than those that do support their preferred conclusion.

Biased Information Search

A biased information search occurs when people only seek out, accept, or pay attention to information that confirms their previously held beliefs (Nickerson, 1998). One meta-analysis indicated people are more likely to expose themselves to information that supports their pre-existing attitudes than information that challenges their preexisting attitudes (Hart et al., 2009). This effect occurs when people make predictions about which outcome or answer is correct: Participants chose information supporting their previous prediction more than information contradicting their previous prediction (Windschitl et al., 2013). People are even biased in their information search after making *arbitrary* predictions (Scherer et al., 2013).

Biased information searches occur in political attitudes and interpersonal relationships—topics relevant to the pandemic. First, people selectively exposed themselves to political messages that aligned with their prior political attitudes (Knobloch-Westerwick et al., 2020). Second, people chose friends most similar to themselves, even when they could choose friends from a diverse group (Bahns et al., 2012). Facebook users sought out other users and communities with beliefs similar to their own and interacted more with posts confirming their preexisting views (Quattrociocchi et al., 2016; Sunstein, 2001). During the pandemic, people who want businesses to open will search for confirming information about other countries that had few business restrictions but a low infection rate—while ignoring disconfirming information about countries that had few business restrictions and high infection rates.

Biased Memory and Selective Recall

Selective recall of information and memory is another type of biased information search. Human memory is often complex, contains contradictory information, and is so large that people can only access a fraction of existing memories at a time (Sanitioso et al., 1990). As such, people are motivated to search for memories consistent with their preexisting attitudes.

Memory can be biased in three ways. First, people can have biased memories because they tend to remember information consistent with existing schemas. People pay attention to information consistent with prior beliefs, and thus they are more likely to encode and recall this information (Frost et al., 2015). Second, biased search of autobiographical memory occurs when people are led to believe certain personality traits are desirable. Sanitioso et al. (1990) led participants to believe either extroverts or introverts were more successful; participants were quicker and more likely to recall autobiographical memories consistent (rather than inconsistent) with the desired trait. Third, people have biased recognition memory because they tend to recognize information more when it is consistent (rather than inconsistent) with previously held beliefs (Frost et al., 2015).

Biased memory effects occur with political beliefs; participants remembered more articles about gun control that supported (rather than refuted) their preexisting gun control beliefs (Frost et al., 2015). Additionally, prior knowledge and beliefs about health issues can influence memory for new health-related information (Kiviniemi & Rothman, 2006). Participants better remembered information about alcohol consumption that supported their beliefs; they also better remembered health behavior recommendations that were framed to make the participant seem healthy (Kiviniemi & Rothman, 2006). During the pandemic, people who opposed large public gatherings might recall and recount gatherings that spread the virus, while forgetting or misremembering gatherings that did not spread the virus.

In sum, people are motivated to seek out, attend to, and remember preferred and preexisting beliefs. This confirmation bias is most often examined through the theoretical lens of cognitive dissonance (Jonas et al., 2001; Schulz-Hardt et al., 2000), as discussed next.

COGNITIVE DISSONANCE

Once a person makes a decision, the person is motivated to make future decisions, hold thoughts, and perform behaviors consistent with the initial decision. Inconsistency might suggest the individual is not smart, ethical, or competent. Eventually, any ambivalence toward the decision vanishes, and the person develops a strong preference for that decision. Unfortunately, this also means that the person will resist changing their mind or admitting they are wrong. This process is called cognitive dissonance (Festinger, 1957). This section addresses the what, why, and how of cognitive dissonance.

What Is Cognitive Dissonance?

Cognitive dissonance refers to a negative state of arousal that occurs when a person holds inconsistent thoughts, attitudes, or beliefs (Festinger, 1957). In one of the earliest of thousands of cognitive dissonance studies, participants who put a lot of effort into joining a group later liked that group and its members better than people who put in less effort (Aronson & Mills, 1959). Increased liking prevents dissonance resulting from putting effort into a group one does not like. This illustrates how cognitive dissonance can change beliefs or attitudes. Perhaps even people who join conspiracy groups denying COVID-19 exists—and paying the high price of ridicule and rejection from friends or family—would later justify their membership and resist leaving the group, even if it becomes obvious that the virus is not a hoax.

In a different dissonance paradigm, some participants were made to feel like hypocrites for advocating condom use but admitting their own failures to do so (Stone et al., 1994). Later, these participants were more likely to buy condoms—and buy *more* condoms—than people who did not experience hypocrisy. This illustrates how cognitive dissonance can change people's health behavior. Perhaps a parent who preaches to her children the importance of handwashing, but forgets to wash her own hands, would later correct this hypocrisy by being extra careful washing her hands and cleaning surfaces to kill viruses.

Another paradigm of cognitive dissonance is belief disconfirmation. When one holds a belief that later turns out to be untrue, the person has to decide whether to change her belief and admit she was wrong or select another dissonance-reducing strategy. In a classic example, a religious group believed that a spaceship would come on a certain day to rescue them from Earth's corruption. Yet this belief was disconfirmed, creating dissonance. The group restructured their beliefs, reasoning that the spaceship had given them a second chance, and they were to dedicate themselves to improving Earth (Festinger et al., 1956). President Trump's son Eric Trump said in May 2020 that the virus was a ploy to prevent his father's reelection, and that the virus would magically go away in November after the election.[1] This did not happen. Someone who had believed this statement could claim Eric Trump was misinformed, reject the outcome, make an excuse for the contradiction, or claim that the contradiction was not real (Harmon-Jones, 2002). Such methods are detailed below, after a discussion of the reasons that dissonance occurs.

Why Does Cognitive Dissonance Happen?

There are many reasons cognitive dissonance occurs. Perhaps the simplest reason is that people prefer positivity rather than negativity—an effect called the Pollyanna principle (Matlin, 2004). People are motivated to avoid negativity (e.g., COVID-19 is deadly) and the associated discomfort. Another explanation suggests that people are motivated to protect themselves from uncomfortable emotions (Pyszczynski et al., 1993). People are skeptical of inconsistent information (e.g., Ask & Granhag, 2007) and search for confirmatory information (Knobloch-Westerwick et al., 2020) to avoid unpleasant emotional states. Indeed, people with more negative emotional states were more likely to engage in confirmation bias (Jonas et al., 2006). A third explanation suggests that people are motivated to reduce cognitive dissonance because inconsistencies threaten their self-image. Cognitive consistency can help protect people's belief that they are smart, consistent, and make good decisions (Tedeschi et al., 1971).

How Is Cognitive Dissonance Reduced?

No matter the motivation, people engage in strategies to reduce negative states of arousal, such as avoiding new inconsistent information or changing their currently held beliefs (Festinger, 1957). A variety of ways are available for people to make their cognitions consistent and reduce their negative emotional state. Take, for example, the dissonant cognitions could be: "I know research says smoking is bad," and "I am a smoker." To reduce this dissonance, smokers have a number of options. First, they can change their behavior and quit smoking. Second, they can minimize the inconsistency by reasoning: "I don't smoke that much, and I'm going to quit soon." Third, they can adopt new cognitions that bolster the general preferred conclusion and reason: "I will do something healthy to offset the smoking." Fourth, they can deny the conflict by thinking: "Smoking isn't really that bad because I know a lot of smokers who never got cancer." Fifth, smokers can justify the contradiction by thinking: "Smoking calms me down and helps me keep thin." This approach acknowledges contradiction and the nonpreferred cognition, but justifies it by offering a greater good (e.g., staying thin). Indeed, smokers know that smoking causes cancer, and this contradictory cognition arouses negative emotions (Fotuhi et al., 2013).

In sum, people are motivated to reduce unpleasant dissonance in a variety of ways (e.g., justification). Cognitive dissonance could also relate to pandemic behaviors, as discussed next.

CONFIRMATION BIAS AND COGNITIVE DISSONANCE EXPLAIN SOME PANDEMIC BEHAVIOR

There are many examples of confirmation bias and cognitive dissonance in the real world, and the pandemic is likely no exception. No previous research, however, has specifically investigated these relationships.

Many pandemic-related behaviors can result from confirmation biases—for good and for bad. Some preferred or preexisting conclusions might be positive from a public health perspective; for instance, a person who prefers to believe that COVID-19 is serious will seek out and believe information communicating that COVID-19 is a threat—and ignore people who claim otherwise. On the other hand, some preferred conclusions might be negative. For instance, a person who prefers to believe that COVID-19 is a hoax could experience numerous negative outcomes, including spreading the virus and conflict (e.g., with people trying to enforce mask mandates). This section offers a number of examples of pandemic-related behavior that can be explained by cognitive dissonance and the three aspects of confirmation bias (interpretation, information search, and memory).

Examples of Confirmation Bias

There are a number of ways a person might demonstrate confirmation bias during the pandemic. First, people might avoid nonpreferred conclusions, for instance, not taking a COVID-19 test because they do not want to receive results that would mean they cannot work, must quarantine, or might die. Instead, a person might interpret their symptoms as "just a cold" and deem a test as unnecessary. Additionally, a person might avoid nonpreferred information from media sources. For instance, a liberal person might avoid the conservative Fox news.

Second, a person might seek out information and sources that confirm preferred conclusions. A person who believes the conspiracy theory that COVID-19 is caused by 5G cell phone towers would seek out *interactions* with people who support such beliefs. Similarly, a person could seek out *justifications* for his preferred conclusion. A person who wants to have a festival, protest, or political rally might latch on to statements such as that from Vice President Mike Pence, who argued that people have a constitutional right to peacefully assemble.[2]

Third, a person might discount or discredit nonpreferred conclusions. For instance, a person who holds stock in a company that is developing a drug to treat COVID-19 will discount research studies showing that the drug does not work in favor of one study that suggests it does work—ignoring the low quality of that one study. Peter Navarro, the White House trade advisor, was accused of such "cherry-picking" studies that supported his preferred conclusion that hydroxychloroquine could treat the virus successfully.[3]

Fourth, a preferred conclusion could lead a person to interpret information consistent with previous beliefs. Conspiracy theories meet needs such as the need to control, explain, and prepare for the future—especially in times of crisis (van Prooijen & Douglas, 2017). People prefer to find a big explanation for big events and thus might hesitate to believe that the virus was developed in nature. Instead, they might prefer to believe that the virus was created in a lab in a global conspiracy involving former President Obama. Such people interpreted a photo of Obama in a lab as evidence of the plot—a myth that was later debunked.[4]

Fifth, preferred conclusions can result in biased memories. President Trump initially denied that he had ever downplayed the threat posed by the virus, despite previous audio recordings of him downplaying the threat. Trump's memory might have been erroneous because he preferred to believe that he had never downplayed the threat.[5]

Examples of Cognitive Dissonance

During the pandemic, a person might experience uncomfortable cognitive dissonance as a result of conflicting thoughts, behaviors, and actions. This dissonance can be reduced in many ways. The first way to reduce such cognitive dissonance is to deny that any dissonance exists. A person might not want to wear a mask even though credible studies have shown masks save lives. The person might deny the conflict by adopting a false belief that masks create risks of carbon dioxide poisoning. Alternately, a person might falsely claim that COVID-19 does not exist. Such beliefs allow the person to discount the experts, thus eliminating the dissonance.

Second, cognitive dissonance can be reduced, not by denying the conflict, but by justifying one's contradictory beliefs. A person might worry about the effect of a shutdown on the economy, yet also worry about the elderly—one of the groups the shutdown would most protect. Dan Patrick, the lieutenant governor of Texas, suggested that he and other senior citizens were willing to risk death because it was important to protect the economy.[6] The importance of the economy thus justifies putting elderly at risk—and reduces any dissonance caused by devaluing the elderly (which might normally contradict one's belief that one is a caring person).

Third, people might justify their behavior by minimizing the nonpreferred cognition. People might understand that they should social distance, yet still continue to see their family and friends. For example, a person might reason: "I won't be there very long, and I feel healthy; thus, it is not really that risky." This justifies the choice to do a risky behavior (visiting friends) by minimizing the conflict between cognitions.

Fourth, cognitive dissonance could lead a person to change one cognition. A person might initially believe COVID-19 is a serious risk but soon tire of the restrictions and want to go out. This person could then adjust their initial belief by thinking, for example: "All of my friends are going out with each other and they're healthy, so the virus must not be that serious."

Fifth, a person might adopt new cognitions to bolster a preferred conclusion. A person who hosts a party 1 week might reason that he will not do anything risky for the next 2 weeks. On balance, the "good" outweighs the "bad," minimizing the conflict between cognitions.

Finally, dissonance-related principles also might explain some pandemic-related behavior. The Pollyanna principle would explain the optimistic perception that everything will go back to normal as soon as there is a vaccine. We naturally prefer positive outcomes, even if the reality is not as optimistic. This preference also allows us to take risks during the pandemic, reasoning that the solution is just around the corner. But what happens when predictions do not come true (i.e., belief disconfirmation)? In February 2020, Donald Trump suggested that the virus would miraculously disappear, likely that April.[7] In April, the virus persisted, and the Las Vegas mayor predicted that the summer heat would kill the virus.[8] The virus did not disappear as predicted. As such, people must take steps, such as forgetting the claim; rationalizing the inconsistency (e.g., because the virus did not disappear, thus it must be a hoax); minimizing the inconsistency (e.g., by rationalizing that, although the virus did not disappear, perhaps it slowed down or will soon disappear); refocusing their attention (e.g., on predictions that a cure will arise); or simply repeating the claim hoping that others will not notice the dissonance. All these are examples of pandemic-related cognitive dissonance.

LESSONS LEARNED: HOW TO PREVENT CONFIRMATION BIAS

One "lesson learned" involves the reduction of confirmation bias by reducing conflicting messages. Contradictory messages from leaders give people many alternate realities to choose from when they are seeking to confirm preferred conclusions. Reducing contradictory messages is of course not easy. Scientific recommendations change as more studies are conducted. For instance, early in the pandemic there was a shortage of medical masks, and the few existing studies showed masks were unneeded. Thus, the message was not to wear masks. But months later, masks were more available, and many studies found that masks would reduce the spread of the virus. Thus, the message changed. People can use the contradictory messages to support their preferred conclusions; for instance, people who prefer not to wear masks will seek out the earlier message and ignore or discount the later message. In addition to "official" messages, it is difficult to control the contradictory—and often false—messages on social media. Debunking fake news is an ongoing topic for social media outlets and research labs. Despite these difficulties, strong leaders can minimize contradictory messages by consulting with each other and with experts to craft a unified message (Chapter 32 discusses leadership during the pandemic).

A second lesson learned suggests that cognitive dissonance could induce people to comply with protective measures. In a dissonance study, half of a group of children were told there was *severe* punishment for playing with a desirable toy (Aronson & Carlsmith, 1963). The other half were told there was *mild* punishment. They were left alone, and no one played with the desired toy. Later, children in the mild punishment condition decreased their liking of the desirable toy more than those in the severe punishment condition. Children in the severe punishment condition had an external reason not to play with the toy, did not experience dissonance, and therefore still desired the toy. However, children in the mild punishment condition internalized that, without the external threat of severe punishment, they must not like the toy. This finding could be applied to government orders to stay home or wear masks. Mild threats (e.g., small fines) lead people to believe they are following these undesirable orders because they want to—not because of a serious external threat (e.g., a large fine). Small fines could encourage people to continue to take precautions even after the government orders are lifted—which could continue to prevent the spread of the virus.

A third lesson learned is that accountability and requiring a justification for decisions reduce bias. Study participants who are seeking information will select both disconfirming and confirming evidence when required to justify their decision (Jonas et al., 2001). Outside the lab, judges often use "bench cards" with checklists to justify their decision-making and, in theory, reduce bias. Perhaps experts, leaders, and doctors should be encouraged to give justifications for their pandemic-related decisions to help reduce bias. Dobler et al. (2019) and Croskerry et al. (2013) offered suggestions (e.g., use of checklists) that could be used to help medical workers make unbiased decisions about diagnoses, drug administration, and who should receive limited medical resources during the COVID-19 pandemic.

A final lesson learned is to design communication about health-related information in a way that increases the likelihood of remembering it, to combat the effects of biased memory. Public health communication should be designed to make disconfirming information highly salient, such as by asking people to thoroughly think through and elaborate on the implications of the information and spend time attending to it (Kiviniemi & Rothman, 2006). All of these lessons could help reduce biased cognitions in order to minimize harm caused by the virus.

FUTURE RESEARCH ON COGNITIVE BIASES AND PANDEMIC-RELATED BEHAVIOR

The main future research ideas are to test the assumptions discussed above. Few if any of these hypotheses have actually been tested in either laboratory or real-world settings. Beyond testing the hypotheses above, some general research questions can shape future study.

Why Do People Differ in Their Preferred Conclusions?

Confirmation bias theory suggests that we have preferred conclusions. But, why do people differ in their preferred conclusions? The pandemic affects everyone, so why do some people prefer to believe COVID-19 is a genuine threat and other people prefer to believe that it is not? Other chapters in this volume offer some suggestions; for instance, a person's preferences might relate to individual differences (Chapter 46); trust in institutions (Chapter 18); trust in news, which differs by political affiliation[9]; or moral beliefs (Chapter 37). Future studies could test these assumptions.

What Other Mechanisms Underlie Confirmation Bias?

Though cognitive dissonance is the most common mechanism used to explain confirmation bias (Jonas et al., 2001; Schulz-Hardt et al., 2000), there could be other explanations. For example, Ask and Granhag (2007) suggested that "need for closure"—the desire to achieve a decisive opinion on a topic—increases susceptibility to confirmation bias. Applying previously identified mechanisms underlying the effects of confirmation bias to pandemic-related behavior could be critical to identify which mechanisms are most common and therefore identify which techniques are best to prevent or reduce bias related to the pandemic.

How Can Biased Cognitive Processing Be Prevented?

Studies should investigate ways to prevent or reduce cognitive biases, such as confirmation bias, and cognitive dissonance. For example, there are ways to prevent people from believing conspiracy theories by encouraging them to think to a time when they would recognize logic flaws, which is more effective than pointing out the flaws. Biases make it hard to change someone's mind, but it might be easier to have the person recognize inconsistencies so they will change their own mind. Another way to prevent cognitive biases is through increasing scientific literacy, as this method helps people recognize fake news (e.g., about the pandemic). Next, there is a large body of research on persuasion techniques and the role of expertise and source credibility in persuasion, but it has yet to be fully combined with the cognitive bias literature to determine if these persuasion methods prevent cognitive biases related to the pandemic.

CONCLUSION

Confirmation bias and cognitive dissonance can explain many pandemic-related behaviors. In order to reduce discomfort produced by dissonance, people engage in confirmation bias, which skews the information and sources people encounter so that their preferred conclusion is not challenged. Future research should study ways to prevent this bias; doing so would help prevent dangerous behaviors in not only a pandemic, but also life more generally.

NOTES

1. https://www.businessinsider.com/eric-trump-coronavirus-disappear-after-elect ion-day-probably-get-worse-2020-5
2. https://thehill.com/homenews/administration/504737-pence-defends-trump- campaign-events-citing-freedom-of-speech-and
3. https://apnews.com/article/0aa783aa734b2ac3d984c5116b3e8039
4. https://apnews.com/article/archive-fact-checking-9051585361
5. https://www.necn.com/news/politics/president-trump/trump-denies-downplay ing-virus-despite-woodward-recording/2323581/
6. https://www.nbcnews.com/news/us-news/texas-lt-gov-dan-patrick-suggests-he- other-seniors-willing-n1167341
7. https://www.cnn.com/interactive/2020/10/politics/covid-disappearing-trump- comment-tracker/index.html
8. https://www.rgj.com/story/news/2020/04/24/las-vegas-mayor-desert-heat-bake- covid-19-science-isnt-so-sure/3024057001/
9. https://reutersinstitute.politics.ox.ac.uk/infodemic-how-people-six-countries-acc ess-and-rate-news-and-information-about-coronavirus

REFERENCES

Aronson, E., & Carlsmith, J. M. (1963). Effect of the severity of threat on the devaluation of forbidden behavior. *Journal of Abnormal and Social Psychology, 66*(6), 584–588. https://doi.org/10.1037/h0039901

Aronson, E., & Mills, J. (1959). The effect of severity of initiation on liking for a group. *Journal of Abnormal and Social Psychology, 59*(2), 177–181. https://doi.org/10.1037/ h0047195

Ask, K., & Granhag, P. A. (2007). Motivational bias in criminal investigators' judgments of witness reliability. *Journal of Applied Social Psychology, 37*(3), 561–591. https:// doi.org/10.1111/j.1559-1816.2007.00175.x

Bahns, A. J., Pickett, K. M., & Crandall, C. S. (2012). Social ecology of similarity: Big schools, small schools and social relationships. *Group Processes & Intergroup Relations, 15*(1), 119–131. https://doi.org/10.1177/1368430211410751

Croskerry, P., Singhal, G., & Mamede, S. (2013). Cognitive debiasing 2: Impediments to and strategies for change. *BMJ Quality & Safety, 22*, ii65–ii72. https://doi.org/ 10.1136/bmjqs-2012-001713

Ditto, P. H., & Lopez, D. F. (1992). Motivated skepticism: Use of differential decision criteria for preferred and nonpreferred conclusions. *Journal of Personality and Social Psychology, 63*(4), 568–584. https://doi.org/10.1037//0022-3514.63.4.568

Dobler, C. C., Morrow, A. S., & Kamath, C. C. (2019). Clinicians' cognitive biases: A potential barrier to implementation of evidence-based clinical practice.

BMJ Evidence-Based Medicine, 24(4), 137–140. https://doi.org/10.1136/bmjebm-2018-111074

Festinger, L. (1957). *A theory of cognitive dissonance*. Stanford University Press.

Festinger, L., Riecken, H. W., & Schacter, S. (1956). *When prophecy fails*. University of Minnesota Press.

Fotuhi, O., Fong, G. T., Zanna, M. P., Borland, R., Yong, H. H., & Cummings, K. M. (2013). Patterns of cognitive dissonance-reducing beliefs among smokers: a longitudinal analysis from the International Tobacco Control (ITC) Four Country Survey. *Tob Control, 22*(1), 52–58. doi:10.1136/tobaccocontrol-2011-050139. Epub 2012 Jan 3. PMID: 22218426; PMCID: PMC4009366.

Frost, P., Casey, B., Griffin, K., Raymundo, L., Farrell, C., & Carrigan, R. (2015). The influence of confirmation bias on memory and source monitoring. *Journal of General Psychology, 142*(4), 238–252. https://doi.org/10.1080/00221309.2015.1084987

Harmon-Jones, E. (2002). A cognitive dissonance theory perspective on persuasion. In M. Pfau & J. Dillard (Eds.), *Handbook of persuasion: Developments in theory and practice* (pp. 99–116). Lawrence Erlbaum Associates.

Hart, W., Albarracín, D., Eagly, A. H., Brechan, I., Lindberg, M. J., & Merrill, L. (2009). Feeling validated versus being correct: A meta-analysis of selective exposure to information. *Psychological Bulletin, 135*(4), 555–588. https://doi.org/10.1037/a0015701

Jonas, E., Graupmann, V., & Frey, D. (2006). The influence of mood on the search for supporting versus conflicting information: Dissonance reduction as a means of mood regulation? *Personality and Social Psychology Bulletin, 32*(1), 3–15. https://doi.org/10.1177/0146167205276118

Jonas, E., Schulz-Hardt, S., Frey, D., & Thelen, N. (2001). Confirmation bias in sequential information search after preliminary decisions: An expansion of dissonance theoretical research on selective exposure to information. *Journal of Personality and Social Psychology, 80*(4), 557–571. https://doi.org/10.1037/0022-3514.80.4.557

Kiviniemi, M. T., & Rothman, A. J. (2006). Selective memory biases in individuals' memory for health-related information and behavior recommendations. *Psychology & Health, 21*(2), 247–272. https://doi.org/10.1080/14768320500098715

Knobloch-Westerwick, S., Mothes, C., & Polavin, N. (2020). Confirmation bias, ingroup bias, and negativity bias in selective exposure to political information. *Communication Research, 47*(1), 104–124. https://doi.org/10.1177/0093650217719596

Lord, C. G., Ross, L., & Lepper, M. R. (1979). Biased assimilation and attitude polarization: The effects of prior theories on subsequently considered evidence. *Journal of Personality and Social Psychology, 37*(11), 2098–2109. https://doi.org/10.1037/0022-3514.37.11.2098

Matlin, M. W. (2004). Pollyanna principle. In R. Pohl (Ed.), *Cognitive illusions: A handbook on fallacies and biases in thinking, judgement and memory* (pp. 255–272). Routledge Press.

Nickerson, R. S. (1998). Confirmation bias: A ubiquitous phenomenon in many guises. *Review of General Psychology, 2*(2), 175–220. https://doi.org/10.1037/1089-2680.2.2.175

Pyszczynski, T., Greenberg, J., Solomon, S., Sideris, J., & Stubing, M. J. (1993). Emotional expression and the reduction of motivated cognitive bias: Evidence from cognitive dissonance and distancing from victims' paradigms. *Journal of Personality and Social Psychology, 64*(2), 177–186. https://doi.org/10.1037/0022-3514.64.2.177

Quattrociocchi, W., Scala, A., & Sunstein, C. R. (2016). Echo chambers on Facebook. *SSRN Electronic Journal.* https://doi.org/10.2139/ssrn.2795110

Sanitioso, R., Kunda, Z., & Fong, G. T. (1990). Motivated recruitment of autobiographical memories. *Journal of Personality and Social Psychology, 59*(2), 229–241. https://doi.org/10.1037/0022-3514.59.2.229

Scherer, A. M., Windschitl, P. D., & Smith, A. R. (2013). Hope to be right: Biased information seeking following arbitrary and informed predictions. *Journal of Experimental Social Psychology, 49*(1), 106–112. https://doi.org/10.1016/j.jesp.2012.07.012

Schulz-Hardt, S., Frey, D., Lüthgens, C., & Moscovici, S. (2000). Biased information search in group decision making. *Journal of Personality and Social Psychology, 78*(4), 655–669. https://doi.org/10.1037//0022-3514.78.4.655

Stone, J., Aronson, E., Crain, A. L., Winslow, M. P., & Fried, C. B. (1994). Inducing hypocrisy as a means of encouraging young adults to use condoms. *Personality and Social Psychology Bulletin, 20*(1), 116–128.

Sunstein, C. R. (2001). *Republic.com.* Princeton University Press.

Taber, C. S., & Lodge, M. (2006). Motivated skepticism in the evaluation of political beliefs. *American Journal of Political Science, 50*(3), 755–769. https://doi.org/10.1111/j.1540-5907.2006.00214.x

Tedeschi, J., Schlenker, B. R., & Bonoma, T. V. (1971). Cognitive dissonance: Private ratiocination or public spectacle? *American Psychologist, 26*(8), 685–695. https://doi.org/10.1037/h0032110

van Prooijen, J.-W., & Douglas, K. M. (2017). Conspiracy theories as part of history: The role of societal crisis situations. *Memory Studies, 10*(3), 323–333. https://doi.org/10.1177/1750698017701615

Windschitl, P. D., Scherer, A. M., Smith, A. R., & Rose, J. P. (2013). Why so confident? The influence of outcome desirability on selective exposure and likelihood judgment. *Organizational Behavior and Human Decision Processes, 120*(1), 73–86. https://doi.org/10.1016/j.obhdp.2012.10.002

FURTHER READING

Ditto, P. H., Munro, G. D., Apanovitch, A. M., Scepansky, J. A., & Lockhart, L. K. (2003). Spontaneous skepticism: The interplay of motivation and expectation in responses to favorable and unfavorable medical diagnoses. *Personality and Social Psychology Bulletin, 29*(9), 1120–1132. https://doi.org/10.1177/0146167203254536

Jonas, E., Traut-Mattausch, E., Frey, D., & Greenberg, J. (2008). The path or the goal? Decision vs. information focus in biased information seeking after preliminary decisions. *Journal of Experimental Social Psychology, 44*(4), 1180–1186. https://doi.org/10.1016/j.jesp.2008.02.009

Knobloch-Westerwick, S. (2015). The selective exposure self- and affect-management (SESAM) model: Applications in the realms of race, politics, and health. *Communication Research, 42*(7), 959–985. https://doi.org/10.1177/0093650214539173

Metzger, M. J., Hartsell, E. H., & Flanagin, A. J. (2020). Cognitive dissonance or credibility? A comparison of two theoretical explanations for selective exposure to partisan news. *Communication Research, 47*(1), 3–28. https://doi.org/10.1177/0093650215613136

Self-Enhancement and Counterproductive COVID-19 Behavior

ETHAN ZELL AND CONSTANTINE SEDIKIDES ■

The global COVID-19 pandemic has had enormous adverse effects on people, communities, and countries across the world. As of this writing (2021), it has resulted in millions of deaths, tens of millions of infections, countless job losses and resulting economic damage, not to mention detriments in mental health and social relationships.[1] These consequences are likely to last a generation. What makes the COVID-19 pandemic especially troubling, however, is that many of its consequences could have been mitigated if people adopted a small set of behaviors, such as social distancing, mask wearing, handwashing, and, more recently, vaccination.[2] Why have so many failed to adopt these simple behaviors and instead acted counterproductively (e.g., had large social gatherings and refused to wear a mask, sanitize, or vaccinate)?

In this chapter, we describe how *self-enhancement*, characterized by unduly positive self-views, explains some of these counterproductive actions. Many people overestimated their hardiness and viewed preventive behaviors as unnecessary. Thus, inflated self-views, which are normative and often beneficial in nonpandemic times, might promote behaviors that exacerbate the consequences of the pandemic. Strategies that curtail self-enhancement and facilitate more realistic self-views of vulnerability might be key to addressing the harsh toll of the pandemic.

SELF-ENHANCEMENT

Self-enhancement is the motive to pursue, preserve, or amplify the positivity of the self-concept. The result is inflated self-views, that is, self-views that are more

Ethan Zell and Constantine Sedikides, *Self-Enhancement and Counterproductive COVID-19 Behavior* In: *The Social Science of the COVID-19 Pandemic*. Edited by: Monica K. Miller, Oxford University Press. © Oxford University Press 2024. DOI: 10.1093/oso/9780197615133.003.0007 positive than objective criteria (e.g., knowledgeable others, experts, validated tests) warrant (Sedikides, 2020). Self-enhancement manifests in a variety of forms: For example, people attribute success internally to themselves but attribute failure externally to others or the environment (self-serving bias); people selectively remember positive information and forget threatening information about themselves (selective self-memory; see Chapter 6 for more on selective memory); and people claim to have knowledge about bogus topics (overclaiming; Sedikides & Alicke, 2019). Here, we focus on one of the most robust and oft-cited forms of self-enhancement: perceiving one's own characteristics as superior to those of average peers.

Better-Than-Average Effect

A common approach in self-enhancement research is to examine how people evaluate their own abilities, attributes, and traits in comparison to their average peer. By definition, the average person cannot be above average. However, a large literature on the *better-than-average effect* (BTAE) demonstrated that people perceive themselves as superior to their average peer (Alicke & Govorun, 2005; Zell et al., 2020). Ironically, they even believe they are less likely than their peers to fall victim to the BTAE (Pronin et al., 2002). The BTAE is a highly robust and replicable phenomenon. It obtains across many attribute and ability dimensions and replicates across many age, cultural, and demographic groups (Sedikides et al., 2014; Zell & Alicke, 2011). The BTAE is considered one of the major pillars of self-enhancement.

Support for the BTAE comes from research that implements four methods. First, research using the *direct* method has participants evaluate themselves in comparison to an average other on a rating scale ("How considerate are you in comparison to the average person?"). A mean rating that is significantly more favorable than the scale midpoint (typically labeled "average") reflects a BTAE. College students in one study evaluated themselves in comparison to the average student across several personality traits (Alicke et al., 1995, Study 1). Participants rated positive traits as more descriptive, and negative traits as less descriptive, of themselves than the average student.

Second, research using the *indirect* method has participants evaluate themselves ("How considerate are you?") and an average person ("How considerate is the average person?") on separate scales. Mean self-ratings and mean average ratings are then compared to determine whether participants rated themselves significantly more (or less) favorably than the average person. In a representative study, college students provided separate evaluations of themselves and the average student across personality traits (Alicke, 1985). Participants' self-evaluations were more flattering than those of the average student.

Third, research using the *forced-choice* method has participants indicate whether they rank above average or below average on a given dimension. When the percentage of participants who select above average significantly exceeds a neutral benchmark of 50%, the BTAE occurs. For example, 65% of Americans in a nationally representative survey rated their intelligence as above average (Heck et al., 2018).

Fourth, research using the *percentile* method has participants indicate the percentage of people they outrank on a given attribute or ability dimension. Given that the 50th percentile means average (assuming a normal distribution), mean ranks that are significantly higher than the 50th percentile reflect a BTAE. Most people place their knowledge and skills above the 50th percentile, including those who rank in the bottom 25% of test takers (Dunning, 2011).

Recently, we meta-analyzed the BTAE literature by aggregating data across 291 samples and over 950,000 participants (Zell et al., 2020). We obtained a large BTAE, with little evidence of publication bias (i.e., the selective publication of statistically significant results), for traits and abilities, positive and negative characteristics, and each of the above four methods. The meta-analysis further established the BTAE as a pillar of self-enhancement.

Unrealistic Optimism

People perceive their future prospects more favorably than those of the average peer, a phenomenon termed unrealistic comparative optimism (Shepperd et al., 2017). Much of this work has focused on excessive optimism regarding the likelihood of negative events, especially adverse health events. For example, people believe that their personal risk of contracting a sexually transmitted disease, having an automobile accident, or being the victim of a crime is lower than the risk of their average peer.

Evidence for unrealistic optimism derives from several methods, including to compare participants' perception of event likelihood with objective estimates of likelihood (Shepperd et al., 2015). Another common method is to examine the perceived likelihood of events for the self relative to an average peer ("How likely is it that you [the average person] will get diabetes?"). If most people have accurate perceptions of event likelihood, mean perceptions of likelihood for the self should not differ from perceptions of likelihood for the average person. Although unique in its emphasis on future self-perception, unrealistic comparative optimism overlaps considerably with the BTAE, so we use the latter as an umbrella term for much of this chapter.

Self-Enhancement Mechanisms

Three cognitive mechanisms contribute to the BTAE (Chambers & Windschitl, 2004). First, people overweigh their own characteristics and underweigh the characteristics of the average person during comparative judgment. Thus, instructing participants to give greater consideration to the average person reduces the BTAE. Second, people place more emphasis on the self than the average person during comparative judgment, in part because the self is focal in comparative judgment questions. Accordingly, the BTAE is reduced when the average person is focal ("How kind is the average person in comparison to you?"). Third, people perceive concrete targets (e.g., people) more favorably than generalized targets such as the average person. Thus, the BTAE is reduced when judging concrete people.

However, as stated, the cognitive mechanisms serve only to attenuate or accentuate the BTAE. As such, the BTAE is fundamentally motivated (i.e., driven by self-enhancement) and is a signature of self-enhancement (Sedikides & Alicke, 2019). For example, the BTAE is larger for abstract versus concrete dimensions, as people define abstract traits in a self-serving manner. Further, the BTAE is larger when examining traits that are personally and culturally important, as people are especially motivated to perceive themselves favorably on these traits. Finally, the BTAE is stronger among those who received negative feedback about their intelligence, suggesting compensation (Brown, 2012).

Critiques of Self-Enhancement

A common critique of the BTAE is that some people who perceive themselves as above average actually are above average. For example, it would be correct for an award-winning scientist to perceive herself as having above average intelligence. Indeed, the BTAE reflects a bias at the group level, and people who perceive themselves as above average might not necessarily be doing so in error. Furthermore, some might publicly state they are above average, when privately they know they are not.

However, neither of these critiques poses a significant challenge to the BTAE. Research using objective measures of personality and ability (e.g., ratings from other people or a standardized test) found that, consistent with the BTAE, a majority of people have inflated self-views (Heck & Krueger, 2015). Moreover, a BTAE emerges even when people are offered financial incentives for providing accurate self-estimates (Williams & Gilovich, 2008). These findings indicate that the BTAE reflects unduly positive self-views. Further, although people are especially prone to exaggerating their prowess when responding publicly, even their private beliefs about their authentic self are inflated (Zhang & Alicke, 2021).

Adaptiveness of Self-Enhancement

Self-enhancement has intrapersonal benefits. A meta-analysis found that self-enhancement is associated with psychological health (higher life satisfaction and positive affect, lower depression and negative affect; Dufner et al., 2019), and that this association is pronounced when self-enhancement is operationalized with the BTAE. Similarly, another meta-analysis revealed that the BTAE was associated with self-esteem and happiness (Zell et al., 2020). The positive association between self-enhancement and psychological health was present across cultures (Dufner et al., 2019; Sedikides et al., 2015).

We know far less about the link between self-enhancement and physical health. On the one hand, self-enhancement might be conducive to improved physical health, given the connection between psychological and physical health. On the other hand, if self-enhancement encourages overconfidence about one's physical health and thereby reduces precautionary behaviors or increases risky behaviors, it could worsen physical health. Thus, although inflated self-beliefs might generally benefit psychological health, they might induce a false sense of security and prompt counterproductive health behaviors.

SELF-ENHANCEMENT AND PANDEMIC BEHAVIOR

Self-enhancement is relevant to many aspects of everyday life, such as overestimation of one's performance at school and work, one's social skills at a party, or one's physical fitness. Little research has examined the link between self-enhancement and pandemic behaviors. Nonetheless, inflated self-beliefs might underlie several maladaptive pandemic behaviors, including failure to socially distance, wear face masks, sanitize, and vaccinate.

Possible Links Between the BTAE and Risky Pandemic Behaviors

The proclivity to perceive oneself as above average might manifest in a variety of ways during the pandemic and result in risky behaviors. First, people might have exaggerated views of their hardiness, believing that their own ability to resist infection is substantially greater than that of their average peer. This belief could lead people to eschew social distancing recommendations or forgo wearing a face mask, under the assumption that such recommendations are excessively strict for them given their superior resistance. Additionally, self-enhancement could undermine vaccination by leading people to assume that they already have the ability to ward off infection.

Second, people might have exaggerated views of their immune system, believing that their own ability to recuperate from the virus is above average. Although self-enhancers recognize that others might suffer from severe symptoms, hospitalization, and even death due to COVID-19, they might be convinced that such outcomes will not occur for them given their superior immune response. As such, mitigation behaviors might be viewed as unnecessary by self-enhancers, as they assume that, even if they get the virus, they will be able to overcome it easily. Relatedly, people might have exaggerated beliefs about the speed with which they will recover from COVID-19, thinking that, although the virus might engender a prolonged struggle for others, they could dispense of it rather quickly.

Third, people might overestimate their COVID-19 knowledge, believing that their own grasp of the causes and consequences of the virus is superior to others. Scientific understanding of COVID-19 and its prevention is evolving, and thus citizens will do well to pursue updated information via credible news outlets, health professionals, and health organizations. However, people who overestimate their knowledge might arrive at a false sense of security. Given that they presume to master everything necessary about the virus, they might fail to pursue updated information about infection rates, death rates, new variants, and recommended preventive behaviors. Further, some might believe they know more than public health experts and therefore eschew scientifically informed advice from them. Indeed, prominent public health professionals have been sharply criticized, and even received death threats, for offering pandemic recommendations that many people find unduly restrictive.[3] Even worse, those who lack knowledge, but believe they have it, might participate in the spread of misinformation that precipitates counterproductive behavior. Donald Trump, who often exalted his pandemic knowledge, mistakenly claimed that the pandemic was nearly over when it was just beginning, downplayed the significant risks of attending large indoor political rallies, and regularly proposed treatments that ranged from ineffective to deadly (e.g., drinking bleach).[4]

Fourth, people might believe they have a superior ability to resist the influence of fake news about COVID-19, when in fact fake news has influenced them. People believe they are less influenced by persuasive messages than others (the third-person effect; Davison, 1983). Many fraudulent messages about COVID-19—for example, that it was intentionally created by the Chinese government, is worsened by use of face masks, or was concocted as an excuse to insert microchips into one's arms—have gone viral on social media.[5,6,7] Although people might think that they can identify and discount dubious information of this sort, they might actually be susceptible to believing it. Moreover, confirmation biases might contribute to the perseverance of false beliefs about the pandemic even after exposure to disproving information (see also Chapter 6).

Possible Links Between Unrealistic Optimism and Risky Pandemic Behaviors

Unrealistic optimism has been documented during the pandemic. For example, students perceive their risk of infection with COVID-19 as lower than that of their average peer (Dolinski et al., 2020; Kulesza et al., 2020). Unrealistic optimism about COVID-19 risk might contribute to counterproductive behaviors, such as gathering in large groups, neglecting to wear masks, and declining to vaccinate.

Unrealistic optimism might even occur among those who have COVID-19 and are undergoing treatment. People can be overly optimistic about the impact of health treatments on their future health, for example, believing that the treatment will contribute to faster or more complete recovery than it actually does (Sweeny & Andrews, 2017). Such beliefs are associated with disappointment and declines in well-being once reality hits. As such, it is crucial for people receiving COVID-19 treatments, such as pharmaceuticals or use of a ventilator, to have accurate expectations regarding the speed of recovery and to recognize potential lingering effects of infection.

Moreover, people might have unrealistic optimism about their country's ability to address COVID-19 and resume normal activities. They might advocate, for example, that COVID-19 is more likely to spread in other countries and therefore poses a greater risk for other countries than their own. Relatedly, people might be convinced that their own country will be able to resume normal (prepandemic) activities more quickly than other countries. Consistent with this perspective, positively distorted beliefs extend from the self to the national group (Zell et al., 2022).

Literature Relevant to the Association Between Self-Enhancement and Pandemic Behavior

The literature on the putative connection between self-enhancement and counterproductive pandemic behavior is nascent. Yet, a few studies have linked dark triad traits (see next paragraph) and assorted antisocial traits to such behaviors. We summarize the relevant findings below (see also Chapter 46 for other traits that relate to pandemic behaviors).

Dark triad traits are narcissism, psychopathy, and Machiavellianism. People high (vs. low) on those traits are less likely to comply with government-mandated rules in regard to COVID-19 (Zajenkowski et al., 2020). Further, people high (vs. low) on narcissism are less likely to engage in preventive behavior (e.g., comply with lockdowns, wash hands; Nowak et al., 2020). Last, people high (vs. low) on antisocial traits (e.g., callousness, deceitfulness) are less likely to comply with preventive measures (Miguel et al., 2021). A thread underlying most of these dark triad or antisocial traits is inflated self-views. Thus, the BTAE might play a role in the observed behavioral noncompliance.

LESSONS LEARNED: CURTAILING SELF-ENHANCEMENT

Lessons from the self-enhancement literature are applicable to the current conundrum. For starters, rendering one accountable for their self-evaluations, that is, requiring them to explain, justify, and defend their self-evaluations to others, curtails self-enhancement (Sedikides et al., 2002). Accountability curbs self-enhancement, in part, by making one aware of their weaknesses. Therefore, one strategy for reducing self-enhancement is to invite people who report inflated perceptions of COVID-19 resistance to defend these beliefs. Having to justify such beliefs to a jury of one's peers might encourage a more balanced perception of personal risk.

Also, having people generate reasons why they might or might not have a particular trait, termed explanatory introspection, curtails self-enhancement (Sedikides et al., 2007). Introspecting on why one might or might not have a particular trait, such as organized or patient, curbs self-enhancement by raising self-uncertainty. Therefore, if a friend, family member, or colleague reports inflated perceptions of their COVID-19 risk, a follow-up "why" question might be useful to nudge the self-enhancer toward a more balanced perspective. Further, those who strongly oppose vaccination might later report more moderate views after being invited to explain and justify their position.

Moreover, providing people with pertinent information about others' behavior might curtail self-enhancement (Kruger et al., 2008). People might assume that they sanitize, socially distance, and wear face masks more than others because they lack accurate information about how others are behaving during the pandemic.[8] Disseminating such information might quell self-enhancement and encourage conformity to social norms. Learning, for example, that most people in one's community are complying with COVID mandates or have been vaccinated could encourage normative behavioral change (local dominance effect; Zell & Alicke, 2010).

Last, messages that induce fear can motivate people to appreciate grievous risks (Tannenbaum et al., 2015), such as those posed by the pandemic (see also Chapters 10 and 14 for more on message construction). Therefore, information campaigns that clearly describe the adverse health effects (some long term) of infection and the difficult treatment regimens they require could awaken some to the urgency of complying with health mandates. In support of this idea, fear-inducing messages were found to be effective at counteracting antivaccination attitudes (Horne et al., 2015). Fear appeals are particularly potent when they are paired with a solution; hence, promoting vaccination alongside fear-inducing messages might be promising, especially if these appeals come from ingroup rather than outgroup members (Hornsey, 2020).

FUTURE RESEARCH ON SELF-ENHANCEMENT AND PANDEMIC BEHAVIOR

Next, we outline research questions regarding self-enhancement and pandemic behavior that are in need of an answer.

Do People Believe Their Resistance to COVID-19 Is Above Average?

As we have shown, people believe they are above average across a wide array of characteristics, abilities, and traits. Thus, it appears likely that people perceive their ability to resist COVID-19, capacity to recuperate from COVID-19, and level of pandemic knowledge as above average. Further, people might exhibit a larger BTAE for pandemic-related dimensions than for other dimensions given the enormous salience and importance of the former. People also moralize pandemic behaviors (e.g., perceive those who wear masks as immoral; Betsch et al., 2020), which could exacerbate the BTAE, given that it is pronounced in the moral domain (Epley & Dunning, 2000). Future studies could test these hypotheses in different age groups and cultures to determine if self-enhancing views of COVID-19 are stronger in some groups than others. People at an elevated risk (older adults, the immunocompromised) or who live in societies with more frequent exposure to pandemics (East Asians) might manifest reduced self-enhancement.[9]

Is Self-Enhancement Regarding COVID-19 Maladaptive?

Evidence indicates that positively distorted views of the self are beneficial for psychological health (Dufner et al., 2019; Sedikides et al., 2015; Zell et al., 2020), but it remains unclear whether such benefits occur during a pandemic. We focused in this chapter on putative links between self-enhancement and counterproductive health behavior, but it is possible that self-enhancement serves an adaptive function as well. For example, self-enhancement might buffer pandemic-related stress or anxiety (Green et al., 2008) and thus help the person abstain from overcautious pandemic behavior (e.g., excessive social isolation or handwashing). As such, research is needed to assess whether inflated views of one's hardiness lead to negligent pandemic behavior that increases one's risk of infection. Field studies could examine the association of self-enhancement with behaviors such as social distancing, wearing face masks, and vaccination. Prospective studies could also test whether self-enhancement in an earlier stage of the pandemic predicted later COVID-19 infection, hospitalization, or death.

Are There Additional Ways to Reduce Self-Enhancement?

The literature suggests that holding people accountable for self-evaluations and encouraging them to explain why they make the particular evaluations they do reduces self-enhancement in ratings of personality and ability (Sedikides et al., 2002, 2007). Thus, future work should explore whether such approaches decrease self-enhancement on COVID-19-related dimensions as well. In addition, future work should examine whether providing information about the pandemic behavior of others calibrates one's self-views and encourages those who are engaging in risky behaviors to conform to group norms. Also, self-enhancement is exacerbated among those who lack skill or knowledge (Dunning, 2011); thus, experiments could test whether increasing people's knowledge of COVID-19 reduces self-enhancement. Finally, future experiments could examine whether inducing empathy decreases self-enhancement, leading to productive pandemic behaviors (Pfattheicher et al., 2020), or whether one's self-enhancement can be used to strengthen productive pandemic behavior ("You need to set an example for others").

CONCLUSIONS

Self-enhancement can explain counterproductive pandemic behaviors, especially those that reflect an overestimation of one's hardiness. People might assume that they are more resistant to infection, and that they would recover more quickly and easily from infection than others. Research is needed to examine whether self-enhancement is maladaptive during the pandemic and, if so, how to encourage more realistic views of health risk.

NOTES

1. https://www.worldometers.info/coronavirus
2. https://www.cnn.com/2021/03/27/politics/covid-war-deaths-preventable
3. https://www.npr.org/sections/coronavirus-live-updates/2020/08/05/899415906
4. https://www.vox.com/coronavirus-covid19/21497221
5. https://www.pbs.org/newshour/politics/why-covid-19-conspiracy-theories-persist
6. https://www.theatlantic.com/politics/archive/2020/10/can-masks-make-you-sicker/616641
7. https://www.bbc.com/news/52847648
8. https://www.ucl.ac.uk/news/2020/dec/majority-feel-they-comply-covid-19-rules-better-others
9. https://www.piie.com/blogs/realtime-economic-issues-watch/lessons-east-asia-and-pacific-taming-pandemic

REFERENCES

Alicke, M. D. (1985). Global self-evaluation as determined by the desirability and controllability of trait adjectives. *Journal of Personality and Social Psychology, 49*(6), 1621–1630. https://doi.org/10.1037/0022-3514.49.6.1621

Alicke, M. D., & Govorun, O. (2005). The better-than-average effect. In M. D. Alicke, D. A. Dunning, & J. I. Krueger (Eds.), *The self in social judgment* (pp. 85–106). Psychology Press.

Alicke, M. D., Klotz, M. L., Breitenbecher, D. L., Yurak, T. J., & Vredenburg, D. S. (1995). Personal contact, individuation, and the better-than-average effect. *Journal of Personality and Social Psychology, 68*(5), 804–825. https://doi.org/10.1037/0022-3514.68.5.804

Betsch, C., Korn, L., Sprengholz, P., Felgendreff, L., Eitze, S., Schmid, P., & Bohm, R. (2020). Social and behavioral consequences of mask policies during the COVID-19 pandemic. *Proceedings of the National Academy of Sciences of the United States of America, 117*(36), 21851–21853. https://doi.org/10.1073/pnas.2011674117

Brown, J. D. (2012). Understanding the better than average effect: Motives (still) matter. *Personality and Social Psychology Bulletin, 38*(2), 209–219. https://doi.org/10.1177/0146167211432763

Chambers, J. R., & Windschitl, P. D. (2004). Biases in social comparative judgments: The role of nonmotivated factors in above-average and comparative-optimism effects. *Psychological Bulletin, 130*(5), 813–838. https://doi.org/10.1037/0033-2909.130.5.813

Davison, W. P. (1983). The third-person effect in communication. *Public Opinion Quarterly, 47*(1), 1–15. https://doi.org/10.1086/268763

Dolinski, D., Dolinska, B., Zmaczynska-Witek, B., Banach, M., & Kulesza, W. (2020). Unrealistic optimism in the time of coronavirus pandemic: May it help to kill, if so-whom: Disease or the person? *Journal of Clinical Medicine, 9*(5), 1464. https://doi.org/10.3390/jcm9051464

Dunning, D. (2011). The Dunning-Kruger effect: On being ignorant of one's own ignorance. *Advances in Experimental Social Psychology, 44*, 247–296. https://doi.org/10.1016/B978-0-12-385522-0.00005-6

Dufner, M., Gebauer, J. E., Sedikides, C., & Denissen, J. J. A. (2019). Self-enhancement and psychological adjustment: A meta-analytic review. *Personality and Social Psychology Review, 23*(1), 48–72. https://doi.org/10.1177/1088868318756467

Epley, N., & Dunning, D. (2000). Feeling "holier than thou": Are self-serving assessments produced by errors in self- or social prediction? *Journal of Personality and Social Psychology, 79*(6), 861–875. https://doi.org/10.1037/0022-3514.79.6.861

Green, J. D., Sedikides, C., & Gregg, A. P. (2008). Forgotten but not gone: The recall and recognition of self-threatening memories. *Journal of Experimental Social Psychology, 44*(3), 547–561. https://doi.org/10.1016/j.jesp.2007.10.006

Heck, P. R., & Krueger, J. I. (2015). Self-enhancement diminished. *Journal of Experimental Psychology: General, 144*(5), 1003–1020. https://doi.org/10.1037/xge0000105

Heck, P. R., Simons, D. J., & Chabris, C. F. (2018). 65% of Americans believe that they are above average in intelligence: Results of two nationally representative surveys. *PLoS One, 13*(7), e0200103. https://doi.org/10.1371/journal.pone.0200103

Horne, Z., Powell, D., Hummel, J. E., & Holyoak, K. J. (2015). Countering antivaccination attitudes. *Proceedings of the National Academy of Sciences of the United States of America, 112*(33), 10321–10324. https://doi.org/10.1073/pnas.1504019112

Hornsey, M. J. (2020). Why facts are not enough: Understanding and managing the motivated rejection of science. *Current Directions in Psychological Science, 29*(6), 583–591. https://doi.org/10.1177/0963721420969364

Kruger, J., Windschitl, P. D., Burrus, J., Fessel, F., & Chambers, J. R. (2008). The rational side of egocentrism in social comparisons. *Journal of Experimental Social Psychology, 44*(2), 220–232. https://doi.org/10.1016/j.jesp.2007.04.001

Kulesza, W., Dolinski, D., Muniak, P., Derakhshan, A., Rizulla, A., & Banach, M. (2020). We are infected with the new, mutated virus UO-COVID-19. *Archives of Medical Science, 16*(6). https://doi.org/10.5114/aoms.2020.99592

Miguel, F. K., Machado, G. M., Pianowski, G., & de Francisco Carvalho, L. (2021). Compliance with containment measures to the COVID-19 pandemic over time: Do antisocial traits matter? *Personality and Individual Differences, 168*, 110346. https://doi.org/10.1016/j.paid.2020.110346

Nowak, B., Brzóska, P., Piotrowski, J., Sedikides, C., Żemojtel-Piotrowska, M., & Jonason, P. K. (2020). Adaptive and maladaptive behaviour during the COVID-19 pandemic: The roles of dark triad traits, collective narcissism, and health beliefs. *Personality and Individual Differences, 167*, 110232. https://doi.org/10.1016/j.paid.2020.110232

Pfattheicher, S., Nockur, L. Böhm, R., Sassenrath, C., & Petersen, N. B. (2020). The emotional path to action: Empathy promotes physical distancing and wearing of face masks during the COVID-19 pandemic. *Psychological Science*, *31*(11), 1363–1373. https://doi.org/10.1177/0956797620964422

Pronin, E., Lin, D. Y., & Ross, L. (2002). The bias blind spot: Perceptions of bias in self versus others. *Personality and Social Psychology Bulletin*, *28*(3), 369–381. https://doi.org/10.1177/0146167202286008

Sedikides, C. (2020). On the doggedness of self-enhancement and self-protection: How constraining are reality constraints? *Self and Identity*, *19*(3), 251–271. https://doi.org/10.1080/15298868.2018.1562961

Sedikides, C., & Alicke, M. D. (2019). The five pillars of self-enhancement and self-protection. In R. M. Ryan (Ed.), *The Oxford handbook of human motivation* (2nd ed., pp. 307–319). Oxford University Press.

Sedikides, C., Gaertner, L., & Cai, H. (2015). On the panculturality of self-enhancement and self-protection motivation: The case for the universality of self-esteem. *Advances in Motivation Science*, *2*, 185–241. https://doi.org/10.1016/bs.adms.2015.04.002

Sedikides, C., Herbst, K. C., Hardin, D. P., & Dardis, G. J. (2002). Accountability as a deterrent to self-enhancement: The search for mechanisms. *Journal of Personality and Social Psychology*, *83*(3), 592–605. https://doi.org/10.1037/0022-3514.83.3.592

Sedikides, C., Horton, R. S., & Gregg, A. P. (2007). The why's the limit: Curtailing self-enhancement with explanatory introspection. *Journal of Personality*, *75*(4), 783–824. https://doi.org/10.1111/j.1467-6494.2007.00457.x

Sedikides, C., Meek, R., Alicke, M. D., & Taylor, S. (2014). Behind bars but above the bar: Prisoners consider themselves more prosocial than non-prisoners. *British Journal of Social Psychology*, *53*(2), 396–403. https://doi.org/10.1111/bjso.12060

Shepperd, J. A., Pogge, G., & Howell, J. L. (2017). Assessing the consequences of unrealistic optimism: Challenges and recommendations. *Consciousness and Cognition*, *50*, 69–78. https://doi.org/10.1016/j.concog.2016.07.004

Shepperd, J. A., Waters, E. A., Weinstein, N. D., & Klein, W. M. P. (2015). A primer on unrealistic optimism. *Current Directions in Psychological Science*, *24*(3), 232–237. https://doi.org/10.1177/0963721414568341

Sweeny, K., & Andrews, S. E. (2017). Should patients be optimistic about surgery? Resolving a conflicted literature. *Health Psychology Review*, *11*(4), 374–386. https://doi.org/10.1080/17437199.2017.1320771

Tannenbaum, M. B., Hepler, J., Zimmerman, R. S., Saul, L., Jacobs, S., Wilson, K., & Albarracín, D. (2015). Appealing to fear: A meta-analysis of fear appeal effectiveness and theories. *Psychological Bulletin*, *141*(6), 1178–1204. https://doi.org/10.1037/a0039729

Williams, E. F., & Gilovich, T. (2008). Do people really believe they are above average? *Journal of Experimental Social Psychology*, *44*(4), 1121–1128. https://doi.org/10.1016/j.jesp.2008.01.002

Zajenkowski, M., Jonason, P. K., Leniarska, M., & Kozakiewicz, Z. (2020). Who complies with the restrictions to reduce the spread of COVID-19? Personality and perceptions of the COVID-19 situation. *Personality and Individual Differences*, *166*, 110199. https://doi.org/10.1016/j.paid.2020.110199

Zell, E., & Alicke, M. D. (2010). The local dominance effect in self-evaluation: Evidence and explanations. *Personality and Social Psychology Review*, *14*(4), 368–384. https://doi.org/10.1177/1088868310366144

Zell, E., & Alicke, M. D. (2011). Age and the better-than-average effect. *Journal of Applied Social Psychology*, *41*(5), 1175–1188. https://doi.org/10.1111/j.1559-1816.2011.00752.x

Zell, E., Stockus, C. A., & Bernstein, M. J. (2022). It's their fault: Partisan attribution bias and its association with voting intentions. *Group Processes & Intergroup Relations*, *25*(4), 1139–1156. https://doi.org/10.1177/1368430221990084

Zell, E., Strickhouser, J. E., Sedikides, C., & Alicke, M. D. (2020). The better-than-average effect in comparative self-evaluation: A comprehensive review and meta-analysis. *Psychological Bulletin*, *146*(2), 118–149. https://doi.org/10.1037/bul0000218

Zhang, Y., & Alicke, M. (2021). My true self is better than yours: Comparative bias in true self judgments. *Personality and Social Psychology Bulletin*, *47*(2), 216–231. https://doi.org/10.1177/0146167220919213

FURTHER READING

Alicke, M. D., & Sedikides, C. (2009). Self-enhancement and self-protection: What they are and what they do. *European Review of Social Psychology*, *20*(1), 1–48. https://doi.org/10.1080/10463280802613866

Alicke, M. D., & Sedikides, C. (Eds.). (2011). *Handbook of self-enhancement and self-protection*. Guilford Press.

Dunning, D., Heath, C., & Suls, J. M. (2004). Flawed self-assessment: Implications for health, education, and the workplace. *Psychological Science in the Public Interest*, *5*(3), 69–106. https://doi.org/10.1111/j.1529-1006.2004.00018.x

Shepperd, J. A., Klein, W. P., Waters, E. A., & Weinstein, N. D. (2013). Taking stock of unrealistic optimism. *Perspectives on Psychological Science*, *8*(4), 395–411. https://doi.org/10.1177/1745691613485247

Reactance Theory, Freedom Seeking, Protesting, and Other COVID-19 Behaviors

JUNGKEUN KIM, JOOYOUNG PARK, RICKY Y. K. CHAN, AND
ROGER MARSHALL ■

INTRODUCTION

Evidence of people's behavioral response to the various restrictions and requirements arising from the COVID-19 pandemic is both obvious and rather more subtle. It is easy to see overt protest and acquiescent behaviors globally in, for example, the frequently reported street protests (Haddad, 2021) and rates of movement-tracing app usage (Statista, 2021).

But more subtle behaviors have also been noted. People typically respond to the COVID-19 pandemic in two distinctive manners. On the one hand, some show so-called safety-seeking behavior under the threat. During the pandemic, these people tend to avoid crowds (J. Kim & Lee, 2020; Park et al., 2021), prefer the middle option over the extreme one when presented with more that two choices (J. Kim, Park, et al., 2021), prefer interactions with robots over humans (S. S. Kim, Kim, et al., 2021), or stockpile necessities such as toilet paper or basic foods (J. Kim et al., 2020). On the other hand, some people also show a pattern contrary to safety behaviors, such as attending a mass social gathering during a pandemic lockdown (Rajput & Chaudhry, 2021); showing a high level of variety seeking even to the extreme of choosing a less preferred option in a multiple-choice situation (J. Kim, 2020); or showing a higher purchase intention for luxury products (e.g., sales of luxury products increased 50% in China during the pandemic; Aloisi & Yu, 2020). These behaviors strongly associate with the important human motivation of *freedom seeking*, in this instance, freedom from the restrictions or limitations

Jungkeun Kim, Jooyoung Park, Ricky Y. K. Chan, and Roger Marshall, *Reactance Theory, Freedom Seeking, Protesting, and Other COVID-19 Behaviors* In: *The Social Science of the COVID-19 Pandemic*. Edited by: Monica K. Miller, Oxford University Press. © Oxford University Press 2024. DOI: 10.1093/oso/9780197615133.003.0008 of self-control driven by the COVID-19 pandemic. Put differently, after the initial shock of COVID-19, policies in most countries were almost ubiquitously enacted to prevent people from working outside the home, traveling to other countries or regions, and keeping a strict distance from others (see Chapter 3 for more on the policies related to COVID-19). These restrictions generated one salient social response: freedom seeking.

Building on reactance theory, this chapter examines people's freedom-seeking behavior during the pandemic and suggests an underlying mechanism. It concludes with practical suggestions and recommendations for future research.

REACTANCE THEORY AND FREEDOM SEEKING

The following sections first provide an explanation of the underlying theoretical constructs under discussion, then provide a set of conditions under which the theoretical mechanisms come into play. This is followed by placing reactance theory into the COVID-19 pandemic milieu, showing how it can explain a significant number of observed behaviors.

Definition and Conditions

People desire to possess the freedom to behave according to their wishes. However, when they feel that their freedom is being threatened, or eliminated, they become motivationally aroused (Brehm, 1989; Clee & Wicklund, 1980). This motivational arousal is called reactance, which is directed toward the restoration of the lost or threatened freedom (Brehm, 1966). Research has conceptualized reactance as a combination of affective and cognitive reactions (Dillard & Shen, 2005; Quick & Stephenson, 2007). That is, reactance is an unpleasant motivational state arising when people experience a threat or loss of freedoms (Zemack-Rugar & Lehmann, 2007). Therefore, reactance theory (Brehm 1966; Brehm & Brehm, 1981) posits that when people believe they are free to engage in a given behavior, they will generate psychological reactance if that freedom is eliminated or threatened. In other words, when faced with limited freedom, they will develop a strong motivational state directed toward re-establishing the threatened or eliminated freedom. Thus, the typical outcomes of psychological reactance are attempts to reassert freedom through behavior.

Boundary Conditions of Reactance Theory

There are conditions under which reactance appears. For reactance to be aroused a person must, obviously, possess the freedom to begin with. Thus, reactance is considered reactive not proactive, as it exists only in "the context of other forces motivating the person to give up the freedom and comply with the threat or elimination" (Brehm & Brehm, 1981, p. 37). Furthermore, the degree of reactance that individuals experience is determined by various factors, not only the expectation that people possess freedom to begin with, but also the importance of the freedom threatened, the proportion of freedoms threatened (Brehm, 1966), and the ease/difficulty of restoring the threatened freedom (Miron & Brehm, 2006).

Uncontrollable events often threaten or eliminate freedom and generally create more reactance than outcomes over which people have control (Wortman & Brehm, 1975). For example, the COVID-19 pandemic eliminates consumers' freedom to shop due to the unavailability of options or restrictions on offline shopping (Akhtar et al., 2020; Kirk & Rifkin, 2020; Naeem, 2021). The importance of restricted freedom also determines the magnitude of reactance (Miron & Brehm, 2006). In general, the more important a particular freedom is, the more reactance one will experience when the freedom is lost or threatened. Some prior work also examined whether the number of restricted freedoms, or their proportions, affect the degree of reactance (e.g., Brehm, 1966). In an experiment, Brehm (1966) asked participants to rate the attractiveness of several movies. Some of the participants were told they would be assigned a movie to watch, while others were told that they would be able to choose which movie they wanted to watch. Half of each of these groups was also informed that there were three movies, and the other half were told there were six movies to choose from. Finally, when it was time for participants to choose or be assigned, they were all told that the movie that participants had ranked the second most attractive earlier was unavailable. Participants then rated the attractiveness of the movies again, and the results showed that those who lost one of three possible choices showed a greater increase in attractiveness of the second-ranked movie than those who lost one of six, indicating that the proportion of restricted freedoms can determine the magnitude of reactance.

Finally, research documented that intended effort, or the extent of motivational arousal, will be proportional to the perceived ease or difficulty of restoring freedom (Miron & Brehm, 2006). Thus, if one believes that it is easy to restore the threatened freedom, little reactance will occur. The classic reactance studies support understanding that if a threatened freedom is perceived as moderately difficult to restore, then the motivation to restore that freedom will be high. This suggests that the severity of a pandemic can influence a person's motivation to restore their freedom threatened by the pandemic or regulations.

Affective, Behavioral, and Cognitive Outcomes Under the Pandemic

Reactance appears in affective, cognitive, and behavioral forms. With regard to affect, when freedom is threatened people usually feel uncomfortable, hostile, and angry toward the responsible agent (Berkowitz, 1973; Brehm, 1966; Brehm & Brehm, 1981; Dillard & Shen, 2005). Behaviorally, people exhibit both direct and indirect forms of restoration. For example, people may directly engage in the restricted behavior. Or, as an indirect form of restoration, people may show derogating or hostile acts toward the message source (Brehm, 1966; Burgoon et al., 2002; Worchel & Brehm, 1971). Studies have also shown how threatened freedom affects cognitive judgments when someone makes a choice. For example, Worchel and Arnold (1973) asked participants to believe that they would be able to choose whether they would listen to a certain speech in an experiment. Later, the participants were informed that the speech had been censored, and that they would not be able to listen to it. Supporting reactance theory, participants desired to listen to the speech that was censored more after realizing that they could not listen to the speech.

These affective, behavioral, and cognitive forms of reactance were prevalent during the COVID-19 pandemic because of governments' measures, such as compulsory mask wearing and restrictions on social gathering (Kirk & Rifkin, 2020). Restrictions on public gathering and the lockdown of offline stores during the pandemic limited individuals' control over the availability of necessities and led to panic buying or stockpiling (i.e., buying more than usual), posing a substantial threat to consumers' purchase liberty (Addo et al., 2020). As psychological reactance theory posits, these new restrictions create affective, cognitive, and behavioral reactance (Brehm, 1966; Brehm & Brehm, 1981). For example, as accumulating evidence supports the importance of face masks in preventing infection, many countries enforced mask wearing in public places (Taylor & Asmundson, 2021). Although the public generally adhere to mask wearing, some citizens exert negative emotions and refuse to wear masks, creating violent antimask rallies throughout the world. Taylor and Asmundson (2021) showed that people who did not wear masks during the COVID-19 pandemic tended to have more negative attitudes about masks as compared to people who wore masks. People who did not wear masks disliked being forced to wear a mask, believed that masks were ineffective, that masks had adverse interpersonal effects, and considered mask wearing an inconvenient habit to form. Similar protests are evident in the reports regarding behavioral reaction to other enforcement measures, such as the commonplace ignoring of personal distancing rules (Kendall-Raynor, 2020), unwillingness to use a tracer app (Hassandoust, 2020), and refusal to accept a vaccine (Dolan, 2021).

Psychological reactance is also evident in consumer choice, which has long been considered a source of personal control (Langer, 1975). A growing body of research has examined consumers' choices made to restore lost freedoms during the pandemic, providing evidence of psychological reactance. Kavvouris et al. (2020) showed that threats to freedom decrease consumer choice or decision confidence and provoke psychological reactance. Boukamcha (2017) argued that resistance to persuasion acts as a defensive, oppositional, and cognitive approach toward psychological consistency and status quo. Consistently, the COVID-19 pandemic eliminates the freedom of consumers' physical shopping choices and decreases their confidence, enhancing consumers' resistance to persuasion. Akhtar et al. (2020) showed that public psychological reactance caused by the COVID-19 pandemic decreased perceived choice confidence but raised perceived choice hesitation, increasing resistance to persuasion.

Consumer research has also observed an indirect form of reactance in consumer choice. Variety seeking refers to the propensity to seek diversity in choices (Kahn & Ratner, 2005). Research documents that decision makers sometimes pursue variety seeking to restore a sense of freedom (Levav & Zhu, 2009). Extending this idea, J. Kim (2020) examined variety seeking during the COVID-19 pandemic. He showed that a viral infection threat positively influenced variety seeking, as it helped restore restricted personal control during the pandemic and thus enhanced freedom. In sum, increasing evidence supports the view that restrictions during the pandemic create diverse affective, behavioral, and cognitive forms of psychological reactance.

LESSONS LEARNED: HOW TO MANAGE FREEDOM SEEKING

The first lesson reactance theory teaches regarding the COVID-19 pandemic is the important role of the perceived threat on behaviors. When people experience a high level of threat, especially during the early period of the pandemic, they show extreme safety-seeking behavior, such as stockpiling or panic buying (J. Kim et al., 2020). When the threat of the virus is attenuated, people rather tend to demonstrate freedom seeking. To prevent such problematic behaviors, a growing body of research highlighted the importance of utilizing the concept of "nudging" to minimize the perceived threat of COVID-19 (J. Kim et al., 2020; Kim, Giroux, et al., 2021). For example, the salience of COVID-19 information could change the perceived level of threat, resulting in a different pattern of safety or freedom seeking (J. Kim et al., 2020). In sum, one easy way to control problematic behaviors resulting from freedom seeking is to provide the public with relevant and adequate information of COVID-19.

The second lesson is about satisfying the restricted freedom with alternatives. The desire for freedom is a fundamental and essential human motivation. People naturally generate a negative response to relatively long-term restrictions or depreciation of self-control. For example, the need to belong (Baumeister & Leary, 2017) and travel motivations (Hsu & Huang, 2008) are difficult for many to suppress, especially over time. In such a situation, alternative, but related, activities could fulfill these motivations. For example, virtual reality-based travel could at least temporarily satisfy the travel motivation (Itani & Hollebeek, 2021). In conclusion, the viral world can provide alternative ways for people to at least partially satisfy their basic freedom-seeking motivation.

Third, the existing literature suggests the importance of understanding individual differences in freedom seeking. For example, early or childhood socioeconomic status (SES) can influence perceived threat using different messages as nudges. Research has shown that controlling the perceived threat of COVID-19 is only effective for those with relatively high (vs. low) childhood SES (J. Kim, Giroux, et al., 2021). Park et al. (2021) also suggested the importance of differences in sensation seeking and need for uniqueness on the preference between crowded and less crowded options under the COVID-19 threat. Specifically, even during the COVID-19 pandemic, people prefer the crowded (vs. less crowded) option as a means of seeking freedom, but only for those who are high in sensation seeking or need for uniqueness. In sum, the tendency to seek freedom will be dramatically different depending on personal characteristics (see Chapter 46 for more on how individual differences affect pandemic behavior).

Next, it is important to make everyone aware that their various compliant behaviors can really make a difference. As expectancy theory posits (Vroom, 1964), people are motivated to behave in a certain way based on the expected result of the chosen behavior. Taking human motivation as a cognitive process that governs choices among alternative forms of voluntary acts, the theory contends that decision makers' eventual behavioral choice depends much on their estimation of the extent to which a given behavior will lead to the desired consequences. This suggests that to encourage compliance with pandemic-related restrictions, policymakers need to widely publicize the benefits associated with this compliance. These benefits may include decreasing infection, hospitalization, and mortality rates. In short, despite the inconvenience and suffering from various pandemic-related restrictions, people should be better informed of the positive impacts of their cooperative efforts to motivate them to cooperate.

Finally, the perception of a threatened loss of freedom and the consequent psychological reactance to it can be reduced, or even avoided altogether, by the careful framing of policymakers' messages. Thus, instead of framing messages as threats to freedom, they can be framed as opportunities to gain freedom. For example, instead of threatening that those who do not accept a COVID-19 vaccination will have their travel restricted, the inoculation should be presented as an opportunity to gain travel freedom. Instead of refusing to allow people without face masks to enter public transport vehicles or shops, the masks should be presented as a device to offer freedom to travel and shop. Even a full lockdown can be portrayed not as a restriction of personal liberty but rather as a route to combat the threatened tyranny of a life-threatening, freedom-restricting, virus.

FUTURE RESEARCH ON REACTANCE THEORY AND PANDEMIC-RELATED BEHAVIOR

First, it is obvious that the COVID-19 pandemic has generated a "new normal." But both the public and researchers are curious about what happens after the pandemic. When the universal application of a vaccine has bought the pandemic under control, will people keep the current "new normal" or, as Kirk and Rifkin (2020) suggested, revert to their old habits? Put differently, will freedom seeking still be so salient after the pandemic? Future research needs to investigate the long-term effect of the rise of freedom seeking due to the COVID-19 pandemic.

Second, even though the behavioral outcomes of safety seeking and freedom seeking are opposed, the outcomes conceptually originate from the same root, the threat of the COVID-19 pandemic. In this situation, it is important to know the moderator(s) determining the direct threat of the COVID-19 pandemic on behavioral consequences. Even though previous research has identified some moderators—such as differences in sensation seeking and need for uniqueness (Park et al., 2021) or childhood SES (J. Kim, Giroux, et al., 2021)—there is still a significant opportunity to investigate keys to better predict individuals' behaviors.

Last, on the premise that government-sponsored persuasive messages could serve as a nudging tool to change the magnitude of people's reactance in the face of pandemic-related restrictions, it would be interesting to further examine the respective communication effectiveness of different persuasive messages among people who exhibit different demographic or psychological characteristics. For instance, when it comes to publicizing the benefits of complying with pandemic-related restrictions, future research should be conducted to explore if emphasizing the benefits of lower infection rate will only work well among the risk averse or aged (vs. risk taking or young). Similarly, it is worth examining if emphasizing the benefit of a faster border reopening will have higher communication effectiveness only among high (vs. low) sensation seekers. By juxtaposing the dimensions of message content and individual-level difference, this stream of research could generate valuable practical insights to help policymakers develop corresponding communication strategies to encourage compliance behaviors among different audience groups during a pandemic period.

CONCLUSION

Reactance theory explains many pandemic-related behaviors. In order to better manage the re-emphasized freedom seeking due to the pandemic, we have suggested the importance of utilizing nudging to control the perceived threat, such as providing alternative methods for satisfying the basic motivation, understanding the importance of individual differences in freedom seeking, and more positive framing of persuasive messages. Future research should be concerned with both attempting to understand postpandemic behaviors regarding freedom seeking and developing a deeper understanding of how to manage the perceived loss of freedoms often accompanying policymakers' social controls when threats to the status quo generate psychological reactance among those threatened.

REFERENCES

Addo, C., Jiaming, F., Kulbo, B., & Liangqiang, L. (2020). COVID-19: Fear appeal favoring purchase behavior towards personal protective equipment. *The Service Industries Journal, 40*(7–8), 471–490. https://doi.org/10.1080/02642069.2020.1751823

Akhtar, N., Nadeem Akhtar, M., Usman, M., Ali, M., & Iqbal Siddiqi, U. (2020). COVID-19 restrictions and consumers' psychological reactance toward offline shopping freedom restoration. *The Service Industries Journal, 40*(13–14), 891–913. https://doi.org/10.1080/02642069.2020.1790535

Aloisi, S., & Yu, S. (2020). Luxury handbags jump in price as brands make up for coronavirus hit. https://www.reuters.com/article/us-health-coronavirus-luxury-prices/luxury-handbags-jump-in-price-as-brands-make-up-for-coronavirus-hit-idUSKBN22Q2UW

Baumeister, R. F., & Leary, M. R. (2017). The need to belong: Desire for interpersonal attachments as a fundamental human motivation. *Interpersonal Development, 117*(3), 57–89. https://doi.org/10.1037/0033-2909.117.3.497

Berkowitz, L. (1973). Reactance and the unwillingness to help others. *Psychological Bulletin, 79*(5), 310–317. https://doi.org/10.1037/h0034443

Boukamcha, F. (2017). The impact of attitudinal ambivalence on information processing and resistance to anti-smoking persuasion. *Journal of Indian Business Research, 9*(1), 2–19. https://doi.org/10.1108/JIBR-02-2016-0010

Brehm, J. W. (1966). *A theory of psychological reactance.* Academic Press.

Brehm, J. W. (1989). Psychological reactance: Theory and applications. In T. K. Surll (Ed.), *NA—Advances in consumer research* (Vol. 16, pp. 72–75). Association for Consumer Research.

Brehm, J. W., & Brehm, S. S. (1981). *Psychological reactance: A theory of freedom and control.* Academic Press.

Burgoon, M., Alvaro, E., Grandpre, J., & Voulodakis, M. (2002). Revisiting the theory of psychological reactance: Communicating threats to attitudinal freedom. In J. P. Dillard & M. W. Pfau (Eds.), *The persuasion handbook: Developments in theory and practice* (pp. 213–232). Sage.

Clee, M. A., & Wicklund, R. A. (1980). Consumer behavior and psychological reactance. *Journal of Consumer Research, 6*(4), 389–405. https://doi.org/10.1086/208782

Dillard, J. P., & Shen, L. (2005). On the nature of reactance and its role in persuasive health communication. *Communication Monographs, 72*(2), 144–168. https://doi.org/10.1080/03637750500111815

Dolan, E. W. (2021, March 13). New study uncovers several factors linked to unwillingness to vaccinate against COVID-19. https://www.psypost.org/2021/03/new-study-uncovers-several-factors-linked-to-unwillingness-to-vaccinate-against-covid-19-60032

Haddad, M. (2021, February 2). Mapping coronavirus anti-lockdown protests around the world. https://www.aljazeera.com/news/2021/2/2/mapping-coronavirus-anti-lockdown-protests-around-the-world/

Hassandoust, F. (2020, December 2). Covid-19 coronavirus: Why people are reluctant to use contact-tracing apps. https://www.nzherald.co.nz/nz/covid-19-coronavirus-why-people-are-reluctant-to-use-contact-tracing-apps/FPDPOW2IHLHOCZ5NDHXHWKV7UM

Hsu, C. H., & Huang, S. (2008). Travel motivation: A critical review of the concept's development. In A. Woodside & D. Martin (Eds.), *Tourism management: Analysis, behaviour and strategy* (pp. 14–27). Wallingford. https://doi.org/10.1079/9781845933234.0014

Itani, O. S., & Hollebeek, L. D. (2021). Light at the end of the tunnel: Visitors' virtual reality (versus in-person) attraction site tour-related behavioral intentions during and post-COVID-19. *Tourism Management, 84*, 104290. https://doi.org/10.1016/j.tourman.2021.104290

Kahn, B. E., & Ratner, R. K. (2005). Variety for the sake of variety? Diversification motives in consumer choice. In S. Ratneshwar & D. G. Mick (Eds.), *Inside consumption: Frontiers of research on consumer motives, goals, and desires* (pp. 102–121). Routledge.

Kavvouris, C., Chrysochou, P., & Thøgersen, J. (2020). "Be careful what you say": The role of psychological reactance on the impact of pro-environmental normative appeals. *Journal of Business Research*, *113*, 257–265. https://doi.org/10.1016/j.jbusres.2019.10.018

Kendall-Raynor, P. (2020, November 2). COVID-19 visiting: Families ignoring social distancing rules "adds to pressures."https://rcni.com/nursing-older-people/newsroom/news/covid-19-visiting-families-ignoring-social-distancing-rules-adds-to-pressures-168616

Kim, J. (2020). Impact of the perceived threat of COVID-19 on variety-seeking. *Australasian Marketing Journal*, *28*(3), 108–116. https://doi.org/10.1016/j.ausmj.2020.07.001

Kim, J., Giroux, M., Gonzalez-Jimenez, H., Jang, S., Kim, S., Park, J., Kim, J., Lee, J., & Choi, Y. K. (2020). Nudging to reduce the perceived threat of coronavirus and stockpiling intention. *Journal of Advertising*, *9*(5), 633–647. https://doi.org/10.1080/00913367.2020.1806154

Kim, J., Giroux, M., Kim, J. E., Choi, Y. K., Gonzalez-Jimenez, H., Lee, J. C., Jang, S., & Kim, S. S. (2021). The moderating role of childhood socioeconomic status on the impact of nudging on the perceived threat of coronavirus and stockpiling intention. *Journal of Retailing and Consumer Services*, *59*, 102362. https://doi.org/10.1016/j.jretconser.2020.102362

Kim, J., & Lee, J. C. (2020). Effects of COVID-19 on preferences for private dining facilities in restaurants. *Journal of Hospitality and Tourism Management*, *45*, 67–70. https://doi.org/10.1016/j.jhtm.2020.07.008

Kim, J., Park, J., Lee, J., Kim, S., Gonzalez-Jimenez, H., Lee, J., Choi, Y. K., Lee, J. C., Jang, S., Franklin, D., Spence, M. T., & Marshall, R. (2021). COVID-19 and extremeness aversion: The role of safety seeking in travel decision making. *Journal of Travel Research*. *61*(4), 837–854. https://doi.org/10.1177/00472875211008252

Kim, S. S., Kim, J., Badu-Baiden, F., Giroux, M., & Choi, Y. (2021). Preference for robot service or human service in hotels? Impacts of the COVID-19 pandemic. *International Journal of Hospitality Management*, *93*, 102795. https://doi.org/10.1016/j.ijhm.2020.102795

Kirk, C. P., & Rifkin, L. S. (2020). I'll trade you diamonds for toilet paper: Consumer reacting, coping and adapting behaviors in the COVID-19 pandemic. *Journal of Business Research*, *117*, 124–131. https://doi.org/10.1016/j.jbusres.2020.05.028

Langer, E. J. (1975). The illusion of control. *Journal of Personality and Social Psychology*, *32*(2), 311–328. https://doi.org/10.1037/0022-3514.32.2.311

Levav, J., & Zhu, R. (2009). Seeking freedom through variety. *Journal of Consumer Research*, *36*(4), 600–610. https://doi.org/10.1086/599556

Miron, A. M., & Brehm, J. W. (2006). Reactance theory—40 years later. *Zeitschrift für Sozialpsychologie*, *37*(1), 9–18. https://doi.org/10.1024/0044-3514.37.1.9

Naeem, M. (2021). Do social media platforms develop consumer panic buying during the fear of Covid-19 pandemic? *Journal of Retailing and Consumer Services*, *58*, 102226. https://doi.org/10.1016/j.jretconser.2020.102226

Park, I., Kim, J., Kim, S., Lee, J., & Giroux, M. (2021). Impact of the COVID-19 pandemic on travelers' preference for crowded versus non-crowded options. *Tourism Management*, *87*, 104398. https://doi.org/10.1016/j.tourman.2021.104398

Rajput, R. B., & Chaudhry, M. N. (2021, April 28). Mass gatherings—Neglected factor in COVID surges seen in India, Pakistan and neighbors. Health Policy Watch. https://

healthpolicy-watch.news/cultural-religious-gatherings-as-a-contributing-factor-of-covid-19-in-four-asian-countries/

Quick, B. L., & Stephenson, M. T. (2007). Further evidence that psychological reactance can be modeled as a combination of anger and negative cognitions. *Communication Research*, *34*(3), 255–276. https://doi.org/10.1177/0093650207300427

Statista. (2021). Adoption of government endorsed COVID-19 contact tracing apps in selected countries as of July 2020.https://www.statista.com/statistics/1134669/share-populations-adopted-covid-contact-tracing-apps-countries/

Taylor, S., & Asmundson, G. J. (2021). Negative attitudes about facemasks during the COVID-19 pandemic: The dual importance of perceived ineffectiveness and psychological reactance. *PloS One*, *16*(2), e0246317. https://doi.org/10.1371/journal.pone.0246317

Vroom, V. H. (1964). *Work and motivation*. John Wiley and Sons.

Worchel, S., & Arnold, S. E. (1973). The effects of censorship and attractiveness of the censor on attitude change. *Journal of Experimental Social Psychology*, *9*(4), 365–377. https://doi.org/10.1016/0022-1031(73)90072-3

Worchel, S., & Brehm, J. W. (1971). Direct and implied social restoration of freedom. *Journal of Personality and Social Psychology*, *18*(3), 294–230. https://doi.org/10.1037/h0031000

Wortman, C. B., & Brehm, J. W. (1975). Responses to uncontrollable outcomes: An integration of reactance theory and the learned helplessness model. In L. Berkowitz (Ed.), *Advances in experimental social psychology* (Vol. 8, pp. 277–336). Academic Press.

Zemack-Rugar, Y., & Lehmann, D. R. (2007). Reducing reactance induced backlash responses to recommendations. In G. Fitzsimons & V. Morwitz (Eds.), *NA—Advances in consumer research* (Vol. 34, pp. 263–264). Association for Consumer Research.

FURTHER READING

Brehm, J. W., & Brehm, S. S. (1981). *Psychological reactance: A theory of freedom and control*. Academic Press.

Kim, J. (2020). Impact of the perceived threat of COVID-19 on variety-seeking. *Australasian Marketing Journal*, *28*(3), 108–116. https://doi.org/10.1016/j.ausmj.2020.07.001

Kim, J., Giroux, M., Gonzalez-Jimenez, H., Jang, S., Kim, S., Park, J., Kim, J., Lee, J., & Choi, Y. K. (2020). Nudging to reduce the perceived threat of coronavirus and stockpiling intention. *Journal of Advertising*, *9*(5), 633–647. https://doi.org/10.1080/00913367.2020.1806154

9

Morality in Times of Crisis

Panic, Grandstanding, Disengagement, and Outrage as Drivers of Pandemic-Related Behavior of Citizens

BILJANA GJONESKA ■

"We have rung the alarm bell loud and clear" read the opening remarks of the official statement by the director-general of the World Health Organization (WHO) on declaring the novel coronavirus disease (COVID-19) a pandemic.[1]

Proclamation of a pandemic represents a delicate task. The word itself is simple in utterance (i.e., form) and definition (i.e., content), yet the very mention of "pandemic" can stir complex psychological responses with unforeseeable consequences (Gilman, 2010). This word resonates deeply in the collective psyche of people, with power to arouse emotionally charged and morally motivated behaviors and a potential to incite political and societal changes (see Chapter 37 of this volume for discussion of how the pandemic could produce changes in society's morals).

In its essence, the label *pandemic* refers to a global spreading of a novel and potentially *lethal disease*.[2] Hence, the very thought of a risky disease with deadly consequences can easily arouse a sense of fear in people. Additionally, this label is used to refer to a *contagion,* one that is enabled through means of human transmission. Thus, it might lead to public blaming and shaming of those who are viewed as potential vectors of the infectious disease. Last, the word *pandemic* represents a disease that *is both widespread and universal,*[3] which could in turn incite public frustration, anger, and commotion, along with a desire for retaliation toward people who are held responsible for the crisis.

The initial reaction to the pandemic was indeed marked by an increased level of alarm, as was forewarned by the WHO's director-general. However, citizens also reported increased levels of fear, anxiety, and depression at the start of the pandemic (Rajkumar, 2020). The dread from the looming danger mounted quickly and became exacerbated in various parts of the world. As a result, waves of *moral panic* (Cohen, 1972) were ignited, marked by overreactions toward individual

Biljana Gjoneska, *Morality in Times of Crisis* In: *The Social Science of the COVID-19 Pandemic.* Edited by: Monica K. Miller, Oxford University Press. © Oxford University Press 2024. DOI: 10.1093/oso/9780197615133.003.0009 people, groups, behaviors, and events that were perceived as social threats. Such exaggerated and disproportional reactions were mostly motivated by a desire to secure safety and to restore a collective sense of stability and order. In certain instances, however, the ensuing moralization and blaming of others could be described as *moral grandstanding* (Tosi & Warmke, 2016) and ascribed to a desire to signal virtue or secure public approval. Regardless of the motivation, these tendencies were at times harmful, producing heated discussions that often gave way to unsubstantiated accusations laced with animosity, thus fueling polarization, tribalism, and political sectarianism among people (Finkel et al., 2020). On occasions, public judgment erupted into *moral outrage* (Crockett, 2017), with open expression of strong negative emotions and a desire to shame and punish people who were perceived as moral transgressors (Davidson et al., 2020) Throughout this public health crisis, there have been instances of *moral disengagement* (Bandura, 1990), marked by suspension of moral principles, as a way to disengage from social responsibility and engage in civil disobedience.

This chapter draws from this most recent pandemic, describing prominent episodes, as a way to tackle relevant questions and contemplate solutions. Specifically, the chapter discusses

- (a) how the spread of the virus coincided with waves of moral panic around the world;
- (b) how the lack of scientific consensus and distrust in public authorities resulted in moral grandstanding and moral disengagement with refusal to comply with health measures; and
- (c) how moral outrage was born as a reaction to those who refuse by those who chose to adhere with the measures.

Crucially, the chapter focuses on some common themes and underlying causes, including the interplay between external (societal) events and internal (group) processes, as well as the inflammatory content, unchecked reactions, and polarized stances that were disseminated on and amplified by the Internet.

MORAL PANIC AS A FIRST RESPONSE TO THE PANDEMIC

The COVID-19 disease started spreading in China, so it was repeatedly and pejoratively labeled as a "Chinese disease" or "Wuhan flu" (Lillo, 2020), while the early fears of infection were most often manifested as fears of people of Asian race and origin (Gao & Sai, 2021; Wang et al., 2021; Xu et al., 2021). Fears were typically expressed as excessive concern, avoidance, stigmatization, and discrimination of targeted groups or individual people, both offline and online (Stechemesser et al., 2020; see Chapter 23 for more on discrimination and hate). On the more sinister end of the spectrum, there were documented instances of hate speech (including verbal harassment) and hate crimes (including physical assaults).[4,5,6,7]

The targets of stigma and discrimination were not fixed; rather, they changed in accordance with the geographic and socioeconomic shifts of the pandemic across different world regions. Lower income countries, resource-poor households, and marginalized people were especially susceptible to "othering," often accused of spreading the "foreign sickness" (Lillo, 2020) and ultimately subjected to unfair treatment (Devakumar et al., 2020).

A collective behavior can be characterized as moral panic when it is marked by the following core features: (a) *concern* over an event that is perceived as a misfortune or an incident (e.g., the COVID-19 pandemic); (b) feelings of animosity and *hostility* toward people who are viewed as responsible for that incident (e.g., Chinese people, who were regarded as primary sources and potential vectors of infection); (c) *consensual regard* of targeted citizens (e.g., negative perception of tourists, foreigners, or nationals of Asian origin); (d) *disproportionality* in the public reaction (e.g., shunning or bullying of targeted citizens); and (e) *volatility* in interest from the public and the media (e.g., shifting of attention toward nationals from other countries that became badly affected in the meantime; Goode & Ben-Yehuda, 1994).

In the initial stages of the pandemic, a decreased sense of security and stability, along with anxiety due to anticipation of scarcity (i.e., shortages, limitations or exhaustion of resources), often produced other waves of panicky behavior, including panic buying (i.e., excessive ordering and purchasing, stockpiling and hoarding of supplies). Nationals of different countries exhibited such behavior even prior to the arrival of the infection in their homelands (Arafat et al., 2020; Islam et al., 2021). The real moral panic, however, ensued after media circulated images and videos of emptied market shelves and distraught customers (Van Bavel et al., 2020). These scenes spread across social networks around the world in a matter of days.[8,9] Signaling imminent danger and *misfortune* (by way of exhaustion of essential goods), these events created some of the initial ripples of what was to become a wave of moral panic. As a result, panicked buyers were regarded with *hostility* (as social deviants and threats), and they were *consensually perceived* as contributing to the disruptions in the supply chain, so they were demonized for their behavior. In addition, they were subjected to unanimous and *disproportional reaction* by the public (with scrutiny, moralization, and public backlash) that quickly receded, with the sudden shift of media's focus (Li, 2021).

MORAL GRANDSTANDING AND DISENGAGEMENT IN RESPONSE TO PUBLIC HEALTH MEASURES

As the infection spread, so did the need for protecting public health. The issue was becoming more pressing as the disease was rapidly progressing and picking up speed around the world. Rising to the challenge, scientific communities across the globe drew on their expertise and put forth their best effort in formulating a response to the pandemic, racing against time and making impressive leaps in the development of vaccines (Callaway, 2020). However, at times (and especially during the early stages of the pandemic), scientific consensus was lacking on certain subjects (e.g., the question of wearing protective face masks) (Feng et al., 2020). This lack of consensus gave rise to heated public debates as well as broad moralization on the necessity to wear a mask in public, which in turn resulted in diminished trust in authorities (see Chapter 18 of this volume). The reasons for moralization, however, often associated with a desire to feel good about oneself, or to look good in front of others, rather than do good for oneself and the community.[10]

In the case of moral grandstanding, impressing members of the ingroup or the wider public (by showing moral superiority, prestige, and knowledge) is mostly achieved at the expense of the outgroups or any potential rival (by silencing, berating, discrediting, and humiliating others). Those who grandstand signal a virtue and seek recognition via different mechanisms: *piling up* (reiterating previously voiced issues on already discussed subject), *ramping up* (making stronger and more exaggerated claims that only intensify with time), *trumping up* (insisting on nonexistent problems), claims of obviousness and *self-evidence* (in the absence of arguments), and finally expression of *strong emotional reactions* with displays of anger, disgust, and contempt regarding the moralized subject (Tosi & Warmke, 2016).

In the context of the pandemic, the issue of mask wearing quickly became a polarizing topic (Lang et al., 2021), one that proved to be very divisive across cultural backgrounds (e.g., from Eastern and Western countries), as well as across party lines (e.g., liberals and conservatives in the United States). For instance, the practice of wearing a mask in some parts of Asia (commonplace even before the start of the pandemic) was both ridiculed and portrayed as aimed at spreading panic among people in Western societies at the early stages of the pandemic (Xu et al., 2021). In the political arena, lack of compliance with mask wearing recommendations by members of one political demographic was labeled as a selfish and criminal act by partisans from the opposing group.[11] In addition to wearing masks, these public debates extended to other health measures that were recommended or enforced by public authorities. In such cases, some people (who valued personal liberty) equated mandates for public health compliance to a form of closeted fascism, openly partaking in moral grandstanding. On the other hand, people in opposing camps (who valued societal duties over personal liberty), responded in equal measure by likening the refusal to comply with health requirements to conspiring to commit murder.[10]

Overall, inconsistent messaging around public health measures, coupled with a flood of misinformation and conspiracy theories, reduced trust in official authorities, to the point where moral grandstanding and open disagreements were at times accompanied by moral disengagement (Maftei & Holman, 2020) and civic disobedience (e.g., in the case of the antimask protests around the world).[12] Early in the pandemic, conditions seemed to be particularly favorable for such behavior as people could easily *displace personal responsibility* (e.g., blame public authorities for the inconsistent messaging) or *diffuse their own responsibility* by marginalizing individual acts of disobedience (e.g., rationalizing actions as conforming to a group of similarly minded individuals). Also, they could *morally justify* their actions as socially acceptable (e.g., by highlighting the need for protection of their civil liberties) or use *euphemistic labeling* (e.g., by qualifying the disease as just another type of flu) to normalize their behavior or even present it in a positive light. Finally, they could also engage in *advantageous comparisons* (relative to someone who was even less compliant with public health measures) or *attribute blame* to infected people (e.g., by ascribing to "just world beliefs" and portraying them as deserving of ill fate) and ultimately *dehumanize* the victims of unfavorable outcomes (Devereux et al., 2021). Indeed, the lack of trust in government and the propensity for moral disengagement have been proven to mediate the relationship between unfavorable personality traits (e.g., emotional instability, psychopathy, and narcissism) and noncompliant behaviors (specifically refusal of social distancing) in Italian respondents during the COVID-19 pandemic (Alessandri et al., 2020). In fact, moral disengagement was found to be the strongest predictor of lower support for pandemic containment measures when compared with two other individual difference variables (just world belief and a locus of control) and when controlling for demographics and pandemic beliefs (Devereux et al., 2021). As "pandemic fatigue" caused by prolonged restrictions started to take hold in the later stages of the contagion (Reicher & Drury, 2021) and the sense of uncertainty about personal health deepened in people, a favorable setting was provided for moral disengagement (Gori & Topino, 2021). On the other hand, growing scientific consensus on many public health issues served as a ballast. For example, mask-wearing behavior gained broader support over time.[13,14] Hence, the majority of citizens in many countries have normalized many of the public health practices and incorporated them in their everyday lives.

MORAL OUTRAGE IN RESPONSE TO CIVIC DISOBEDIENCE

Moral outrage was born predominantly as a reaction directed toward the minority who refused and originating with the majority who chose to adhere with the mask-wearing practices or other public health measures. It was often expressed as "blaming, naming, and shaming"[15] or simply "corona shaming"[16] of people, who were perceived to violate moral norms, ethical principles or professional standards, and engage in improper practices (Davidson et al., 2020). People have received extremely high levels of public attention for their (supposedly) unacceptable behaviors, and they were called derogatory terms, publicly humiliated, or even "lynched" by the masses. Most of the moral outrage in the COVID-19 age has happened online (Crockett, 2017), dominating cyberspace and spreading across social networks like wildfire. It was facilitated by the Internet, which has provided a venue that is free of charge (or at low material cost), convenient (effortless and accessible), and quite safe (private and anonymous) for expressing personal anger and frustration (please refer to the following section for more details).

However, there were also instances when virtual outrage manifested in the physical world. For example, a series of attacks on telecommunication engineers and masts were registered across different continents.[17,18] These were fueled by conspiracy theories about a theorized link between 5G mobile technology and the enhanced spread of COVID-19 (Jolley & Paterson, 2020). Such allegations have produced an inverted perception, whereby random and ordinary workers (i.e., the engineers) were regarded as conspirators and violators of moral norms and physically assaulted as a result. This is an illustrative example of collective behaviors that can be morally motivated, but are not necessarily and morally justified.

THE VIRAL NATURE OF MORAL CONTAGIONS

The discussed behavioral phenomena (moral panic, grandstanding, outrage, and disengagement) shared one important commonality: They all mirrored the real contagion with COVID-19, unfolding as virtual contagions themselves. Namely, both the real and the virtual contagions were viral in essence, with the former labeled as "viral" due to the cause (i.e., the etiological agent that is the SARS-CoV-2 [severe acute respiratory syndrome coronavirus 2 [COVID-19] virus), while the latter labeled as "going viral" in reference to the consequences (i.e., the unchecked spread of inflammatory content on the Internet). The academic community has already emphasized the role of social media platforms in the viral spread of moral and emotional contents (Brady et al., 2020; Crockett, 2017; Finkel et al., 2020; Rost et al., 2016). Information can travel fast and cover vast distances across social networks because they represent both dense and diverse social circles. The "nodes" in the online network are in fact people, while the close (or distant) "links" represent bonds with close (or distant) contacts, including partners, relatives, friends, colleagues, and acquaintances (Christakis & Fowler, 2011). Overall, modern social networks are designed to enhance the human propensity to be attracted by moral and emotional content and to get engaged in dissemination of such content as a means of communication and association with ingroups or as a way to "gossip, preen, manipulate and ostracize" outgroups.[19] The interpersonal communication starts to resemble a virtual contagion when the content (i.e., information, beliefs, attitudes, initiatives) starts to flow across the network like a "highly infectious virus" itself, and people start to behave like "vectors" (i.e., intercepting, receiving, and disseminating the content) without necessarily mounting much in the way of a defense, a critical stance, or inhibition. In such cases, the pronounced responsiveness toward affective and moralized stimuli is also coupled with diminished willingness for rational and premeditated or emotional yet empathetic responses (Crockett, 2017). As a result, online interactions in the virtual sphere become saturated with hyperbolic moral language (comments with moral overtones and conversations with undercurrents of moralization), constant judgments, blaming, and accusations.

In times of the COVID-19 crisis, morally motivated behaviors of citizens contributed greatly to an already heated atmosphere and sparked *online firestorms*

(Pfeffer et al., 2014) within a matter of days or hours in some cases. These behaviors might not always function as defensive strategies, but they were certainly offensive to others, targeting outgroups with the aim to avoid, restrain, exclude and isolate (in moral panic), discredit, degrade and humiliate (in moral grandstanding), punish, or intimidate and retaliate (in moral outrage) or maybe even harm (in moral disengagement). While primarily practiced online, these moral behaviors often crossed the virtual/physical world boundary, with very serious repercussions and consequences.

DISCUSSION AND CONCLUSIONS

This chapter provides a chronological account of important events during the COVID-19 crisis: the official proclamation of the pandemic, the academic response to it, and the implementation of public health measures. The described sequence of events are also linked to subsequent behavioral responses of citizens that were amplified through interactions on the social platforms: moral panic (with discrimination of people of Asian origins and hostile response toward panic buyers); grandstanding (with polarized disagreements regarding some of the public health measures); disengagement (manifested as noncompliance with the public health measures or public acts of civil disobedience); and outrage (in response to civil disobedience).

In the framework of this chapter, the described *moral and social psychological phenomena* are presented as nicely delineated from each other. For instance, moral disengagement is primarily related to cognitive strategies that are employed in decision-making processes, while moral outrage is primarily related to expression of negative emotions (i.e., anger, disgust, and contempt). In practice, however, there was a considerable overlap between the motivations and reactions of people and in the behavioral manifestation of some of these phenomena. One such example are the waves of moral panic that were originally initiated by fear, but sometimes evolved into hurricanes of moral outrage, crushing people's destinies with open displays of hostility and violence. Also, one of the defining features of moral grandstanding is associated with the expression of strong negative emotions, which is again reminiscent of moral outrage. When such coupling happened, some of the phenomena became amplified, while the negative consequences became multiplied manifold (see Chapter 34 for more on how moral cognition can affect pandemic outcomes).

In addition, the described *sequence of collective behaviors* seemingly resembles a negative-feedback loop (i.e., *circulus vitiosus*)[20] that seems to be perpetually reinforced (i.e., *ad infinitum*).[21] In reality, however, many of these behaviors happened at different or parallel points in time, and many remained limited to narrow geographical contexts. The implications in any case are wide (pertaining to different pandemics or even different types of massive crises) and potentially damaging (for lives of individual people, groups, collectives, or even the whole society). Importantly, the victims of the negative outcomes were also causes for such consequences. People themselves are the main obstacle for prevention, as summarized in a seminal work from the past pandemic with influenza A virus (Soper, 1919) and reiterated after one century, at the time of the present pandemic with the novel coronavirus (Van Bavel et al., 2020). By becoming "hosts" (who passively tolerate or actively endorse); "transmitters" (who blindly disseminate or passionately propagate); or even "superspreaders" (e.g., influential people with a large follower base) of highly virulent misinformation and conspiracy theories about COVID-19, people serve as enforcers of the negative loop and perpetual drivers of harmful collective behaviors, marked by grouping and overreaction against others who are perceived as threatening enemies (in the case of the moral panic), competing outgroups (moral grandstanding), moral transgressors (moral outrage), or dehumanized victims (in the case of the moral disengagement). This chapter is a "cautionary tale" of sorts, showing that behaviors labeled as "moral" might easily serve immoral purposes, and that "wisdom of the crowd" is not always wise. Hence, strategies that would restore the original meaning of those words or phrases, and help improve the containment of massive crises, should mainly be aimed at (a) reducing susceptibility toward unchecked and inflammatory content on social platforms and (b) reducing competition between people. The former strategy is aimed to improve the critical thinking of people, and it entails accuracy reminders that direct attention of social media users to the truthfulness of the messages preceding the acts of reading or sharing (Pennycook et al., 2020; Pennycook & Rand, 2021), forewarning of possible misinformation or preemptive refutation of misinformation before the actual encountering (Basol et al., 2021; van der Linden et al., 2020), as well as active debunking of potent fake news and conspiracy theories (Lewandowsky et al., 2020). The latter strategy is aimed to induce empathy and foster cooperation via creating a sense of shared identity and togetherness in times of crisis (Van Bavel et al., 2020, 2021).

This chapter represents an important scholarly contribution because it takes into account each of the prevalent and morally motivated behaviors, but paints a picture that is bigger than the sum of its parts. Future research could benefit from an integrated conceptual framework that will incorporate all these interrelated phenomena, model their interactions as well as ensuing behavioral reactions, and test them in experimental settings. Also, observational studies and longitudinal examinations (at starting and ending points or at different times and "waves" of the pandemic) might prove beneficial for gaining insight on the mechanisms and the course of these phenomena, improving the expectations and prognostics of people, and enhancing the overall preparedness of nations to deal with crises.

Moral panic, grandstanding, outrage, and disengagement represent collective behavioral constituents of all modern societies and an integral part of our deeply interconnected lives. They were also defining factors of our collective response to the COVID-19 pandemic thus far. They can become even more pronounced with the advancement of the Internet and might serve as aggravating (rather than correcting) forces in handling of massive crises. Proper scholarly attention can help toward better understanding, preparedness, balance, and control of our collective response to future massive crises.

NOTES

1. [7]https://www.who.int/director-general/speeches/detail/who-director-general-s-opening-remarks-at-the-media-briefing-on-covid-19---11-march-2020
2. [7]https://www.who.int/csr/disease/swineflu/frequently_asked_questions/pandemic/en/
3. [7]https://www.cdc.gov/csels/dsepd/ss1978/lesson1/section11.html
4. [7]https://abcnews.go.com/US/fbi-warns-potential-surge-hate-crimes-asian-americans/story?id=69831920
5. [7]https://www.theguardian.com/world/2020/may/13/anti-asian-hate-crimes-up-21-in-uk-during-coronavirus-crisis
6. [7]https://media.nature.com/original/magazine-assets/d41586-020-01009-0/d41586-020-01009-0.pdf
7. [7]https://www.hrw.org/news/2020/05/12/covid-19-fueling-anti-asian-racism-and-xenophobia-worldwide
8. [7]https://www.straitstimes.com/multimedia/photos/in-pictures-panic-buying-around-the-world-amid-fears-over-coronavirus-outbreak
9. [7]https://time.com/5804722/coronavirus-fear-contagious/
10. [7]https://www.forbes.com/sites/emilychamleewright/2020/07/22/in-a-pandemic-we-need-philosophers-too/
11. [7]https://philarchive.org/archive/ARATPO-6
12. [7]https://www.theguardian.com/world/2020/oct/18/covid-in-europe-protests-czech-republic-ireland-toughen-rules
13. [7]https://www.ipsos.com/en-us/news-and-polls/more-people-say-theyre-wearing-masks-protect-themselves-covid-19-march
14. [7]https://morningconsult.com/2020/07/30/covid-face-masks-polling-update/
15. [7]https://www.theguardian.com/science/2020/apr/04/pandemic-shaming-is-it-helping-us-keep-our-distance
16. [7]https://www.theguardian.com/society/2020/apr/18/duty-or-score-settling-rights-and-wrongs-of-corona-shaming
17. [7]https://www.businessinsider.com/coronavirus-violence-feared-as-5g-conspiracy-theories-reach-us-abc-2020-5
18. [7]https://www.businessinsider.com/17-cell-towers-have-been-vandalized-in-new-zealand-since-lockdown-began-2020-5
19. [7]https://www.theatlantic.com/magazine/archive/2019/12/social-media-democracy/600763/
20. [7]https://dictionary.cambridge.org/dictionary/english/vicious-circle
21. [7]https://dictionary.cambridge.org/dictionary/english/ad-infinitum

REFERENCES

Alessandri, G., Filosa, L., Tisak, M. S., Crocetti, E., Crea, G., & Avanzi, L. (2020). Moral disengagement and generalized social trust as mediators and moderators of rule-respecting behaviors during the COVID-19 outbreak. *Frontiers in Psychology, 11,* 2102. https://doi.org/10.3389/fpsyg.2020.02102

Arafat, S. M. Y., Kar, S. K., Marthoenis, M., Sharma, P., Hoque Apu, E., & Kabir, R. (2020). Psychological underpinning of panic buying during pandemic (COVID-19). *Psychiatry Research, 289,* 113061. https://doi.org/10.1016/j.psychres.2020.113061

Bandura, A. (1990). Selective activation and disengagement of moral control. *Journal of Social Issues*, *46*(1), 27–46. https://doi.org/10.1111/j.1540-4560.1990.tb00270.x

Basol, M., Roozenbeek, J., Berriche, M., Uenal, F., McClanahan, W. P., & Linden, S. van der. (2021). Towards psychological herd immunity: Cross-cultural evidence for two prebunking interventions against COVID-19 misinformation. *Big Data & Society*, *8*(1), 20539517211013868. https://doi.org/10.1177/20539517211013868

Brady, W. J., Crockett, M. J., & Van Bavel, J. J. (2020). The MAD model of moral contagion: The role of motivation, attention, and design in the spread of moralized content online. *Perspectives on Psychological Science: A Journal of the Association for Psychological Science*, *15*(4), 978–1010. https://doi.org/10.1177/1745691620917336

Callaway, E. (2020). The race for coronavirus vaccines: A graphical guide. *Nature*, *580*(7805), 576–577. https://doi.org/10.1038/d41586-020-01221-y

Christakis, N., & Fowler, J. H. (2011). *Connected: The amazing power of social networks and how they shape our lives*. Little, Brown Spark.

Cohen, S. (1972). *Folk devils and moral panics: The creation of the mods and rockers*. McGibbon & Kee.

Crockett, M. J. (2017). Moral outrage in the digital age. *Nature Human Behaviour*, *1*(11), 769–771. https://doi.org/10.1038/s41562-017-0213-3

Davidson, P. M., Padula, W. V., Daly, J., & Jackson, D. (2020). Moral outrage in COVID-19: Understandable but not a strategy. *Journal of Clinical Nursing*, *29*(19–20), 3600–3602. https://doi.org/10.1111/jocn.15318

Devakumar, D., Shannon, G., Bhopal, S. S., & Abubakar, I. (2020). Racism and discrimination in COVID-19 responses. *The Lancet*, *395*(10231), 1194. https://doi.org/10.1016/S0140-6736(20)30792-3

Devereux, P. G., Miller, M. K., & Kirshenbaum, J. M. (2021). Moral disengagement, locus of control, and belief in a just world: Individual differences relate to adherence to COVID-19 guidelines. *Personality and Individual Differences*, *182*, 111069. https://doi.org/10.1016/j.paid.2021.111069

Feng, S., Shen, C., Xia, N., Song, W., Fan, M., & Cowling, B. J. (2020). Rational use of face masks in the COVID-19 pandemic. *The Lancet. Respiratory Medicine*, *8*(5), 434–436. https://doi.org/10.1016/S2213-2600(20)30134-X

Finkel, E. J., Bail, C. A., Cikara, M., Ditto, P. H., Iyengar, S., Klar, S., Mason, L., McGrath, M. C., Nyhan, B., Rand, D. G., Skitka, L. J., Tucker, J. A., Van Bavel, J. J., Wang, C. S., & Druckman, J. N. (2020). Political sectarianism in America. *Science (New York, NY)*, *370*(6516), 533–536. https://doi.org/10.1126/science.abe1715

Gao, G., & Sai, L. (2021). Opposing the toxic apartheid: The painted veil of the COVID-19 pandemic, race and racism. *Gender, Work & Organization*, *28*(S1), 183–189. https://doi.org/10.1111/gwao.12523

Gilman, S. L. (2010). Moral panic and pandemics. *The Lancet*, *375*(9729), 1866–1867. https://doi.org/10.1016/S0140-6736(10)60862-8

Goode, E., & Ben-Yehuda, N. (1994). Moral panics: Culture, politics, and social construction. *Annual Review of Sociology*, *20*, 149–171. https://doi.org/10.1146/annurev.so.20.080194.001053

Gori, A., & Topino, E. (2021). Across the COVID-19 waves; assessing temporal fluctuations in perceived stress, post-traumatic symptoms, worry, anxiety and civic moral disengagement over one year of pandemic. *International Journal of Environmental Research and Public Health*, *18*(11), 5651. https://doi.org/10.3390/ijerph18115651

Islam, T., Pitafi, A. H., Arya, V., Wang, Y., Akhtar, N., Mubarik, S., & Xiaobei, L. (2021). Panic buying in the COVID-19 pandemic: A multi-country examination. *Journal of Retailing and Consumer Services*, *59*, 102357. https://doi.org/10.1016/j.jretcon ser.2020.102357

Jolley, D., & Paterson, J. L. (2020). Pylons ablaze: Examining the role of 5G COVID-19 conspiracy beliefs and support for violence. *The British Journal of Social Psychology*, *59*(3), 628–640. https://doi.org/10.1111/bjso.12394

Lang, J., Erickson, W. W., & Jing-Schmidt, Z. (2021). #MaskOn! #MaskOff! Digital polarization of mask-wearing in the United States during COVID-19. *PLoS One*, *16*(4), e0250817. https://doi.org/10.1371/journal.pone.0250817

Lewandowsky, S., Cook, J., Ecker, U. K. H., Albarracín, D., Amazeen, M. A., Kendeou, P., Lombardi, D., Newman, E. J., Pennycook, G., Porter, E. Rand, D. G., Rapp, D. N., Reifler, J., Roozenbeek, J., Schmid, P., Seifert, C. M., Sinatra, G. M., Swire-Thompson, B., van der Linden, S., . . . Zaragoza, M. S. (2020). The debunking handbook. Databrary. https://www.doi.org/10.17910/b7.1182

Li, S. (2021). Toilet paper thrones and heated tweets: Applying moral panic and social network theory to responses over panic buying during COVID-19. *International Journal of Social Science and Humanity*, *11*(2), 35–39. https://doi.org/10.18178/ijssh.2021.V11.1035

Lillo, A. (2020). COVID-19, the beer flu; or, the disease of many names. *Lebende Sprachen*, *65*(2), 411–438. https://doi.org/10.1515/les-2020-0021

Maftei, A., & Holman, A.-C. (2020). Beliefs in conspiracy theories, intolerance of uncertainty, and moral disengagement during the coronavirus crisis. *Ethics & Behavior*, *32*(1), 1–11. https://doi.org/10.1080/10508422.2020.1843171

Pennycook, G., McPhetres, J., Zhang, Y., Lu, J. G., & Rand, D. G. (2020). Fighting COVID-19 misinformation on social media: Experimental evidence for a scalable accuracy-nudge intervention. *Psychological Science*, *31*(7), 770–780. https://doi.org/10.1177/0956797620939054

Pennycook, G., & Rand, D. G. (2021). The psychology of fake news. *Trends in Cognitive Sciences*, *25*(5), 388–402. https://doi.org/10.1016/j.tics.2021.02.007

Pfeffer, J., Zorbach, T., & Carley, K. M. (2014). Understanding online firestorms: Negative word-of-mouth dynamics in social media networks. *Journal of Marketing Communications*, *20*(1–2), 117–128. https://doi.org/10.1080/13527266.2013.797778

Rajkumar, R. P. (2020). COVID-19 and mental health: A review of the existing literature. *Asian Journal of Psychiatry*, *52*, 102066. https://doi.org/10.1016/j.ajp.2020.102066

Reicher, S., & Drury, J. (2021). Pandemic fatigue? How adherence to COVID-19 regulations has been misrepresented and why it matters. *BMJ*, *372*, n137. https://doi.org/10.1136/bmj.n137

Rost, K., Stahel, L., & Frey, B. S. (2016). Digital social norm enforcement: Online firestorms in social media. *PLoS One*, *11*(6), e0155923. https://doi.org/10.1371/journal.pone.0155923

Soper, G. A. (1919). The lessons of the pandemic. *Science*, *49*(1274), 501–506. https://doi.org/10.1126/science.49.1274.501

Stechemesser, A., Wenz, L., & Levermann, A. (2020). Corona crisis fuels racially profiled hate in social media networks. *EClinicalMedicine*, *23*, 100372. https://doi.org/10.1016/j.eclinm.2020.100372

Tosi, J., & Warmke, B. (2016). Moral grandstanding. *Philosophy & Public Affairs*, *44*(3), 197–217. https://doi.org/10.1111/papa.12075

Van Bavel, J. J., Baicker, K., Boggio, P. S., Capraro, V., Cichocka, A., Cikara, M., Crockett, M. J., Crum, A. J., Douglas, K. M., Druckman, J. N., Drury, J., Dube, O., Ellemers, N., Finkel, E. J., Fowler, J. H., Gelfand, M., Han, S., Haslam, S. A., Jetten, J., . . . Willer, R. (2020). Using social and behavioural science to support COVID-19 pandemic response. *Nature Human Behaviour*, 4(5), 460–471. https://doi.org/10.1038/s41 562-020-0884-z

Van Bavel, J. J., Cichocka, A., Capraro, V., Sjåstad, H., Nezlek, J. B., Pavlović, T., Alfano, M., Gelfand, M. J., Azevedo, F., Birtel, M. D., Cislak, A., Lockwood, P., Ross, R. M., Abts, K., Agadullina, E., Amodio, D. M., Apps, M. A. J., Aruta, J. J. B. R., Besharati, S, . . . Boggio, P. (2021). National identity predicts public health support during a global pandemic: Results from 67 nations. *Nature Communications, 13*, 517. https://doi.org/10.31234/osf.io/ydt95

van der Linden, S., Roozenbeek, J., & Compton, J. (2020). Inoculating against fake news about COVID-19. *Frontiers in Psychology*, 11, 566790. https://doi.org/10.3389/fpsyg.2020.566790

Wang, S., Chen, X., Li, Y., Luu, C., Yan, R., & Madrisotti, F. (2021). "I'm more afraid of racism than of the virus!": Racism awareness and resistance among Chinese migrants and their descendants in France during the COVID-19 pandemic. *European Societies, 23*(Suppl.), S721–S742. https://doi.org/10.1080/14616696.2020.1836384

Xu, J., Sun, G., Cao, W., Fan, W., Pan, Z., Yao, Z., & Li, H. (2021). Stigma, discrimination, and hate crimes in Chinese-speaking world amid COVID-19 pandemic. *Asian Journal of Criminology, 16*(1), 51–74. https://doi.org/10.1007/s11417-020-09339-8

FURTHER READING

Bandura, A. (1990). Mechanisms of moral disengagement. In Walter Reich (ed.), *Origins of terrorism: Psychologies, ideologies, theologies, states of mind* (pp. 161–191). Cambridge University Press.

Brady, W. J., & Crockett, M. J. (2019). How effective is online outrage? *Trends in Cognitive Sciences, 23*(2), 79–80. https://doi.org/10.1016/j.tics.2018.11.004

Brady, W. J., Wills, J. A., Burkart, D., Jost, J. T., & Van Bavel, J. J. (2019). An ideological asymmetry in the diffusion of moralized content on social media among political leaders. *Journal of Experimental Psychology. General, 148*(10), 1802–1813. https://doi.org/10.1037/xge0000532

Garland, D. (2008). On the concept of moral panic. *Crime, Media, Culture, 4*(1), 9–30. https://doi.org/10.1177/1741659007087270

Tosi, J., & Warmke, B. (2020). *Grandstanding: The use and abuse of moral talk*. Oxford University Press.

10

Temporal Discounting, Uncertainty, and COVID-19

MATTIA NESE, GRETA RIBOLI, VALENTINA SASSI, GIANNI BRIGHETTI, AND ROSITA BORLIMI ■

Unprecedented community containment measures were taken following the out-break of COVID-19 in Europe in early 2020. The success in reducing the number of infections relied largely on the compliance of citizens with stay-home orders. The severity of restrictions and the uncertainty linked to their duration and effectiveness represented a great challenge for the people involved. The pressure of fundamental needs against the risk of infection (or infecting other people) created a psycholog-ical tension that could put at risk individual and public health. In some cases, when the satisfaction of immediate needs (e.g., spending time with family) has more value than protecting your health until the emergency has passed and overcomes the perceived likelihood of infection, safety behaviors (e.g., social distancing) could be abandoned. These cases are well described by what psychologists define as temporal discounting and probability discounting. In other words, people tend to prefer immediate or larger rewards over delayed or smaller ones. Also, they tend to prefer more likely rewards compared to more uncertain ones.

This chapter discusses the phenomenon of discounting healthy behaviors and its potential impact on compliance with containment measures during the COVID-19 pandemic.

DELAY AND PROBABILITY DISCOUNTING

Every choice people make potentially involves the representation of the subjective value of the gain associated with each option. When scrolling through the menu at the restaurant, people might compare the dishes based on the taste they expect

Mattia Nese, Greta Riboli, Valentina Sassi, Gianni Brighetti, and Rosita Borlimi, *Temporal Discounting, Uncertainty, and COVID-19* In: *The Social Science of the COVID-19 Pandemic*. Edited by: Monica K. Miller, Oxford University Press.
© Oxford University Press 2024. DOI: 10.1093/oso/9780197615133.003.0010

and order the one they think will have the best taste. However, while some rewards are immediate, others are delayed, and time can modify people's representation of gains during decision-making. The most common examples used to show this effect refer to monetary rewards. For example, when offered two monetary rewards that differ in amount but not in the time until their receipt, one typically would choose the larger amount, whereas when offered two rewards of the same amount that would be received at different times, one typically would choose the one that is available sooner. Similarly, when offered two monetary rewards of the same amount that differ in the probability that they will be actually received, one typically would choose the more probable (Green et al., 2013).

However, the relationship between the value of the reward and the time and probability of its receipt can create tension that makes decisions a lot less straightforward. People often choose smaller, sooner rewards instead of greater, future rewards; for example, when offered to choose between $100 now or $105 in a year people would typically choose the first option. Although it could be considered an *irrational* choice from an economic perspective, as the objective value of the second option is larger than the immediate one, from a psychological perspective people tend to decrease the value of a reward when this is delayed in time. As in this example, if the delay to its receipt is long enough, the subjective (i.e., present) value of the larger reward actually might be less than that of the smaller, immediate reward. This tendency has been called *temporal discounting* (also known as *time discounting* or *delay discounting*; Odum, 2011a). Analogously, if the likelihood to receive a large reward is low enough, individuals might choose smaller but more likely rewards (i.e., *probability discount*). The value of the reward at different hypothetical delays can be modeled as a curve whose steepness represents the magnitude of the temporal discount. The steeper the curve, the higher the discount of the reward will be over time.

These principles have been widely studied in the context of behavioral economics as they explain how decisions are made in the context of monetary rewards (e.g., when choosing between financial investments with different amounts of profits and probability). However, a steep delay discounting has been associated with drug abuse, smoking, gambling, obesity, risky sexual behaviors, preventive health behaviors, and personal safety (Odum et al., 2020). In all these cases, people engage maladaptive behaviors that are detrimental in the long term while potentially rewarding in the short term. For example, a smoker might smoke a cigarette now thinking about the immediate pleasure it gives despite being aware of the damage it can do to health over time. Similarly, a person with obesity might eat an extra slice of cake, underestimating the effect of overeating on health in the long term. This happens because future representations tend to be more abstract than immediate rewards, which are represented more concretely and vividly (Trope & Liberman, 2003; Vaidya & Fellows, 2017). Also, the nondeterministic nature of some behaviors (e.g., smoking) toward future adverse health conditions (e.g., cancer) might contribute to weakening the perceived risk.

Empirical studies on delay discounting led some authors to conclude that people can be differentiated based on their tendency to discount the probability of future events: Risk-averse people tend to devalue positive outcomes more steeply as these cease to be sure and become more uncertain, and, on the other side, people who expose themselves to risky conditions tend to underestimate information about the probability of negative outcomes. Whether the tendency to delay discount is the product of a stable trait linked to personality or a transient state depending on the circumstances (e.g., the type of choice) is a key element to understand how it can be modified to disengage maladaptive behaviors. Temporal discounting occurs as both a state and a trait characteristic, although it might also be the result of the combination of the two (Odum, 2011b).

The contextual factors that can lead to underestimating future rewards concern the nature of the reward itself. For example, temporal discounting might be steeper for rewards that act as unconditional reinforcements and are perishable (e.g., food, alcohol, and drugs) compared to money, which shows a less steep discounting over time.

On the other hand, considering temporal discounting as a trait, regardless of the context or the nature of the evaluated object, opens up to the potential role of genes (Gray et al., 2019; Mitchell, 2011). Some researchers tried to determine the relative importance of genetic predisposition in delay discounting by conducting laboratory experiments on rodents (Beckwith & Czachowski, 2014; Linsenbardt et al., 2017), as well as research on twins. For example, Anokhin and colleagues (2011) examined the differences in delay discounting rates between monozygotic and dizygotic twins. While monozygotic twins result from the fertilization of a single egg and share all of their genes, dizygotic twins result from the fertilization of two separate eggs during the same pregnancy and share half of their genes. In both cases, a correlation was found in the delay discounting trend among the twins, which was more pronounced in monozygotic twins. This suggests that there is a genetic component.

Moreover, several studies investigated the brain areas involved in the phenomenon of delay discounting: thalamus; sensory cortex; parietal cortex; insula; temporal lobe; cingulate cortex; prefrontal cortex; motor cortex; and basal ganglia (see Frost & McNaughton, 2017, for a review). Delay discounting, then, appears to emerge from the interaction of different neural systems rather than being a simple calculation carried out in a single region of the brain.

DISCOUNTING HEALTHY BEHAVIORS

Temporal and probability discounting can have important consequences when applied to health decision-making. A steeper temporal discounting of future benefits for health is associated with a wide range of maladaptive behaviors (Amlung et al., 2019; Bickel et al., 2019), such as substance abuse (Barlow et al., 2017); poor health behavior; unhealthy food consumption (Garza et al., 2016); obesity (Amlung et al., 2016; Barlow et al., 2016); infrequent physical activity; not wearing sunscreen (Daugherty & Brase, 2010); texting while driving (Hayashi et al., 2016); pathological gambling (Steward et al., 2017); and risky sexual behaviors (Johnson & Bruner, 2012).

Delay and probability discounting might not only facilitate engaging in maladaptive behaviors but also be associated with adherence to the therapeutic prescriptions. Moreover, higher rates of discounting based on treatment risks are associated with poor treatment adherence. When choosing to undergo treatment, patients with multiple sclerosis evaluate the probability of long-term benefits against the probability of side effects in the short term (Bruce et al., 2016). Interesting research on cancer survivors showed that higher delay discounting rates are associated with more alcohol consumption, cigarette smoking, other tobacco use, tanning booth use, and, conversely, greater adherence to annual primary care visits; on the contrary, lower delay discounting rates are associated with several important healthy lifestyle behaviors (Sheffer et al., 2018).

Temporal and probability discounting can affect the cognitive processes during health decision-making and facilitate maladaptive behaviors and poor treatment adherence, with negative consequences for people's health. Therefore, it is important to ask if and how these phenomena might impact both individual and public health in the context of the pandemic, where the global population is called to adopt protective behaviors and adhere to severe restrictions.

DELAY DISCOUNTING AND PANDEMIC

The rapid spread of COVID-19 in early 2020 led many nations to implement containment measures aimed at limiting infection, such as washing hands frequently, the use of face masks, social distancing, and avoiding going out from home if not strictly necessary,[1] along with the closure of all schools and nonessential activities (i.e., lockdown) during the peaks of contagion (see Chapter 3 for summary of pandemic-related policies).

In light of the above information, compliance with prevention guidelines could be modeled as an intertemporal risk–benefit trade-off framework. That is, people who tend to discount future uncertain benefits in favor of immediate ones might be less compliant with protective norms. In this case, the future benefit would be not exposing themselves or others to COVID-19, while the immediate rewards would be doing those activities that bring gratification (e.g., social contact, sport).

In order to better describe the situation caused by the pandemic during the first months of 2020, we now focus on the case of Italy, as it was the first Western country to report a widespread outbreak of COVID-19 at the end of February 2020. The rapid increase of hospitalizations led the Italian government to take dramatic containment measures. On March 9, 2020, a decree of the Italian prime minister declared a nationwide lockdown meant to reduce the probability of the person-to-person spread of disease linked to social aggregation. The decree (named "I Stay at Home") included community-wide containment measures that affected the daily life of the population at all levels in an unprecedented way. According to this, people were not allowed to leave their homes except for the following proven necessities: going to work, buying food, helping other people with special needs, and receiving medical care. The violation of the restrictions was sanctioned with a fine. The companies producing nonindispensable goods (48.8% of the total) were forced to close their facilities. It is estimated that 7,784,000 people (33.3% of the total workers) either began to work remotely from their houses or stopped working completely (Italian National Institute of Statistics, March 31, 2020). Most of the public spaces involving the gathering of people (e.g., schools, restaurants, shops, hotels) were closed.

When the first lockdown began, nobody was able to predict its duration as its end was exclusively tied to a significant drop in transmission rate, hospitalizations, and deaths. People were called to comply with restrictions and protective behaviors without knowing how long this could last or whether the containment measures would be effective. How long could people give up their everyday life before they would consider their needs more valuable than their health?

Our research group (Nese et al., 2020) surveyed the Italian population using different scenarios in which the hypothetical probability of contracting COVID-19 and the hypothetical duration of the lockdown were manipulated. Participants were asked to estimate their adherence to social isolation at different moments (today, at 7, 14, 30, 60, 90, and 180 days from now) at three hypothetical risk levels (10%, 50%, 90% of likelihood of contracting the COVID-19). Each scenario was presented using the following question: "Interrupting the isolation in . . . days in your area would give you a . . .% chance of contracting COVID-19. How acceptable do you think the decision to terminate the isolation is?" and participants answered on a scale from 1 (totally unacceptable) to 5 (totally acceptable).

We found that, when the risk of contagion was relatively low (e.g., 10%), the level of adherence tended to decrease as the number of containment days increased, thus confirming the tendency to devalue the long-term benefits typical of delay discounting. The same tendency was still observable although much weaker when the risk was higher (i.e., 50% and 90%). The respondents showed a discounting pattern of compliance over time similar to those found in past studies (Lawless et al., 2013), with a stronger discounting rate in case of a low likelihood of contracting COVID-19. This index did not seem to vary according to sex or age, although female participants reported greater anxiety and intolerance to uncertainty. Also, participants were asked to rate the importance of psychological needs: meeting partners and friends, going to work, recreational activities, and physical activity. These were thought to be associated with the temporal discounting rate. Surprisingly, only the reported importance of outdoor physical activity was associated with a steeper discounting of adherence to social isolation. However, some of the other needs (e.g., meeting friends and partners) were more or less relevant depending on the age groups of the sample, potentially hiding their effect on the general self-reported compliance trends. Notably, the need to meet others has been associated with the severity of anxiety symptoms.

In general, humans take the volatility of the reward environment into account in an optimal manner to adjust decision-making, and this process is supported by the activation of a specific brain region (i.e., the anterior cingulate cortex; Behrens et al., 2007). It means that when in uncertain situations, the salience of new information is evaluated and integrated with past knowledge to produce more accurate predictions of future outcomes. Thus, the adherence to containment measures might be subject to changes due to the availability of new information. For example, the perception of risk associated with the infection might have been modulated over time by the improvement of medical treatment during hospitalization, the appearance of new variants of the virus, and better knowledge of the spread dynamics. In line with these considerations, Lloyd and colleagues (2020) reported that those who adapted more quickly to new information were better equipped to change their behavior in response to public health measures. People who gave priority to recent information might therefore exhibit better adaption to novel health guidelines, allowing them to adjust behaviors more easily. On the contrary, a slower update of beliefs might have constrained the compliance to lockdown measures.

In the context of the COVID-19 pandemic, the increased messaging about the number of infections and the risks for health might be driving healthy behaviors and pro-health beliefs at first, but it could also be responsible for the high levels of anxiety reported since the beginning of the lockdown and fail to inform decision-making when excessive or prolonged in time, especially for vulnerable groups (Barari et al., 2020).

To our knowledge, our research was the first to apply the concept of delay discounting to safety behaviors during the COVID-19 epidemic. The only other example of research about delay discounting applied to other epidemics regards a certain number of studies about risky sexual behavior and HIV transmission, showing that sexual discounting (preference for immediate unprotected sex) strongly affects HIV sexual risk behavior. Other studies in line with our research are being published, focusing on specific behaviors (Johnson & Bruner, 2012). For example, Byrne and colleagues (2021) reported that people who are more inclined to make risky choices are also less compliant to appropriate mask-wearing behavior and social distancing recommendations.

LESSONS LEARNED: HOW TO PROMOTE COMPLIANCE OVER TIME

When disposing of public health measures that involve severe restrictions like those during the COVID-19 lockdown, policymakers should always consider the psychological variables that could negatively affect adherence to protective behaviors. Temporal and probability discount greatly affect health decision-making and should be carefully monitored in order to maximize the effects of containment measures.

These considerations have practical implications for the management of public health communications (see also Chapter 14 for more on pandemic-related messages). For example, communicating data about the number of infections with a certain optimism might reassure the population about the effectiveness of containment measures. However, we showed that perceived risk has a major impact on the intention to comply with containment measures in the future. Therefore, underlining the health risks associated with COVID-19 might positively affect compliance. However, it is important to note that this does not mean catastrophizing communication inducing fear would be an effective strategy, as it could contribute to enhancing psychological distress, especially among more vulnerable groups (see Chapter 20 for more on mental health during the pandemic). As shown, the negative effects of the lockdown on mental health represent not only a priority target for interventions but also a potential obstacle for an efficient update of information that could weaken adherence to protective behaviors.

As lockdowns were often contingent on the severity of the contagion and their duration is often unpredictable, public communication should focus on the safety criteria rather than announcing ending dates and subsequently prolong the lockdown if safety criteria are not met in time,[2] as these messages contribute to increasing uncertainty about the future that could have negative effects on compliance in the present.

Also, policymakers should carefully consider the psychological cost of each restriction oriented to preserve public health. Compliance with containment measures could be weakened if the psychological cost overcomes the perceived health benefits. For example, people might want to practice outdoor sport for its beneficial effects on physical and mental health even when not allowed if they believe that the risk of spreading the virus by doing it is low.

FUTURE RESEARCH ON TEMPORAL DISCOUNTING AND PANDEMIC-RELATED BEHAVIOR

Although research on the temporal and probability discounting of health has provided us with much useful information, there are still several questions to be answered in the future.

For example, the majority of studies about delay discounting used hypothetical outcomes; given a set of choices or situations, the participants were required to imagine what they think they would prefer or do. Whether people's subjective statements about hypothetical scenarios—like those used in the aforementioned studies, for example ("It is totally unacceptable to violate isolation with a 50% chance of contracting COVID-19)—can predict actual behaviors over time is still debated. However, there is evidence that humans consider hypothetical and real rewards in the same way when making decisions; several studies did not find differences in the tendency to discount the value of a reward when comparing real monetary rewards (i.e., participants were actually paid the chosen amount) and hypothetical ones (i.e., participants were asked to choose based on what they think they would prefer). Future studies should investigate the extent to which subjective statements about future healthy behaviors translate into actions during the pandemic.

Another important element to consider is the impact that mass communications might have on risk perception, which in turn greatly influence the discounting of security behaviors. Future studies could investigate the effects that the communication of certain information (e.g., the number of reported cases of infection or the discovery of a dangerous variant of the virus) and the manner in which it is communicated on the temporal discounting of compliance with containment measures and safety behaviors. This would help predict people's future reactions to risk-related communications and could improve awareness of the effects of mass communications on compliance with containment measures during future pandemics.

CONCLUSION

Delay and probability discounting can negatively affect health decision-making. People tend to devaluate future positive outcomes (e.g., protecting themselves and others from contracting COVID-19) and prefer immediate gratifications (e.g., meeting other people violating the restrictions) when they perceive a low risk for themselves and when they cannot accurately estimate the likelihood of future events. In order to promote adherence to protective behaviors and containment measures during the COVID-19 pandemic, it is crucial to adopt strategies that minimize the impact of discounting without increasing mental distress.

NOTES

1. https://www.who.int/docs/default-source/coronaviruse/who-china-joint-mission-on-covid-19-final-report.pdf
2. https://www.theguardian.com/world/2021/may/31/end-of-england-covid-lockdown-on-21-june-increasingly-in-doubt

REFERENCES

Amlung, M., Marsden, E., Holshausen, K., Morris, V., Patel, H., Vedelago, L., Naish, K. R., Reed, D. D., & McCabe, R. E. (2019). Delay discounting as a transdiagnostic process in psychiatric disorders: A meta-analysis. *JAMA Psychiatry*, *76*(11), 1176–1186. https://doi.org/10.1001/jamapsychiatry.2019.2102

Amlung, M., Petker, T., Jackson, J., Balodis, I., & MacKillop, J. (2016). Steep discounting of delayed monetary and food rewards in obesity: A meta-analysis. *Psychological Medicine*, *46*(11), 2423–2434. https://doi.org/10.1017/S0033291716000866

Anokhin, A. P., Golosheykin, S., Grant, J. D., & Heath, A. C. (2011). Heritability of delay discounting in adolescence: A longitudinal twin study. *Behavior Genetics*, *41*(2), 175–183. https://doi.org/10.1007/s10519-010-9384-7

Barari, S., Caria, S., Davola, A., Falco, P., Fetzer, T., Fiorin, S., Hensel, L., Ivchenko, A., Jachimowicz, J., King, G., Kraft-Todd, G., Ledda, A., MacLennan, M., Mutoi,

L., Pagani, C., Reutskaja, E., Roth, C., & Raimondi Slepoi, F. (2020). Evaluating COVID-19 public health messaging in Italy: Self-reported compliance and growing mental health concerns. medRxiv [Preprint]. https://gking.harvard.edu/covid-italy

Barlow, P., McKee, M., Reeves, A., Galea, G., & Stuckler, D. (2017). Time-discounting and tobacco smoking: A systematic review and network analysis. *International Journal of Epidemiology, 46*(3), 860–869. https://doi.org/10.1093/ije/dyw233

Barlow, P., Reeves, A., McKee, M., Galea, G., & Stuckler, D. (2016). Unhealthy diets, obesity and time discounting: A systematic literature review and network analysis. *Obesity Reviews, 17*(9), 810–819. https://doi.org/10.1111/obr.12431

Beckwith, S. W., & Czachowski, C. L. (2014). Increased delay discounting tracks with a high ethanol-seeking phenotype and subsequent ethanol seeking but not consumption. *Alcoholism: Clinical and Experimental Research, 38*(10), 2607–2614. https://doi.org/10.1111/acer.12523

Behrens, T. E., Woolrich, M. W., Walton, M. E., & Rushworth, M. F. (2007). Learning the value of information in an uncertain world. *Nature Neuroscience, 10*(9), 1214–1221. https://doi.org/10.1038/nn1954

Bickel, W. K., Athamneh, L. N., Basso, J. C., Mellis, A. M., DeHart, W. B., Craft, W. H., & Pope, D. (2019). Excessive discounting of delayed reinforcers as a trans-disease process: Update on the state of the science. *Current Opinion in Psychology, 30*, 59–64. https://doi.org/10.1016/j.copsyc.2019.01.005

Bruce, J. M., Bruce, A. S., Catley, D., Lynch, S., Goggin, K., Reed, D., Lim, S.-L., Strober, L., Glusman, M., Ness, A. R., & Jarmolowicz, D. P. (2016). Being kind to your future self: Probability discounting of health decision-making. *Annals of Behavioral Medicine, 50*(2), 297–309. https://doi.org/10.1007/s12160-015-9754-8

Byrne, K. A., Six, S. G., Anaraky, R. G., Harris, M. W., & Winterlind, E. L. (2021). Risk-taking unmasked: Using risky choice and temporal discounting to explain COVID-19 preventative behaviors. *PLoS One, 16*(5), e0251073. https://doi.org/10.1371/journal.pone.0251073

Daugherty, J. R., & Brase, G. L. (2010). Taking time to be healthy: Predicting health behaviors with delay discounting and time perspective. *Personality and Individual Differences, 48*(2), 202–207. https://doi.org/10.1016/j.paid.2009.10.007

Frost, R., & McNaughton, N. (2017). The neural basis of delay discounting: A review and preliminary model. *Neuroscience and Biobehavioral Reviews, 79*, 48–65. https://doi.org/10.1016/j.neubiorev.2017.04.022

Garza, K. B., Ding, M., Owensby, J. K., & Zizza, C. A. (2016). Impulsivity and fast-food consumption: A cross-sectional study among working adults. *Journal of the Academy of Nutrition and Dietetics, 116*(1), 61–68. https://doi.org/10.1016/j.jand.2015.05.003

Gray, J. C., Sanchez-Roige, S., de Wit, H., Mackillop, J., & Palmer, A. A. (2019). Genomic basis of delayed reward discounting. *Behavioural Processes, 162*, 157–161. https://doi.org/10.1016/j.beproc.2019.03.006

Green, L., Myerson, J., Oliveira, L., & Chang, S. E. (2013). Delay discounting of monetary rewards over a wide range of amounts. *Journal of the Experimental Analysis of Behavior, 100*(3), 269–281. https://doi.org/10.1002/jeab.45

Hayashi, Y., Miller, K., Foreman, A. M., & Wirth, O. (2016). A behavioral economic analysis of texting while driving: Delay discounting processes. *Accident; Analysis & Prevention, 97*, 132–140. https://doi.org/10.1016/j.aap.2016.08.028

Italian National Institute of Statistics (2020, March 31). *Esame del disegno di legge A.S. 1766 Conversione in legge del decreto-legge 17 marzo 2020, n. 18.* https://www.istat.it/it/files/2020/03/Aggiornamento_MemoriaAS-1766_rev31marzo.pdf

Johnson, M. W., & Bruner, N. R. (2012). The Sexual Discounting Task: HIV risk behavior and the discounting of delayed sexual rewards in cocaine dependence. *Drug and Alcohol Dependence, 123*(1–3), 15–21. https://doi.org/10.1016/j.drugalc dep.2011.09.032

Lawless, L., Drichoutis, A. C., & Nayga, R. M. (2013). Time preferences and health behaviour: A review. *Agricultural and Food Economics, 1*(1), 17. https://doi.org/10.1186/2193-7532-1-17

Linsenbardt, D. N., Smoker, M. P., Janetsian-Fritz, S. S., & Lapish, C. C. (2017). Impulsivity in rodents with a genetic predisposition for excessive alcohol consumption is associated with a lack of a prospective strategy. *Cognitive, Affective and Behavioral Neuroscience, 17*(2), 235–251. https://doi.org/10.3758/s13415-016-0475-7

Lloyd, A., McKay, R., Hartman, T. K., Vincent, B. T., Murphy, J., Gibson-Miller, J., . . . & Mason, L. (2021). Delay discounting and under-valuing of recent information predict poorer adherence to social distancing measures during the COVID-19 pandemic. *Scientific Reports, 11*(1), 19237. https://doi.org/10.1038/s41598-021-98772-5

Mitchell, S. H. (2011). The genetic basis of delay discounting and its genetic relationship to alcohol dependence. *Behavioural Processes, 87*(1), 10–17. https://doi.org/10.1016/j.beproc.2011.02.008

Nese, M., Riboli, G., Brighetti, G., Sassi, V., Camela, E., Caselli, G., Sassaroli, S., & Borlimi, R. (2020). Delay discounting of compliance with containment measures during the COVID-19 outbreak: A survey of the Italian population. *Journal of Public Health (Berl.), 30*, 503–511. https://doi.org/10.1007/s10389-020-01317-9

Odum, A. L. (2011a). Delay discounting: I'm a k, you're a k. *Journal of the Experimental Analysis of Behavior, 96*(3), 427–439. https://doi.org/10.1901/jeab.2011.96-423

Odum, A. L. (2011b). Delay discounting: Trait variable? *Behavioural Processes, 87*(1), 1–9. https://doi.org/10.1016/j.beproc.2011.02.007

Odum, A. L., Becker, R. J., Haynes, J. M., Galizio, A., Frye, C. C. J., Downey, H., Friedel, J. E., & Perez, D. M. (2020). Delay discounting of different outcomes: Review and theory. *Journal of the experimental Analysis of Behavior, 113*(3), 657–679. https://doi.org/10.1002/jeab.589

Sheffer, C. E., Miller, A., Bickel, W. K., Devonish, J. A., O'Connor, R. J., Wang, C., Rivard, C., & Gage-Bouchard, E. A. (2018). The treasure of now and an uncertain future: Delay discounting and health behaviors among cancer survivors. *Cancer, 124*(24), 4711–4719. https://doi.org/10.1002/cncr.31759

Steward, T., Mestre-Bach, G., Fernández-Aranda, F., Granero, R., Perales, J. C., Navas, J. F., Soriano-Mas, C., Baño, M., Fernández-Formoso, J. A., Martín-Romera, V., Menchón, J. M., & Jiménez-Murcia, S. (2017). Delay discounting and impulsivity traits in young and older gambling disorder patients. *Addictive Behaviors, 71*, 96–103. https://doi.org/10.1016/j.addbeh.2017.03.001

Trope, Y., & Liberman, N. (2003). Temporal construal. *Psychological Review, 110*(3), 403–421. https://doi.org/10.1037/0033-295X.110.3.403

Vaidya, A. R., & Fellows, L. K. (2017). The neuropsychology of decision-making: A view from the frontal lobes. In J.-C. Dreher & L. Tremblay (Eds.), *Decision neuroscience: An integrative perspective* (pp. 277–289). Elsevier Academic Press. https://doi.org/10.1016/B978-0-12-805308-9.00022-1

FURTHER READING

Green, L., Myerson, J., & Vanderveldt, A. (2014). Delay and probability discounting. In F. K. McSweeney & E. S. Murphy (Eds.), *The Wiley Blackwell handbook of operant and classical conditioning* (pp. 307–337). Wiley Blackwell. https://doi.org/10.1002/9781118468135.ch13

Mazur, J. E. (1987). An adjusting procedure for studying delayed reinforcement. In M. L. Commons, J. E. Mazur, J. A. Nevin, & H. Rachlin (Eds.), *The effect of delay and of intervening events on reinforcement value* (pp. 55–73). Lawrence Erlbaum Associates.

11

An Objectification Theory Lens for Understanding Compliance With COVID-19 Safety Measures

ELVIRA PRUSACZYK, MEGAN EARLE, BECKY CHOMA, AND
RACHEL CALOGERO ∎

At the start of the COVID-19 pandemic, governments and health organizations worldwide recommended numerous safety guidelines for people to follow, including instructions for prolonged handwashing, wearing masks, and social distancing. Such safety measures were crucial for slowing the spread of COVID-19, a highly contagious and deadly virus. Despite the feats of rapid vaccine development, vaccines rolled out relatively slowly. Moreover, it remained unclear whether being fully vaccinated protected against all COVID-19 variants or prevented spread to others. As such, the World Health Organization (WHO) recommended safety precautions even for fully vaccinated individuals.[1] Thus, widespread behavioral change remained the leading way to slow the spread of COVID-19, even into the second year of the pandemic. Problematically, however, people have varied drastically in the degree to which they follow COVID-19 safety measures. Such variation is attributable to several factors, including personal politics (Choma et al., 2021), belief in science (Stosic et al., 2021), and gender. For instance, public opinion polls and research consistently showed that women (vs. men) complied more with COVID-19 safety measures.[2] In this chapter, we explore gender differences, specifically between women and men, in COVID-19 safety measure compliance using objectification theory (Fredrickson & Roberts, 1997) as a lens.

Research on objectification theory (e.g., see Calogero et al., 2011) demonstrated that people who frequently experience sexual objectification (e.g., sexual harassment) are more likely to adopt an observer's perspective of their bodies, that is, self-objectify. Self-objectification, in turn, is associated with higher levels of safety

Elvira Prusaczyk, Megan Earle, Becky Choma, and Rachel Calogero, *An Objectification Theory Lens for Understanding Compliance With COVID-19 Safety Measures* In: *The Social Science of the COVID-19 Pandemic*. Edited by: Monica K. Miller, Oxford University Press. © Oxford University Press 2024. DOI: 10.1093/oso/9780197615133.003.0011 anxiety or diffuse and nonspecific hypervigilance toward potential threats to one's body (Calogero et al., 2021). Safety anxiety, in turn, has been found to restrict people's freedom of movement in public spaces, presumably to reduce potential exposures to sexual harm (Calogero et al., 2021). In a novel extension of objectification theory to a pandemic context, we summarize our new research showing that safety anxiety also predicted greater compliance with COVID-19 safety measures (Earle et al., 2021). Further, we found that women scored higher than men in sexual and self-objectification, safety anxiety, and safety measure compliance. Thus, men's lower adherence to safety measures might stem from their lower levels of sexual and self-objectification and, therefore, less preoccupation with their physical safety. In this way, both gender and sexual objectification processes predicted pandemic-related behavior. The purpose of this chapter is to introduce a novel framework for understanding gender differences in compliance with COVID-19 safety measures and provide concrete recommendations for research and social policy concerning disease-specific safety vigilance and increasing men's safety measure compliance.

GENDER DIFFERENCES IN COVID-19 OUTCOMES

Since the onset of the pandemic, scholars have observed robust gender differences concerning COVID-19-related outcomes. For instance, relative to women, men tend to experience greater COVID-19 symptom severity and are 2.4 times more likely to die from COVID-19 (Jin et al., 2020; Scully et al., 2020). In an analysis of 38 countries where sex-disaggregated data were available, a male bias in COVID-19 mortality rates emerged in 37 of the 38 countries (Scully et al., 2020). As one possible explanation, scholars speculated that women (vs. men) exhibit stronger immune system responses, which underlie their higher survival rates.[3] Importantly, gender differences extend beyond symptomatology and mortality outcomes. U.S. polls and studies also showed that women were more likely than men to comply with COVID-19 safety measures, such as following guidelines for frequent handwashing, social distancing, and wearing masks.[4] Thus, a male bias exists for not only COVID-19 morbidity and mortality rates but also poorer adherence with COVID-19 safety behaviors. Given the importance of compliance with safety measures for reducing the risk of contracting and spreading COVID-19, identifying the reasons underlying the gender difference in compliance is essential.

Several studies revealed that men are more likely than women to downplay the severity of COVID-19 symptoms and adopt an irresponsible or cavalier attitude toward preventive measures, including stay-home orders (Griffith et al., 2020). These attitudes, in turn, are thought to reduce men's adherence to COVID-19 safety guidelines (see Griffith et al., 2020). Moreover, scholars have pinpointed masculine norms as partly explaining the gender difference. For instance, Palmer and Peterson (2020) found that men scored higher than women in masculine toughness (i.e., the expectation that men show toughness), with masculine toughness predicting adverse reactions to wearing masks. Given the strong link between intentions and behavior (Sheeran, 2002), men who endorse masculine norms and exhibit negative attitudes toward masks are probably less likely to wear them or engage in other safety measures that make them look "weak" (for more on gender norms, see Chapter 12).

This chapter introduces another potential factor that can help explain the gender difference in COVID-19 safety measure compliance, namely, safety anxiety. Safety anxiety is the preoccupation with threats to one's safety that arises from experiences of sexual and self-objectification (see Calogero et al., 2021). Recent research demonstrated the role of safety anxiety in connection to varied risk-reducing behaviors (e.g., Calogero et al., 2021; Earle et al., 2021). Below, we first provide an overview of objectification theory. We then review our research demonstrating the link between safety anxiety and compliance with COVID-19 safety measures, followed by a discussion of gender differences in objectification theory processes that might help to illuminate gender differences in compliance.

OBJECTIFICATION THEORY

Objectification theory (Fredrickson & Roberts, 1997) is a framework for understanding the harmful effects of being regularly sexually objectified. Sexual objectification experiences involve the depiction, consumption, or treatment of people as sexual objects rather than whole human beings. Some examples of sexual objectification include being the target of leering and ogling, sexual comments and jokes, or sexual assault. Relative to men, women are more likely to experience sexual objectification (e.g., Smith et al., 2018). Studies showed that frequent exposure to sexual objectification socialized targets to self-objectify. The operationalization of self-objectification has evolved in recent years. According to Lindner and Tantleff-Dunn (2017), and their corresponding Self-Objectification and Beliefs Scale (SOBBS) scale, self-objectification involves two dimensions: internalization of an observer's perspective on the body (e.g., "I often think about how my body must look to others") and treating the body as representing the self (e.g., "My body is what gives me value to other people"). In response to sexual objectification, targets, predominantly women, begin to see themselves and their own bodies through the perspective of an observer's sexually objectifying gaze (i.e., the internalized observer dimension) and regard their self-worth as based on their physical appearance (i.e., body-as-self dimension) and how they look to others. Self-objectification, in turn, predicts a cascade of negative subjective experiences, including greater body shame, greater appearance anxiety, and lower self-esteem; ultimately, these processes are linked to the development of sexual dysfunction, disordered eating, self-harm, substance abuse, and depression (e.g., see Calogero et al., 2011; Moradi & Huang, 2008). In other words, sexual objectification can predict a downstream of negative consequences that disproportionately affect women.

In recent research, Calogero and colleagues (2021) examined safety anxiety as another downstream component of objectification theory (Fredrickson & Roberts, 1997). Conceived as a response to the threat of sexual violence that is implied in routine encounters of sexual objectification, Calogero et al. developed and validated a scale to assess safety anxiety as a diffuse and nonspecific tendency to be hypervigilant to, and worried about, potential threats to one's safety. They demonstrated links between sexual and self-objectification and increased safety anxiety across five samples of women, with safety anxiety further predicting restricted movement in public spaces. Although men also experience sexual objectification and might feel anxious about their personal safety, research has shown that women make adaptions to their routines and lifestyle because of safety concerns to a much greater degree than men do (Fisher et al., 1995). Although costly to one's freedom of mobility, limiting one's movement in public is a risk-reducing behavior that might be perceived as a necessary precaution to protect against sexual objectification and violence.

COVID-19 Safety Compliance Behavior as an Outcome of Objectification Processes

In a novel extension of objectification theory, we (Earle et al., 2021) tested whether chronic safety anxiety would generalize to predict greater adherence with COVID-19 safety guidelines. In general, hypervigilance is a chronic state that involves excessive monitoring of one's surroundings, even when threat is absent (Richards et al., 2014). Those who tend to be hypervigilant routinely and broadly scan their environments for potential signs of danger, in turn detecting emergent threats better than nonanxious people (for a review, see Richards et al., 2014). Of relevance, encounters of sexual objectification condition women to be generally and diffusely hypervigilant to possible environmental threats to their physical safety. By implication, chronic safety anxiety also involves broad attentional processing of *any* potential bodily danger and theoretically should extend to detecting the threat of contracting COVID-19. As such, we expected that chronic hypervigilance regarding one's safety would generalize to predict greater adherence with COVID-19 safety guidelines, given that these behaviors protect one's body from danger. To test our extended objectification theory model in a pandemic context, in our Earle et al. (2021) article, we conducted analyses on a sample of 489 U.S. participants, where 51.1% identified as cisgender women and 48.9% identified as cisgender men.[*] On average, participants were approximately 41 years old. Regarding racial identity, 75.5% of participants identified as White, 8.8% as Black, 14% as Asian, 4.3% as Latin American, and 0.4% as another race. As such, our sample generally approximated the nationally representative demographics of the U.S. population. By mid-April 2020, almost 2 million COVID-19

---

[*]. Participants who did not self-identify as men or women ($n = 4$) were excluded from analyses.

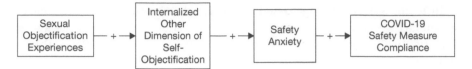

Indirect Effects Observed:
Sexual objectification → Self-Objectification → Safety Anxiety
Self-Objectification → Safety Anxiety → COVID-19 Safety Measure Compliance

Note. In Earle et al. (2021), the links between more frequent sexual objectification and greater COVID-19 safety measure compliance were accounted for by increased self-objectification (internalized other dimension) and safety anxiety in a significant two-step mediation process.

Figure 11.1 Visualization of objectification theory model with COVID-19 safety measure compliance as an outcome. (Adapted from Earle et al., 2021.)

cases were confirmed worldwide, including over 120,000 deaths.[5] Data were collected in April 2020 when approximately one third of all COVID-19 cases worldwide were in the United States, and government officials began disseminating COVID-19 safety guidelines.

For a conceptual visualization of the overall pattern of results, see Figure 11.1, which was adapted from Earle et al. (2021). As illustrated, the links between stranger harassment (i.e., sexual objectification) and COVID-19 safety measure compliance were explained by the internalized other dimension of self-objectification and safety anxiety. Specifically, and as expected, a significant two-step mediation model was observed. First, more frequent stranger harassment predicted higher self-objectification on the internalized other dimension and, in turn, increased hypervigilance about one's safety. Second, higher self-objectification on the internalized other predicted increased safety anxiety, which in turn predicted greater compliance with COVID-19 safety precautions. Put simply, complying with COVID-19 safety measures occurred more frequently for those conditioned by sexual objectification to observe their bodies and be vigilant about their physical safety. Therefore, the alertness and prevention-focused mindset involved in chronically and widely scanning one's environment for danger to one's body seems to facilitate adopting various risk-reducing behaviors, not just those concerning the risk of sexual violence. Someone less conditioned to be concerned about threats to their physical safety would be less oriented toward noticing the potential hazards in their environment and, therefore, engage in preventive behaviors like COVID-19 safety compliance less often.

Gender Differences in Our Extended Objectification Theory Model

In Earle et al. (2021), we also examined gender differences in the model's variables. Consistent with past research and objectification theory (Fredrickson & Roberts, 1997; Smith et al., 2018), our analyses revealed that, in general, women (vs. men) were more likely to report sexual objectification experiences (i.e., stranger harassment) and self-objectification (i.e., internalized other dimension). Moreover, women were also more likely than men to experience chronic safety anxiety and to report increased compliance with COVID-19 safety measures. Having higher levels of sexual harassment, self-objectification, safety anxiety, and COVID-19 safety compliance, we concluded that women (vs. men) complied more with COVID-19 safety guidelines in part because they were socialized to a greater extent by sexual and self-objectification to worry about and monitor their safety. In other words, women's lived experiences in a society that regularly harms them disproportionately promoted a trait-like level of hypervigilance that encouraged them to adopt risk-reducing behaviors in the face of an impending physical threat. By implication, men's lower adherence to safety precautions is partly due to worrying less about external threats to their safety before the pandemic (due to having lower levels of sexual objectification and self-objectification) and therefore complying with COVID-19 safety measures less frequently. Ultimately, women's hypervigilance about their safety helps to identify and protect themselves against novel dangers, and likely explains (in part) why women (vs. men) were also more compliant with safety measures during other pandemics like the severe acute respiratory syndrome (SARS) (e.g., Jin et al., 2020) outbreak.

LESSONS LEARNED

Given that one can contract COVID-19 anywhere (both within and outside one's home), the hypervigilance characterizing safety anxiety is adaptive for encouraging frequent adherence to safety measures. Regularly engaging in physical distancing, handwashing, and wearing masks is a disruption to one's usual way of life. Unless people are cautious about all the possible chances for contracting COVID-19, they will miss out on opportunities to protect themselves against COVID-19. Women, relative to men, are especially likely to engage in COVID-19 safety measures, being more vigilant about their physical safety due to regular encounters of sexual objectification and the threat of sexual violence by men. Thus, gender and sexual objectification processes are relevant predictors of people's compliance with COVID-19 safety measures. These findings point to potential suggestions for social policy recommendations. Rather than promoting safety anxiety, which ultimately stems from the harms of sexual and self-objectification to disproportionately affect women, we propose that government efforts to increase compliance with disease-specific precautionary measures should focus on (1) fostering disease-specific safety vigilance and (2) targeting men to increase their compliance with these measures. Below we detail these recommendations.

First, at least as part of an early pandemic response, governments should promote COVID-19-specific safety vigilance among citizens to encourage compliance with safety measures. This recommendation is consistent with objectification theory in that hypervigilance stemming from bodily threat can encourage the adoption of risk-reducing behaviors. In stark contrast to this advice, in March 2020, (former) U.S. President Donald Trump downplayed the deadliness of COVID-19, comparing it to the flu and suggesting it would go away with warmer weather, despite evidence to the contrary.[6] Relatedly, research suggested that messages from local and national government leaders were associated with community cases of COVID-19 (see Grossman et al., 2020). For instance, compared to Ohio, wherein the governor took a cautious approach emphasizing the risks of COVID-19, the governor in Florida followed Trump's approach and downplayed the risks of COVID-19. An empirical analysis suggested that the cases of community spread were much higher in Florida than Ohio, in association with downplaying the severity of COVID-19 (Yano, 2020). Presumably, by not highlighting and emphasizing the dangers of COVID-19, citizens' concerns and vigilance about the virus were relatively lower, and thus their compliance inadequate, accelerating the spread of COVID-19. As such, regular and clear communication regarding the risks of COVID-19 is necessary, including information about the effectiveness of safety measures for reducing the spread of COVID-19.

Important to consider, however, is that hypervigilance waxes and wanes. Long-term compliance with restrictive safety measures is not sustainable, with research providing evidence in 14 countries for behavioral compliance fatigue related to COVID-19 specifically. That is, people's initial levels of compliance gradually reduced over time, likely due to the chronic fatigue of having to comply with high-cost rules and regulations constantly (see Petherick et al., 2021). Not only is long-term compliance hard to maintain, but prolonged stress and hypervigilance are harmful to mental and physical health (e.g., Cohen et al., 2012), highlighting the need for multifaceted and changing government responses. Perhaps as an early pandemic response, fostering COVID-19-specific hypervigilance alongside a lockdown is the most effective way to slow the spread of COVID-19 and prevent follow-up waves. Indeed, Ngonghala and colleagues (2020) used mortality data to forecast that the combination of COVID-19 precautionary measures and prolonged lockdowns can effectively halt follow-up surges of COVID-19 cases, but only if people comply with safety measures (e.g., wearing masks). Thus, an initial government response that broadcasts educational messages to increase citizens' safety vigilance alongside a prolonged lockdown could curb the spread of COVID-19, saving lives and substantially alleviating the burden on hospitals treating COVID-19 patients. Such a response would only be effective if done quickly and at the beginning of a pandemic, as long-term solutions relying on promoting hypervigilance might backfire as some citizens begin to struggle with compliance fatigue.

Second, given that men (vs. women) are overall less likely to comply with COVID-19 safety guidelines, an additional strategy for governments to consider is to target men specifically in separate educational campaigns. Given that our data were based on largely White, cisgender, and (presumably) heterosexual men, the focus of educational strategies should be on higher status or more socially privileged men.[†] Indeed, men of color, gay men, or transgender men are more likely to experience the threat of harm and sexual objectification in their daily lives (e.g., see Flores et al., 2018; Teunis, 2007) and therefore might have higher safety anxiety and COVID-19 safety measure compliance than nonmarginalized men. One way to help increase (socially privileged) men's safety anxiety or COVID-19-specific safety vigilance, and therefore their compliance with safety measures, could be to highlight their higher morbidity and mortality rates (see Chapter 33 for more on terror management theory and mortality salience). Overall, men's risks for contracting, suffering, and dying from COVID-19 are higher than women's, and efforts to increase awareness about these increased risks might help to foster concern and worry, at least for some men. A result could be a less cavalier attitude about the risks of COVID-19.

However, a potential concern surrounding this strategy includes compensatory toughness among some men who endorse toxic masculinity norms. Men who endorse masculine norms of toughness might downplay their risks even further, resisting safety measure compliance due to fears of appearing weak. As such, messages could communicate that men who wear masks or practice social distancing are performing civic duties, helping to protect citizens and their loved ones. Although we must be careful about upholding systems of masculinity, it might be a fruitful and effective strategy in a crisis to portray safety measure compliance as attractive, courageous, and resilient, a strategy that could appeal to masculinity-endorsing men and arguably to others. An alternative and potentially more effective strategy could be to develop and distribute educational campaigns that broadly focus on conditioning socially privileged men to be more mindful about the social spaces that they occupy, behaviors that women (and presumably other marginalized group members) are typically better at employing.[‡] By promoting greater mindfulness and awareness of their environments, socially privileged men might be better able to identify potential sources for contracting COVID-19 and thus comply more frequently with safety precautions.

FUTURE RESEARCH IDEAS

Given that sexual objectification might condition men and women to respond differently to a novel viral threat, by implication it is likely relevant for predicting responses to future infectious diseases. In past pandemics, such as the SARS outbreak of 2003, men (vs. women) were also more likely to exhibit higher morbidity and mortality rates and lower compliance with safety measures (Jin et al., 2020).

---

†. For the remainder of the chapter, we refer to men with these specific demographic characteristics as socially privileged.

‡. Marginalized group members are more likely to experience sexual objectification and harm and, thus, theoretically more likely to exhibit safety anxiety and risk-reducing behaviors. Future research could test these claims.

Future research could continue to document gender differences in compliance with safety measures, determine other potential reasons, and document when and why strategies are effective for narrowing the gender difference in compliance. In this vein, future research could empirically validate our proposed strategies of targeting men in educational campaigns. Does educating men about their elevated morbidity and mortality risks help to increase their compliance? Are education effects stronger for some men relative to others? Can mindfulness increase compliance? Determining when interventions work and for whom is essential for developing varied strategies to increase compliance with safety measures. For instance, if more socially privileged men who endorse masculine norms are resistant to messages conveying harm, future research could determine which educational messages are more effective for increasing their safety measure compliance.

Importantly, future research could also pinpoint ways to maintain compliance even when disease-specific safety anxiety reduces. As discussed above, fostering mindfulness of one's physical environment might encourage compliance and might even be helpful when hypervigilance wanes over time. Mindfulness is the present-moment awareness or attention to one's internal and external environment, with nonreactivity to one's thoughts, emotions, and actions.[7] In the context of sexual objectification, mindfulness training can be tailored to help people focus on where they are concerning others in their physical environments, rather than seeing themselves through an observer's perspective.[§] Although the result would likely be less safety anxiety, compliance with disease-specific precautions might nonetheless increase given the nonjudgmental and nonreactive focus and responsiveness to one's environment. In effect, disease-specific precautions could be maintained without the intense feelings of threat or anxiety that typically encourage risk-reducing behaviors in people who are higher in hypervigilance. A mindfulness strategy should also be effective outside of a sexual objectification context by generally cultivating awareness and responsiveness to the safety measures needed to be safe in one's environment. Thus, although some anxiety and worry are likely required to adopt health-relevant behaviors, daily mindfulness habits might encourage compliance with such behaviors over time without the negative mental and physical health consequences of chronic hypervigilance. Future research could test whether mindfulness is a helpful strategy for encouraging and maintaining people's compliance with disease-specific precautions.

Important to also consider is that cultural or regional differences could affect relations between objectification-relevant variables and risk-reducing behaviors (see Chapter 16 for more on cultural aspects of the pandemic). Countries vary in both COVID-19 prevalence and government guidelines for reducing the spread of COVID-19. Perhaps in countries with inconsistent or weak safety measure

---

§. Reducing the incidence of sexual objectification, to begin with, is integral. Such an approach requires large-scale systemic and societal reform to target the systems of sexism that promote and maintain sexual harms against women. This goal is necessary to accomplish alongside personal-level strategies.

protocols, a wider gender difference in safety measure compliance exists. When people have more opportunities to avoid compliance, they tend to be less compliant. Thus, in countries with weak safety guidelines combined with high masculine or binary gender norms, some men might be particularly likely to avoid safety guidelines to display their "toughness." Future research could test these claims, identifying the countries and regions that might benefit most from educational campaigns.

More generally, the gender differences observed in Earle et al. (2021) might depend on a country's overall level of institutionalized sexism and prevalence of sexual objectification. Based on reported cases, WHO estimated that about 36% of women worldwide are subjected to sexual violence by partners or nonpartners, and strangers sexually assault 7.2% of women.[8] However, variation exists within and between countries. Of data extracted from 79 countries and two territories, the reported prevalence of sexual violence against women by their partners was highest in African, Eastern Mediterranean, and South-East Asia regions and lowest in higher income countries such as Switzerland, Denmark, Sweden, or Finland. By implication, countries lower in sexual violence could, in turn, exhibit narrower gender differences in both safety anxiety and disease-specific safety measure compliance. This is because the processes that tend to make women disproportionately vigilant to threat would be fewer, presumably helping to narrow the gender differences in compliance. Future work could test these claims and consider how processes of objectification, safety anxiety, and risk-reducing behaviors operate across cultural contexts. Understanding these differences could also help illuminate which strategies are effective and in what regions of the world.

CONCLUSIONS

Despite never being applied to a pandemic context, we have shown that objectification theory is a helpful framework for understanding compliance with COVID-19 safety measures. We provide evidence that men (primarily those socially privileged in status) and women differ in their compliance levels, introducing safety anxiety as one potential reason about why. Governments are responsible for intervening and maintaining citizens' compliance with safety measures throughout a pandemic. Understanding the possible reasons underlying the gender difference in compliance can help policymakers develop and deliver effective interventions, using resources wisely in the face of financial constraint. Doing so will serve as a roadmap for government responses in future pandemics, particularly as leaders wait for vaccines and instead rely on instilling behavioral change to slow the spread of a virus.

NOTES

1.   https://www.who.int/news-room/q-a-detail/coronavirus-disease-(covid-19)-vacci nes?topicsurvey=v8kj13)&gclid=EAIaIQobChMI16Od4ZPl8AIVwW5vBB06cgTE EAAYASAAEgLW8vD_BwE

2. https://voxeu.org/article/gender-differences-covid-19-perception-and-compliance
3. https://theconversation.com/covid-19s-deadliness-for-men-is-revealing-why-rese
    archers-should-have-been-studying-immune-system-sex-differences-years-ago-
    138767
4. https://www.pewresearch.org/fact-tank/2020/04/07/younger-americans-view-coro
    navirus-outbreak-more-as-a-major-threat-to-finances-than-health/
5. https://www.who.int/docs/default-source/coronaviruse/situation-reports/20200
    415-sitrep-86-covid-19.pdf?sfvrsn=c615ea20_6
6. https://www.forbes.com/sites/tommybeer/2020/09/10/all-the-times-trump-compa
    red-covid-19-to-the-flu-even-after-he-knew-covid-19-was-far-more-deadly/?sh=
    65d5d1f5f9d2
7. https://www.mindful.org/what-is-mindfulness/
8. https://www.who.int/news-room/fact-sheets/detail/violence-against-women

REFERENCES

Calogero, R. M., Tantleff-Dunn, S., & Thompson, J. K. (2011). *Self-objectification in women: Causes, consequences, and counteractions.* American Psychological Association.

Calogero, R. M., Tylka, T. L., Siegel, J. A., Pina, A., & Roberts, T. A. (2021). Smile pretty and watch your back: Personal safety anxiety and vigilance in objectification theory. *Journal of Personality and Social Psychology, 121*(6), 1195–1222. https://doi.org/10.1037/pspi0000344

Choma, B. L., Hodson, G., Sumantry, D., Hanoch, Y., & Gummerum, M. (2021). Ideological and psychological predictors of COVID-19-related collective action, opinions, and health compliance across three nations. *Journal of Social and Political Psychology, 9*(1), 123–143. https://doi.org/10.5964/jspp.5585

Cohen, S., Janicki-Deverts, D., Doyle, W. J., Miller, G. E., Frank, E., Rabin, B. S., & Turner, R. B. (2012). Chronic stress, glucocorticoid receptor resistance, inflammation, and disease risk. *Proceedings of the National Academy of Sciences of the United States of America, 109*(16), 5995–5999. https://doi.org/10.1073/pnas.1118355109

Earle, M., Prusaczyk, E., Choma, B., & Calogero, R. (2021). Compliance with COVID-19 safety measures: A test of an objectification theory model. *Body Image, 37,* 6–13. https://doi.org/10.1016/j.bodyim.2021.01.004

Fisher, B. S., Sloan, J. J., & Wilkins, D. L. (1995). Fear and perceived risk of victimization in an urban university setting. In B. S. Fisher & J. J. Sloan (Eds.), Campus crime: Legal, social and policy perspectives (pp. 179–209). Charles C Thomas.

Flores, M. J., Watson, L. B., Allen, L. R., Ford, M., Serpe, C. R., Choo, P. Y., & Farrell, M. (2018). Transgender people of color's experiences of sexual objectification: Locating sexual objectification within a matrix of domination. *Journal of Counseling Psychology, 65*(3), 308. https://doi.org/10.1037/cou0000279

Fredrickson, B. L., & Roberts, T. A. (1997). Objectification theory: Toward understanding women's lived experiences and mental health risks. *Psychology of Women Quarterly, 21*(2), 173–206. https://doi.org/10.1111/j.1471-6402.1997.tb00108.x

Griffith, D. M., Sharma, G., Holliday, C. S., Enyia, O. K., Valliere, M., Semlow, A. R., Stewart, E. C., & Blumenthal, R. S. (2020). Men and COVID-19: A biopsychosocial approach to understanding sex differences in mortality and recommendations for practice and policy interventions. *Preventing Chronic Disease, 17*, E63. https://doi.org/10.5888/pcd17.200247

Grossman, G., Kim, S., Rexer, J. M., & Thirumurthy, H. (2020). Political partisanship influences behavioral responses to governors' recommendations for COVID-19 prevention in the United States. *Proceedings of the National Academy of Sciences of the United States of America, 117*(39), 24144–24153. https://doi.org/10.1073/pnas.2007835117

Jin, J. M., Bai, P., He, W., Wu, F., Liu, X. F., Han, D. M., Liu, S., & Yang, J. K. (2020). Gender differences in patients with COVID-19: Focus on severity and mortality. *Frontiers in Public Health, 8*, 152. https://doi.org/10.3389/fpubh.2020.00152

Lindner, D., & Tantleff-Dunn, S. (2017). The development and psychometric evaluation of the Self-Objectification Beliefs and Behaviors Scale. *Psychology of Women Quarterly, 41*(2), 254–272. https://doi.org/10.1177/0361684317692109

Moradi, B., & Huang, Y. P. (2008). Objectification theory and psychology of women: A decade of advances and future directions. *Psychology of Women Quarterly, 32*(4), 377–398. https://doi.org/10.1111/j.1471-6402.2008.00452.x

Ngonghala, C. N., Iboi, E. A., & Gumel, A. B. (2020). Could masks curtail the post-lockdown resurgence of COVID-19 in the US? *Mathematical Biosciences, 329*, 108452. https://doi.org/10.1016/j.mbs.2020.108452

Palmer, C. L., & Peterson, R. D. (2020). Toxic mask-ulinity: The link between masculine toughness and affective reactions to mask wearing in the COVID-19 era. *Politics & Gender, 16*(4), 1044–1051. https://doi.org/10.1017/S1743923X20000422

Petherick, A., Goldszmidt, R. G., Andrade, E. B., Furst, R., Pott, A., & Wood, A. (2021). *A worldwide assessment of COVID-19 pandemic-policy fatigue.* SSRN. http://dx.doi.org/10.2139/ssrn.3774252

Richards, H. J., Benson, V., Donnelly, N., & Hadwin, J. A. (2014). Exploring the function of selective attention and hypervigilance for threat in anxiety. *Clinical Psychology Review, 34*(1), 1–13. https://doi.org/10.1016/j.cpr.2013.10.006

Scully, E. P., Haverfield, J., Ursin, R. L., Tannenbaum, C., & Klein, S. L. (2020). Considering how biological sex impacts immune responses and COVID-19 outcomes. *Nature Reviews Immunology, 20*(7), 442–447. https://doi.org/10.1038/s41577-020-0348-8

Sheeran, P. (2002). Intention–behavior relations: A conceptual and empirical review. *European Review of Social Psychology, 12*(1), 1–36. https://doi.org/10.1080/14792772143000003

Smith, S. G., Zhang, X., Basile, K. C., Merrick, M. T., Wang, J., Kresnow, M., Chen, J. (2018). The National Intimate Partner and Sexual Violence Survey (NISVS): 2015 data brief—Updated release. National Center for Injury Prevention and Control, Centers for Disease Control and Prevention.

Stosic, M. D., Helwig, S., & Ruben, M. A. (2021). Greater belief in science predicts mask-wearing behavior during COVID-19. *Personality and Individual Differences, 176*, 110769. https://doi.org/10.1016/j.paid.2021.110769

Teunis, N. (2007). Sexual objectification and the construction of Whiteness in the gay male community. *Culture, Health & Sexuality, 9*(3), 263–275. https://doi.org/10.1080/13691050601035597

Yano, M. (2020). Covid-19 pandemic and politics: The cases of Florida and Ohio. Research Institute of Economy, Trade and Industry (RIETI). https://ideas.repec.org/p/eti/dpaper/20040.html

FURTHER READING

Calogero, R. M. (2012). Objectification theory, self-objectification, and body image. In T. F. Cash (Ed.), *Encyclopedia of body image and human appearance* (Vol. *2*, pp. 574–580). Academic Press.

Roberts, T. A., Calogero, R. M., & Gervais, S. (2018). Objectification theory: Continuing contributions to feminist psychology. In C. Travis & J. White (Eds.), *APA handbook of the psychology of women* (Vol. *1*: History, theory, and battlegrounds, pp. 249–272). American Psychological Association.

12

Could Gender-Related Norms Predict Compliance With COVID-19 Prevention Behaviors?

Negative Impacts of Masculine Social Norms

METE SEFA UYSAL, EMIR ÜZÜMÇEKER, AND SARA VESTERGREN ■

Research in both public health and psychology have demonstrated men's risky health behaviors. For example, men score higher than women in relation to prevalence of smoking,[1] alcohol intake,[2] cardiovascular risk factors such as unhealthy eating behaviors and sedentary lifestyle (Albrektsen et al., 2016), reckless driving and traffic injuries (Sengoelge et al., 2018), substance use and not seeking medical care (Ragonese et al., 2019), not using condoms and sexual risk taking (Jacques-Aviñó et al., 2019). Further, male violence based on masculine norms and defining *real manhood* in many countries is one of the most important factors in morbidity and mortality for both men and women (Krug et al., 2002).

While current gendered masculine norms reinforce men's (especially heterosexual cis men's) superior social status in the gender system, they also reinforce the lower status for other genders and sexual identities (e.g., women, nonbinaries). Although we acknowledge that gendered social norms (including masculine and feminine norms) mostly affected women and sexual minorities, including nonbinaries, transgenders, and homosexuals, adversely through discrimination, inequalities, and male violence, we argue that the ways that masculine norms harm cis men also need to be explored. The current gender status system could cause cis men to behave in ways that harm their own mental and physical health (see Courtenay, 2000; Wong et al., 2017). We discuss masculine gender norms and cis men's harmful health behavior in the context of the COVID-19 pandemic.

Mete Sefa Uysal, Emir Üzümçeker, and Sara Vestergren, *Could Gender-Related Norms Predict Compliance With COVID-19 Prevention Behaviors?* In: *The Social Science of the COVID-19 Pandemic.* Edited by: Monica K. Miller, Oxford University Press.
© Oxford University Press 2024. DOI: 10.1093/oso/9780197615133.003.0012

Throughout the COVID-19 pandemic, men have had higher mortality rates compared to women,[3] similar to the severe acute respiratory syndrome (SARS) and Middle Eastern respiratory syndrome (MERS) outbreak (Karlberg et al., 2004). Moreover, a meta-analysis showed that severity of COVID-19 infection (requiring an intensive treatment unit) was three times higher for men than women (Peckman et al., 2020). For every 10 women, 11 men are hospitalized, 18 need intensive care, 13 to 15 die, but only 8 are tested for the infection.[4] Hence, even though men are more likely to have severe infection and more likely to die from the COVID-19 virus, they are less likely than women to get tested. We believe that these data indicate the importance of discussing social psychological factors related to gender rather than only focusing on biological factors (see also Chapter 11 for discussion of how objectification of women can result in gender differences in COVID-19 behaviors). We argue that three prominent social psychology theories (i.e., *focus theory of normative conduct* [FTNC], *social identity approach*, and *social role theory*) focusing on different aspects of gendered social norms could offer some explanation for these disparities. In this chapter, we outline each of the three theories with a focus on health behavior implications and then end with a summarizing theoretical discussion in relation to COVID-19 behaviors and what avenues to explore next.

FOCUS THEORY OF NORMATIVE CONDUCT

The FTNC was developed by Cialdini and colleagues to overcome the conceptual ambivalence in the literature on norms (Cialdini et al., 1991). While some social scientists consider norms as indispensable for understanding human behavior, others question the explanatory power of the concept. Cialdini and colleagues (1991) argued that norms are defined in inconsistent ways and concluded that there are two types of norms that influence behavior: injunctive and descriptive. Injunctive norms are the norms that state whether a behavior is approved or not. In contrast, descriptive norms refer to the behaviors people exhibit, as conceptualized in the seminal work of Muzaffer Sherif (1936). In other words, while injunctive norms are what people think one *ought to do*, descriptive norms are *what they actually do*. Finally, the contextual salience of these norms (i.e., the focus of normative conduct) determines the normative influence on behavior.

To assess their new conceptualization in a natural setting, Cialdini and colleagues (1991) conducted a series of experiments in the context of littering behavior. Their studies indicated that the presence of descriptive norms, that is, the knowledge that other people litter, increased littering behavior. Moreover, even though people knew that littering was not accepted (injunctive), they still littered when they thought that others where littering (descriptive). Thus, descriptive and injunctive norms influence behavior in different, and sometimes conflicting, ways. Similar results have been demonstrated in research on various types of behavior, such as college student drinking (Lee et al., 2007), healthy eating (Staunton et al., 2014), pro-environmental behaviors (Fornara et al., 2011), ingroup favoritism

(Iacoviello et al., 2017), and support to refugees (Yitmen & Verkuyten, 2020). In short, FTNC provides a well-supported framework for researching and understanding the influence of social norms on behavior.

There is a considerable literature on the relationship between health behaviors and social norms (Reid et al., 2011), documenting that both positive and negative behaviors are influenced by both descriptive and injunctive norms, albeit in complex ways. The survey study by Park et al. (2009) on college students' drinking intentions is a good example. They investigated how descriptive and injunctive norms of the university and the United States are related to college students' drinking. Park et al. showed that all types of norms are uniquely associated with students' intentions of drinking. Using a similar method, Smith-McLallen and Fishbein (2008) examined the relationship between descriptive/injunctive norms and six types of cancer-related behavior. They found that while injunctive norms predicted intentions for prostate and colon cancer screening, getting a monogram, and healthy eating, descriptive norms only predicted dieting.

In addition to the cross-sectional surveys, some researchers have employed a longitudinal methodology to infer causal relations. For example, Voogt and colleagues (2013) conducted a 4-year study with 428 adolescents exploring descriptive and injunctive reference group norms and problem drinking. Their results indicated that both descriptive and injunctive norms predicted future problem drinking behavior, providing strong support for the causal influence of norms. In a similar vein, Napper and colleagues (2016) found that perceived friend and parental approval of marijuana use (injunctive norms) predicted later behavior (marijuana use), although perceived descriptive norms did not emerge as a predictor for marijuana use.

There are also studies using experimental design to demonstrate the interaction between descriptive and injunctive norms, particularly how they influence health behaviors when they contradict. Stok (2014) exposed adolescents to norms about fruit eating. While exposure to descriptive norms increased the level of fruit intake, exposure to injunctive norms decreased fruit consumption, suggesting a reactive behavior by adolescents. Additionally, Staunton and colleagues (2014) explored the effect of exposure to negative descriptive norms on healthy eating intentions. When no descriptive norm was salient, exposure to injunctive norms caused no change on intentions. Interestingly, when participants were exposed to negative descriptive norms (i.e., it is uncommon for other students to eat healthily), exposure to injunctive norms decreased their intentions to eat healthily.

These studies, taken together, suggest the importance of descriptive norms on injunctive norms and how these two types of norms interact. In addition to the unique contributions of descriptive and injunctive norms to health behaviors, previous research pointed out the complexity of their interaction. Moreover, researchers should consider the valence of the norms (i.e., negative vs. positive norms) to implicate more concrete predictions of social norms' effects on health behaviors. In times of crises like the COVID-19 pandemic, the interaction between the valence of the norms (i.e., positive or negative) and type of norms (i.e., descriptive or injunctive) becomes more important to motivate adherence to public health measures: (a) positive descriptive norms (e.g., news and discourses on how many people are vaccinated for convincing vaccine hesitant); (b) negative descriptive norms (e.g., science communication statements about just a few people actually stockpiling during the lockdown against the news that boost the panic buying); (c) positive injunctive norms (e.g., leaders' discourses how people appreciated mutual aid groups and their acts for solidarity and communal coping); and (d) negative injunctive norms (e.g., collective anger and responses against group-based inequalities of medical supply, including COVID-19 vaccines). Hence, the answer to what kind of social norms would be effective is embedded in the social context. In brief, these norms and their interactions with other variables are not contested choices, rather they are opportunities. Last but not least, the way people relate to norms, such as what norms we perceive as important, is connected to the way people see ourselves and others, our concept of the self and others through social categorization and social identification.

SOCIAL IDENTITY APPROACH

The basis of the social identity approach (Tajfel, 1982; Tajfel & Turner, 1979; Turner et al., 1987) is the assumption that group memberships make significant contributions to one's self-definition. Specifically, social identity was defined as the perception of belonging to a social category or group accompanied by an emotional significance and value attribution to that group membership (Tajfel, 1978). Shared emotions, values, opinions, and experiences help to build this kind of sense of belonging and strengthen the perception of being a member of a social group. Hence, they reinforced the "we-ness" by creating and embedding ingroup (and perceived outgroup) norms.

People define themselves not only by their unique personal characteristics and interpersonal relationships (*I*), but also by the collective characteristics they feel they belong to (*we*). Reicher (2001) agreed with this distinction made by the social identity approach, but claimed that this distinction has led to a misunderstanding. According to Reicher, all the selves of an individual are fundamentally social and related to a group context. Even for the personal self, one needs a reference point to others to define oneself, and this reference point is thereby social and hence needs a perception of a social category or a group of people. For example, if an important part of a person's personal identity is male related, such as strong and tough, the person will need to compare the self with others to define the self as male and to understand what it means to be a male.

Relatedly, some social categories and group memberships, such as gender, are so salient in our daily lives that they can become seen as individual characteristics and individual behaviors. However, these behaviors and attitudes might be collective behaviors as a result of self-categorization processes, congruent with the idea that collective behaviors become possible only if there is a shared social identity. For instance, environmentalists think and behave with the norm boundaries of what it means to be an environmentalist. This could entail changing the consumption to a more environmentally friendly diet in line with the perception of the self-concept of an environmentalist (Vestergren et al., 2019). Similarly, many daily behaviors, including health behaviors, are greatly influenced by gender identity because it is salient in most social contexts and gender norms are very established. Thereby, men might think and behave within the framework and norm boundaries of what it means to be a *real* man, which could entail carrying out risky behaviors for both physical and mental health. Hence, shared social identities such as gender identities provide definitions of appropriate and possible conduct and in turn enable people to act collectively in normative ways according to ingroup norms such as gender norms. These gender norms are closely related to the social roles that are assigned to binary gender categories, men and women.

SOCIAL ROLE THEORY

Social role theory (Eagly & Wood, 2012) focuses on binary stereotypes for gender roles. Accordingly, gender roles have formed with stereotypes embedded in the narratives of "typical" man and woman as well as their roles and positions in the society that flow from the deep-seated division of labor and socialization. As a result of these stereotypes, women are expected to take care of the household and children while men are breadwinners. Moreover, gender roles prescribe that women are communal, warm, and caregivers, while masculine gender roles prescribe that men are agentic, tough, and beyond some emotional responses (Levant et al., 2006). Gender roles not only prescribe behaviors, but also proscribe behaviors discouraging people to disobey these roles. For example, men should not display weakness, such as anxiety, distress, or hesitation.

Related social roles and norms of gender make connections between construction of masculinity and men's risky health behaviors. Brannon (1976) described showing no emotion, staying calm and solid in crisis, and taking risks as crucial steps of the construction of masculinity. The socialization into masculinity has been demonstrated in multinational studies conducted with children, showing that boys are expected to prove their toughness and never display traits or emotions associated with femininity; further, boys who do not conform to the masculinity contract are bullied by their peers (Blum et al., 2017). We believe that these reflect destructive aspects of masculine norms, among adults and children, and are part of the explanation of why men might be less inclined to follow health measures and exhibit more risky health behaviors during the COVID-19 pandemic (see also Salali et al., 2021).

As a result of masculine social norms and roles, men display more risky health behaviors such as smoking and drinking, less preventive health measures such as mask-wearing and handwashing,[5,6] and less healthcare seeking during the pandemic (see Betron et al., 2020). Moreover, there is a risk that psychological exhaustion and mental health problems among men remain unrecognized because men are more likely to hide their emotions and stress, consistent with social role theory. It is important to emphasize that the COVID-19 pandemic increased not only medical and psychological problems, but also structural issues and economic concerns,[7] and men have been more affected by financial worries than women (Harth & Mitte, 2020). This is consistent with masculine norms prescribing men to be successful breadwinners. When men fulfill the traditional masculine norms and face difficulties regarding responsibilities of these roles, psychological distress arises (Syrda, 2020). During lockdowns in which many workplaces are closed, most men who see their main function as going to work and making money for their family within the framework of masculine roles and shared male identity might have not only experienced psychological stress due to economic hardship but also struggled with the dysfunction of being unable to fulfill their masculine duties.

Hence, masculinity can be seen as a construct that harms the physical and psychological health of cis men as much as the identities it leaves out such as women, nonbinaries, and transgenders. We suggest that these negative effects manifest themselves as risky health behaviors of men during social and health crises such as the COVID-19 pandemic at the intersection of the norms, identities, and roles. In the next section, we elaborate the important points that need to be address by further works.

DISCUSSION, LESSONS LEARNED, AND FUTURE RESEARCH

There are a few areas to be discussed in relation to gender, masculinity, and the COVID-19 pandemic. In this chapter we emphasize three areas: the importance of gendered-related norms, the need for a more critical and intersectional perspective, and neglecting gender complexities by using binary gender categorization.

First, based on previous literature and theoretical contributions, we believe that different effects of different types of social norms need to be discussed in terms of the role of gender-related norms in the pandemic. According to social role theory, health behaviors related to gender norms are reinforced by both injunctive and descriptive social norms. However, FTNC studies showed that injunctive norms could be a stronger predictor for health behaviors than descriptive norms (e.g., Napper et al., 2016; Smith-McLallen & Fishbein, 2008). We believe that these findings could be consistent with premises of social role theory and the social identity approach. Stereotypes are generally described as people's expectations about behaviors of members who are a part of a particular social group. As the social identity approach suggests, stereotypes serve a crucial function in offering a framework for identification. Although these stereotypes include a fluidity and context dependence for almost all group memberships, gender appears as an exception and is considered as a primary feature that should be performed identically by representatives of this social group across situations (Ellemers, 2018). As norms are affected by our salient identity, what *one ought to do* (injunctive norm) is based on our reference framework that stems from our perception of the shared social identity. Moreover, what one ought to do as a male is more often salient than what one ought to do as a representative of any other group or category, and gender identity is often intersectional with other social identities. In turn, the tendency for risky behaviors can be salient throughout social contexts even if *what people do* (descriptive norm) is different from this reference framework. Hence, the difference between *what people think one ought to do* and *what they do* might be salient in terms of gender norms, especially in time of crises such as the COVID-19 pandemic. In turn, *what people think one ought to do* can become a facilitator for health-related behaviors. Further research focusing on these disparities is needed. The effects on behavior should be carefully studied when types of gender norms related to health behavior contradict each other. In other words, for instance, when what people think one ought to do implies a protective health behavior but what they do implies risky health behavior, individuals' tendency for behavior should be tested in different contexts.

Second, we argue that there is a need to develop a more critical and intersectional social psychological perspective that goes beyond the singular identity approaches on the role of identity and social norms related to shared identity in health behaviors. Although social psychology research investigates the role of a particular identity, some scholars criticize these singular approaches and point out the intersectionality of multiple identities (see, e.g., Greenwood, 2012; Ostrove & Brown, 2018). While conducting research on gender norms, the use of singular approaches and overlooking the intersectionality of real-world identities related to gender issues could cause two interrelated and important limitations. First, singular approaches ignore that people have both advantaged and disadvantaged identities (e.g., White and woman or man and gay) and make a reductive deduction based on the one-to-one impact of other particular identities. We believe that social psychology research on gender-related norms and health behavior can benefit from other areas that include the complex intersectionality, such as collective action research on allyship (e.g., Selvanathan et al., 2020; Subašić et al., 2018; Tropp & Uluğ, 2019). For instance, men who identify themselves as allies of women or the feminist movement might be more aware of their privileges and stereotypes. This might affect their fulfillment of masculine social roles and norms when these norms contain a risk for their health. For instance, pro-feminist men who are more aware of gender privileges are less hesitant to wear masks, which is considered as a weakness.[8] Similarly, they might be less likely to endorse the conspiracy theories about COVID-19 vaccines that are strongly associated with masculinities (e.g., *vaccines cause infertility*). Hence, we believe that more work that incorporates both gender and ally identification and focuses the role of their intersectionality on men's health behavior is needed.

Finally, social psychological research on gender-related norms often applies a binary gender categorization as a consequence of adopting the singular approaches. Trying to capture the impact of single gender identity in a particular and noncontextual time point causes researchers to neglect the fluidity, performativity, and intersectionality of gender identity. We argue that by disregarding the importance of these dimensions, researchers are also disregarding ecological validity because gender is a spectrum or maybe even a matrix. We need to acknowledge that researchers do not have efficient conceptualization of what gender is and of how people identify with a gender. Even so, researchers often still measure gender as they measure other social identities, such as national or political identity. As such, theorizations related to *gender identity* might be based on false construction or axiom both ontologically and epistemologically. For instance, conceptualizing gender as identity will have different consequences than conceptualizing gender as performance (see Butler, 2006). Hence, acknowledging this conceptual limitation and making room for different types of gender construction in social sciences and philosophy allow social psychology and other fields to become more inclusive and provide a wider perspective. Subsequently, through reflexivity in our research, researchers should argue and apply the acknowledgment that not every individual is affected by static masculine norms because every person is positioned in a different place in the gender system and status quo. In the short term (until psychology has more valid conceptualization[s] for gender), considering the role of intersectionality of multiple identities might be the most effective way to further explore the relationship between gender-related social norms and health behaviors and should be included in discussions and management of COVID-19.

CONCLUSION

Gender disparities in COVID-19 mortality and intensive treatment unit rates cannot be explained with only biological approaches. Instead, social psychological factors such as gendered social norms, gender identification, and gender role endorsement should be examined. Reports showed that men displayed more risky health behaviors both before and during the pandemic (e.g., Betron et al., 2020; Sengoelge et al., 2018). Masculine gender norms cause cis men to behave in ways that harm their own mental and physical health. In the name of "real manhood," men avoid wearing masks and healthcare seeking. To deepen our understanding of the adverse effects of traditional masculine norms on men's health behaviors, future research should be more inclusive, consider intersectionality, and utilize the FT NC, social identity approach, and social role theory.

NOTES

1. https://blogs.worldbank.org/opendata/men-smoke-5-times-more-women
2. https://www.who.int/publications/m/item/gender-health-and-alcohol-use
3. https://www.eurekalert.org/pub_releases/2020-04/f-css042420.php
4. https://globalhealth5050.org/the-sex-gender-and-covid-19-project/
5. "Real men don't wear masks": The link between masculinity and face coverings: https://www.independent.co.uk/life-style/face-masks-men-masculinity-coronavirus-lockdown-boris-johnson-b1077119.html
6. https://www.nytimes.com/2020/03/17/us/women-men-hand-washing-coronavirus.html

7. https://www.worldbank.org/en/news/feature/2020/06/08/the-global-economic-outlook-during-the-covid-19-pandemic-a-changed-world
8. See Note 5.

REFERENCES

Albrektsen, G., Heuch, I., Løchen, M. L., Thelle, D. S., Wilsgaard, T., Njølstad, I., & Bønaa, K. H. (2016). Lifelong gender gap in risk of incident myocardial infarction: The Tromsø Study. *JAMA Internal Medicine, 176*(11), 1673–1679. https://doi.org/10.1001/jamainternmed.2016.5451

Betron, M., Gottert, A., Pulerwitz, J., Shattuck, D., & Stevanovic-Fenn, N. (2020). Men and COVID-19: Adding a gender lens. *Global Public Health, 15*(7), 1090–1092. https://doi.org/10.1080/17441692.2020.1769702

Blum, R. W., Mmari, K., & Moreau, C. (2017). It begins at 10: How gender expectations shape early adolescence around the world. *The Journal of Adolescent Health, 61*(4 Suppl), S3–S4. https://doi.org/10.1016/j.jadohealth.2017.07.009

Brannon, R. (1976). The male sex role: Our culture's blueprint of manhood, and what it's done for us lately. In D. S. David & R. Brannon (Eds.), *The forty-nine percent majority: The male sex role* (pp. 14–32). Addison-Wesley.

Butler, J. (2006). *Gender trouble*. Routledge.

Cialdini, R. B., Kallgren, C. A., & Reno, R. R. (1991). A focus theory of normative conduct: A theoretical refinement and reevaluation of the role of norms in human behavior. *Advances in Experimental Social Psychology, 24*, 201–234. https://doi.org/10.1016/S0065-2601(08)60330-5

Courtenay, W. H. (2000). Constructions of masculinity and their influence on men's well-being: A theory of gender and health. *Social Science & Medicine, 50*(10), 1385–1401. https://doi.org/10.1016/S0277-9536(99)00390-1

Eagly, A. H., & Wood, W. (2012). Social role theory. In P. A. M. Van Lange, A. W. Kruglanski, & E. T. Higgins (Eds.), *Handbook of theories of social psychology* (p. 458–476). Sage Publications. https://doi.org/10.4135/9781446249222.n49

Ellemers, N. (2018). Gender stereotypes. *Annual Review of Psychology, 69*(1), 275–298. https://doi.org/10.1146/annurev-psych-122216-011719

Fornara, F., Carrus, G., Passafaro, P., & Bonnes, M. (2011). Distinguishing the sources of normative influence on proenvironmental behaviors: The role of local norms in household waste recycling. *Group Processes & Intergroup Relations, 14*(5), 623–635. https://doi.org/10.1177/1368430211408149

Greenwood, R. M. (2012). Standing at the crossroads: An intersectional approach to women's social identities and political consciousness. In S. Wiley & T. A. Revenson (Eds.), *Social categories in everyday experience* (pp. 103–129). American Psychological Association.

Harth, N. S., & Mitte, K. (2020). Managing multiple roles during the COVID-19 lockdown: Not men or women, but parents as the emotional "loser in the crisis." *Social Psychological Bulletin, 15*(4), 1–17. https://doi.org/10.32872/spb.4347

Iacoviello, V., Berent, J., Frederic, N. S., & Pereira, A. (2017). The impact of ingroup favoritism on self-esteem: A normative perspective. *Journal of Experimental Social Psychology, 71*, 31–41. https://doi.org/10.1016/j.jesp.2016.12.013

Jacques-Aviñó, C., García de Olalla, P., González Antelo, A., Fernández Quevedo, M., Romaní, O., & Caylà, J. A. (2019). The theory of masculinity in studies on HIV. A systematic review. *Global Public Health*, *14*(5), 601–620. https://doi.org/10.1080/17441692.2018.1493133

Karlberg, J., Chong, D. S., & Lai, W. Y. (2004). Do men have a higher case fatality rate of severe acute respiratory syndrome than women do? *American Journal of Epidemiology*, *159*(3), 229–231. https://doi.org/10.1093/aje/kwh056

Krug, E. G., Dahlberg, L. L., Mercy, J. A., Zwi, A. B., & Lozano, R. (2002) . *World report on violence and health*. World Health Organization. https://iris.who.int/handle/10665/42495

Lee, C. M., Geisner, I. M., Lewis, M. A., Neighbors, C., & Larimer, M. E. (2007). Social motives and the interaction between descriptive and injunctive norms in college student drinking. *Journal of Studies on Alcohol and Drugs*, *68*(5), 714–721. https://doi.org/10.15288/jsad.2007.68.714

Levant, R. F., Good, G. E., Cook, S. W., O'Neil, J. M., Smalley, K. B., Owen, K., & Richmond, K. (2006). The normative Male Alexithymia Scale: Measurement of a gender-linked syndrome. *Psychology of Men & Masculinity*, *7*(4), 212–224. https://doi.org/10.1037/1524-9220.7.4.212

Napper, L. E., Kenney, S. R., Hummer, J. F., Fiorot, S., & Labrie, J. W. (2016). Longitudinal relationships among perceived injunctive and descriptive norms and marijuana use. *Journal of Studies on Alcohol and Drugs*, *77*(3), 457–463. https://doi.org/10.15288/jsad.2016.77.457

Ostrove, J. M., & Brown, K. T. (2018). Are allies who we think they are?: A comparative analysis. *Journal of Applied Social Psychology*, *48*(4), 195–204. https://doi.org/10.1111/jasp.12502

Park, H. S., Klein, K. A., Smith, S., & Martell, D. (2009). Separating subjective norms, university descriptive and injunctive norms, and U.S. descriptive and injunctive norms for drinking behavior intentions. *Health Communication*, *24*(8), 746–751. https://doi.org/10.1080/10410230903265912

Peckman, H., de Gruijter, N. M., Raine, C., Radziszewska, A., Ciurtin, C., Wedderburn, L. R., Rosser, E. C., Webb, K., & Deakin, C. T. (2020). Male sex identified by global COVID-19 meta-analysis as a risk factor for death and ITU admission. *Nature Communications*, *11*, 6317. https://doi.org/10.1038/s41467-020-19741-6

Ragonese, C., Shand, T., & Barker, G. (2019). Masculine norms and men's mental health: Making the connections. Promundo-US.

Reicher, S. (2001). The psychology of crowd dynamics. In M. A. Hogg & R. S. Tindale (Ed.), *Blackwell handbook of social psychology: Group processes* (pp. 182–208). Blackwell Publishers.

Reid, A. E., Cialdini, R. B., & Aiken, L. S. (2011). Social norms and health behavior. In A. Steptoe, K. Freedland, J. R. Jennings, M. M. Llabre, S. B. Manuck, & E. J. Susman (Eds.), *Handbook of behavioral medicine: Methods and applications* (pp. 263–274). Springer Science + Business Media.

Salali, G. D., Uysal, M. S., & Bevan, A. (2021). Adaptive function and correlates of anxiety during a pandemic. Research Square. https://doi.org/10.21203/rs.3.rs-271498/v1

Selvanathan, H. P., Lickel, B., & Dasgupta, N. (2020). An integrative framework on the impact of allies: How identity-based needs influence intergroup solidarity and social movements. *European Journal of Social Psychology*, *50*(6), 1344–1361. https://doi.org/10.1002/ejsp.2697

Sengoelge, M., Laflamme, L., & El-Khatib, Z. (2018). Ecological study of road traffic injuries in the eastern Mediterranean region: Country economic level, road user category and gender perspectives. *BMC Public Health 18*(1), 236. https://doi.org/10.1186/s12889-018-5150-1

Sherif, M. (1936). *The psychology of social norms*. Harper & Brothers.

Smith-McLallen, A., & Fishbein, M. (2008). Predictors of intentions to perform six cancer-related behaviours: Roles for injunctive and descriptive norms. *Psychology, Health & Medicine, 13*(4), 389–401. https://doi.org/10.1080/13548500701842933

Staunton, M., Louis, W. R., Smith, J. R., Terry, D. J., & McDonald, R. I. (2014). How negative descriptive norms for healthy eating undermine the effects of positive injunctive norms. *Journal of Applied Social Psychology, 44*(4), 319–330. https://doi.org/10.1111/jasp.12223

Stok, F. M. (2014). Don't tell me what I should do, but what others do: The influence of descriptive and injunctive peer norms on fruit consumption in adolescents. *British Journal of Health Psychology, 19*(1), 52–64. https://doi.org/10.1111/bjhp.12030

Subašić, E., Hardacre, S., Elton, B., Branscombe, N. R., Ryan, M. K., & Reynolds, K. J. (2018). "We for she": Mobilising men and women to act in solidarity for gender equality. *Group Processes and Intergroup Relations, 21*(5), 707–724. https://doi.org/10.1177/1368430218763272

Syrda, J. (2020). Spousal relative income and male psychological distress. *Personality and Social Psychology Bulletin, 46*(6), 976–992. https://doi.org/10.1177/0146167219883611

Tajfel, H. (Ed.). (1978). *Differentiation between social groups: Studies in the social psychology of intergroup relations*. Academic Press.

Tajfel, H. (1982). *Social identity and intergroup relations*. Cambridge University Press.

Tajfel, H., & Turner, J. C. (1979). An integrative theory of intergroup conflict. In W. G. Austin & S. Worchel (Eds.), *The social psychology of intergroup relations* (pp. 33–48). Brooks/Cole.

Tropp, L. R., & Uluğ, Ö. M. (2019). Are White women showing up for racial justice? Intergroup contact, closeness to people targeted by prejudice, and collective action. *Psychology of Women Quarterly, 43*(3), 335–347. https://doi.org/10.1177/0361684319840269

Turner, J. C., Hogg, M. A., Oakes, P. J., Reicher, S. D., & Wetherell, M. S. (1987). *Rediscovering the social group: A self-categorization theory*. Basil Blackwell.

Vestergren, S., Drury, J., & Chriac, E. H. (2019). How participation in collective action changes relationships, behaviours, and beliefs: An interview study of the role of inter- and intragroup processes. *Journal of Social and Political Psychology, 7*(1), 76–99. https://doi.org/10.5964/jspp.v7i1.903

Voogt, C. V., Larsen, H., Poelen, E. A. P., Kleinjan, M., & Engels, R. C. M. E. (2013). Longitudinal associations between descriptive and injunctive norms of youngsters and heavy drinking and problem drinking in late adolescence. *Journal of Substance Use, 18*(4), 275–287. https://doi.org/10.3109/14659891.2012.674623

Wong, Y. J., Ho, M.-H. R., Wang, S.-Y., & Miller, I. S. K. (2017). Meta-analyses of the relationship between conformity to masculine norms and mental health-related outcomes. *Journal of Counseling Psychology, 64*(1), 80–93. https://doi.org/10.1037/cou0000176

Yitmen, Ş., & Verkuyten, M. (2020). Support to Syrian refugees in Turkey: The roles of descriptive and injunctive norms, threat, and negative emotions. *Asian Journal of Social Psychology, 23*(3), 293–301. https://doi.org/10.1111/ajsp.12400

13

Cooperation and Acting for the Greater Good During the COVID-19 Pandemic

VALERIO CAPRARO, PAULO S. BOGGIO, ROBERT BÖHM, MATJAŽ PERC, AND HALLGEIR SJÅSTAD ∎

INTRODUCTION

As we write this, the novel coronavirus has led to the greatest pandemic since the "Spanish flu" a century ago (1918–1920). Termed *COVID-19*, the new pandemic has so far infected more than 170 million people worldwide, with a preliminary death rate exceeding 3 million. At all stages of the collective effort to defeat the virus, *cooperation* is essential. In this book chapter, we therefore outline some key characteristics of successful cooperation before we suggest how such principles can inform effective interventions during the current pandemic and future health crises requiring large-scale behavior change.

COVID-19: A COOPERATIVE SUPERCHALLENGE

In response to the COVID-19 pandemic and future pandemics, *cooperation* is essential. Cooperation is required in many areas, including identifying the initial threat; sharing relevant information; implementing policy interventions to initiate large-scale behavior change and "flatten the infection curve" (e.g., lockdowns of society in critical periods, mask wearing, improved physical hygiene and social distancing; see Chapters 3 and 5 for more on COVID-19 policies); developing evidence-based vaccines that are both safe and effective; distributing the vaccines as soon as they are ready; and finally, making sure that the majority of the public

Valerio Capraro, Paulo S. Boggio, Robert Böhm, Matjaž Perc, and Hallgeir Sjåstad, *Cooperation and Acting for the Greater Good During the COVID-19 Pandemic* In: *The Social Science of the COVID-19 Pandemic*. Edited by: Monica K. Miller, Oxford University Press. © Oxford University Press 2024. DOI: 10.1093/oso/9780197615133.003.0013 actually decide to take the vaccine. When facing a global pandemic like COVID-19, none of these stages can succeed without effective cooperation because each stage requires a combination of personal costs and social coordination to achieve a greater goal. This makes psychology, behavioral economics, and social science a relevant starting point for how to approach the problem (Van Bavel et al., 2020).[1]

Just like many other domains in social life, the COVID-19 pandemic represents a "public goods dilemma": When most people cooperate most of the time, the larger group can succeed at defeating the virus. If a sufficiently large minority refuses to cooperate, however, the problem could persist or get much worse. In our understanding, "cooperation" is characterized by the willingness to incur personal costs to help someone else, in which mutual cooperation generates a greater sum of resources and better outcomes than each party could achieve alone (Henrich & Henrich, 2007; Nowak, 2006).

The ideal form of cooperation is often referred to as positive-sum interaction, as the total benefits outweigh the costs in the long run (Axelrod & Hamilton, 1981; Morgenstern & Von Neumann, 1953; Trivers, 1971). When people perceive a given situation this way, they are likely to engage in helping behavior (Ent et al., 2020). However, as cooperation involves an immediate cost and the greater reward is usually delayed or uncertain, there is always a risk that freeriding could overturn the initial willingness to share resources and help each other (Aleta et al., 2020; Chinazzi et al., 2020; Van Bavel et al., 2020; Wang et al., 2016). For instance, mask wearing in public spaces is an effective intervention to reduce infection spread (Mitze et al., 2020), but the greatest benefit appears to manifest for the people surrounding the mask-wearing person. When it comes to social distancing and adherence to public lockdowns, young people have probably made the largest sacrifice by implementing the greatest changes in their daily lives (which normally is very social at that age), whereas the elderly and people with pre-existing health conditions have received the greatest benefits from these interventions as they are at highest mortality risk. Another important example regards vaccine uptake. Clearly, vaccination during a pandemic should be quite attractive to people because it allows getting back to "normal" even for those with low risk of severe infection, who are nevertheless affected by the behavioral regulations imposed on them. However, this happens only if the majority of other people get vaccinated as well. Moreover, compared to other vaccines against well-known diseases, newly developed vaccines could be perceived as less trustworthy, and misinformation around COVID-19 may further undermine vaccination intentions (see Chapter 36 for more on COVID-19-related misinformation; Dodd et al., 2021; Freeman et al., 2021; Gozum, 2021; Kaplan & Milstein, 2021; Loomba et al., 2021). This combination of personal costs and social benefits suggests that vaccination also has a prosocial value (Betsch et al., 2015; Korn et al., 2020). In line with this view, Wells et al. (2020) found that polio vaccination in Israel was mainly attributable to prosocial motivation. Finally, practices of physical hygiene (e.g., handwashing and sneezing on one's sleeves) and information seeking have also been shown to correlate with prosocial behavior during the COVID-19 pandemic (Boggio et al., 2021; Campos-Mercade et al., 2021).

In light of these reflections on the cooperative nature of pandemic responses, we take a closer look at the underlying logic of successful cooperation based on relevant research from economic games and real-life scenarios.

THE FUNDAMENTAL MECHANISMS OF COOPERATIVE BEHAVIOR

First, we outline some key principles of cooperative behavior in general. We focus on kin selection, direct reciprocity, indirect reciprocity, cost and benefit of cooperation, norms, social heuristics, leadership, network reciprocity, and higher order network reciprocity.

Kin Selection

Humans (and other animals) are more likely to incur personal costs to help genetic relatives than nongenetic cooperation partners. Due to the principle of "inclusive fitness," genetic self-interest motivates people to secure not only their own survival, but also the survival and well-being of relatives sharing similar genes (Hamilton, 1964). In consequence, people are more likely to cooperate when it is clear that it will benefit their loved ones. Even simple cues that suggest genetic kinship increase cooperation in public goods games (Krupp et al., 2008).

Direct Reciprocity

Direct reciprocity is a form of "tit-for-tat" strategy in repeated interactions between the same individuals over time. This is a widely observed pattern: People are strongly motivated to return favors and previous helping behavior and, conversely, to defect from future cooperation with individuals who have violated their trust in the past (Cialdini, 2009; Gouldner, 1960; Nowak, 2006). So-called end-game effects refer to the common drop in cooperation toward the end of repeated interactions, meaning that when there is no possibility for future reciprocity, people tend to cooperate less. On the other hand, the "shadow of the future" typically increases cooperation (Bó, 2005; Camera & Casari, 2009; Van Lange et al., 2011), and even just thinking about the future makes people more willing to share resources with others (Sjåstad, 2019).

Indirect Reciprocity

Indirect reciprocity represents a form of social learning in which third parties may punish or reward cooperators or defectors through reputational information (Fehr, 2004; Gächter & Falk, 2002; Milinski et al., 2001; Nax et al., 2015;

Nowak & Sigmund, 1998, 2005). Recent research has confirmed that reputation is a powerful motive in social decision-making, as people often assume they are being observed by potential cooperation partners even when they make anonymous choices (Jordan & Rand, 2020). Thinking about the future can amplify this reputational concern further (Vonasch & Sjåstad, 2021). One implication is that whenever people's behavior is observable and identifiable to others, cooperative behavior tends to increase. Conversely, when people are less visible or perhaps not identifiable at all, adaptive group functioning tends to suffer and decline (Baumeister et al., 2016).

Cost and Benefit of Cooperation

The definition of cooperation itself suggests that cooperation rates might depend negatively on the cost of cooperation and positively on the benefit created. Experiments on the one-shot prisoner's dilemma have confirmed that people are more likely to cooperate when the cost of cooperation decreases (Engel & Zhurakhovska, 2014) and when the benefit of cooperation increases (Capraro et al., 2014). This suggests that also making salient the social benefits (or downplaying the costs) of cooperation may increase cooperative behavior. For example, Dal Bó and Dal Bó (2014) found that having people read a "utilitarian message" that makes salient that cooperating maximizes the group payoff increases cooperation in the iterated prisoner's dilemma.

Norms

Cooperative behavior is also driven by a desire to follow a norm (Biziou-van-Pol et al. 2015; Capraro & Rand, 2018; Kimbrough & Vostroknutov, 2016; see Capraro & Perc, 2021, for a review). This suggests that making salient the normative value of an action can increase cooperative behavior. Accordingly, making people read the Golden Rule increases cooperative behavior in the iterated prisoner's dilemma (Dal Bó & Dal Bó, 2014) and asking people to report what they think is the morally right thing to do, or what they think others think is the morally right thing, increases cooperation in the one-shot prisoner's dilemma (Capraro et al., 2019).

Social Heuristics

The social heuristics hypothesis states that people internalize heuristics that are successful in everyday interactions and use them in situations where they do not possess enough cognitive resources to compute their payoff maximizing strategy. Because most of our real-life interactions are repeated, this framework predicts that people tend to internalize cooperative heuristics (Rand et al., 2014). Accordingly, promoting intuition tends to increase cooperative behavior in one-shot economic games played in the lab (Rand, 2016), especially among inexperienced subjects (Rand et al., 2014) and those who trust those around them (Rand & Kraft-Todd, 2014). Although this finding has also been criticized (Kvarven et al., 2020), scholars agree that nudging people to rely on their emotion increases cooperative behavior (Kvarven et al., 2020; Levine et al., 2018; Rand, 2016; see Capraro, 2019, for a review).

Leadership

The role of leaders is fundamental to promote collective changes, especially when they are costly for the individual person (see Chapter 32 for more on COVID-19 and leadership). When there is ambiguity about what is the right thing to do in a given situation, as could happen during a public health crisis, people might look to leaders to find out how to behave. The experimental literature using economic games has demonstrated that good examples by leaders can improve cooperation (Haigner & Wakolbinger, 2010), whereas poor examples can decrease cooperation (Moxnes & Van der Heijden, 2003). Moreover, "leading by example" has a greater positive effect than leading by words on cooperation in a public goods game (Dannenberg, 2015). That said, trust in leaders is a key moderator (see Chapter 18 for more on trust). For example, during the Ebola outbreak, trust in institutions was associated with the decisions to abide by social distancing mandates in Liberia (Blair et al., 2017) and vaccination mandates in Congo (Vinck et al., 2019).

Group Selection

The human population is obviously divided in groups (e.g., nations). This group structure could lead to the evolution of cooperation as follows: Assume that a group made by cooperators grows faster than a group made by defectors. If there are constraints on the total population size, then smaller, defective, groups could become extinct as cooperative groups grow larger. This logic could lead to the evolution of cooperation, despite the centrifugal within-group forces that drive individuals toward defection (Nowak, 2006). Group selection is psychologically based on group identity. This suggests that making group identity salient could increase cooperative behavior (Dawes et al., 1988).

Network Reciprocity

Modern human societies are built on social networks (Christakis & Fowler, 2009). Although these networks change over time (Holme & Saramäki, 2012; Perc & Szolnoki, 2010), they nevertheless introduce a limited interaction range to our existence that significantly shapes our cooperative behavior (see Chapter 19 for more on social networks and the pandemic). In fact, an important mechanism for cooperation is *network reciprocity* (Nowak & May, 1992), which stands for the fact that a limited interaction range facilitates the formation of compact clusters of cooperators that are in this way protected against invading defectors. This basic mechanism can be enhanced further if the degree distribution of the social network is strongly heterogeneous (Gómez-Gardeñes et al., 2007; Santos & Pacheco, 2005), if there is a set or community structure (Fotouhi et al., 2019; Tarnita et al., 2009), or if the evolution unfolds on two or more network layers that mutually support cooperative clusters (Battiston et al., 2017; Fotouhi et al., 2018; Fu & Chen, 2017; Gómez-Gardeñes et al., 2012; Wang et al., 2012). This adds to a long line of mechanisms for cooperation on networks, ranging from simple coevolutionary rules that could affect the structure of the interaction network; the teaching activity of individual people, their reputation, mobility, or age (Santos et al., 2006); to various forms of heterogeneity that arises as a consequence of these rules or is inherently present in a population (Amaral et al., 2016; Perc & Szolnoki, 2008; Santos et al., 2008, 2012; see Perc et al., 2017, for a review).

Higher Order Network Reciprocity

Despite the wealth of important insights concerning cooperation on networks, an important unsolved problem remained accounting for cooperation in groups, such as for example in the public goods game (Archetti & Scheuring, 2012; Perc et al., 2013). The simplest remedy was to consider members of a group to be all the players that are pairwise connected to a central player (Santos et al., 2008; Szolnoki et al., 2009). However, because the other players are further connected in a pairwise manner, one would also need to consider all the groups in which the central player is a member but is not central. Evidently, classical networks do not provide a unique procedure for defining a group. Moreover, members of the same group are commonly not all directly connected with one another, which prevents strategy changes among them. These facts used to posit a lack of common theoretical foundation for studying the evolution of cooperation in networked groups. Without knowing who is connected to whom in a group, it was also impossible to implement fundamental mechanisms that promote cooperation.

Recently, a solution came in the form of higher order networks, where, unlike in classical networks (Latora et al., 2017), a link can connect more than just two people (Battiston et al., 2020). Thus, higher order networks naturally account for structured group interactions, wherein a group is made up of all players that are connected by a hyperlink (Berge, 1984). The public goods game on a uniform hypergraph corresponds to the replicator dynamics in the well-mixed limit, thus providing a formal theoretical foundation to study cooperation in networked groups (Alvarez-Rodriguez et al., 2021). Moreover, the presence of hubs and the coexistence of interactions in groups of different sizes can critically boost cooperation (Perc et al., 2017).

HOW TO PROMOTE COOPERATION DURING A PANDEMIC

Now we focus more specifically on what type of interventions could support a cooperative response to the COVID-19 pandemic. Specifically, our focus is on message-based interventions intended to promote social distancing, physical hygiene, mask wearing, vaccine uptake, and information seeking. We consider these behaviors because they are key to fight the COVID-19 pandemic, and they have all been shown to correlate with prosocial behavior and intentions (Boggio et al., 2021; Campos-Mercade et al., 2021; Coroiu et al., 2020; Jordan et al., 2020; Lu et al., 2021; Nivette et al., 2021). We focus on message-based interventions because they represent a powerful means to reach the population and induce collective changes because they can be displayed in the street through posters and screens or reach people inside their homes through social media, television, and radio.

Social Distancing

Five studies found that prosocial messages are more effective than proself messages at increasing intentions to practice social distancing: Deslatte (2020) found that public health frames increase intentions to avoid unnecessary travels; Pfattheicher et al. (2020) reported that inducing empathy increases intentions to practice social distancing; Lunn et al. (2020) found that prosocial messages highlighting that violating social distancing rules can lead to the infection of others increased intentions to practice social distancing; Heffner et al. (2020) found that a prosocial message increased willingness to self-isolate; Cucchiarini et al. (2021) established that nudging the injunctive norm positively affected intentions to comply with physical isolation, especially among people with low-risk perception. On the other hand, two studies found that messages that highlighted that the coronavirus was a threat to people's community did not increase intentions to practice social distancing, compared to the baseline or to proself messages (Capraro & Barcelo, 2020; Jordan et al., 2020). A third study found that priming prosocial motivations, through messages highlighting that we can stop the spread only if we work together, did not affect intentions to practice social distancing (Favero & Pedersen, 2020).

Some works tested messages highlighting consequences on close others, or kinship. Christner et al. (2020) found that moral judgments and empathy for loved ones were associated with intentions to practice social distancing, beyond self-oriented factors. However, Capraro and Barcelo (2020) found that a close prosocial message highlighting that the coronavirus is a "threat to your family" did not increase intentions to practice social distancing compared to the baseline or a proself message.

Abu-Akel et al. (2021) explored the role of different spokespersons on people's intentions to share a message calling for social distancing. Across six countries, they found that Dr. Anthony Fauci reached the highest level of resharing, followed by government spokespersons, and popular celebrities. This is in line with correlational work finding that trust in experts is associated with intentions to comply with social distancing, more than trust in institutions (Ahluwalia et al., 2021; Jørgensen et al., 2021).

Physical Hygiene

Despite the aforementioned positive correlation between prosociality and physical hygiene (Boggio et al., 2021; Campos-Mercade et al., 2021; Jordan et al., 2020), prosocial messages have not promoted intentions of washing hands properly (Hacquin et al., 2020). One potential explanation for this lack of effect might be saturation: Jordan et al. (2020) found that a prosocial message that highlighted that the coronavirus is a "threat to your community" was more effective at increasing intentions to engage in preventive measures, including physical hygiene, than a proself message highlighting that the coronavirus was a "threat to you" only in the early stage of pandemics but not in later ones.

As far as we know, there have been no studies exploring the effect of close prosocial messages. We believe this to be an important direction for future work. Because practices of physical hygiene tend to benefit those who are in close contact, it is possible that making salient the benefit to close others, or kinship, is more effective at promoting this particular kind of behavior.

Mask Wearing

Several prosocial messages increase intentions to wear a face mask. Capraro and Barcelo (2020) found that telling people that the coronavirus is a "threat to your community" increased intentions to wear a face covering, compared to telling them that the coronavirus was a "threat to you." They also explored other messages based on kinship ("threat to your family") and on group identity ("threat to your country"), but they did not significantly increase intentions to wear a face mask. Van der Linden and Savoie (2020) found that a prosocial message highlighting that those who do not wear a face mask can infect people with whom they come into contact increased intentions to wear a face mask, compared to a proself message highlighting that those who do not wear a face mask could take the virus from those with whom they come into contact. Pfattheicher et al. (2020) found that inducing empathy by having people read a text regarding a woman with a rare immune disease being affected by the coronavirus increased intentions to wear a face mask.

There has also been one work testing the effect of messages manipulating intuitive and deliberative decision-making. Capraro and Barcelo (2021) found that telling people to "rely on their reasoning" increased their intentions to wear a face covering, compared to telling them to "rely on their emotion" and also compared to the baseline.

Vaccine Uptake

Some works showed that prosocial intentions matter and can be used to increase vaccine uptake during a pandemic. A theoretical framework, known as the 5C model, lists "collective responsibility," defined as a willingness to protect others and contribute to the elimination of infectious diseases, as one of the key determinants of the decision to vaccinate (Betsch et al., 2018). Specifically related to COVID-19, Jung and Albarracín (2021) found that concern for others is more likely to relate to COVID-19 vaccination intentions in areas with low (vs. high) social density, potentially due to a greater perceived prosocial benefit of one's vaccination on others. Pfattheicher et al. (in press) found that people with knowledge about and belief in herd immunity as well as empathy for those most vulnerable to the virus were more motivated to get vaccinated against COVID-19. In a second study, Pfattheicher and colleagues found that providing information about herd immunity and inducing empathy promoted vaccination intentions. Schwarzinger et al. (2021) found that vaccine hesitancy was lower when the benefits associated with herd immunity were made salient. However, there have also been studies finding no effect of prosocial information on intentions to get vaccinated (Freeman et al., 2021; Sprengholz et al., in press). In particular, Freeman et al. (2021) tested the effect of 10 message-based interventions on intentions to get vaccinated, including a message that highlighted the collective benefits of vaccination and a message that highlighted the individual benefit. They found that information type had no effect among people who were already willing to get vaccinated or doubtful. However, among people who were strongly hesitant, highlighting the individual benefit increased vaccination intentions more than highlighting the collective benefit of not getting ill and of not transmitting the virus. Yet, there is also experimental evidence that strong material individual benefits, in the form of monetary rewards for getting vaccinated or fines for not getting vaccinated in case of compulsory/mandatory vaccination, could cause psychological reactance, specifically among people with negative attitudes toward vaccination (Betsch & Böhm, 2016; Sprengholz et al., in press).

Seeking and Understanding Official Information

Despite the positive correlation between prosocial behavior in economic experiments and information seeking during the COVID-19 pandemic (Campos-Mercade et al., 2021), two experiments found that prosocial messages did not increase seeking and understanding official information beyond proself messages. Banker and Park (2020) found that a prosocial frame ("protect your community") was actually less effective than a proself frame ("protect yourself") in eliciting clicks on a Facebook post containing official recommendations; whereas a close prosocial frame ("protect your loved ones") was equally effective as the proself frame. Bilancini et al. (2020) tested the effect of three norm-based posters (see also Chapter 12 for more on norms and COVID-19). The first poster contained a message designed to nudge the personal norm, "do what you think is right"; the second one contained a message designed to nudge the descriptive norm, "do what you think others are doing"; the third one contained a message designed to nudge the injunctive norm, "do what you think others approve of." The authors found that none of them increased understanding of official governmental rules, as measured through comprehension questions, compared to the baseline.

SUGGESTED INTERVENTIONS, LESSONS LEARNED, AND FUTURE RESEARCH

As in catastrophes or other epidemics, the new coronavirus pandemic reveals something fundamental of our species: the ability to cooperate and help others even at a cost to ourselves. Zaki (2020), when describing this human characteristic, used the term *compassion catastrophe*. Humans are living the pandemic, or in other words: participating in a tragic and deadly social and biological experiment. As in many naturalistic research, a lot can be learned by observing the behavior of people and groups in the face of this tragedy. Examples from around the world show people's ability to organize spontaneously to help those in greatest need— ranging from donations of food and medications, making masks, to even phone calls to those who live alone. At the same time, clandestine parties are observed with people flocking without protection as are demonstrations against vaccination, among other examples. Thus, a fundamental question is how to foster cooperative behaviors for the protection against and combat of the pandemic. In this chapter, we reviewed the literature, both general and then with a special focus on message-based interventions intended to promote cooperative response to COVID-19.

As can be seen, one of the most important aspects for promoting coping behaviors to COVID-19, present in both correlational and experimental studies, was prosociality. Consistently, individual profiles of greater prosociality, or experimental manipulations fostering participant's prosociality, were associated with or resulted in greater support and adherence to several protective behaviors to COVID-19.

In specific and common to the studies, there is generally greater support for the use of masks both for more prosocial people and after presenting prosocial messages in comparison to less prosocial people or more proself messages. Such data are important information for the promotion of public policies to combat pandemics because the use of a mask is one of the main tools for protecting oneself and others, but depends on its widespread use in the whole community to be effective. Laboratory studies as well as analysis of the effects of mandatory masking policies have shown significant declines in the spread of SARS-CoV2 (severe acute respiratory syndrome coronavirus 2) (Brooks & Butler, 2021). Thus, investment in campaigns promoting prosocial behaviors associated with the use of masks seems to be effective in changing the population's behavior and positively impacting the control of the pandemic.

But in addition to the positive effect on the use of masks, prosociality and empathy also promoted important changes to face the pandemic, namely physical distancing and reduction of unnecessary travel. However, this has not been observed in some studies, signaling the need for further research evaluating the effect of prosocial messages on physical isolation. In this context, messages sent by expert leaders are more effective than those sent by governmental officials and celebrities. This suggests that people trust experts more than they trust politicians or celebrities, a finding that was confirmed also by correlational evidence. This could be a useful suggestion for policymakers.

The effectiveness of prosocial messages is less conclusive when it comes to physical hygiene, vaccine uptake, and information seeking. General, distant, prosocial messages do not seem to increase practices of physical hygiene. Because physical hygiene benefits people in close proximity, it is possible that close prosocial messages, highlighting the benefit to kinship or close others, might be more effective. Future work could test this hypothesis. The evidence regarding the effect of prosocial messages on intentions to get vaccinated is mixed, with some studies showing a positive effect, while others finding a null effect. At the same time, some studies found that proself messages were more effective, at least among strongly hesitant people. This suggests the existence of important moderators. Given this mixed evidence, policymakers should consider and test the potential positive and negative behavioral consequences of message-based interventions for vaccination before implementing them at large. Finally, information seeking is a relatively unexplored territory. We believe this to be an important gap in the scientific literature because the way citizens seek and understand official information is key to combat the pandemic as it prevents the spread of misinformation or the access to unofficial, often contradictory, information. There is some evidence that close prosocial messages, norm-based messages, and proself messages have similar effects in promoting information seeking; thus, further work should explore the effectiveness of different mechanisms.

Most message-based interventions are built on a handful of mechanisms that support cooperation: kin selection, group selection, cost and benefits of cooperation. However, these are not the only mechanisms known to be associated with cooperative behavior. For example, several forms of reciprocity (direct, indirect, network, higher order network) are known to promote cooperative behavior under certain circumstances. New studies could test such effects on behaviors necessary to face the pandemic, for example, evaluating aspects such as reciprocity and reputation in the use of a mask in contexts that manipulate experimental variables such as the level of relationship between people (family, friends, strangers) and the degree of cooperation of each participant (cooperatives and freeriders). Future research should attempt to integrate epidemic models with social dilemmas on higher order networks to obtain even more realistic insights into what it takes to resolve the dilemma of epidemic control (Glaubitz & Fu, 2020). A deep understanding of behavioral change in disease control and prevention, and in particular large-scale human cooperation, is urgently needed and will surely help to better inform pandemic response in the future.

The role of leadership is also relatively underexplored, as we found only one paper testing the effect of spokesperson. Studies that evaluate the types of leadership as well as the messages that each one brings to their respective populations can teach us important lessons for facing future pandemics. Similarly, just one work tested message-based interventions aimed at increasing group identity. Because Van Bavel et al. (2022) found that national identity is one of the main predictors of social distancing and physician hygiene, future work should explore the effect of message-based interventions grounded on national identity or other group identities.

In sum, society emerged from this pandemic with some lessons and some challenges. It is evident how humans are able to respond cooperatively to tragic situations such as the new coronavirus pandemic. But it is also evident that researchers need to know more about how to keep cooperatives cooperating and, very importantly, encourage cooperative behavior in freeriders.

ACKNOWLEDGMENTS

Paulo S. Boggio was supported by Coordenação de Aperfeiçoamento de Pessoal de Nível Superior—Brasil (CAPES—Programa Institucional de Internacionalização), grant 88887.310255/2018–00 (PSB)—National Council for Scientific and Technological Development grant 309905/2019-2 (PSB).

Matjaž Perc was supported by the Slovenian Research Agency (grant nos. P1-0403 and J1-2457).

NOTE

1.   The full list of references is available at: https://psyarxiv.com/65xmg/

REFERENCES

Abu-Akel, A., Spitz, A., & West, R. (2021). The effect of spokesperson attribution on public health message sharing during the COVID-19 pandemic. *PLoS ONE, 16,* e0245100.

Ahluwalia, S. C., Edelen, M. O., Qureshi, N., & Etchegaray, J. M. (2021). Trust in experts, not trust in national leadership, leads to greater uptake of recommended actions during the COVID-19 pandemic. *Risk, Hazards & Crisis in Public Policy.*

Aleta, A., Martin-Corral, D., y Piontti, A. P., Ajelli, M., Litvinova, M., Chinazzi, M., . . . & Moreno, Y. (2020). Modelling the impact of testing, contact tracing and household quarantine on second waves of COVID-19. *Nature Human Behaviour, 4,* 964–971.

Alvarez-Rodriguez, U., Battiston, F., de Arruda, G. F., Moreno, Y., Perc, M., & Latora, V. (2021). Evolutionary dynamics of higher-order interactions in social networks. *Nature Human Behaviour.*

Amaral, M. A., Wardil, L., Perc, M., & da Silva, J. K. (2016). Evolutionary mixed games in structured populations: Cooperation and the benefits of heterogeneity. *Physical Review E, 93,* 042304.

Archetti, M., & Scheuring, I. (2012). Game theory of public goods in one-shot social dilemmas without assortment. *Journal of Theoretical Biology, 299,* 9–20.

Axelrod, R., & Hamilton, W. D. (1981). The evolution of cooperation. *Science, 211,* 1390–1396.

Banker, S., & Park, J. (2020). Evaluating prosocial COVID-19 messaging frames: Evidence from a field study on Facebook. *Judgment and Decision Making, 15,* 1037–1043.

Battiston, F., Cencetti, G., Iacopini, I., Latora, V., Lucas, M., Patania, A., . . . & Petri, G. (2020). Networks beyond pairwise interactions: Structure and dynamics. *Physics Reports, 874,* 1–92.

Battiston, F., Perc, M., & Latora, V. (2017). Determinants of public cooperation in multiplex networks. *New Journal of Physics, 19,* 073017.

Baumeister, R. F., Ainsworth, S. E., & Vohs, K. D. (2016). Are groups more or less than the sum of their members? The moderating role of individual identification. *Behavioral and Brain Sciences, 39,* 1–56.

Berge, C. (1984). *Hypergraphs: combinatorics of finite sets.* Elsevier.

Betsch, C., & Böhm, R. (2016). Detrimental effects of introducing partial compulsory vaccination: experimental evidence. *The European Journal of Public Health, 26,* 378–381.

Betsch, C., Böhm, R., & Chapman, G. B. (2015). Using behavioral insights to increase vaccination policy effectiveness. *Policy Insights from the Behavioral and Brain Sciences, 2,* 61–73.

Betsch, C., Schmid, P., Heinemeier, D., Korn, L., Holtmann, C., & Böhm, R. (2018). Beyond confidence: Development of a measure assessing the 5C psychological antecedents of vaccination. *PloS One, 13,* e0208601.

Bilancini, E., Boncinelli, L., Capraro, V., Celadin, T., Di Paolo, R. (2020). The effect of norm-based messages on reading and understanding COVID-19 pandemic response governmental rules. *Journal of Behavioral Economics for Policy, 4*(Special Issue 1), 45–55.

Biziou-van-Pol, L., Haenen, J., Novaro, A., Occhipinti Liberman, A., & Capraro, V. (2015). Does telling white lies signal pro-social preferences? *Judgment and Decision Making, 10,* 538–548.

Blair, R. A., Morse, B. S., & Tsai, L. L. (2017). Public health and public trust: Survey evidence from the Ebola virus disease epidemic in Liberia. *Social Science & Medicine, 172,* 89–97.

Bó, P. D. (2005). Cooperation under the shadow of the future: Experimental evidence from infinitely repeated games. *American Economic Review, 95*(5), 1591–1604.

Boggio, P. S., et al. (in preparation). The pandemic is a time for moral actions: Individual's morality predicts support of collective action to fight the pandemic in an international sample.

Brooks, J. T., & Butler, J. C. (2021). Effectiveness of mask wearing to control community spread of SARS-CoV-2. *JAMA, 325,* 998–999.

Camera, G., & Casari, M. (2009). Cooperation among strangers under the shadow of the future. *American Economic Review, 99,* 979–1005.

Campos-Mercade, P., Meier, A. N., Schneider, F. H., & Wengström, E. (2021). Prosociality predicts health behaviors during the COVID-19 pandemic. *Journal of Public Economics, 195,* 104367.

Capraro, V. (2019). The dual-process approach to human sociality: A review. SSRN 3409146.

Capraro, V., & Barcelo, H. (2020). The effect of messaging and gender on intentions to wear a face covering to slow down COVID-19 transmission. *Journal of Behavioral Economics for Policy, 4*(Special Issue 2), 45–55.

Capraro, V., & Barcelo, H. (2021). Telling people to "rely on their reasoning" increases intentions to wear a face covering to slow down COVID-19 transmission. *Applied Cognitive Psychology*.

Capraro, V., Jagfeld, G., Klein, R., Mul, M., & Van De Pol, I. (2019). Increasing altruistic and cooperative behaviour with simple moral nudges. *Scientific Reports, 9*, 11880.

Capraro, V., Jordan, J. J., & Rand, D. G. (2014). Heuristics guide the implementation of social preferences in one-shot prisoner's dilemma experiments. *Scientific Reports, 4*, 6790.

Capraro, V., & Perc, M. (2021). Mathematical foundations of moral preferences. *Journal of the Royal Society Interface, 18*, 20200880.

Capraro, V., & Rand, D. G. (2018). Do the right thing: Experimental evidence that preferences for moral behavior, rather than equity or efficiency per se, drive human prosociality. *Judgment and Decision Making, 13*, 99–111.

Chinazzi, M., Davis, J. T., Ajelli, M., Gioannini, C., Litvinova, M., Merler, S., . . . & Vespignani, A. (2020). The effect of travel restrictions on the spread of the 2019 novel coronavirus (COVID-19) outbreak. *Science, 368*, 395–400.

Christakis, N. A., & Fowler, J. H. (2009). *Connected: The surprising power of our social networks and how they shape our lives*. Little Brown Spark.

Christner, N., Sticker, R. M., Söldner, L., Mammen, M., & Paulus, M. (2020). Prevention for oneself or others? Psychological and social factors that explain social distancing during the COVID-19 pandemic. *Journal of Health Psychology*.

Cialdini, R. B. (2009). *Influence: Science and practice* (Vol. 4). Pearson Education.

Coroiu, A., Moran, C., Campbell, T., & Geller, A. C. (2020). Barriers and facilitators of adherence to social distancing recommendations during COVID-19 among a large international sample of adults. *PloS One, 15*(10), e0239795.

Cucchiarini, V., Caravona, L., Macchi, L., Perlino, F. L., & Viale, R. (2021). Behavioral changes after the COVID 19 lockdown in Italy. *Frontiers in Psychology, 12*, 617315.

Dal Bó, E., & Dal Bó, P. (2014). "Do the right thing": The effects of moral suasion on co-operation. *Journal of Public Economics, 117*, 28–38.

Dannenberg, A. (2015). Leading by example versus leading by words in voluntary con-tribution experiments. *Social Choice and Welfare, 44*, 71–85.

Dawes, R. M., Van De Kragt, A. J., & Orbell, J. M. (1988). Not me or thee but we: The impor-tance of group identity in eliciting cooperation in dilemma situations: Experimental manipulations. *Acta Psychologica, 68*, 83–97.

Deslatte, A. (2020). To shop or shelter? Issue framing effects and social-distancing preferences in the COVID-19 pandemic. *Journal of Behavioral Public Administration, 3*, 1–13.

Dodd, R. H., Pickles, K., Nickel, B., Cvejic, E., Ayre, J., Batcup, C., . . . & McCaffery, K. J. (2021). Concerns and motivations about COVID-19 vaccination. *The Lancet Infectious Diseases, 21*, 161–163.

Engel, C., & Zhurakhovska, L. (2014). Conditional cooperation with negative externalities–An experiment. *Journal of Economic Behavior & Organization, 108*, 252–260.

Ent, M. R., Sjåstad, H., von Hippel, W., & Baumeister, R. F. (2020). Helping behavior is non-zero-sum: Helper and recipient autobiographical accounts of help. *Evolution and Human Behavior, 41*, 210–217.

Favero, N., & Pedersen, M. J. (2020). How to encourage "Togetherness by Keeping Apart" amid COVID-19? The ineffectiveness of prosocial and empathy appeals. *Journal of Behavioral Public Administration, 3*, 1–18.

Fehr, E. (2004). Don't lose your reputation. *Nature, 432*, 449–450.

Fotouhi, B., Momeni, N., Allen, B., & Nowak, M. A. (2018). Conjoining uncooperative societies facilitates evolution of cooperation. *Nature Human Behaviour, 2*, 492–499.

Fotouhi, B., Momeni, N., Allen, B., & Nowak, M. A. (2019). Evolution of cooperation on large networks with community structure. *Journal of the Royal Society Interface, 16*, 20180677.

Freeman, D., Loe, B. S., Yu, L. M., Freeman, J., Chadwick, A., Vaccari, C., . . . & Lambe, S. (2021). Effects of different types of written vaccination information on COVID-19 vaccine hesitancy in the UK (OCEANS-III): A single-blind, parallel-group, randomised controlled trial. *The Lancet Public Health*.

Fu, F., & Chen, X. (2017). Leveraging statistical physics to improve understanding of co-operation in multiplex networks. *New Journal of Physics, 19*, 071002.

Gächter, S., & Falk, A. (2002). Reputation and reciprocity: Consequences for the labour relation. *Scandinavian Journal of Economics, 104*, 1–26.

Glaubitz, A., & Fu, F. (2020). Oscillatory dynamics in the dilemma of social distancing. *Proceedings of the Royal Society A, 476*, 20200686.

Gómez-Gardeñes, J., Campillo, M., Floría, L. M., & Moreno, Y. (2007). Dynamical orga-nization of cooperation in complex networks. *Physical Review Letters, 98*, 108103.

Gómez-Gardeñes, J., Reinares, I., Arenas, A., & Floría, L. M. (2012). Evolution of coop-eration in multiplex networks. *Scientific Reports, 2*, 620.

Gouldner, A. W. (1960). The norm of reciprocity: A preliminary statement. *American Sociological Review*, 161–178.

Gozum, I. E. A. (2021). Common good and public service as vital components for gov-ernment officials in promoting COVID-19 vaccination. *Journal of Public Health*.

Hacquin, A. S., Mercier, H., & Chevallier, C. (2020). Improving preventive health behaviors in the COVID-19 crisis: A messaging intervention in a large nationally representative sample. PsyArXiv Preprints. https://psyarxiv.com/nyvmg/

Haigner, S. D., & Wakolbinger, F. (2010). To lead or not to lead: Endogenous sequencing in public goods games. *Economics Letters, 108*, 93–95.

Hamilton, W. D. (1964). The genetical evolution of social behaviour. II. *Journal of Theoretical Biology, 7*, 17–52.

Heffner, J., Vives, M. L., & FeldmanHall, O. (2020). Emotional responses to prosocial messages increase willingness to self-isolate during the COVID-19 pandemic. *Personality and Individual Differences, 170*, 110420.

Henrich, N., & Henrich, J. P. (2007). *Why humans cooperate: A cultural and evolutionary explanation*. Oxford University Press.

Holme, P., & Saramäki, J. (2012). Temporal networks. *Physics Reports, 519*, 97–125.

Jordan, J. J., & Rand, D. G. (2020). Signaling when no one is watching: A reputation heuristics account of outrage and punishment in one-shot anonymous interactions. *Journal of Personality and Social Psychology, 118*, 57–88.

Jordan, J. J., Yoeli, E., & Rand, D. (2020, April 3). Don't get it or don't spread it? Comparing self-interested versus prosocially framed COVID-19 prevention mes-saging. PsyArXiv. https://psyarxiv.com/yuq7x

Jørgensen, F. J., Bor, A., & Petersen, M. B. (2021). Compliance without fear: Predictors of protective behavior during the first wave of the COVID-19 pandemic. *British Journal of Health Psychology, 26*, 679–696.

Jung, H., & Albarracín, D. (2021). Concerns for others increases the likelihood of vaccination against influenza and COVID-19 more in sparsely rather than densely populated areas. *Proceedings of the National Academy of Sciences of the United States of America, 118*, e2007538118.

Kaplan, R. M., & Milstein, A. (2021). Influence of a COVID-19 vaccine's effectiveness and safety profile on vaccination acceptance. *Proceedings of the National Academy of Sciences of the United States of America, 118*(10), e2021726118.

Kimbrough, E. O., & Vostroknutov, A. (2016). Norms make preferences social. *Journal of the European Economic Association, 14*, 608–638.

Korn, L., Böhm, R., Meier, N. W., & Betsch, C. (2020). Vaccination as a social contract. *Proceedings of the National Academy of Sciences of the United States of America, 117*, 14890–14899.

Krupp, D. B., Debruine, L. M., & Barclay, P. (2008). A cue of kinship promotes cooperation for the public good. *Evolution and Human Behavior, 29*, 49–55.

Kvarven, A., Strømland, E., Wollbrant, C., Andersson, D., Johannesson, M., Tinghög, G., . . . & Myrseth, K. O. R. (2020). The intuitive cooperation hypothesis revisited: a meta-analytic examination of effect size and between-study heterogeneity. *Journal of the Economic Science Association, 6*, 26–42.

Latora, V., Nicosia, V., & Russo, G. (2017). *Complex networks: Principles, methods and applications.* Cambridge University Press.

Levine, E. E., Barasch, A., Rand, D., Berman, J. Z., & Small, D. A. (2018). Signaling emotion and reason in cooperation. *Journal of Experimental Psychology: General, 147*, 702–719.

Loomba, S., de Figueiredo, A., Piatek, S. J., de Graaf, K., & Larson, H. J. (2021). Measuring the impact of COVID-19 vaccine misinformation on vaccination intent in the UK and USA. *Nature Human Behaviour, 5*, 337–348.

Lu, J. G., Jin, P., & English, A. S. (2021). Collectivism predicts mask use during COVID-19. *Proceedings of the National Academy of Sciences of the United States of America, 118*.

Lunn, P. D., Timmons, S., Barjaková, M., Belton, C. A., Julienne, H., & Lavin, C. (2020). Motivating social distancing during the Covid-19 pandemic: An online experiment. *Social Science & Medicine,* 113478.

Milinski, M., Semmann, D., Bakker, T. C., & Krambeck, H. J. (2001). Cooperation through indirect reciprocity: image scoring or standing strategy? *Proceedings of the Royal Society: Biological Sciences, 268*, 2495–2501.

Mitze, T., Kosfeld, R., Rode, J., & Wälde, K. (2020). Face masks considerably reduce COVID-19 cases in Germany. *Proceedings of the National Academy of Sciences of the United States of America, 117*, 32293–32301.

Morgenstern, O., & Von Neumann, J. (1953). *Theory of games and economic behavior.* Princeton University Press.

Moxnes, E., & Van der Heijden, E. (2003). The effect of leadership in a public bad experiment. *Journal of Conflict Resolution, 47*, 773–795.

Nax, H. H., Perc, M., Szolnoki, A., & Helbing, D. (2015). Stability of cooperation under image scoring in group interactions. *Scientific Reports, 5*, 12145.

Nivette, A., Ribeaud, D., Murray, A., Steinhoff, A., Bechtiger, L., Hepp, U., . . . & Eisner, M. (2021). Non-compliance with COVID-19-related public health measures among young adults in Switzerland: Insights from a longitudinal cohort study. *Social Science & Medicine, 268*, 113370.

Nowak, M. A. (2006). Five rules for the evolution of cooperation. *Science, 314*, 1560–1563.

Nowak, M. A., & May, R. M. (1992). Evolutionary games and spatial chaos. *Nature, 359*, 826–829.

Nowak, M. A., & Sigmund, K. (1998). Evolution of indirect reciprocity by image scoring. *Nature, 393*, 573–577.

Nowak, M. A., & Sigmund, K. (2005). Evolution of indirect reciprocity. *Nature, 437*, 1291–1298.

Perc, M., Gómez-Gardenes, J., Szolnoki, A., Floría, L. M., & Moreno, Y. (2013). Evolutionary dynamics of group interactions on structured populations: A review. *Journal of the Royal Society Interface, 10*, 20120997.

Perc, M., Jordan, J. J., Rand, D. G., Wang, Z., Boccaletti, S., & Szolnoki, A. (2017). Statistical physics of human cooperation. *Physics Reports, 687*, 1–51.

Perc, M., & Szolnoki, A. (2010). Coevolutionary games—A mini review. *BioSystems, 99*, 109–125.

Perc, M., & Szolnoki, A. (2008). Social diversity and promotion of cooperation in the spatial prisoner's dilemma game. *Physical Review E, 77*, 011904.

Pfattheicher, S., Nockur, L., Böhm, R., Sassenrath, C., & Petersen, M. B. (2020). The emotional path to action: Empathy promotes physical distancing during the COVID-19 pandemic. *Psychological Science*, 31, 1363–1373.

Pfattheicher, S., Petersen, M. B., & Böhm, R. (In press). Information about herd immunity through vaccination and empathy promote COVID-19 vaccination intentions. *Health Psychology*. PsyArXiv Preprints. https://doi.org/10.31234/osf.io/wzu6k

Rand, D. G. (2016). Cooperation, fast and slow: Meta-analytic evidence for a theory of social heuristics and self-interested deliberation. *Psychological Science, 27*, 1192–1206.

Rand, D. G., & Kraft-Todd, G. T. (2014). Reflection does not undermine self-interested prosociality. *Frontiers in Behavioral Neuroscience, 8*, 300.

Rand, D. G., Peysakhovich, A., Kraft-Todd, G. T., Newman, G. E., Wurzbacher, O., Nowak, M. A., & Greene, J. D. (2014). Social heuristics shape intuitive cooperation. *Nature Communications, 5*, 3677.

Santos, F. C., & Pacheco, J. M. (2005). Scale-free networks provide a unifying framework for the emergence of cooperation. *Physical Review Letters, 95*, 098104.

Santos, F. C., Pacheco, J. M., & Lenaerts, T. (2006). Cooperation prevails when individuals adjust their social ties. *PLoS Computational Biology, 2*, 1284–1290.

Santos, F. C., Pinheiro, F. L., Lenaerts, T., & Pacheco, J. M. (2012). The role of diversity in the evolution of cooperation. *Journal of Theoretical Biology, 299*, 88–96.

Santos, F. C., Santos, M. D., & Pacheco, J. M. (2008). Social diversity promotes the emergence of cooperation in public goods games. *Nature, 454*, 213–216.

Schwarzinger, M., Watson, V., Arwidson, P., Alla, F., & Luchini, S. (2021). COVID-19 vaccine hesitancy in a representative working-age population in France: A survey experiment based on vaccine characteristics. *The Lancet Public Health*, 6(4), e210–e221.

Sjåstad, H. (2019). Short-sighted greed? Focusing on the future promotes reputation-based generosity. *Judgment and Decision Making, 14*, 199–213.

Sprengholz, P., Betsch, C., & Böhm, R. (In press). Reactance revisited: Consequences of mandatory and scarce vaccination in the case of COVID-19. *Applied Psychology: Health & Well-Being.*

Szolnoki, A., Perc, M., & Szabó, G. (2009). Topology-independent impact of noise on cooperation in spatial public goods games. *Physical Review E, 80,* 056109.

Tarnita, C. E., Antal, T., Ohtsuki, H., & Nowak, M. A. (2009). Evolutionary dynamics in set structured populations. *Proceedings of the National Academy of Sciences of the United States of America, 106,* 8601–8604.

Trivers, R. L. (1971). The evolution of reciprocal altruism. *The Quarterly Review of Biology, 46,* 35–57.

Van Bavel, J. J., Baicker, K., Boggio, P. S., Capraro, V., Cichocka, A., Cikara, M., . . . & Willer, R. (2020). Using social and behavioural science to support COVID-19 pandemic response. *Nature Human Behaviour, 4,* 460–471.

Van Bavel, J. J., et al. (2022). National identity predicts public health support during a global pandemic: Results from 67 nations. *Nature Communications, 13,* 517. https://pubmed.ncbi.nlm.nih.gov/35082277/

Van der Linden, C., & Savoie, J. (2020). Does collective interest or self-interest motivate mask usage as a preventive measure against COVID-19? *Canadian Journal of Political Science, 53,* 391–397.

Van Lange, P. A., Klapwijk, A., & Van Munster, L. M. (2011). How the shadow of the future might promote cooperation. *Group Processes & Intergroup Relations, 14,* 857–870.

Vinck, P., Pham, P. N., Bindu, K. K., Bedford, J., & Nilles, E. J. (2019). Institutional trust and misinformation in the response to the 2018–19 Ebola outbreak in North Kivu, DR Congo: A population-based survey. *The Lancet Infectious Diseases, 19*(5), 529–536.

Vonasch, A. J., & Sjåstad, H. (2021). Future-orientation (as trait and state) promotes reputation-protective choice in moral dilemmas. *Social Psychological and Personality Science, 12,* 383–391.

Wang, Z., Bauch, C. T., Bhattacharyya, S., d'Onofrio, A., Manfredi, P., Perc, M., . . . & Zhao, D. (2016). Statistical physics of vaccination. *Physics Reports, 664,* 1–113.

Wang, Z., Szolnoki, A., & Perc, M. (2012). Evolution of public cooperation on interdependent networks: The impact of biased utility functions. *Europhysics Letters, 97,* 48001.

Wells, C. R., Huppert, A., Fitzpatrick, M. C., Pandey, A., Velan, B., Singer, B. H., . . . & Galvani, A. P. (2020). Prosocial polio vaccination in Israel. *Proceedings of the National Academy of Sciences of the United States of America, 117,* 13138–13144.

Zaki, J. (2020). Catastrophe compassion: Understanding and extending prosociality under crisis. *Trends in Cognitive Sciences, 24,* 587–589.

14

Crafting Effective Messages to Encourage COVID-19 Vaccination

PAUL G. DEVEREUX, SARAH Y. T. HARTZELL, AND MOLLY M. HAGEN ∎

Understanding a population's response to a pandemic is an area in which social science should be at the forefront. Much of the response needed to combat the severe acute respiratory syndrome coronavirus 2 (SARS-CoV-2) virus involves individual behavior such as wearing masks and getting vaccinated against the virus, yet these behaviors must be performed by the collective to be effective, so an understanding of group behavior is also needed. Although most U.S. citizens want the vaccine[1] and millions have been vaccinated to date, researchers have learned the importance of group differences in behavioral responses as there are large gaps in willingness to be vaccinated along various group identities. For example, Republicans, rural Americans, and Black Americans are among the groups most hesitant to receive vaccines.[2] There are different reasons for resistance among these groups; therefore, messages to encourage vaccinations need to be tailored to the particular concerns within groups identified as vaccine hesitant.

The resistance to get vaccinated will make it difficult to achieve mass protection from the virus and reduce its impact. Social scientists, and psychologists specifically, study how people perceive risks and interpret messages; they also study how the message source influences the recipient's response (see Chapter 17 in this volume). Fortunately, there are a number of empirically supported approaches to utilize during this current pandemic. For example, the large numbers of people who are vaccinated will influence others to get vaccinated as humans do what they see other people doing and what they think is popular. The lack of serious adverse reactions to the vaccine will be helpful as concerns about side effects are

Paul G. Devereux, Sarah Y. T. Hartzell, and Molly M. Hagen, *Crafting Effective Messages to Encourage COVID-19 Vaccination*
In: *The Social Science of the COVID-19 Pandemic.* Edited by: Monica K. Miller, Oxford University Press.
© Oxford University Press 2024. DOI: 10.1093/oso/9780197615133.003.0014

associated with lower adherence (Tedla & Bautista, 2016). People's desires to return to "normal" life before the pandemic is also a strong motivator.[3] Relatedly, that vaccines are accessible and affordable is critical for their uptake and equity.

In response to the misinformation being spread about the virus, Tedros Adhanom Ghebreyesus, the director-general of the World Health Organization (WHO) stated: "We're not just fighting an epidemic; we're fighting an infodemic" (Department of Global Communications, 2020). WHO explained an infodemic is an "excessive amount of information about a problem, which makes it difficult to identify a solution" (Department of Global Communications, 2020). All the misinformation and conspiracy theories during a pandemic can lead to public health messages to be perceived as false and can lead to distrust for public health officials (see Chapter 18 for more on trust, Chapter 36 for more on misinformation, and Chapter 31 on conspiracy theories).

In this chapter, we describe the messaging used in vaccination attempts in history and describe theories that are relevant for crafting messages.

HISTORICAL INOCULATIONS AND EFFECTIVE MESSAGING CAMPAIGNS

Applying the lens of social science to past mass inoculation events is crucial for identifying effective approaches for increasing vaccine uptake. Social science studies of historical inoculation campaigns showed that developing effective messaging to promote vaccination uptake is complex: social norms, religious beliefs, trust, vaccine knowledge, and many other factors impact how effective inoculation campaigns are in a given community. In this section, we examine the successes and failures of past mass inoculation events and discuss how lessons from these examples can be applied to crafting effective messages to encourage COVID-19 vaccination today.

The World's First Immunization Campaign

In 1661, the Chinese Emperor K'ang His promoted smallpox inoculation by having his children inoculated and publishing a letter in royal support of inoculation (Glynn & Glynn, 2005). Since this first documented example, subsequent campaigns have demonstrated that effective messaging incorporates building community trust, and that personal/familial use of vaccines by high-powered people is one way to do that. Also, because smallpox inoculation was not new to India when Edward Jenner's vaccine arrived there, attempts to replace it with Jenner's vaccination encountered more resistance than in other areas of the world—illustrating how failure to integrate the unique circumstances of communities (i.e., local knowledge and religious contexts) in messaging can impede vaccine uptake (Mark & Rigau-Pérez, 2009).

Jenner's inoculation method spread to English colonies in North America and was publicly endorsed by Thomas Jefferson, George Washington, and Benjamin

Franklin (Stern & Markel, 2005). After Benjamin Franklin's son died of smallpox, he helped to write and distribute a pamphlet for free in 1759: "Some Account of the Success of Inoculation for the Small-Pox in England and America: Together with Plain Instructions By which any Person may be enabled to perform the Operation and conduct the Patient through the Distemper." Franklin's actions are an early demonstration of the importance of using clear and accessible language in messaging campaigns, and that affordable or free healthcare services can increase utilization.

Despite widespread use and some government-mandated inoculations, the use of Jenner's smallpox vaccine by King Charles IV of Spain in the Spanish Empire from 1803–1810 is considered by many to be "the world's first immunization campaign" (Mark & Rigau-Pérez, 2009). King Charles IV used his royal fleet to transport and administer Jenner's inoculation to combat smallpox in the Americas. Characteristics of this expedition that marked it the world's first vaccination campaign, and that relate to effective messaging campaigns today, include collaborating with ecclesiastic authorities to deliver messages, using financial benefits of vaccination to show that benefits outweigh the costs, and adapting operational plans for where campaigns would be undertaken based on local political developments and disease outbreaks in real time (Mark & Rigau-Pérez, 2009).

Edward Jenner used an 8-year-old boy for experimentation to develop his vaccine, and for the vaccination campaign in the Americas, 22 orphan children were infected with cowpox in order to transport the virus needed for inoculation to the Americas (Glynn & Glynn, 2005; Mark & Rigau-Pérez, 2009). Given that vaccine campaigns started with child experimentation, that infectious diseases are most common today in impoverished/developing countries (e.g., HIV vaccine trials in sub-Saharan Africa), and that throughout various periods in U.S. history Black Americans have been the target of unethical medical experimentation (e.g., the Tuskegee syphilis experiment and the case of Henrietta Lacks), it is crucial that vaccine development be carried out in strictly ethical manners, and that subsequent vaccine campaigns encourage vaccine uptake by using transparent messaging that ensures vaccines were developed ethically (see Chapter 18 for more on trust in the medical field). This topic is explored further with examples of how distrust, including distrust regarding the moral integrity/hidden purposes of vaccines, can negatively impact vaccine uptake in the subsequent sections on polio and MMR (measles, mumps, and rubella) vaccine campaigns.

Smallpox eradication was achieved almost 200 years after Jenner's publication of his inoculation, following the WHO's smallpox eradiation campaign from 1967 to 1980 and the 1977 World Health Assembly's resolution to pursue, "Health for all by the year 2000." Lessons learned include messages of universal political commitment, of vaccine equity regardless of income, and in particular, and of eradication rather than simply individual or community-level protection; all are beneficial for increasing vaccine uptake (Henderson, 1987). In addition to high publicity and noble goals, public health practitioners learned during this period that educational rather than simply motivational messages can be effective in prompting people to act, but specifically when using tailored programs to train local people to conduct messaging in their own communities.

Lessons Learned From Polio Campaigns

The first polio vaccine was introduced in the mid-1900s and due to mass inoculations, the disease was quickly brought under control in industrialized countries. However, unlike smallpox, polio was never eradicated worldwide: Vaccine uptake (in addition to availability) was a challenge in developing countries, and these challenges reinforce the lessons that messages are more effective when they build trust, honor the religious and political characteristics of the communities in which they are delivered, have noble and equitable goals, and are delivered by community health workers.

The Kick Polio Out of Africa campaign was launched in the late 1990s when polio had been eradicated from most countries outside of Africa and the Middle East. Nelson Mandela launched the campaign, the African Football Confederation helped to promote it, and community health workers distributed messages in local door-to-door campaigns to great success (Jegede, 2007). As of August 2020, the African region has been certified free of wild poliovirus and has not seen a single case in 4 years. Nigeria was one of the last countries in the Africa region to be declared polio free. Shortly after the Kick Polio Out of Africa campaign was launched, major setbacks occurred in Nigeria, where 45% of cases worldwide and 80% of cases among African countries were being reported. Political and religious leaders in northern Nigeria called for their communities to boycott the vaccine due to fears that the vaccines were contaminated with antifertility agents and could cause HIV and AIDS (Jegede, 2007). These calls to boycott were largely heeded. The northern Nigeria polio vaccine boycott underscores the importance of considering the local political context of individual communities in inoculation campaigns. Because President Babangida's administration had set a birth limit of four children per woman in the 1980s, and people often could not access even the most basic medicines at their local health clinics, the door-to-door campaigns for free polio immunizations were seen as aggressive and suspicious. The upfront work to communicate with, and hear from, local political and religious leaders was not carried out effectively, resulting in organized action to impede polio vaccinations in the area.

Messaging Amid Misinformation: The case of MMR

Implementing inoculation campaigns that address community-specific political/religious factors, educate the public, and train community health workers to deliver information to diverse and rural communities has been successful for the MMR vaccine in some communities where polio campaigns had been met with resistance (Sarma et al., 2019). Yet, several developed countries that accepted the polio and smallpox vaccines during mid-20th century with little hesitancy have since become increasingly skeptical of mass vaccination campaigns. Vaccine hesitancy is not new, and the importance of building community trust has been understood since the very first vaccine campaign, but the rise of antivaccination beliefs in developed countries is much newer, and childhood vaccination coverage rates are declining despite vaccination being safe, affordable, and easily available (Pluviano et al., 2019). The misperception that the MMR vaccine increases autism represents one of the first big shifts toward vaccine hesitancy in developed countries.

Developing effective messages to improve MMR vaccination rates is an important area of ongoing social science research. Unfortunately, to date, randomized clinical trials that test the effectiveness of various messaging approaches for reversing/preventing antivaccination beliefs have provided more evidence on what not to do than on what to do. For example, Nyhan and colleagues (2014) randomly assigned over 1,700 parents to one of four interventions providing parents with (1) information on the lack of evidence linking MMR and autism, (2) information on the dangers of diseases prevented by the MMR vaccine, (3) images of children with diseases prevented by the vaccine, or (4) a narrative on an infant who almost died of measles. They found that none of the interventions reduced vaccine misperceptions, but that relative to the control group, the images of sick children increased beliefs in the MMR vaccine/autism link and the narrative about an infant in danger increased beliefs in serious vaccine side effects. Another method to promote vaccine uptake amid misinformation is "myths-versus-facts" messaging, whereby information that contrasts false vaccine beliefs is provided alongside the misperceptions. However, this method has also been shown to backfire and increase, rather than decrease, MMR vaccine misconceptions (Pluviano et al., 2019).

To date, evidence is scant on what information should be included in public health messages aimed at combatting vaccine misinformation. However, learning from previous mass inoculation campaigns about the importance on not only on *what is said* but *by _whom_* it is said has provided useful information for inoculation campaigns on *what _not_ to say* to successfully promote vaccine uptake to prevent disease.

WHY TALK ABOUT THEORIES?

When interventions to try to change human behavior are developed, they should be grounded in a theory (see Chapters 41–47 for more on COVID-19 research). Research suggested that these interventions can lead to more effective public health interventions for behavior change (Glanz & Bishop, 2010). Think of a theory as the bones that make up the skeleton structure of a human body—it provides the support and keeps everything else, like the muscles, organs, and skin (think of this as the intervention) upright and functional. Without the bones, the rest of the body would not be so effective, and this highlights how theories can provide the extra support to interventions. This chapter focuses on just a few theories (the health belief model [HBM], social learning theory [SLT], and social network theory [SNT]) that can be applied to reduce the transmission of misinformation and the ramifications from the infodemic.

Health Belief Model

The central idea behind the HBM is that people are motivated to change their behavior if a threat of a disease is perceived (Skinner et al., 2015). The other constructs of the HBM are perceived susceptibility, perceived severity, self-efficacy, cues to action, and perceived benefits and barriers. Perceived susceptibility is the belief that a person has about the likelihood of getting the disease or condition (Skinner et al., 2015). Perceived severity is the belief about how serious contracting the disease or condition would be if it were left untreated (Skinner et al., 2015). Both combine to create the perceived threat. For perceived threat to be high, perceived susceptibility and perceived severity must also be high. Cues to action are personal and social triggers that lead to behavior change (Skinner et al., 2015). Self-efficacy is the belief a person has that they feel confident they can perform the recommended behavior. Finally, research has shown that the perceived benefits and barriers can have an independent effect on the recommended behavior (Skinner et al., 2015). The perceived benefits are the beliefs of the advantages of performing the recommended behavior (e.g., getting vaccinated will prevent me from getting ill), whereas the perceived barriers are the obstacles that might prevent a person from performing the recommended behavior (e.g., cost, time, disapproval from others).

Public health interventions could use the HBM to create a campaign highlighting things that could increase a person's perceived susceptibility to the virus, like messages to highlight the number of people who have gotten COVID-19, and stress how people of all ages are susceptible. For perceived severity, messages could highlight how severe someone's health can get when they contract COVID-19. An example of applicability would be a television advertisement of a young adult who is not abiding by social distancing guidelines (i.e., wearing a face mask, staying 6 feet apart, not congregating in large social gatherings), then contracts COVID-19 (susceptibility) and showcases the person in a hospital unit on an oxygen tank (severity). Alternatively, using the HBM to try to increase the perceived benefits of performing a behavior could be accomplished by showing how getting vaccinated would prevent this outcome.

Social Learning Theory

According to SLT, a person will observe and interact with other people and their environment, which influences their behaviors (Bandura, 1977). SLT has a wider array of applicability and can be used for intermittent and lifelong behaviors.

A classic example of SLT is the 1960s Bobo doll experiment (Bandura, 1977). For this experiment, the researchers wanted to show how observational learning plays a role in children's behaviors. The children observed an overly aggressive adult, a passive adult, or did not see an adult role model at all (Bandura, 1977). Then, the researchers observed the children to examine their treatment of the doll. The researchers found that the children exposed to the aggressive adult would also act overly aggressively to the doll (Bandura, 1977). This study suggested the importance of observational learning with behavior change; children were imitating aggression from observing adults' behaviors.

Public health interventions could use SLT to change intermittent and lifelong health behaviors regarding COVID-19. An example of applying SLT to increasing the uptake of the COVID-19 vaccine would be public health officials working with influencer YouTubers, who create a YouTube video of their experience receiving the COVID-19 vaccination. The video would show the process of receiving the vaccine and the YouTuber's side effects. People who follow the YouTuber's channel will be more inclined to receive the COVID-19 vaccination because they want to model the behavior of someone they admire.

Social Network Theory

When using SNT, scholars view networks as a set of nodes that have ties connecting the nodes together (see Chapter 19 in this volume for more on social networks). To better understand this, imagine a person's social network. Within that social network the person has nodes consisting of family members, friends, classmates, teachers, and more. The ties connecting a node to the person is the type of relationship they have with that specific network member (i.e., the person can have a friendship, romantic relationship, or professional relationship linking one person to another). These nodes then have other ties connecting to other nodes (consider someone who has a tie to their father and their father has a tie to his friend, which inadvertently creates a tie from the original person to their father's friend). These ties to another node are still connected to the original person, but the tie to that node is not as strong as some of the ones directly tied to himself or herself. All these connections are important and even a node indirectly tied to a person might be an invaluable source. For example, perhaps someone is searching for a job and that person's mom mentions she heard her hairdresser talking about how her son has a position that needs to be filled. It is from the indirect tie that the person learned about a job opportunity.

Public health officials could use SNT to invoke collective change in health behaviors in groups of people; ideally, the change would spread through social networks. An example would be if public health officials created online community discussion boards where people could discuss their experiences through the COVID-19 pandemic and strategies targeted at improving a person's health during this time. The discussion board would be run by a moderator who would have knowledge on the COVID-19 pandemic and could provide advice to participants in the discussion board. The idea is the discussion board would facilitate a social network that people could utilize to feel supported during the pandemic. As people become engrained in the social network, ideally they might be more susceptible to suggestions from the moderator about social distancing guidelines and receiving the COVID-19 vaccination.

Moving Beyond Individual-Level Theories to Community-Based Approaches

The theories discussed above are especially helpful for understanding how people interpret messages and respond to them. However, they are less focused on the community context in which the messages need to be communicated. Some of the most effective public health interventions, regardless of topic, are those that have more community input and target levels beyond the individual person, such as neighborhoods or worksites.

The importance of knowing the public's values, beliefs, and concerns as well as having people who are members of the community involved and using trusted leaders deliver the messages will also increase adoption of intended behaviors. As was seen with the smallpox and other vaccination efforts, support from community leaders is critical. How a community is defined depends on the public health issue. In this case, there are differences in vaccination hesitancy across not only cultural, racial/ethnic, or political lines, but also differences even between regions with higher and lower vaccination rates. That is, an approach tailored to those who are hesitant to receive the vaccine might be very different in an area with low compliance compared to messages to reach the few holdouts in an area where many people already comply (Krpan et al., 2021). There are several community engagement approaches to a public health intervention like mass vaccinations. In this chapter, we focus on one specific to research approaches.

Community-Based Participatory Research

Community-based participatory research (CBPR) is an approach to "scientific inquiry conducted in communities in which community members, persons affected by the condition or issue under study and other key stakeholders in the community's health have the opportunity to be full participants in each phase of the work, including conception, design, conduct, analysis, interpretation, conclusions and communication of results" (Education Network to Advance Cancer Clinical Trials [ENACCT] and Community-Campus Partnerships for Health [CCPH], 2008, p. 5). CBPR promotes a co-learning and empowering process that attends to social inequalities, builds on strengths and resources within the community (Israel et al., 2003), works through established structures, and helps ensure culturally appropriate research. CBPR also helps to ensure that researchers know the language literacy, vernacular, and preferred source for information in the community, which all improve message impact. CBPR practitioners know the community's values and are more likely to develop messages with empathy for the community. Empathy for concerns about the safety of vaccines is used in the approach taken by the Ad Council,[4] whose messages are very clear that it is understandable to be concerned and to have questions about the vaccine. With this approach, it is hoped that the community will be more receptive to hearing answers to their concerns.

Community-based participatory research is a tool to use in the design of large-scale intervention studies. CBPR techniques allow for more effective interventions by including those impacted by the public health issue early in the design of the intervention and including them in its delivery and importantly sharing in its benefits. For example, partnering with African American churches, a CBPR approach was used to disseminate accurate information about the pandemic to about 12,000 church members (Brewer et al., 2020). This example highlights how vaccination messages might be disseminated through existing structures and trusted locations like a church, but other communities might trust other sources, such as community agencies, popular businesses, or large employers in the community.

Although CBPR is a research approach and can answer questions about the best intervention for increasing vaccination rates within a community, the technique belongs to a broader tack of community engagement practices used in public health. These practices can also help overcome the distrust of outsiders and experts and help fight the misinformation about vaccines. Additionally, these community engagement approaches often lead to long-lasting partnerships (Faridi et al., 2007) that will be important to have established before the next public health crisis.

LESSONS LEARNED AND FUTURE RESEARCH

As discussed above, history shows that people will resist public health messaging, and therefore researchers need to be ready with messages tailored to particular communities to combat vaccine hesitancy and distrust. The public's mistrust of scientific experts and the consumption of nonscientific media sources to access information about the virus (Hagen et al., 2021) fuels misinformation and anxiety and will hamper future vaccination efforts. To combat this, researchers must become more engaged with the nonscientific community. Rather than just collecting data from participants in a community, it is important to share results with those who are impacted by the research. Knowledge is power, and researchers should share their power. These actions will promote trust of researchers and help create relationships that can be leveraged in the next crisis.

Evidence has shown that some messages are more effective than others. Treating people with respect and empathy and acknowledging that it is okay to have questions is helpful. Messages containing altruism and hope are more effective than negative ones in encouraging vaccination (Chou & Budenz, 2020). It is also important to use scientific evidence in our messaging, especially in addressing concerns about vaccinations.[5]

As a broad direction for the future, researchers need to move beyond the laboratory and study more real-world situations using participants beyond college student samples. There have been only a few randomized trials that have successfully changed what people think and feel about vaccines, with only minimal effectiveness (Brewer et al., 2017). Relatedly, using more CBPR approaches will help with the applicability of the research findings to real-world circumstances. More intervention research trying to apply what has been learned so far will also inform basic, more traditional lab-based research as which theories do and do not hold up when applied to an existing problem will become clearer.

Studies that investigate the behaviors of people during this pandemic will provide valuable data from this case study, especially studies about how people process messages (see Chapter 17 in this volume). What messages work for which populations rather than a one-size-fits-all approach will continue to be needed. For example, Wood and Schulman (2021) have developed tailored messages based on vaccine hesitancy level. Survey data that identify community concerns and views are important in this regard, but so is studying social media and other sources of information because this is such a common outlet for information (Hagen et al., 2021). Using methods beyond self-reports such as observational studies in which real behavior in real situations is examined are needed as well (Baumeister et al., 2007).

Although meeting the rigorous standards for published research as part of the peer review process should not be bypassed, researchers should be quicker in disseminating their findings so gaps in vaccination rates can be identified and addressed as soon as possible. Finally, for future efforts, teaching students how to speak to media and discuss research in a way that is understandable to lay audiences will be helpful, as will employing social media to communicate directly with the public. In these ways, the understanding and impact of the science of messaging can be improved to be better prepared for the next pandemic.

In conclusion, there are helpful lessons learned by examining past public health vaccination efforts that can be applied to the current pandemic. Combating mistrust and misinformation while working directly with communities and providing consistent messaging will be needed for COVID-19 vaccination efforts just as was needed in the past. Researchers can help by carefully choosing which theories to study and then identifying which are more effective in influencing behavior during the pandemic.

NOTES

1. https://news.gallup.com/poll/349580/support-vaccination-proof-varies-activ ity.aspx
2. https://www.kff.org/coronavirus-covid-19/poll-finding/kff-covid-19-vaccine-moni tor-march-2021/

3. https://debeaumont.org/changing-the-covid-conversation/vaccineacceptance/
4. https://www.adcouncil.org/our-impact/covid-vaccine/our-covid-19-vaccine-retrospective
5. See Note 3.

REFERENCES

Bandura, A. (1977). *Social learning theory*. Prentice-Hall.

Baumeister, R. F., Vohs, K. D., & Funder, D. C. (2007). Psychology as the science of self-reports and finger movements: Whatever happened to actual behavior? *Perspectives on Psychological Science, 2*(4), 396–403. https://doi.org/10.1111/j.1745-6916.2007.00051.x

Brewer, N. T., Chapman, G. B., Rothman, A. J., Leask, J., & Kempe, A. (2017). Increasing vaccination: Putting psychological science into action. *Psychological Science in the Public Interest, 18*(3), 149–207. doi:10.1177/1529100618760521. PMID: 29611455.

Brewer, L. C, Asiedu G. B., Jones C., Richard M., Erickson J., Weis J., Abbenyi, A., Brockman, T. A., Sia, I. G., Wieland, M. L., White, R. O., & Doubeni, C. A. (2020). Emergency preparedness and risk communication among African American churches: Leveraging a community-based participatory research partnership COVID-19 Initiative. *Preventing Chronic Disease, 17*, 200408. https://dx.doi.org/10.5888/pcd17.200408

Chou, W. S., & Budenz, A. (2020). Considering emotion in COVID-19 vaccine communication: Addressing vaccine hesitancy and fostering vaccine confidence. *Health Communication, 35*(14), 1718–1722. https://doi.org/10.1080/10410236.2020.1838096

Department of Global Communications. (2020). UN tackles "infodemic" of misinformation and cybercrime in COVID-19 crisis. https://www.un.org/en/un-coronavirus-communications-team/un-tackling-%E2%80%98infodemic%E2%80%99-misinformation-and-cybercrime-covid-19

Education Network to Advance Cancer Clinical Trials (ENACCT) and Community-Campus Partnerships for Health (CCPH). (2008). *Communities as partners in cancer clinical trials: Changing research, practice and policy*. Silver Spring. http://www.inspireresearch.org/resources/guide/enaact-report-communities-partners-cancer-clinical-trials-changing-research-practice

Faridi Z., Grunbaum J. A., Gray B. S., Franks A., & Simoes, E. (2007). Community-based participatory research: Necessary next steps. *Preventing Chronic Disease, 4*(3), A70.

Glanz, K., & Bishop, D. B. (2010). The role of behavioral science theory in development and implementation of public health interventions. *Annual Review of Public Health, 31*, 399–418. https://doi.org/10.1146/annurev.publhealth.012809.103604

Glynn, I., & Glynn, J. (2005). *The life and death of smallpox* (p. 385). Cambridge, U.K.

Hagen, M. M., Hartzell, S. Y. T., & Devereux, P. G. (2021). Social media use and COVID-19: A cross-sectional study examining health behaviors, knowledge, and mental health among University of Nevada, Reno Students. *Health Behavior Research, 37*(2), 103–127.

Henderson, D. A. (1987). Principles and lessons from the smallpox eradication programme. *Bulletin of the World Health Organization, 65*, 535–546. https://www.ncbi.nlm.nih.gov/pmc/articles/PMC2491023/

Israel, B. A., Schulz A. J., Parker E. A., Becker A. B., Allen A. J., & Guzman J. R. (2003). Critical issues in developing and following community based participatory research principles In M. Minkler & N. Wallerstein (Eds.), *Community-based participatory research for health* (pp. 53–76). Jossey-Bass.

Jegede, A. (2007). What led to the Nigerian boycott of the polio vaccination campaign? *PLoS Medicine, 4*(3), e73. https://doi.org/10.1371/journal.pmed.0040073

Krpan, D., Makki, F., Saleh, N., Brink, S. I., & Klauznicer, H. V. (2021). When behavioural science can make a difference in times of COVID-19. *Behavioural Public Policy, 5*(2), 153–179. https://doi.org/10.1017/bpp.2020.48

Mark, C., & Rigau-Pérez, J. (2009). The world's first immunization campaign: The Spanish smallpox vaccine expedition, 1803–1813. *Bulletin of the History of Medicine, 83*, 63–94. https://www.jstor.org/stable/44448715

Nyhan, B., Reifler, J., Richey, S., & Freed, G. L. (2014). Effective messages in vaccine promotion: A randomized trial. *Pediatrics, 133*(4), e835–e842. https://doi.org/10.1542/peds.2013-2365

Pluviano, S., Watt, C., Ragazzini, G., & Della Sala, S. (2019). Parents' beliefs in misinformation about vaccines are strengthened by pro-vaccine campaigns. *Cognitive Processing, 20*, 325–331. https://doi.org/10.1007/s10339-019-00919-w

Sarma, H., Budden, A., Luies, S. K. Lim, S. S., Shamsuzzaman, M., Sultana, T., Rajaratnam, J. K., Craw, L., Banwell, C., Wazed Ali, M., & Jasim Uddin, M. (2019). Implementation of the world's largest measles-rubella mass vaccination campaign in Bangladesh: A process evaluation. *BMC Public Health, 19*, 925. https://doi.org/10.1186/s12889-019-7176-4

Skinner, C. S., Tiro, J., & Champion, V. L. (2015). The health belief model. In K. Glanz, B. K. Rimer, & K. Viswanath (Eds.), *Health behavior: Theory, research, and practice* (5th ed.) (pp. 75–94). Jossey-Bass.

Stern, A. M., & Markel, H. (2005). The history of vaccines and immunization: Familiar patterns, new challenges. *Health Affairs, 24*(3), 611–621. https://doi.org/10.1377/hlthaff.24.3.611

Tedla, Y. G., & Bautista, L. E. (2016). Drug side effect symptoms and adherence to antihypertensive medication. *American Journal of Hypertension, 29*(6), 772–779. https://doi.org/10.1093/ajh/hpv185

Wood, S., & Schulman, K. (2021). Beyond politics—Promoting Covid-19 vaccination in the United States. *New England Journal of Medicine, 384*(7), e23. https://doi.org/10.1056/NEJMms2033790

FURTHER READING

Larson, H. J. (2020). A call to arms: Helping family, friends and communities navigate the COVID-19 infodemic. *Nature Reviews, 20*, 449–450. https://doi.org/10.1038/s41577-020-0380-8.

National Academies of Sciences, Engineering, and Medicine. (2020). *A framework for equitable allocation of vaccine for the novel coronavirus.* https://www.nationalacademies.org/our-work/a-framework-for-equitable-allocation-of-vaccine-for-the-novel-coronavirus

Volpp, K. G., Loewenstein, G., & Buttenheim, A. M. (2020). Behaviorally informed strategies for a national COVID-19 vaccine promotion program. *JAMA*, *325*(2), 125–126. https://doi:10.1001/jama.2020.24036

Wieland M. L., Asiedu G. B., Lantz K., Abbenyi A., Njeru J. W., Osman A., Goodson, M., Ahmed, L. E., Molina, L. E., Doubeni, C. A., Sia, I. G., & Rochester Healthy Community Partnership COVID-19 Task Force. (2020). Leveraging community engaged research partnerships for crisis and emergency risk communication to vulnerable populations in the COVID-19 pandemic. *Journal of Clinical and Translational Science*, *5*(1), 1–21. https://doi.org/10.1017/cts.2020.47

15

Party Polarization and COVID-19

JENNIFER LIN AND JAMES N. DRUCKMAN ■

On the morning of September 11, 2001, little did the people of New York City, much less the country, know that their attitudes toward their neighbors and country were about to change. The terrorist attacks on the World Trade Center and Pentagon left a lasting rally-around-the-flag effect; it led to increased support of Democrats and Republicans for then (Republican) President George W. Bush (Kam & Ramos, 2008). These attacks, thus, suggest that external threats to the country tend to unite citizens (Carlin & Love, 2016; Levendusky, 2018). The onset of the COVID-19 pandemic led many to speculate a similar uniting. An early article stated: "The pandemic not only highlights a common identity with individuals all facing the same risk, but could also foster a sense of shared fate. By highlighting an overarching identity, politicians, the media and opinion leaders could help reduce political division around the issue" (van Bavel et al., 2020, p. 464). By most accounts, though, this unity never occurred, and instead, the country ostensibly became even more divided by partisanship. The precise dynamics, however, are more subtle than most recognize: Our goal here is to unravel this subtlety to explore the relationship between partisan affective polarization and COVID-19 reactions in the United States. This helps explain how partisanship in general and polarization more specifically shaped pandemic opinions and behaviors.

We start with a discussion of the different types of polarization. Here, we chiefly focus on affective polarization, which is the extent to which one likes their own party relative to how much they dislike the other party (Iyengar et al., 2012). We then discuss political communication during COVID-19 as a key lever for partisan reactions. Next, we turn to data on partisan differences in COVID-19 response; this evidence not only is extensive but also leaves unclear whether affective polarization in fact played a role. To address that question, we present trends on polarization from the onset of the pandemic, which show surprisingly that affective polarization declined. Then, we describe a study that showed—despite the decline in affective polarization—it

Jennifer Lin and James N. Druckman, *Party Polarization and COVID-19* In: *The Social Science of the COVID-19 Pandemic*. Edited by: Monica K. Miller, Oxford University Press. © Oxford University Press 2024.
DOI: 10.1093/oso/9780197615133.003.0015

still played a central role in driving partisan responses. We conclude with a discussion about lessons learned and some suggestions of ways to temper polarization during crises.

POLARIZATION: THE CONCEPT, TRENDS OVER THE COURSE OF TIME, AND POSSIBLE CONSEQUENCES

Ideological polarization occurs when parties move toward the extreme ends of the liberal-conservative scale and become more homogeneous. For example, Democrats become increasingly liberal and like one another, and Republicans become increasingly conservative and also like one another (Hetherington, 2001). In the United States, this pattern describes Congress (McCarty, 2019; McCarty et al., 2006); over the past 50 years, members of Congress have been increasingly moving to the extremes and becoming homogeneous, based on their observed floor votes. However, this movement to the extremes is not as prevalent among the public (Fiorina, 2017; Lelkes, 2016). What is prevalent, however, is another type of polarization: affective polarization. This refers to the process by which partisans have become more negative toward the opposing party, relative to their positive feelings toward their own party. A common measure of affective polarization is a feeling thermometer that asks individuals to rate the parties from 0 (very cold) to 100 (very warm). Lower ratings on this scale indicate greater animosity, and higher ratings indicate greater friendliness, with 50 being a neutral rating (Druckman & Levendusky, 2019; Iyengar et al., 2012). While it is unclear if the members of Congress are becoming increasingly affectively polarized, partisan animosity has been growing in the public during the same time that ideological polarization has been growing in the halls of government (Finkel et al., 2020; Groenendyk, 2018).

What causes affective polarization, and what are its effects? In terms of the latter, affective polarization has led to an increase in levels of observed social discrimination (Gift & Gift, 2015), dehumanization of out-partisans (Martherus et al., 2021), and decreased support for government institutions when the out-party is in office (Hetherington & Rudolph, 2015). In terms of causes of affective polarization, it stems from social and ideological sorting present in American politics today, media echo chambers, and the aforementioned ideological elite divide (Finkel et al., 2020). It also stems from the moralization of politics (Garrett & Bankert, 2020). People who are more likely to perceive issues as right or wrong are more likely to display animosity toward those who do not moralize politics in the same lens as they do. Finally, vitriolic elite rhetoric plays a role in driving both affective polarization and its consequences (e.g., Gentzkow et al., 2019; Lau et al., 2017). Given the role of rhetoric in affective polarization, we next turn to a discussion of political communication during COVID-19.

POLITICAL COMMUNICATION DURING
THE COVID-19 PANDEMIC

In times of crises, people often turn to the experts for guidance. During the COVID-19 pandemic, the public health experts partnered with political leaders to communicate best practices to prevent the spread of the disease. However, in a polarized era, these messages ended up being quite distinct based on party.

Even at the start of the lockdowns in March 2020, Democrat politicians were more eager to tell the public to observe social distancing guidelines and wear a face mask (or other facial covering during times of mask shortages) while in public (Lipsitz & Pop-Eleches, 2020). Contrary to this tone, Republican politicians, led by then-President Donald Trump, were less enthusiastic about these measures and consequentially were more likely to downplay the severity of the pandemic and less eager to push the people to abide by these rules. Moreover, Democrat politicians emphasized the importance of delivering aid to affected workers. In contrast, Republicans focused more on aid to small businesses, preserving national unity, and attacking China, for whom they blamed the source of the virus (Lipsitz & Pop-Eleches, 2020).

These partisan rhetorical differences were echoed in the media, which politicized the pandemic at levels that exceeded that of climate change (Hart et al., 2020). The rhetorical divide also manifested on Twitter (Green et al., 2021). Using a corpus of tweets scraped from both office-sponsored and personal accounts managed by members of the 116th Congress, Green et al. (2021) identified tweets that discussed the ongoing COVID-19 pandemic. They used these tweets to then predict the partisanship of the sender. The results suggest that members of Congress polarized quickly with the onset of the pandemic. Political elites differed in not only how they discussed the issue but also how frequently. Democrats tended to discuss the issue more frequently and started doing so earlier in the pandemic. They also were more likely to discuss issues such as aid to affected workers and emphasize public health. Republicans tended to focus more on national unity, China, and businesses.

Beyond Twitter, research into local county websites on COVID-19 guidance issued by the elites also demonstrated partisan differences (Hansen et al., 2020). Here, each county website was coded between April 17 and April 24, 2020, for whether or not it (a) mentioned COVID-19 and (b) provided tips for visitors for how to stay safe during the pandemic. Even when controlling for COVID prevalence, counties that voted for Clinton in 2016 (the partisanship measure) were more likely to mention and provide safety guidance for their residents compared to those who voted for Trump in 2016.

PARTISAN ATTITUDES AND BEHAVIORS DURING
THE PANDEMIC

Here we look at partisan differences in attitudes and behaviors during the pandemic. Differences emerged immediately, with the most salient being abiding by the stay-at-home orders and social distancing. This was shown by tracking social distancing and mobility with data from SafeGraph (Allcott et al., 2020; Gollwitzer et al., 2020). SafeGraph is a proprietary data source that tracks cell phone mobility and provides data at the census block group level. By comparing the user's starting location and the duration that they are out with their final location at the end of the day, the data predict the rate that people in a given area are likely to travel or stay at home on any given day. Allcott et al. (2020) demonstrated that Democrats were more likely to abide by the social distancing orders. Similarly, Gollwitzer et al. (2020) compared compliance to stay-at-home orders between Democrat and Republican counties. After most states implemented these orders on March 23, 2020, the gap between residents in Democrat and Republican counties abiding by these orders increased rather than decreased. In line with Allcott et al.'s (2020) findings, residents in Democrat counties were more likely, relative to Republican counties, to shelter in place and observe these guidelines (also see Clinton et al., 2021).

For the most part, people follow the lead of the politicians they trust, and partisanship plays a big role in this. One instance is in social distancing (Bisbee & Lee, 2022). In a study of Trump-supporting countries, Bisbee and Lee (2022) found that adherence to the social distancing recommendations were highest when the former President endorsed the seriousness of the virus, but this was not adhered to when Trump downplayed the virus in his speeches and other public statements.

Partisan differences were not limited to movement. Gadarian et al. (2021) showed that Democrats were more likely to alter their personal behaviors, such as mask wearing and more frequent handwashing. Additionally, Republicans and Democrats differed in their attitudes toward government policies. Republicans were less likely to support movement across international borders and were more likely to endorse proposals that involved trade restrictions during the pandemic. On the contrary, Democrats were more likely to support free trade and measures that would cut taxes during the pandemic. Democrats were also more likely to endorse provisions to cut the cost of testing and healthcare associated with COVID-19. Partisans also differed by their blame attribution about the virus. Graham and Singh (2023) demonstrated that Republicans were less likely to attribute blame toward Donald Trump for his handling of the pandemic, while Democrats attributed more blame. This pattern grew as the pandemic continued.

Party differences also manifested in interpretations of the COVID-19 pandemic. The COVID States Project conducted surveys each month from April 2020 to April 2021 to identify the attitudes and behaviors during the pandemic. Each survey contained items on attitudes and behaviors during the pandemic, including attitudes toward policies to curb the spread of the virus and intentions to get the COVID vaccine. Additionally, each survey fielded respondents from each state plus the District of Columbia. With each survey, the COVID States team released a series of reports covering the core findings on each topic from the data. More details on the project can be found online (https://covidstates.org/). Table 15.1 highlights some of the key partisan differences found in some of the reports. The numbers reported in this table correspond with the report in which the findings were presented (see the project website). Table 15.1 shows that experiences with the economy or education are relatively similar for partisans. However, trust in key institutions to handle the pandemic, support for policies aimed at curbing the spread of the disease, and vaccine acceptance were distinct for members of both parties.

Interestingly, the table reveals a deep partisan divide regarding Dr. Fauci, director of the U.S. National Institute of Allergy and Infectious Diseases, who became a central scientific advisory figure during the pandemic. He became highly politicized, with Democrats being far more likely to trust him to handle the virus compared to their Republican counterparts. While not in the table, the project found much less polarization when it came to general trust in scientists, doctors, researchers, the Centers for Disease Control and Prevention, and hospitals to stop the spread. Nonetheless, data made clear that vaccines even split the parties, with more Republicans saying that they are going to wait or just not receive the vaccine at all.

AFFECTIVE POLARIZATION DURING COVID-19

Partisan divisions led many to presume that affective polarization grew during COVID-19. That is, partisans came to cherish their party more and hold even more animus for the other party; after all, the partisan elite rancoring and vast partisan differences in responses suggest discord. Yet, interestingly, the extant data suggest otherwise. Boxell et al. (2022) identified several data sources that tracked levels of affective polarization at the start of the pandemic. Perhaps their most impressive source of data came from NationScapes, which cover more than 300,000 interviews between July 2019 and July 2020. These data included a measure that asked respondents to rate their favorability toward each of the parties (on 4-point scales)—items akin to the aforementioned thermometer ratings. As redisplayed in Figure 15.1, it shows that affective polarization in fact declined after the first COVID-19 death in the United States. The authors reported the same trend in three of five other data sources, with the other two showing neither a decline nor an increase. They also presented results from a survey experiment in which people were primed to think about the start of COVID-19, and this also lowered out-party animus. Thus, despite two thirds of the respondents in the survey experiment expressing a belief that the country had become more divided during COVID-19, it seems, from Figure 15.1, that it was the George Floyd murder and not COVID-19 that sparked an increase in affective polarization.

Related evidence came from Rodriguez and colleagues (2020), who showed that the country did not polarize on various political issues (distinct from those in Table 15.1). They found no evidence that the onset of COVID-19 led to divides in attitudes on welfare, delaying elections, deploying the National Guard, banning domestic travel, and use of cell phones to track behaviors.

In sum, even though the elite rhetoric and partisan attitudes/behaviors with regard to COVID-19 revealed a sharp divide, affective polarization itself did

Table 15.1 Partisan Differences in Experiences During the COVID-19 Pandemic (Results From the COVID States Project)

Topic	Partisan Differences	COVID States Project Report Number (Release Month, Year)
Economic hardships	- Lost a job: 17% Democrats, 14% Republicans - Unable to pay rent: 14% Democrats, 10% Republicans - Took a pay cut: 19% Democrats, 15% Republicans	30 (December 2020)
Education	-Somewhat or very concerned with quality of education: 73% Democrats, 61% Republicans	38 (January 2021)
Trust in institutions	- 60% Democrats and 24% Republicans trusted Anthony Fauci a lot - 4% Democrats and 46% Republicans trusted Donald Trump a lot - 36% Democrats and 5% Republicans trusted Joe Biden a lot	13 (September 2020)
COVID policies	- Asking people to stay home and avoid gatherings: 96% Democrats and 72% Republicans somewhat or strongly approved - Requiring most businesses to close: 78% Democrats, 40% Republicans - Canceling major sports and entertainment events: 90% Democrats, 65% Republicans - Limiting restaurants to carry-out only: 89% Democrats, 56% Republicans - Restricting international travel to the United States: 92% Democrats, 85% Republicans - Restricting travel within the United States: 82% Democrats, 57% Republicans - Prohibit K–12 schools from teaching in person: 85% Democrats, 48% Republicans	25 (November 2020)
Vaccine acceptance	- Would not get the vaccine: 11% Democrats, 30% Republicans - Would get the vaccine after most people they know: 13% Democrats, 17% Republicans	43 (March 2021)

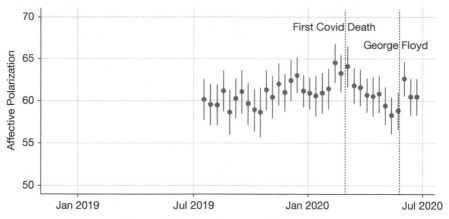

Figure 15.1 Affective polarization during the onset of the COVID-19 pandemic. (From Boxell et al., 2022.)

not seem to increase. There seemed to be somewhat of a feeling of "we are all in this together." In fact, even President Trump's approval level depolarized (Boxell et al., 2022)—although nothing comparable to Bush's after 9/11. This might seem puzzling, but it reflects a distinction between the *extent* of polarization and the *consequences* of polarization. The extent of it might have even declined as people recognized a shared sense of threat. But at the same time, the issues concerning COVID-19 were politicized, leading to the aforementioned partisan variations.

THE CONSEQUENCES OF AFFECTIVE POLARIZATION DURING COVID-19

There remains a question of whether affective polarization itself shaped COVID-19 responses, even if the level of polarization itself shrunk. This is a difficult question to answer because if one observes a correlation between affective polarization levels and COVID-19 attitudes or behaviors, one of three possible dynamics may be at work. It could be that affective polarization shapes reactions, that reactions are leading to polarization, or that some third variable such as exposure to partisan media determines both affective polarization and reactions. Druckman et al. (2021) offered a way around this. Specifically, they had conducted a survey that included measures of affective polarization in the summer of 2019, a half year before the emergence of COVID-19. They then returned to these same respondents in April 2020, once COVID-19 had spread and shut down economies. They were able to re-interview nearly 75% of the respondents, asking about the extent to which they worried about COVID-19; which COVID-19 behaviors they practiced (e.g., washing hands, wearing masks, staying at home, ordering groceries); and their opposition or support for various restrictive policies (e.g., stay-at-home orders). Because the affective polarization measures were taken well before COVID-19 existed as an issue, the authors could be confident that COVID-19 did not affect polarization levels. The authors also measured a host of potential confounding variables, such as media exposure, partisan identity strength, and social media behaviors, to control for factors that could shape both affective polarization and COVID-19 reactions. In short, the design allowed for a test of whether affective polarization—aside from party—shaped COVID-19 attitudes and behaviors.

The authors found clear evidence that affective polarization—specifically animus toward the out-party—shaped COVID-19 worry, behaviors, and policy support (also see Druckman et al., 2021). We redisplay their results in Figure 15.2 (taken from Druckman et al., 2021, p. 31). The figure reports the marginal change in the given outcome for a change in party animosity for Democrats and Republicans. For instance, when it comes to worry about COVID-19, an increase in partisan animosity did not alter Democrats' worry (the effect encompasses 0), but it led Republicans to become less worried. We also see that it led to more behaviors and policy support for Democrats and less policy support for Republicans. The overall results made clear that partisan animosity—not just party differences—played a role in shaping COVID-19 responses.

This matters because it suggests that the partisan divisions we presented above may stem, at least partially, from affective polarization. The idea is that those who are more affectively polarized are motivated to differentiate themselves from the other party they dislike. When they see the clear elite party cues concerning COVID-19 (see above discussion), they then act in concert with their party and against the other party. Affective polarization acts as a mechanism for elite influence and underlying partisan divides. It shows these divides stem from nonsubstantive considerations (i.e., feelings about the parties), which itself may be concerning. That said, Druckman et al. (2021) reported that the impact of

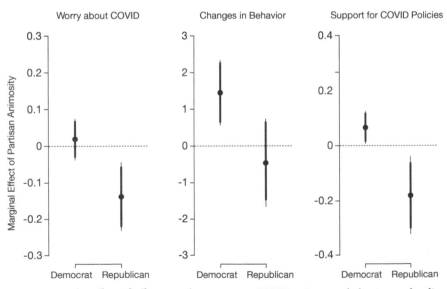

Figure 15.2 The effect of affective polarization on COVID-19 worry, behavior, and policy support. [From Druckman et al., 2021.]

affective polarization was muted in counties with high COVID-19 case counts; in those areas, the threat of COVID-19 led people to depart from their partisan motivations and engage in more accuracy-oriented thinking.

LESSONS FOR POLARIZATION FROM THE COVID-19 PANDEMIC

What lessons has this pandemic taught us, and how can we move forward from here? For one, the evidence makes clear that, unlike 9/11, partisanship emerged as a major factor in driving COVID-19 response. Even though this was a health crisis, it politicized and partisanship became central. This is clear in political communications, partisan differences in attitudes, and affectively polarized responses. That said, that affective polarization levels did not simultaneously increase makes clear that one needs to distinguish levels of polarization from its effect. Second, these results have implications for our understanding of political geography. In the early days of the pandemic, Republican-led states seemed to have had fewer cases, but this pattern reversed course in early June. Republican states increasingly had a heavier caseload compared to their Democratic counterparts (Neelon et al., 2021). While this likely stemmed in part from the more rural, less dense nature of Republican states, it also may have been a reflection of the patterns discussed in this chapter, such that Republicans tended to have relaxed their adherence to the guidelines earlier than Democrats (Kempler, 2021). Indeed, population density alone could not explain the stark monotonic rise in Republican states relative to Democratic states. It was the partisan politics surrounding the resulting attitudes toward the pandemic and the subsequent divide in behaviors that led Republican states to see increased caseloads by the middle of the pandemic.

Beyond the effects observed in caseloads, the pandemic made clear that elite messaging is crucial for addressing a crisis as massive as COVID-19. According to a Pew Research Center survey (Funk & Tyson, 2021), trust in the COVID-19 vaccine is a significant predictor of whether someone would take the vaccine (see Chapter 18 for more on trust related to the pandemic). Beyond that, the belief that vaccines will help the country emerge from the pandemic differs significantly by party. Democrats are more likely to believe that the vaccine will significantly help the economy compared to the Republican counterparts. Consequently, as displayed in Table 15.1, Republicans were more likely to be vaccine resistant compared to Democrats (Lazer et al., 2021). Bokemper et al. (2020) reported that Democrats were more likely to want to take the vaccine if people who they trust, such as Dr. Anthony Fauci, endorsed the vaccine. The vaccine partisan divide not only demonstrated how quickly novel events can be politicized (Druckman et al., 2021) but also provided an opportunity to explore what can be done to mitigate the results. Pink and colleagues (2021) provided a hint related to messaging campaigns by political elites. From their survey experiment, they found that if Republican elites endorsed a vaccine, Republican identifiers in the public would be more likely to want to get vaccinated. The reason why Republicans seemed to be more hesitant to get the vaccine is because of the messages that their leaders had been communicating (and/or their lack of public endorsement for the vaccine). Clearly, elite messages can be even more powerful in pushing people to solve novel crises such as getting vaccinated from COVID-19. This is an example of those on top, even the most partisan of politicians, having a group of supporters who would listen to their recommendations. If the elites agree and provide similar messages, the gap between partisans narrows and becomes a greater reflection of the "we are in this together" sentiment. After all, Republicans and Democrats alike found COVID-19 to be the most important problem facing the country in the lead-up to the 2020 presidential election (Baum et al., 2020). For leaders, the willingness to be on the same page or to at least be collegial to one another, despite differences in political beliefs, can reduce affective polarization in the public (Huddy & Yair, 2021). In a time of a novel crisis, that is what the country needs most.

For future research, it is important to understand the ways to temper the jump to politicize novel issues that drive partisans apart. Additionally, it is important for researchers to understand ways to bring partisans together rather than exacerbate a crisis when partisans are interpreting the situation differently and behaving differently as a result. The work that we present in this chapter considers these topics from the top down, addressing the need for elites to come together so that the people will do the same. In future research, we can consider bottom-up approaches to mitigating affective polarization, to increase tolerance and cooperation among people from opposing parties. With a better understanding of how partisans can build trust and tolerance toward each other during the so-called normal times, it can perhaps become easier to apply this knowledge to times of crisis.

CONCLUSION

We provided an overview of the partisan differences in attitudes and behaviors during the COVID-19 pandemic. We demonstrated a sharp partisan divide in elite rhetoric, with Democrats expressing more care toward affected workers and Republicans highlighting the need for unity and strength in standing up to China. We also showed these partisan divides carried over to citizens. For example, Republicans tended to loosen their observance to social distancing guidance earlier than Democrats. Alternatively, Democrats were more likely to endorse tax cuts during the pandemic and to ensure that healthcare costs associated with COVID-19 were decreased. Even though levels of polarization did not increase during the pandemic, the clear partisan divides may have exacerbated inefficiencies in pandemic response, including those related to patchwork policies across the nation and incomplete vaccine uptake.

REFERENCES

Allcott, H., Boxell, L., Conway, J., Gentzkow, M., Thaler, M., & Yang, D. (2020). Polarization and public health: Partisan differences in social distancing during the coronavirus pandemic. *Journal of Public Economics, 191*, 104254. https://www.nber.org/papers/w26946

Baum, M. A., Lin, J., Gitomer, A., Quintana, A., Ognyanova, K., Green, J., Lazer, D., Druckman, J. N., Perlis, R. H., Santillana, M., Chwe, H., & Simonson, M. (2020). The state of the nation: A 50-state COVID-19 survey, report 21: Most important problems facing the country today. COVID States Project. https://osf.io/q3av7/

Bisbee, J., & Lee, D. (2022). *Objective Facts and Elite Cues: Partisan Responses to COVID-19. The Journal of Politics, 84*(3), 1278–1291.

Bokemper, S. E., Huber, G. A., Gerber, A. S., James, E. K., & Omer, S. B. (2020). Timing of COVID-19 vaccine approval and endorsement by public figures. *Vaccine, 39*(5), 825–829. https://doi.org/10.1016/j.vaccine.2020.12.048

Boxell, L., Conway, J., Druckman, J. N., & Gentzkow, M. (2022). *Affective polarization did not increase during the COVID-19 pandemic. Quarterly Journal of Political Science 17*(4), 491–512.

Carlin, R. E., & Love, G. J. (2016). Political competition, partisanship and interpersonal trust in electoral democracies. *British Journal of Political Science, 48*(1), 115–139. https://doi.org/10.1017/S0007123415000526

Clinton, J., Cohen, J., Lapinski, J., & Trussler, M. (2021). Partisan pandemic: How partisanship and public health concerns affect individuals' social mobility during COVID-19. *Science Advances, 7*(2), eabd7204. https://doi.org/10.1126/sciadv.abd7204

Druckman, J. N., Klar, S., Krupnikov, Y., Levendusky, M., & Ryan, J. B. (2021). How affective polarization shapes Americans' political beliefs: A study of response to the COVID-19 pandemic. *Journal of Experimental Political Science, 8*(3), 223–234. https://doi.org/10.1017/XPS.2020.28

Druckman, J. N., Klar, S., Krupnikov, Y., Levendusky, M., & Ryan, J. B. (2021). Affective polarization, local contexts and public opinion in America. *Nature Human Behaviour, 5*(1), 28–38. https://doi.org/10.1038/s41562-020-01012-5

Druckman, J. N., & Levendusky, M. S. (2019). What do we measure when we measure affective polarization? *Public Opinion Quarterly, 83*(1), 114–122. https://doi.org/10.1093/poq/nfz003

Finkel, E. J., Bail, C. A., Cikara, M., Ditto, P. H., Iyengar, S., Klar, S., Mason, L., McGrath, M. C., Nyhan, B., Rand, D. G., Skitka, L. J., Tucker, J. A., van Bavel, J. J., Wang, C. J., & Druckman, J. N. (2020). Political sectarianism in America. *Science, 370*(6516), 533–536. https://doi.org/10.1126/science.abe1715

Fiorina, M. P. (2017). *Unstable majorities: Polarization, party sorting, and political stalemate*. Hoover Press.

Funk, C., & Tyson, A. (2021). Growing share of Americans say they plan to get a COVID-19 vaccine—or already have. Pew Research Center Science & Society. https://www.pewresearch.org/science/2021/03/05/growing-share-of-americans-say-they-plan-to-get-a-covid-19-vaccine-or-already-have/

Gadarian, S. K., Goodman, S. W., & Pepinsky, T. B. (2021). Partisanship, health behavior, and policy attitudes in the early stages of the COVID-19 pandemic. *PloS One, 16*(4), e0249596. https://doi.org/10.1371/journal.pone.0249596

Garrett, K. N., & Bankert, A. (2020). The moral roots of partisan division: How moral conviction heightens affective polarization. *British Journal of Political Science, 50*(2), 621–640. https://doi.org/10.1017/S000712341700059X

Gentzkow, M., Shapiro, J. M., & Taddy, M. (2019). Measuring group differences in high-dimensional choices: Method and application to congressional speech. *Econometrica, 87*(4), 1307–1340. https://doi.org/10.3982/ECTA16566

Gift, K., & Gift, T. (2015). Does politics influence hiring? Evidence from a randomized experiment. *Political Behavior, 37*(3), 653–675. https://doi.org/10.1007/s11109-014-9286-0

Gollwitzer, A., Martel, C., Brady, W. J., Pärnamets, P., Freedman, I. G., Knowles, E. D., & van Bavel, J. J. (2020). Partisan differences in physical distancing are linked to health outcomes during the COVID-19 pandemic. *Nature Human Behaviour, 4*(11), 1186–1197. https://doi.org/10.1038/s41562-020-00977-7

Graham, M. H., & Singh, S. (2023). Partisan selectivity in blame attribution: Evidence from the COVID-19 pandemic. *American Political Science Review,* 1–19.

Green, J., Edgerton, J., Naftel, D., Shoub, K., & Cranmer, S. J. (2021). Elusive consensus: Polarization in elite communication on the COVID-19 pandemic. *Science Advances, 6*(28), eabc2717. https://doi.org/10.1126/sciadv.abc2717

Groenendyk, E. (2018). Competing motives in a polarized electorate: Political responsiveness, identity defensiveness, and the rise of partisan antipathy. *Political Psychology, 39*, 159–171. https://doi.org/10.1111/pops.12481

Hansen, M. A., Johansson, I., Sadowski, K., Blaszcynski, J., & Meyer, S. (2020). The partisan impact on local government dissemination of COVID-19 information: Assessing U.S. county government websites. *Canadian Journal of Political Science/Revue Canadienne de Science Politique, 54*(1), 150–162. https://doi.org/10.1017/S0008423920000918

Hetherington, M. J. (2001). Resurgent mass partisanship: The role of elite polarization. *American Political Science Review, 95*(3), 619–631. https://doi.org/10.1017/S0003055401003045

Hetherington, M. J., & Rudolph, T. J. (2015). *Why Washington won't work: Polarization, political trust, and the governing crisis.* University of Chicago Press.

Huddy, L., & Yair, O. (2021). Reducing affective polarization: Warm group relations or policy compromise? *Political Psychology, 42*(2), 291–309. https://doi.org/10.1111/pops.12699

Iyengar, S., Sood, G., & Lelkes, Y. (2012). Affect, not ideology: A social identity perspective on polarization. *Public Opinion Quarterly, 76*(3), 405–431. https://doi.org/10.1093/poq/nfs038

Kam, C. D., & Ramos, J. M. (2008). Joining and leaving the rally: Understanding the surge and decline in presidential approval following 9/11. *Public Opinion Quarterly, 72*(4), 619–650. https://doi.org/10.1093/poq/nfn055

Kempler, C. (2021). Link found between state governors' political parties and COVID-19 case and death rates. https://hub.jhu.edu/2021/03/11/covid-death-rate-governor-politics/

Lau, R. R., Andersen, D. J., Ditonto, T. M., Kleinberg, M. S., & Redlawsk, D. P. (2017). Effect of media environment diversity and advertising tone on information search, selective exposure, and affective polarization. *Political Behavior, 39*(1), 231–255. https://doi.org/10.1007/s11109-016-9354-8

Lazer, D., Ognyanova, K., Baum, M., Druckman, J., Green, J., Gitomer, A., Simonson, M., Perlis, R. H., Santillana, M., Quintana, A., Lin, J., & Uslu, A. (2021). *The state of the nation: A 50-state COVID-19 survey, report 43: COVID-19 vaccine rates and attitudes among Americans. COVID States Project.* https://osf.io/rnw8z/

Lelkes, Y. (2016). Mass polarization: Manifestations and measurements. *Public Opinion Quarterly, 80*(S1), 392–410. https://doi.org/10.1093/poq/nfw005

Levendusky, M. S. (2018). When efforts to depolarize the electorate fail. *Public Opinion Quarterly, 82*(3), 583–592. https://doi.org/10.1093/poq/nfy036

Lipsitz, K., & Pop-Eleches, G. (2020). The partisan divide in social distancing. SSRN. https://papers.ssrn.com/sol3/papers.cfm?abstract_id=3595695

Martherus, J. L., Martinez, A. G., Piff, P. K., & Theodoridis, A. G. (2021). Party animals? Extreme partisan polarization and dehumanization. *Political Behavior, 21*(43), 517–540. https://doi.org/10.1007/s11109-019-09559-4

McCarty, N. (2019). *Polarization: What everyone needs to know.* Oxford University Press.

McCarty, N., Poole, K. T., & Rosenthal, H. (2006). *Polarized America: The dance of ideology and unequal riches.* MIT Press.

Neelon, B., Mutiso, F., Mueller, N. T., Pearce, J. L., & Benjamin-Neelon, S. E. (2021). Associations between governor political affiliation and COVID-19 cases and deaths in the United States. *American Journal of Preventative Medicine, 61*(1), 115–119. https://doi.org/10.1016/j.amepre.2021.01.034

Pink, S., Chu, J., Druckman, J.N., Rand D.G., & Willer, R. (2021). Elite party cues increases vaccination intentions among Republicans. *Proceedings of the National Academy of Science, 118*(32), e2106559118.

Rodriguez, C., Gadarian, S. K., Goodman, S. W., & Pepinsky, T. (2020). Morbid polarization: Exposure to COVID-19 and partisan disagreement about pandemic response. *Political Psychology 43*(6), 1169–1189. https://doi.org/10.1111/pops.12810

Van Bavel, J. J., Baicker, K., Boggio, P. S., Capraro, V., Cichocka, A., Cikara, M., Crockett, M. J., Crum, A. J., Douglas, K. M., Druckman, J. N., Drury, J., Dube, O., Ellemers, N., Finkel, E. J., Fowler, J. H., Gelfand, M., Han, S., Haslam, S. A., Jetten, J., . . . & Willer, R. (2020). Using social and behavioural science to support COVID-19 pandemic response. *Nature Human Behaviour, 4*(5), 460–471. https://doi.org/10.1038/s41562-020-0884-z

FURTHER READING

Finkel, E. J., Bail, C. A., Cikara, M., Ditto, P. H., Iyengar, S., Klar, S., Mason, L., McGrath, M. C., Nyhan, B., Rand, D. G., Skitka, L. J., Tucker, J. A., van Bavel, J. J., Wang, C. J., & Druckman, J. N. (2020). Political sectarianism in America. *Science, 370*(6516), 533–536. https://doi.org/10.1126/science.abe1715

Hetherington, M. J., & Rudolph, T. J. (2015). *Why Washington won't work: Polarization, political trust, and the governing crisis.* University of Chicago Press.

Iyengar, S., Lelkes, Y., Levendusky, M., Malhotra, N., & Westwood, S. J. (2019). The origins and consequences of affective polarization in the United States. *Annual Review of Political Science, 22*, 129–146. https://doi.org/10.1146/annurev-polisci-051117-073034

Iyengar, S., & Westwood, S. J. (2014). Fear and loathing across party lines: New evidence on group polarization. *American Journal of Political Science, 59*(3), 690–707. https://doi.org/10.1111/ajps.12152

Klein, E. (2020). *Why we're polarized*. Simon Schuster.

Lelkes, Y., & Westwood, S. J. (2016). The limits of partisan prejudice. *Journal of Politics, 79*(2), 485–501. https://doi.org/10.1086/688223

Mason, L. (2018). *Uncivil agreement: How politics became our identity*. University of Chicago Press.

Moore-Berg, S. L., Ankori-Karlinsky, L.-O., Hameiri, B., & Bruneau, E. (2020). Exaggerated meta-perceptions predict intergroup hostility between American political partisans. *Proceedings of the National Academy of Sciences of the United States of America, 117*(26), 14864–14872. https://doi.org/10.1073/pnas.2001263117

16

How Will Collective-Level Dynamics Influence the Spread of COVID-19?

SHINOBU KITAYAMA ∎

Throughout the last year and a half, the world has witnessed an unprecedented spread of the novel coronavirus disease (COVID-19). Some fear that its magnitude could eventually be comparable to that of the 1918 flu pandemic, which killed more than 50 million people worldwide. As the virus's onslaught unfolded, I began to feel that social and behavioral scientists must join forces in the fight against the pandemic. In particular, I wondered whether massive variation in countries' vulnerability to the virus might shed light on the core mechanisms underlying its transmission. This thought might not be too far-fetched; even though the infectious disease is caused by a virus—a biological agent composed of DNA—the virus's behavior is nearly entirely contingent on human behavior (Habersaat et al., 2020; Quammen, 2012; Van Bavel et al., 2020). Thus, social and behavioral sciences might have a lot to offer. Relevant regulatory agencies, including the Centers for Disease Control and Prevention in the United States, must heed social and behavioral science insights when formulating their policies and regulations.

In this chapter, I address three issues that strike me as particularly important as we face the challenge of managing the current and future pandemics. I argue that the collective-level dynamics of (a) complacency induction, (b) egocentric versus prosocial motivations, and (c) culture and social relations powerfully influence the spread of infectious diseases, including COVID-19. I draw heavily on my first-hand experiences in the United States, where I live. However, I hope my discussion carries relevance for readers elsewhere. I conclude with evidence-based policy recommendations.

Shinobu Kitayama, *How Will Collective-Level Dynamics Influence the Spread of COVID-19?* In: *The Social Science of the COVID-19 Pandemic.* Edited by: Monica K. Miller, Oxford University Press. © Oxford University Press 2024.
DOI: 10.1093/oso/9780197615133.003.0016

PLURALISTIC IGNORANCE AND COMPLACENCY

Any cursory observation would suggest that people's behavior during the pandemic depends on their ability and willingness to recognize COVID-19 as a threat. Once people perceive this threat as urgent, they will be alarmed. They will then try to cope with the threat. For example, they might sacrifice some conveniences and wear face masks or socially isolate themselves. The problem, however, is that there is nothing concrete about the threat of infectious disease. The threat is often invisible until it is too late when many people have already been infected and hospitalized. These days (in the middle of 2021) in the United States, it is not uncommon to see infected people in their hospital beds express their regret of having declined to be vaccinated, for example.

There are multiple reasons why people fail to recognize the threat they face. However, there is one mechanism that cuts across them. People are motivated to elaborate on information that serves their motivational goals while discounting information that does not (Kunda, 1990). For example, people often seek to maintain their self-image as strong and confident (Taylor & Brown, 1988). Indeed, they might be accused of being an alarmist or being too worrying and weak when they took warnings from medical experts seriously. They might therefore be motivated to perceive the warnings as hearsay. Moreover, social media often provides misleading information that assures people of their safety and invincibility (see Tsao et al., 2021, for a review). People might be motivated to believe such information since they find it quite comforting and assuring. Such motivated reasoning processes lead to complacency (see also Chapter 6).

To illustrate, by February 2020, many residents I met in New York City already knew about the spread of COVID-19 in Asia and Europe. They had been informed of earlier infections in the area. The first death in the city was to emerge in the first week of March. Nevertheless, most residents failed to act, seemingly feeling safe and protected. With the benefit of hindsight, this calmness seems like complacency, which indeed eventually haunted many of them. Motivated reasoning is an important part of why such complacency comes about. This reasoning could be particularly potent, especially during the pandemic since there are abundant cues in the environment that suggest that the situation is safe and manageable. Some of the most powerful cues of this sort come from inactions of other people.

Miller and Prentice (1994) argued that people often believe that everyone else feels safe because they do not show any signs of discomfort or anxiety. Consistent with the notion of the fundamental attribution error (Ross, 1977), they infer others' internal states directly from their behaviors. Rarely do they consider the possibility that the others might be hiding their anxiety. Crucially, they do not show any signs of discomfort or anxiety, not because they do not feel them but rather because they find others not showing them. In the context of the current pandemic, everyone might well have suspected a real threat. However, a vast majority refrained from acting proactively to cope with the threat precisely because they witnessed others' inaction and judged that the situation was somehow manageable. The irony is that the error in judgment (i.e., the perceived safety of the situation) was based precisely on the inaction of other people, who were guided by the same judgment error. Thus, this collective failure to calibrate each other's anxiety, called pluralistic ignorance (Allport, 1924), leads to a collective failure to act properly.

In all likelihood, the people who gathered at Florida bars or Southern California beaches in summer 2020 or those riders who blasted their Harley-Davidsons all the way to Sturgis, South Dakota, during the second week of August 2020, were complacent. Also, many Americans, nearly a half of them, who have so far declined to receive COVID vaccines, are equally complacent. Their complacency, however, was not simply due to a failure to understand the reality of the pandemic. To the contrary, their perception of that reality might have been systematically distorted by a little bit of innocuous pretension or even civility—a desire not to be seen as alarmist or as weak or feeble. The resulting distortion of reality might have made it seem completely rational not to worry much about COVID-19, which unfortunately led to the virus's spread in various communities.

THE TRAGEDY OF THE COMMONS: SELF-PROTECTION VERSUS THE PROTECTION OF A COMMUNITY

No matter how prone individuals might be to complacency, they will eventually recognize a real threat if people around them start to fall prey to the disease and begin to die. When the threat is duly recognized, however, another collective dynamic enters and makes it hard to organize risk-mitigating actions.

Since a virus spread is in a community, any risk-mitigating actions must take place at the community level. Mask wearing is ineffective if not practiced by most people in a community. Likewise, social distancing does not mean much unless exercised by most people in the community. However, the effectiveness of these actions is often not obvious for each of the individuals involved. Moreover, these actions are often experienced as inconveniences. Thus, even when such actions are recommended or even required by the state, there might arise a temptation not to follow such recommendations or requirements.

For example, consider the practice of wearing a mask in public. At the individual level, it could be an annoyance. This adverse reaction to mask wearing could be rather strong in contemporary mainstream American culture. According to Masaki Yuki and colleagues, the mouth is a "window to the soul" for Americans (Yuki et al., 2007). The use of the mouth is instrumental in American society for communication, including emotional expression. According to Yuki et al. (2007), it is eyes, rather than the mouth, that are the window for the soul for Asians. Indeed, for Americans, "big smile" signifies a superb soul behind it. A recent study showed that in North American contexts, loan officers are more likely to approve loans to those with big smiles (Park et al., 2020). Such an effect is absent in Taiwan. In North America, then, a request to cover up the mouth could threaten the core of one's identity. In line with this reasoning, in the United States throughout the pandemic, the simple, practical decision to wear a face mask was moralized and portrayed as a matter of individual freedom. Not surprisingly, many Americans persistently refused to cover up their mouths in public, to the detriment of the public welfare. This occurred even though the use of face masks is demonstrably effective in containing the spread of COVID-19 (Lyu & Wehby, 2020).

This discussion illustrates a conflict between personal interest and the public good. This conflict has been studied under the rubric of the tragedy of the commons (Hardin, 1968), which refers to a collapse of the public good (e.g., a virus-free environment) when every individual in the community acts by narrowly focusing on his or her own personal interest (e.g., not wearing a mask or avoiding vaccination).

One important implication of the current analysis is that risk-mitigating actions, including mask wearing, during the pandemic might depend on cultural ideologies of individualism and collectivism. The ideology of individualism holds that each person's autonomy and freedom are to be weighed more heavily even at the expense of the collective good (Markus & Kitayama, 1991; Triandis, 1995). This ideology gives an unalloyed endorsement of self-interest (Miller, 1999). Since risk-mitigating actions, such as mask wearing, protect the collective at the expense of personal conveniences, they might be less common in individualistic societies than in collectivist societies.

Consistent with this analysis, Lu et al. (2021) showed that a validated country-wise index of collectivism (vs. individualism) by Hofstede (1980) predicted both the average intention to wear masks and the perceived proportion of others who wore masks. Specifically, in comparison to many other cultures that are arguably more collectivistic, including East Asian cultures such as China and Japan, the prevalence of mask wearing in the United States was much less. As important, individualism versus collectivism varies within the United States (Vandello & Cohen, 1999). If cultural values prioritizing collective welfare promote mask wearing, then we might expect mask wearing to be more common in U.S. states that are relatively high in collectivism (or low in individualism). Lu and colleagues (2021, Study 1a) tested this analysis using a large data set collected by *The New York Times* and Dynata ($N = 248,941$). The participants were asked: "How often do you wear a mask in public when you expect to be within 6 feet of another person?" Their mean response on a 5-point scale (ranging between 0 = never and 4 = always) by state is shown in Figure 16.1. As can be seen, the self-reported mask wearing increased by state-level collectivism. The authors controlled for several potential confounds, including state-wise COVID-19 severity, state-level government stringency, political affiliation, education level, population density, state-level tightness vs. looseness of social norms.

It appears as though many Americans—especially those in relatively more individualistic states (e.g., Mountain West states, such as Montana and Wyoming)—maximized their practical convenience and their psychological welfare by not covering their mouths. This behavior, however, has come at a grave cost for the collective. Individuals are protected only insofar as most others in the community wear masks. If a majority choose not to wear a mask, then they will not be protected even if they wear a mask. Unfortunately, again and again, many Americans prioritized their personal convenience or preference while ignoring collective consequences of doing so.

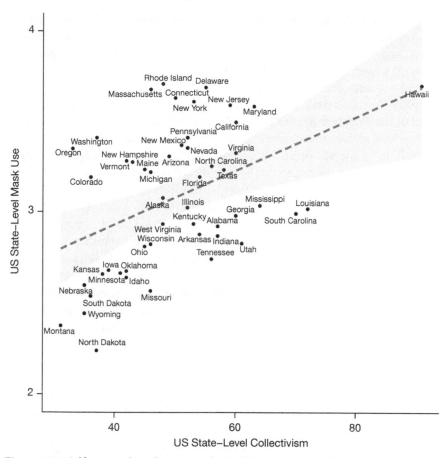

Figure 16.1 Self-reported mask usage in the 50 U.S. states assessed between July 2 and July 14, 2020. (Adopted from Lu et al., 2021, *Proceedings of the American Academy of Sciences.* Reproduced with permission.)

In an article published in the *New York Times* in August 2020,[1] David Leonhardt attributed the U.S. failure to contain COVID-19 to two major factors. One is the lack of adequate federal leadership (see Chapter 32 on leadership in the pandemic). Notably, consistent with my analysis above, as the other culprit he highlighted American individualism. Leonhardt drew our attention to the seemingly selfish behaviors of many Americans, including the refusal to wear masks. As discussed above, unlike more communal, interdependent worldviews based on collectivism, the individualist ideology may therefore be more likely to promote and legitimize self-interested behavior (Betsch et al., 2017).

CULTURE AND SOCIAL RELATIONS

Although the values of independence and interdependence, or equivalently in-dividualism and collectivism, are important, this consideration will have to be

combined with additional considerations to draw a fuller picture. One particularly important consideration concerns the form of social relations this ideology
fosters. Many infectious diseases, including COVID-19, transmit through social
contact. It follows that their spread should depend on the nature of social networks.
If social networks are relatively open, the risk of transmission should increase,
whereas if they are relatively closed, the risk may be contained. One prominent
aspect of individualism lies in the liberation of individuals from socially ascribed
relationships, such as social roles and kinship. People in individualistic countries
are likely to be socially open. Each person is thought to be independent, even
in the domain of social relations. They are therefore encouraged to choose their
acquaintances, friends, and spouses freely. This ideology, an interpersonal extension of the enlightenment idea of the social contract (Rousseau, 1762), has been
ingrained into the matrix of social relations in the United States. American social
relations tend to be highly mobile. If socialized in this cultural milieu, people naturally become socially open, seeking new relations beneficial to the self.

Bear in mind that individualism lends itself to relational mobility, but the two
constructs are distinct (Thomson et al., 2018). One primary reason for the imperfect alignment between the two comes from the fact that some cultures are collectivist in the sense of prioritizing social relations over individual freedom and
choice, and yet, precisely because of this, they are relationally mobile, motivating
their residents to cultivate wide-ranging social relations. One prominent example
is found in Latin America. Evidence is emerging that Latin Americans are highly
expressive of social positive emotions, such as friendly feelings and feelings of
closeness (Salvador et al., in press). They are therefore highly amicable (Campos
& Kim, 2017), which likely predispose the residents of the cultural region to be
socially open. Yet, this form of social openness results from the value placed on
social relations.

Despite this exception to the hypothesized link between individualism and
relational mobility, it still stands that Americans are relationally mobile. I am
grateful to many American friends and colleagues who initially welcomed me as a
new foreign student some decades ago. I am now so happy to interact with many
American students, who constantly challenge me as their intellectual equal for
open intellectual discussions. Social networks in the United States are very open.
I love this aspect of the culture. Ironically, however, this very positive attribute of
individualism could be a liability during the pandemic. Social openness may have
contributed to the spread of COVID-19.

Earlier in 2020 when the pandemic began to unfold, my research team decided
to test the above possibility (Salvador et al., 2020). We adopted a measure of social openness of a community (the degree to which people freely choose partners
of social interaction), called relational mobility. This measure is available for 39
countries across the globe (Thomson et al., 2018). We asked whether the relational
mobility might predict each country's vulnerability to COVID-19.

In testing the cross-cultural differences in the vulnerability to COVID-19, one
important consideration is to preempt the potential effect of cultural variations in
reporting bias. For example, some cultures may be more transparent than others

when reporting infections or deaths. It is also possible that different cultures have varying criteria in defining any given symptoms or deaths as caused by or related to COVID-19. Another important artifact source is the timing of the data we analyzed since the pandemic started at different times in different countries. For example, infections might look more frequent in one country than in another merely because the spread had started earlier in the first country than in the second. Further, one might also worry about the potential effects of various restrictions enforced by the government, which could vary across countries. In addition, it is important to keep in mind that relational mobility could be related to various country-level variables, including individualism versus collectivism and tightness versus looseness of social norms. Further, various demographic variables, such as the average age of each country, its wealth, and its population size, may also influence the spread of the disease. To draw firm conclusions about the potential effect of relational mobility on the spread of COVID-19, we must address all these concerns.

Salvador et al. (2020) overcame this challenge by examining how quickly COVID-19 infections and deaths increased in the first 30 days of country-wise outbreaks. It is possible that all sorts of biases, including reporting biases and diagnostic criteria, influence the number of infections and deaths. However, these biases are unlikely to change systematically within a short period, say, just 30 days. In this way, we excluded these biases. Moreover, we defined the beginning of this testing period as a day on which 100 infections or one death occurred. In this way, we controlled for any cross-cultural variations in the timing of outbreaks. As important, by focusing on the very initial period of an outbreak, we could effectively eliminate any effects of top-down governmental restrictions since they were rarely instituted quickly enough to influence what happened during the first 30 days. Finally, we controlled for individualism versus collectivism, tightness versus looseness of social norms, and various demographic variables, including medium age, gross domestic product, and population size.

Figure 16.2a shows the daily count of confirmed cases on log scale in each country over the first 30 days of country-wise outbreaks. As can be seen, on average, the rate of daily increase is greater in countries that were relatively high in relational mobility. Figure 16.2b plots the slope by relational mobility. As can be seen, the slope systematically became steeper as the country-level relational mobility increases. As shown in Figures 16.2c and 16.2d, we closely replicated the pattern in the analysis of COVID-related deaths. Last, we obtained these findings while controlling for various variables, including individualism versus collectivism, tightness versus looseness, and demographic variables.

It is noteworthy that in this analysis, there was no effect of individualism versus collectivism. The absence of any effects of individualism versus collectivism might be puzzling given its strong impacts on mask wearing (as discussed previously). However, in this work, we looked at the spread of COVID-19 in an initial phase of country-wise outbreaks. Therefore, it stands to reason that the primary determinant of this spread was the social network parameter of relational mobility. Cultural ideologies such as individualism and collectivism might come into play

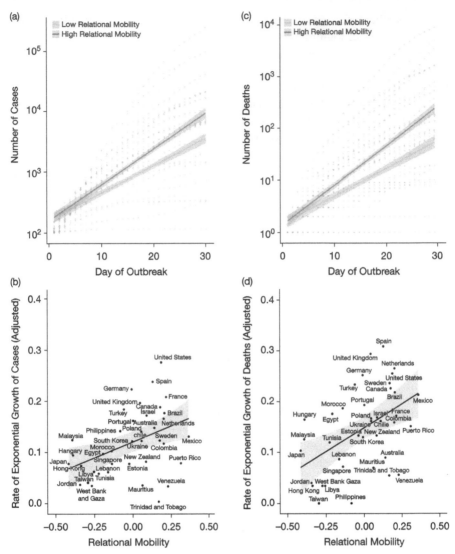

Figure 16.2 The spread of COVID-19 in the first 30 days of country-wise outbreaks by relational mobility. a. The growth curve of the number of confirmed cases. b. The growth rate of confirmed cases in each of the countries by relational mobility. c. The growth curve of the number of deaths. d. The growth rate of deaths in each of the countries by relational mobility. (Adapted from Salvador et al., 2020, *Psychological Science*.)

only later, when people decided whether they would engage in risk-mitigating actions, such as mask wearing.

The effect of relational mobility on the spread of COVID-19 during the initial period of country-wise outbreaks was indeed substantial. As can be seen in Figures 16.2c and 16.2d, the United States is very high—one of the highest—in relational mobility. In our estimation, if the United States had been much less open—say, as little as Japan, one of the least open of the 39 countries tested—U.S. deaths at the end of the 30-day period would have been 8.2% (281) of the actual number reported (3,417).

CONCLUSIONS

In this chapter, I summarized the evidence that collective-level human cognition, motivation, and behavior exert profound influences on the spread of COVID-19. My argument was threefold. First, I showed how individuals' decision to act as if they were not feeling anxious induced a false sense of safety in others. When everyone acts that way even when they feel anxious, everyone ends up believing that the others are feeling safe even though everyone is anxious. This collective-level process of pluralistic ignorance induces complacency at the community level. To fight against this collective bias, community leaders must put in extra effort to encourage people to express their anxiety and explain why this expression is not a sign of weakness or moral deficit (Schroeder & Prentice, 1998). A community-level norm of frank disclosure of anxiety and other feelings would be an important step toward breaking people's failure to see how others really feel (Miller & McFarland, 1987).

Second, when there is a conflict between personal interest and the public good, the public good might often be ignored, especially in individualistic societies. When individuals act to promote their self-interest, they often contribute to the decline of the public good. For example, wearing a mask is uncomfortable and, in fact, not always consequential at the individual level. Nevertheless, if everyone in a community ends up not wearing a mask in public spaces, small effects can accumulate to propagate the virus at the community level. This collective-level dynamic, called the tragedy of commons, is yet another important mechanism contributing to the spread of the virus. To fight against this collective bias, it is essential for the leaders of collectives, whether the collectives are a nation, state, or municipality, to send constant messages highlighting the essential role of the collective as a source of pride and the identity of each member of the collective (Van Bavel et al., 2022). However, to make this strategy work, it would be crucial to build trust in both government and science by being transparent. There must be a constant effort to develop strong social norms for prosocial preventive actions (Habersaat et al., 2020; Van Bavel et al., 2022) (see Chapter 13 on prosocial behavior in COVID-19).

The third collective-level dynamic discussed was related to the second but distinct. There are multiple ways in which individualism can be a risk factor during pandemics. As a constellation of values and practices prioritizing freedom and autonomy over collective good, individualism may be directly linked to the tragedy of commons discussed above. However, just as important, individualism is often related to relatively loose enforcement of social norms (Gelfand et al., 2011). When such loose normative enforcement occurs in relationships, individualism may be expected to entail relatively free and normatively unconstrained choices of who to interact with. Thus, people in individualistic countries tend to be socially more open, increasing the chance of direct social contact with many strangers, which is a direct risk of spreading the virus during a pandemic.

To fight against this, policymakers may use individual incentives for engaging in behaviors that go against their individualistic intuitions and motivations. For example, mask wearing must be rewarded. Or, as some U.S. states have done, the government may offer incentives to take the vaccination. Eventually, however, it may be necessary to breed a community spirit grounded in each person's identity as a proud member of the collective of which they are part (Van Bavel et al., 2022).

The 21st century is said to be an era of infectious disease (Quammen, 2012). Humans will face increasingly frequent assaults from infectious viruses of nonhuman animal origin. This increase is inevitable, given expanding global human mobility, combined with more frequent contact with nonhuman animals resulting from a population explosion and industrialization. Challenging and problematic as this prospect might be, it also presents great opportunities for social and behavioral scientists to explore ways to preempt human misery and possibly enhance human welfare. This effort, in turn, may inform basic theories of our field. As Kurt Lewin noted decades ago: "There is nothing as practical as a good theory" (1943, p. 118). I hope this chapter will contribute in some small ways to this dialectic of applied and basic research.

ACKNOWLEDGMENT

This chapter is based on an Association of Psychological Science (APS) Presidential Column in the October 2020 issue of *APS Observer*.

REFERENCES

Allport, F. H. (1924). *Social psychology*. Houghton Mifflin.

Betsch, C., Böhm, R., Korn, L., & Holtmann, C. (2017). On the benefits of explaining herd immunity in vaccine advocacy. *Nature Human Behaviour*, *1*(3), 0056. https://doi.org/10.1038/s41562-017-0056

Campos, B., & Kim, H. S. (2017). Incorporating the cultural diversity of family and close relationships into the study of health. *American Psychologist*, *72*(6), 543. https://doi.org/10.1037/amp0000122

Cohen, D., & Kitayama, S. (Eds.). (2018). *Handbook of cultural psychology* (2nd ed.). The Guilford Press.

Gehring, W. J., Liu, Y., Orr, J. M., & Carp, J. (2011, December 15). The error-related negativity (ERN/Ne). In E. S. Kappenman & S. J. Luck (Eds.), *The Oxford handbook of event-related potential components* (pp. 232–292). Oxford Academic. https://doi.org/10.1093/oxfordhb/9780195374148.013.0120

Gelfand, M. J., Raver, J. L., Nishii, L., Leslie, L. M., Lun, J., Lim, B. C., Duan, L., Almaliach, A., Ang, S., Arnadottir, J., Aycan, Z., Boehnke, K., Boski, P., Cabecinhas, R., Chan, D., Chhokar, J., D'Amato, A., Ferrer, M., Fischlmayr, I. C., . . . Yamaguchi, S. (2011). Differences between tight and loose cultures: A 33-nation study. *Science*, *332*(6033), 1100–1104. https://doi.org/10.1126/science.1197754

Habersaat, K. B., Betsch, C., Danchin, M., Sunstein, C. R., Böhm, R., Falk, A., Brewer, N. T., Omer, S. B., Scherzer, M., Sah, S., Fischer, E. F., Scheel, A. E., Fancourt, D., Kitayama, S., Dubé, E., Leask, J., Dutta, M., MacDonald, N. E., Temkina, A., . . . Butler, R. (2020). Ten considerations for effectively managing the COVID-19 transition. *Nature Human Behaviour, 4*(7), 677–687. https://doi.org/10.1038/s41 562-020-0906-x

Hardin, G. (1968). The tragedy of the commons. *Science, 162,* 1243–1248.

Hofstede, G. (1980). *Culture's Consequences: International Differences in Work-Related Values.* SAGE.

Kunda, Z. (1990). The case for motivated reasoning. *Psychological Bulletin, 108*(3), 480–498. https://doi.org/10.1037/0033-2909.108.3.480

Lewin, K. (1943). Psychology and the process of group living. *The Journal of Social Psychology, 17*(3), 113–131.

Lu, J. G., Jin, P., & English, A. S. (2021). Collectivism predicts mask use during COVID-19. *Proceedings of the National Academy of Sciences of the United States of America, 118*(23), e2021793118. https://doi.org/10.1073/pnas.2021793118

Lyu, W., & Wehby, G. L. (2020). Community use of face masks and COVID-19: Evidence from a natural experiment of state mandates in the US. *Health Affairs, 39*(8), 1419–1425. https://doi.org/10.1377/hlthaff.2020.00818

Markus, H. R., & Kitayama, S. (1991). Culture and the self: Implications for cognition, emotion, and motivation. *Psychological Review, 98*(2), 224.

Miller, D. T. (1999). The norm of self-interest. *American Psychologist, 54*(12), 1053–1060.

Miller, D. T., & McFarland, C. (1987). Pluralistic ignorance: When similarity is interpreted as dissimilarity. *Journal of Personality and Social Psychology, 53*(2), 298–305. https://doi.org/10.1037/0022-3514.53.2.298

Miller, D. T., & Prentice, D. A. (1994). Collective errors and errors about the collective. *Personality & Social Psychology Bulletin, 20*(5), 541–550.

Park, B., Genevsky, A., Knutson, B., & Tsai, J. (2020). Culturally valued facial expressions enhance loan request success. *Emotion, 20*(7), 1137–1153. https://doi.org/10.1037/ emo0000642

Quammen, D. (2012). *Spillover: Animal infections and the next human pandemic.* W. W. Norton & Company.

Ross, L. (1977). The intuitive psychologist and his shortcomings: Distortions in the attribution process. *Advances in Experimental Social Psychology, 10,* 173–220. https:// doi.org/10.1016/S0065-2601(08)60357-3

Rousseau, J.-J. (1762). *The social contract, or principles of political rights.*

Salvador, C. E., Berg, M. K., Yu, Q., Martin, A. S., & Kitayama, S. (2020). Relational mobility predicts faster spread of COVID-19: A 39-country study. *Psychological Science, 31,* 1236–1244.

Salvador, C. E., Idrovo Carlier, S., Ishii, K., Torres Carlier, C., Nanakdewa, K., Savani, K., San Martin, A., & Kitayama, S. (in press). Emotionally expressive interdependence in Latin America: Triangulating through a comparison of three cultural regions. *Emotion.* https://doi.org/10.31234/osf.io/pw4yk

Schroeder, C. M., & Prentice, D. A. (1998). Exposing pluralistic ignorance to reduce alcohol use among college students. *Journal of Applied Social Psychology, 28*(23), 2150–2180. https://doi.org/10.1111/j.1559-1816.1998.tb01365.x

Taylor, S. E., & Brown, J. D. (1988). Illusion and well-being: A social psychological perspective on mental health. *Psychological Bulletin, 103*(2), 193–210.

Thomson, R., Yuki, M., Talhelm, T., Schug, J., Kito, M., Ayanian, A. H., Becker, J. C., Becker, M., Chiu, C., Choi, H.-S., Ferreira, C. M., Fülöp, M., Gul, P., Houghton-Illera, A. M., Joasoo, M., Jong, J., Kavanagh, C. M., Khutkyy, D., Manzi, C., . . . Visserman, M. L. (2018). Relational mobility predicts social behaviors in 39 countries and is tied to historical farming and threat. *Proceedings of the National Academy of Sciences of the United States of America, 115*(29), 7521–7526. https://doi.org/10.1073/pnas.171 3191115

Triandis, H. C. (1995). *Individualism & collectivism* (pp. xv, 259). Westview Press.

Tsao, S.-F., Chen, H., Tisseverasinghe, T., Yang, Y., Li, L., & Butt, Z. A. (2021). What social media told us in the time of COVID-19: A scoping review. *Lancet Digital Health, 3*(3), e175–e194. https://doi.org/10.1016/S2589-7500(20)30315-0

Van Bavel, J. J., Baicker, K., Boggio, P. S., Capraro, V., Cichocka, A., Cikara, M., Crockett, M. J., Crum, A. J., Douglas, K. M., Druckman, J. N., Drury, J., Dube, O., Ellemers, N., Finkel, E. J., Fowler, J. H., Gelfand, M., Han, S., Haslam, S. A., Jetten, J., . . . Willer, R. (2020). Using social and behavioural science to support COVID-19 pandemic response. *Nature Human Behaviour, 3*, 460–471. https://doi.org/10.1038/s41 562-020-0884-z

Van Bavel, J. J., Cichocka, A., Capraro, V., Sjåstad, H., Nezlek, J. B., Alfano, M., . . . Hudecek, M. F. C. (2022). National identity predicts public health support during a global pandemic: Results from 67 nations. *Nature Communications, 13*, 517. https://www.nature.com/articles/s41467-021-27668-9

Vandello, J. A., & Cohen, D. (1999). Patterns of individualism and collectivism across the United States. *Journal of Personality and Social Psychology, 77*(2), 279–292.

Yuki, M., Maddux, W. W., & Masuda, T. (2007). Are the windows to the soul the same in the East and West? Cultural differences in using the eyes and mouth as cues to recognize emotions in Japan and the United States. *Journal of Experimental Social Psychology, 43*(2), 303–311. https://doi.org/10.1016/j.jesp.2006.02.004

17

The Role of Attitude Strength in Addressing the COVID-19 Pandemic

JOSEPH J. SIEV, MENGRAN XU, ANDREW LUTTRELL, AND RICHARD E. PETTY ■

Health professionals might have imagined that it would be relatively easy in the midst of a global pandemic to convince members of society to take relatively simple steps to protect their own lives and those of others. Yet, in the United States and elsewhere, vehement opposition to seemingly easy behaviors like mask wearing developed, and vaccine hesitancy in some segments of the population threatened to undermine reaching herd immunity. This chapter addresses how health communicators might go about influencing strong attitudes and provides insight into the features of attitudes that help them guide behavior, with special attention paid to health-relevant actions.

ATTITUDE STRENGTH

Strong attitudes are typically defined by their consequences. That is, strong attitudes, like strong people, are durable (stable over time and resistant to change) and impactful (biasing thoughts and influencing behavior; Krosnick & Petty, 1995; Petty et al., 2023). There are several specific attributes of attitudes that indicate whether or not they are likely to produce these consequences (Luttrell & Sawicki, 2020). For example, the more an attitude has a moral basis, is held with certainty, or lacks ambivalence, the stronger it tends to be (see Chapters 9 and 10 on morality and uncertainty). Attitude strength is separate from the attitude itself. Thus, two people could both rate the desirability of a COVID-19 vaccine as an 8

Joseph J. Siev, Mengran Xu, Andrew Luttrell, and Richard E. Petty, *The Role of Attitude Strength in Addressing the COVID-19 Pandemic* In: *The Social Science of the COVID-19 Pandemic*. Edited by: Monica K. Miller, Oxford University Press.

on a 1-to-10 scale, but one person might have more confidence that their attitude is correct than another. Although the individual attitude attributes (like certainty and moral basis) are imperfect indicators of strength and can interact with each other to determine outcomes (cf. Visser et al., 2006), we treat the most common strength indicators similarly in this chapter because despite some differences, their similarities are more striking.

As noted, one of the core challenges in dealing with human behavior in a pandemic is that some people, those with the strongest attitudes, are resistant to attitude and behavior change (Petty & Krosnick, 1995). Thus, it becomes important to understand how to influence these deeply entrenched attitudes if they are contrary to the public interest. The first part of this chapter discusses two ways we have found that can be effective in making strong attitudes more open to change: (1) targeting the strength basis of the attitude with a message-matching strategy and (2) presenting recipients with a two-sided rather than the traditional one-sided communication. The second part of the chapter explains the role that attitude strength plays in determining behavior. In most instances, the stronger the attitude is, the more it guides behavior. However, as we explain, in some instances that might be especially likely to occur in threatening contexts (e.g., during a pandemic), the opposite can occur (Petty et al., 2023). In short, this chapter documents the importance of understanding the role that attitude strength can play in attempts to influence people's attitudes and behaviors related to COVID-19.

CHANGING STRONG ATTITUDES

People are reluctant to change their strongly held attitudes because it can arouse dissonance (Festinger, 1957; see Chapter 6). We describe two methods of changing strong attitudes. The first focuses on matching the message content to the reason the attitude is strong. The second focuses on providing a two-sided rather than a one-sided message.

Overcoming Resistance With Personalized Matching

One reason people resist changing their strong attitudes to a message is that the message arguments are misaligned with the attitudes' bases. Much research in persuasive communication has documented evidence for "matching effects" (Teeny et al., 2021): Messages are often more effective when they are tailored to some aspect of the recipient. Although these effects can take many forms, a common type of matching occurs when a message targets the attitude's underlying basis. If a message can be tailored to the reason an attitude is strong, it can undermine the resistance that is typical.

MATCHING TO ATTITUDE STRENGTH ATTRIBUTES
Consider the challenge of changing moralized attitudes. Although such attitudes often resist social influence (Luttrell et al., 2016), our research suggested that

messages that speak directly to moral concerns can be effective. In a series of studies, Luttrell et al. (2019) presented counterattitudinal messages to samples of pro-recycling and pro-marijuana legalization respondents. Participants were randomly assigned to read either a message containing moral arguments or one containing pragmatic arguments. In addition, all participants rated the extent to which their attitudes had a moral basis (Skitka, 2010). An interaction between message type and moral basis on attitudes revealed that, when people read pragmatic arguments, the typical effect of moralization emerged: greater moralization produced more resistance to change. However, when people read moral arguments, resistance was reduced. In fact, among people with highly moralized views, the moral arguments led to more attitude change than the pragmatic arguments.

A similar kind of moral matching has been demonstrated in the context of the COVID-19 pandemic. Prior health communication research has shown that other-focused messages (e.g., arguing to adopt a health practice to protect one's community) are often better at influencing people to adopt health practices such as handwashing (Grant & Hofmann, 2011), quitting smoking (Lipkus et al., 2013), and getting vaccinated (Kelly & Hornik, 2016) than are self-focused messages (i.e., protecting oneself; see Chapter 13 on cooperation). Because people typically perceive other-focused appeals to be moral arguments, we hypothesized and found that other-focused messages were rated as more persuasive and produced greater intentions to practice social distancing when an audience moralized public health (Luttrell & Petty, 2021).

Notably, it is important to present the right kinds of moral arguments. Consistent with research showing that politically liberal and conservative people differ in the moral values that they prioritize (Graham et al., 2013), a growing literature has shown that different moral arguments appeal to liberal and conservative audiences (Feinberg & Willer, 2019; see Chapter 37 on moral foundations). In accord with this more specific matching proposal, a recent set of studies found that arguments for wearing face masks were more persuasive to liberal audiences when they were framed in terms of fairness and avoiding harm as opposed to patriotism and purity (Trentadue & Luttrell, in press).

The basic principle of personalized matching can be broadly applied to other attitude strength features besides morality. For example, people are often less likely to change attitudes they feel certain about (e.g., Bassili, 1996) in part because they pay less attention to a message when they already feel confident (Tiedens & Linton, 2001). However, if a message appeals directly to confidence (Tormala et al., 2008), it can undermine resistance by increasing the motivation to think about the message. Similarly, if one's attitude is strong because it is based on considerable thought, a message framed to appeal to high thinkers can be more successful than one framed for those who do not like to think (See et al., 2009; Wheeler et al., 2005).

WHY MATCHING UNDERMINES RESISTANCE

There are several reasons why tailoring a message to strength attributes can be persuasive according to the elaboration likelihood model of persuasion (Petty

& Cacioppo, 1986). When people are relatively unmotivated or unable to think about a message, matching can act as a simple cue that the message's conclusion should be accepted because the conclusion seems correct (i.e., it matches the way the person thinks about the issue and feels right). However, when thinking is high, matched messages can be more persuasive because their arguments are evaluated in a biased way and actually seem stronger (Luttrell et al., 2019). When thinking is unconstrained, matching can motivate people to process the message content, leading to greater persuasion when that content is compelling but less persuasion when the content is weak (see Teeny et al., 2021, for a detailed review of matching effects).

Future research on matching should investigate the longer term consequences of matching effects that operate by different mechanisms. In addition, new ways in which messages can be tailored to strength-related attitude features should be studied. For example, perhaps health messages that directly contend with attitude importance, accessibility, or univalence (all strength attributes) could counteract the resistance these variables typically confer.

Overcoming Resistance With Two-Sided Messages

As just discussed, the extent to which a message connects to the reason one's attitude is strong can help undermine resistance. However, it is not always possible to construct compelling matched messages. Thus, it is important to consider other ways to influence deeply held views. In a series of studies, Xu and Petty (2022) found that messages containing arguments in favor of the advocated position as well as a few arguments in opposition, *two-sided messages*, can be more effective at persuading those with strongly held attitudes than messages that contain only arguments in favor of the advocated position, *one-sided messages*.

EVIDENCE FOR THE EFFECTIVENESS OF TWO-SIDED MESSAGES

Past research on message sidedness had shown that sometimes two-sided messages can have a persuasive advantage, but this depended on various other factors, such as the intelligence and educational levels of the recipients (Hovland et al., 1949). One important feature of two-sided messages is that they provide some acknowledgment that the side opposite to the side advocated has some merit. Thus, people with strong attitudes might especially appreciate their side being acknowledged and could reciprocate by being open to the advocate's position. Acknowledging the recipient's opinion is conceptually similar to doing a favor for the recipient. Based on the norm of reciprocity (Cialdini et al., 1992), if another person does a favor for us, then we should do the same. So, if a speaker seems open to the recipient's position, the recipient should be open to the speaker's view. Importantly, acknowledging a person's strongly held opinion should be analogous to doing a larger favor and therefore produce greater reciprocation.

To test this hypothesis, in one study Xu and Petty (2022) used the topic of mask wearing in the context of COVID-19. Participants first rated their attitude toward the topic, and only those who had a negative or slightly positive attitude toward mask wearing were included. To gauge the strength of their attitudes, participants' perceived moral basis was assessed. Next, everyone was randomly presented with a one- or two-sided message arguing that the public should always wear face coverings when they leave home during the pandemic. Then, participants responded to measures of openness to change, attitudes about mask wearing, and intentions to wear a mask when they left home. For each measure, a two-way interaction between moral basis and message sidedness emerged. As the moral basis of participants' attitudes increased, the two-sided message became increasingly more effective than the one-sided communication. Thus, this study demonstrated that using two-sided (vs. one-sided) messages can be a more effective influence tool as attitude strength (indexed by moral basis) increases. Finally, this study also provided evidence for the proposed reciprocity mechanism because a measure of how much recipients appreciated that the speaker acknowledged their view mediated the impact of the independent variables on openness, attitudes, and intentions.

To ensure the robustness of this effect, conceptual replications were conducted using additional topics (e.g., gun control) with success. In addition to using other topics, further research demonstrated that it was not sufficient to merely present a two-sided message, but that the recipient's side needed to be acknowledged with respect. In one study, Xu and Petty (2022) manipulated the quality of the arguments presented on the second side (i.e., the side acknowledging the recipient's position). Results indicated that that a two-sided message elicited more appreciation and was more effective than a one-sided message among those with morally based attitudes only when the second side was presented with strong arguments. When weak arguments for the other side were provided, the two-sided message was no more effective than the one-sided communication.

Finally, although the initial studies on two-sided messages used moral basis as the method of indexing attitude strength, the same results were shown when different attitude strength indicators were examined. In one study, Xu and Petty (in press) presented participants with a one- or two-sided message that challenged their current views on appropriate dental hygiene practices. To measure attitude strength, the certainty with which participants held their positions was assessed. Again, it was observed that, as certainty in the participants' position increased, the two-sided message became increasingly more impactful over the one-sided communication. In yet another demonstration, participants received a message asking them to consider the views of the political party opposite to their own. Strength of party identification was used as the indicator of attitude strength. Results similar to those just reported were obtained. Finally, the interaction between message sidedness and attitude strength was also replicated when the advocacy was for people to shift from their existing consumer brand (e.g., from an iPhone to an Android) and the measure of attitude strength was brand loyalty (see Xu et al., 2023).

FUTURE RESEARCH DIRECTIONS
For future research, it is important to continue examining exactly what elements are needed in the second side of a two-sided message for it to be more effective

than a one-sided communication. For example, although a strong acknowledgment of the other side was effective, can the acknowledgment be too strong? And, should the acknowledgment of the other side occur at the beginning of the message or at the end (as in the reviewed studies)? Last, in future work, it would be of interest for researchers to explore the role of additional mechanisms beyond perceived appreciation. For example, a two-sided message might reduce psychological reactance (Brehm, 1966; see Chapter 8 for more on reactance) or might produce a type of self-affirmation (Steele, 1988; see Chapter 7 for more on self-enhancement), and this affirmation could render people more open to counterattitudinal messages.

ASSURANCE VERSUS COMPENSATION EFFECTS OF ATTITUDE STRENGTH

Having discussed methods of influencing strong attitudes, we now consider when attitudes are most likely to result in behavior. In general, attitudes tend to be more predictive of behavior when they are strong—when based in morality or held with high certainty (Petty & Krosnick, 1995). That is, attitudes often best predict behavior when people feel *assured* about them. However, as described shortly, people can sometimes be more motivated to act on their attitudes precisely because they lack assurance in either themselves or their attitudes. Weaker attitudes are most in need of defending and might be most likely to produce compensatory behavior if this weakness is threatening for some reason. Before turning to our research on assured versus compensatory attitude-behavior consistency (ABC) and considering its implications for compliance with public health directives, we first provide some context by describing two other forms of *assured versus compensatory attitude effects*.

Assured Versus Compensatory Conviction

The distinction between assured versus compensatory attitude effects was first evident in work on attitudinal *conviction*. Conviction is conceptualized as possessing *extreme* attitudes and is frequently assessed by measuring an attitude's *polarization*, or distance from a bipolar scale's neutral midpoint (Abelson, 1995). Assured conviction occurs when feeling confident increases attitude polarization. For example, Baron et al. (1996) showed that increasing confidence (assurance) in a person's attitude by having others agree with it (social consensus) versus providing no statement of agreement led people's attitudes to become more extreme.

In contrast, compensatory conviction occurs when experiencing a threat increases attitude polarization because of a desire for confidence. For example, McGregor et al. (2001) demonstrated that having people experience threatening uncertainty from writing about a difficult personal dilemma versus a nonthreatening situation led them to express more confidence and take more extreme positions on various unrelated political issues. Interestingly, this did not occur when participants repaired their sense of assurance by affirming their personal values prior to completing the measures (Steele, 1988). In sum, both feeling assured and feeling threat can enhance attitude confidence and extremity.

Assured Versus Compensatory Thought Validation

Just as assured and compensatory conviction can stem from feelings of confidence and threat, respectively, similar phenomena occur with respect to people's decision to rely on their own thoughts, which can polarize attitudes. Assured thought validation occurs when making people feel confident increases their thought reliance, whereas compensatory thought validation occurs when making people feel threatened increases it. When people rely on their positive thoughts more, their attitudes become more extreme in a favorable direction, and vice versa for negative thoughts.

In the initial study on assured thought validation, Petty et al. (2002) exposed people to messages presenting strong or weak arguments and assessed the participants' thoughts in response to the message. The confidence participants had in their thoughts was manipulated by telling them either that others had similar thoughts (social validation/high confidence) or not. Demonstrating assured thought validation, people used their thoughts more in the high confidence condition. This was evident because attitudes were more consistent with the quality of the arguments presented (i.e., more favorable when arguments were strong and less favorable when weak) when participants were in the high than the low confidence condition (see Briñol & Petty, 2022, for a review).

However, feeling threatened can also produce thought validation. In one study illustrating this compensatory validation, Moreno et al. (in press) exposed participants to the resume of a job candidate whose qualifications were compelling or lacking. Participants were then randomly assigned to write about what it would feel like to get COVID-19 (threatening uncertainty) or what it would feel like to feel very cold (mild uncertainty; Pyszczynski et al., 2015), after which their attitudes toward the job candidate were assessed (see Chapter 33 on terror management theory). Consistent with a compensatory thought validation effect, participants in the threatening uncertainty (vs. mild uncertainty) condition relied on their thoughts more, reporting attitudes that were more consistent with the job candidates' qualifications (i.e., more polarized). In sum, both feeling assured and feeling threatened can enhance thought confidence and reliance, resulting in more extreme attitudes (see also, Briñol et al., 2015).

Assured Versus Compensatory Attitude-Behavior Consistency

Much like people can compensate for feelings of threat by showing greater reliance on their thoughts to guide their attitudes, they can also compensate by showing greater reliance on their attitudes to guide their behavior. This third type of compensation, ABC, can take two forms. First, people who experience a threat to themselves, such as interpersonal rejection or concern about getting COVID, can demonstrate a *fluid compensatory ABC effect* (cf. Heine et al., 2006) by acting on their attitudes in a domain that is not relevant to the threat (see Chapter 47 on threat). This outcome would parallel the research on compensatory conviction and thought validation just described in that people respond to a self-threat by affirming their attitudes in a domain different from the threat. Though conceptually sensible, this type of compensatory ABC has not yet been demonstrated in the literature.

A second form of compensatory ABC occurs when people who experience threatening uncertainty about a particular attitude can attempt to compensate by acting on that very same attitude (Siev et al., 2022; see also Sawicki & Wegener, 2018). This *attitude-specific compensatory ABC* outcome results in people being more willing to act on weak (e.g., uncertain, ambivalent) than strong (e.g., certain, univalent) attitudes and contrasts with the common and well-known assured ABC pattern in which the opposite occurs.

ATTITUDE-SPECIFIC COMPENSATORY ABC

Recent research has pointed to conditions under which attitude-specific compensatory versus assured ABC is more likely. First, whereas increasing attitude certainty tends to increase ABC when feelings of threat are minimal, increasing attitude uncertainty can increase ABC when people experience the uncertainty as threatening in some way. Second, attitude-specific compensatory ABC may also be more likely when particular kinds of behavior are involved. For example, considering engaging in extreme behaviors (e.g., violent actions) is more likely to prompt compensation than considering more moderate behaviors because: (1) considering extreme behaviors suggests the possibility of additional threats (e.g., bodily harm) that could make attitude uncertainty more aversive and/or (2) engaging in extreme behaviors can offer a compelling response to attitude uncertainty because it sends a strong signal to oneself and others about commitment to one's attitude. Extreme behaviors (much like extreme attitudes) can signal conviction because they are unusual and cannot be attributed to social norms (Kelley, 1973).

To test these ideas, in one study conducted during the COVID-19 pandemic (Siev et al., 2022), participants reported their attitudes about social distancing, certainty in those attitudes, and interest in engaging in a moderate form of attitude-consistent behavior (avoiding crowds to prevent viral spread) as well as a more extreme form (fighting someone who disagreed with their views). A regression analysis including all three variables produced a significant three-way interaction among attitudes, certainty, and behavioral extremity (Figure 17.1). To understand this interaction, the data were analyzed separately for each kind of behavior. Significant two-way interactions between attitudes and certainty were obtained for both moderate and extreme behavior. Whereas greater attitude certainty enhanced attitudinal prediction of moderate behavior (assured ABC, top

panel, Figure 17.1), lower certainty was associated with greater attitudinal prediction of extreme behavior (attitude-specific compensatory ABC, bottom panel,
Figure 17.1).

Contextual threat was also assessed by asking how concerned participants
were that they or someone close to them would become seriously ill with
COVID-19. We reasoned that being unsure about one's attitude toward social distancing would be more disconcerting when COVID-19 seemed threatening. An analysis including this measure as an additional predictor revealed
that the assured ABC effect was most pronounced when those relatively low in
contextual threat considered moderate behaviors, and the compensatory ABC
effect was most pronounced when those relatively high in contextual threat
considered extreme behaviors. These findings suggest that whether ABC is
assured or compensatory can depend on contextual factors (external threats)
and properties of the behavior (extremity; see Siev et al., 2023, for additional
studies).

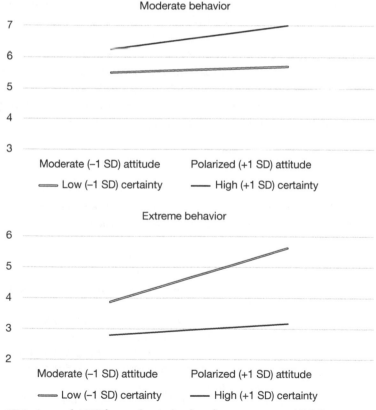

Figure 17.1 Assured ABC for moderate (top) and compensatory ABC for extreme
(bottom) behaviors.

IMPLICATIONS AND FUTURE RESEARCH

All of the compensatory effects described are possible and even likely during a pandemic because of the salient threats such conditions present. Thus, those expressing the most vehement pandemic-related opinions and the strongest behavioral commitment to them might paradoxically be people who actually feel some underlying attitudinal uncertainty and experience these doubts as threatening. Future research inspired by our findings might consider whether, when addressing audiences who generally favor mitigation efforts, emphasizing the threats posed by the virus would increase compliance among those harboring doubts about the issue. When addressing those who oppose mitigation policies, however, alleviating threats as much as possible could help reduce at least the most confrontational and extreme forms of defiant behavior.

SUMMARY AND CONCLUSIONS

We have examined the role that attitude strength plays in influencing behavior, especially as it relates to the COVID-19 pandemic and health communication more generally. We first addressed how particularly strong attitudes might be influenced and provided evidence for two techniques: (1) matching messages to the strength basis of the attitude and (2) providing two- rather than one-sided messages. We then reviewed how extreme attitudes could result from not only assurance but also threat and how behavior is sometimes more likely to be guided by attitudes held with certainty but sometimes by attitudes held with doubt. The behavioral challenges presented by the COVID-19 pandemic are complex, and the science of persuasion continues to generate novel findings that can help address them. Nonetheless, there are still new insights to be uncovered.

REFERENCES

Abelson, R. P. (1995). Attitude extremity. In R. E. Petty & J. A. Krosnick (Eds.), *Attitude strength: Antecedents and consequences* (pp. 25–41). Erlbaum.

Baron, R. S., Hoppe, S. I., Kao, C. F., Brunsman, B., Linneweh, B., & Rogers, D. (1996). Social corroboration and opinion extremity. *Journal of Experimental Social Psychology, 32*(6), 537–560. https://doi.org/10.1006/jesp.1996.0024

Bassili, J. N. (1996). Meta-judgmental versus operative indexes of psychological attributes: The case of measures of attitude strength. *Journal of Personality and Social Psychology, 71*(4), 637–653. https://doi.org/10.1037/0022-3514.71.4.637

Brehm, J. W. (1966). *A theory of psychological reactance.* Academic Press.

Briñol, P., & Petty, R. E. (2022). Self-validation theory: An integrative framework for understanding when thoughts become consequential. *Psychological Review, 129*(2), 340–367. https://doi.org/10.1037/rev0000340

Briñol, P., Petty, R. E., & DeMarree, K. (2015). Being threatened and being a threat can increase reliance on thoughts: A self-validation approach. In P. J. Carroll, R. M. Arkin, & A. Wichman (Eds.), *Handbook of personal security* (pp. 37–54). Psychology Press.

Cialdini, R. B., Green, B. L., & Rusch, A. J. (1992). When tactical pronouncements of change become real change: The case of reciprocal persuasion. *Journal of Personality and Social Psychology, 63*(1), 30–40. https://doi.org/10.1037/0022-3514.63.1.30

Feinberg, M., & Willer, R. (2019). Moral reframing: A technique for effective and persuasive communication across political divides. *Social and Personality Psychology Compass, 13*(12), e12501. https://doi.org/10.1111/spc3.12501

Festinger, L. (1957). *A theory of cognitive dissonance.* Stanford University Press.

Graham, J., Haidt, J., Koleva, S., Motyl, M., Iyer, R., Wojcik, S. P., & Ditto, P. H. (2013). Moral foundations theory: The pragmatic validity of moral pluralism. *Advances in Experimental Social Psychology, 47*, 55–130. https://doi.org/10.1016/B978-0-12-407236-7.00002-4

Grant, A. M., & Hofmann, D. A. (2011). It's not all about me: Motivating hand hygiene among health care professionals by focusing on patients. *Psychological Science, 22*(12), 1494–1499. https://doi.org/10.1177/0956797611419172

Heine, S. J., Proulx, T., & Vohs, K. D. (2006). The meaning maintenance model: On the coherence of social motivations. *Personality and Social Psychology Review, 10*(2), 88–110. https://doi.org/10.1207/s15327957pspr1002_1

Hovland, C. I., Lumsdaine, A. A., & Sheffield, F. D. (1949). *Experiments on mass communication.* Princeton University Press.

Kelley, H. H. (1973). The processes of causal attribution. *American Psychologist, 28*(2), 107–128. https://doi.org/10.1037/h0034225

Kelly, B. J., & Hornik, R. C. (2016). Effects of framing health messages in terms of benefits to loved ones or others: An experimental study. *Health Communication, 31*(10), 1284–1290. https://doi.org/10.1080/10410236.2015.1062976

Krosnick, J. A., & Petty, R. E. (1995). Attitude strength: An overview. In R. E. Petty & J. A. Krosnick (Eds.), *Attitude strength: Antecedents and consequences* (pp. 1–24). Erlbaum.

Lipkus, I. M., Ranby, K. W., Lewis, M. A., & Toll, B. (2013). Reactions to framing of cessation messages: Insights from dual-smoker couples. *Nicotine & Tobacco Research, 15*(12), 2022–2028. https://doi.org/10.1093/ntr/ntt091

Luttrell, A., & Petty, R. E. (2021). Evaluations of self-focused versus other-focused arguments for social distancing: An extension of moral matching effects. *Social Psychological and Personality Science, 12*(6), 946–954. https://doi.org/10.1177/1948550620947853

Luttrell, A., Petty, R. E., Briñol, P., & Wagner, B. C. (2016). Making it moral: Merely labeling an attitude as moral increases its strength. *Journal of Experimental Social Psychology, 65*, 82–93. https://doi.org/10.1016/j.jesp.2016.04.003

Luttrell, A., Philipp-Muller, A. Z., & Petty, R. E. (2019). Challenging moral attitudes with moral messages. *Psychological Science, 30*(8), 1136–1150. https://doi.org/10.1177/0956797619854706

Luttrell, A., & Sawicki, V. (2020). Attitude strength: Distinguishing predictors versus defining features. *Social and Personality Psychology Compass, 14*(8), e12555. https://doi.org/10.1111/spc3.12555

McGregor, I., Zanna, M. P., Holmes, J. G., & Spencer, S. J. (2001). Compensatory conviction in the face of personal uncertainty: Going to extremes and being oneself. *Journal of Personality and Social Psychology, 80*(3), 472–488. https://doi.org/10.1037/0022-3514.80.3.472

Moreno, L., Paredes, B., Horcajo, J., Briñol, P, See, Y. H., DeMarree, K., & Petty, R. E. (in press). The effects of perceived COVID-19 threat on compensatory conviction, thought reliance, and attitudes. *European Journal of Social Psychology.* https://doi. org/10.1002/ejsp.2976

Petty, R. E., Briñol, P., & Tormala, Z. L. (2002). Thought confidence as a determinant of persuasion: The self-validation hypothesis. *Journal of Personality and Social Psychology, 82*(5), 722–741. https://doi.org/10.1037/0022-3514.82.5.722

Petty, R. E., & Cacioppo, J. T. (1986). The elaboration likelihood model of persuasion. *Advances in Experimental Social Psychology, 19,* 123–205. https://doi.org/10.1016/ S0065-2601(08)60214-2

Petty, R. E., & Krosnick, J. A. (Eds.). (1995). *Attitude strength: Antecedents and consequences.* Erlbaum.

Petty, R. E., Siev, J. J., & Briñol, P. (2023). Attitude strength: What's new? *The Spanish Journal of Psychology, 26,* e4, 1–13. https://doi.org/10.1017/SJP.2023.7

Pyszczynski, T., Solomon, S., & Greenberg, J. (2015). Thirty years of terror management theory: From genesis to revelation. *Advances in Experimental Social Psychology, 52,* 1–70. https://doi.org/10.1016/bs.aesp.2015.03.001

Sawicki, V., & Wegener, D. T. (2018). Metacognitive reflection as a moderator of attitude strength versus attitude bolstering: Implications for attitude similarity and attraction. *Personality and Social Psychology Bulletin, 44*(5), 638–652. https://doi.org/ 10.1177/0146167217744196

See, Y. H. M., Petty, R. E., & Evans, L. M. (2009). The impact of perceived message complexity and need for cognition on information processing and attitudes. *Journal of Research in Personality, 43*(5), 880–889. https://doi.org/10.1016/j.jrp.2009.04.006

Siev, J. J., Petty, R. E., & Briñol, P. (2022). Attitudinal extremism. In A. W. Kruglanski, C. Kopetz, & E. Szumowska (Eds.). *The psychology of extremism: A motivational perspective* (pp. 34–65). Taylor & Francis.

Siev, J. J., Petty, R. E., Paredes, B., & Briñol, P. (2023). Behavioral extremity moderates the association between certainty in attitudes about Covid and willingness to engage in mitigation-related behaviors. *Social and Personality Psychology Compass, e12767,* 1–11. https://doi.org/10.1111/spc3.12767

Skitka, L. J. (2010). The psychology of moral conviction. *Social and Personality Psychology Compass, 4*(4), 267–281. https://doi.org/10.1111/j.1751-9004.2010.00254.x

Steele, C. M. (1988). The psychology of self-affirmation: Sustaining the integrity of the self. *Advances in Experimental Social Psychology, 21,* 261–302. https://doi.org/ 10.1016/S0065-2601(08)60229-4

Teeny, J. D., Siev, J. J., Briñol, P., & Petty, R. E. (2021). A review and conceptual framework for understanding personalized matching effects in persuasion. *Journal of Consumer Psychology, 31*(2), 382–414. https://doi.org/10.1002/jcpy.1198

Tiedens, L. Z., & Linton, S. (2001). Judgment under emotional certainty and uncertainty: The effects of specific emotions on information processing. *Journal of Personality and Social Psychology, 81*(6), 973–988. https://doi.org/10.1037/ 0022-3514.81.6.973

Tormala, Z. L., Rucker, D. D., & Seger, C. R. (2008). When increased confidence yields increased thought: A confidence-matching hypothesis. *Journal of Experimental Social Psychology, 44*(1), 141–147. https://doi.org/10.1016/j.jesp.2006.11.002

Trentadue, J., & Luttrell, A. (in press). Advocating for mask-wearing across the aisle: Support for moral reframing in health communication. *Health Communication.* https://doi.org/10.1080/10410236.2022.2163535

Visser, P. S., Bizer, G. Y., & Krosnick, J. A. (2006). Exploring the latent structure of strength-related attitude attributes. *Advances in Experimental Social Psychology, 38*, 1–67. https://doi.org/10.1016/S0065-2601(06)38001-X

Wheeler, S. C., Petty, R. E., & Bizer, G. Y. (2005). Self-schema matching and attitude change: Situational and dispositional determinants of message elaboration. *Journal of Consumer Research, 31*(4), 787–797. https://doi.org/10.1086/426613

Xu, M., Deng, X., & Petty, R. E. (2023). How two-sided messages increase brand switching interest among brand-loyal customers of competitive brands. Unpublished manuscript.

Xu, M., & Petty, R. E. (2022). Two-sided messages promote openness for morally-based attitudes. *Personality and Social Psychology Bulletin, 48*(8), 1151–1166. https://doi.org/10.1177/0146167220988371

Xu, M., & Petty, R. E. (in press). Two-sided messages promote openness for a variety of deeply entrenched attitudes. *Personality and Social Psychology Bulletin.* https://doi.org/10.1177/01461672221128113

FURTHER READING

Petty, R. E., Briñol, P., Fabrigar, L. R., & Wegener, D. T. (2019). Attitude structure and change. In E. J. Finkel & R. F. Baumeister (Eds.), *Advanced social psychology: The state of the science* (2nd ed., pp. 117–156). Oxford University Press.

Rucker, D. D., Tormala, Z. L., Petty, R. E., & Briñol, P. (2014). Consumer conviction and commitment: An appraisal-based framework for attitude certainty. *Journal of Consumer Psychology, 24*(1), 119–136. https://doi.org/10.1016/j.jcps.2013.07.001

Skitka, L. J., Hanson, B. E., Morgan, G. S., & Wisneski, D. C. (2021). The psychology of moral conviction. *Annual Review of Psychology, 72*, 347–366. https://doi.org/10.1146/annurev-psych-063020-030612

18

Trust in the Medical Profession

Reflections From the COVID-19 Pandemic

A. CHRISTINE EMLER AND BRIAN H. BORNSTEIN ■

Among the many unique features of the COVID-19 pandemic is the prominent, and arguably preeminent, role of the medical profession. Medical professionals have been extensively involved in understanding and explaining to the public the nature of the illness, health risks, and prophylactic measures; conducting (along with basic scientists) research on treatments and vaccines; treating infected persons; and administering vaccines. To be sure, medical professionals have performed the same functions during other recent public health threats, such as HIV/AIDS, Ebola, severe acute respiratory syndrome coronavirus 2 (SARS-CoV-1), and Zika. Yet to find something comparable to the current pandemic, one would arguably have to go back to the polio epidemic of the early mid-20th century (Kurlander, 2020). Then as now, much of people's response to the public health threat has been driven by their underlying attitudes toward the medical profession (see Chapter 17 for more on attitudes related to the pandemic).

Americans generally have a positive attitude toward their healthcare providers; that is, for the most part, people like and trust their doctors and nurses (e.g., nursing repeatedly ranks as the most trusted profession in Gallup polls; see https://www.advisory.com/daily-briefing/2020/01/10/nurse-trusted). However, their attitudes toward the healthcare *system*[1]—the diffuse conglomeration of public and private institutions, such as hospitals, health maintenance organizations (HMOs), health insurance companies, and government health departments at the county, state, and federal levels—are a good deal more nuanced. For example, significant differences exist as a function of individual trusters' own characteristics, especially their race and ethnicity, reflecting historic inequalities in the healthcare profession's treatment of minorities. To complicate the picture further, many actors within the healthcare system are themselves medical or allied professionals who provide health services (e.g., physicians, nurses, therapists, and technicians

A. Christine Emler and Brian H. Bornstein, *Trust in the Medical Profession* In: *The Social Science of the COVID-19 Pandemic*. Edited by: Monica K. Miller, Oxford University Press. © Oxford University Press 2024.
DOI: 10.1093/oso/9780197615133.003.0018

with various areas of expertise), but others are not (e.g., hospital, health department, and insurance company administrators).

In this chapter, we reflect on the phenomenon of trust in the medical profession through two intersecting lenses: the theoretical and empirical literature on trust in institutions and the unique circumstances created by the COVID-19 pandemic. These concepts underlying trust will help explain some pandemic-related behavior (e.g., vaccine hesitancy). The first section applies general principles of trust in institutions to the "normal" healthcare context. We then draw on the experiences of healthcare providers, healthcare administrators, and laypeople during the pandemic to discuss the ways in which the healthcare context during the pandemic has been distinctly abnormal. The third section reviews lessons learned during the pandemic so far, and we conclude in the final section with a discussion of next steps—both practical (i.e., how to build and repair trust) and empirical (i.e., needed research).

TRUST IN HEALTHCARE GENERALLY

Trust is a diffuse construct that has been defined in myriad ways and studied from diverse disciplinary perspectives (see, e.g., McEvily & Tortoriello, 2011; Shockley et al., 2016). It can be defined, broadly, as "a psychological state comprising the intention to accept vulnerability based upon positive expectations of the intentions or behavior of another" (Rousseau et al., 1998, p. 395); importantly, the "other" can be a person (e.g., trusting one's spouse) or an institution (e.g., trusting the county health department; see, generally, Bornstein & Tomkins, 2015), and because institutions are necessarily made up of individual people, the two overlap (e.g., trusting Congress vs. specific Congresspersons). Interpersonal trust and institutional trust interact in a bidirectional manner; for example, the more one trusts one's primary care provider, the more one is likely to trust the HMO/practice/hospital/system that employs that provider and vice versa. However, the institution itself persists as an entity despite turnover in personnel. Our focus in this chapter is on the healthcare system and medical profession (between which we do not distinguish for present purposes) as institutions.

Different models of trust in institutions propose various factors that, in addition to the truster's propensity to trust, comprise an institution's (or individual person's) perceived trustworthiness (some of the literature refers to these factors as "dimensions" or "constructs"; see, generally, McEvily & Tortoriello, 2011; PytlikZillig et al., 2016). A widely used model proposed by Mayer et al. (1995; see also Schoorman et al., 2015) distinguishes three key (ABI) factors: ability, perceptions that the trustee has the requisite competence and knowledge; benevolence, perceptions that the trustee is caring and concerned toward the truster; and integrity, perceptions of the trustee's moral character (e.g., honesty, fairness, and absence of bias). Absolute levels of the ABI factors will of course vary across trusters, across target institutions, across domains within an institution (e.g., a county health department might be seen as having high ability for managing an infectious disease but low ability for managing gun violence),[2] and over time (e.g., Americans' trust in many institutions, including the medical establishment, has declined in recent years; Twenge et al., 2014).

What do the ABI factors mean with respect to the healthcare system? The more trustworthy it is, the more that people, who are actual or potential consumers (i.e., patients), perceive it to have the expertise to diagnose, treat, and prevent illness (ability); act in patient-consumers' best interests (benevolence); and treat them fairly and impartially or without bias (integrity). The vulnerability aspect of trust is also essential in the healthcare context, as people are rarely more vulnerable than when their health is threatened—even more so if they are already sick (Campos-Castillo et al., 2016).

Most of the research on trust in healthcare focuses on trust in a specific provider, rather than healthcare institutions (Campos-Castillo et al., 2016). That research shows mixed results when looking at provider demographics (e.g., Nazione et al., 2019; Schoenthaler et al., 2014), but significant and persistent differences as a function of patient demographics. Specifically, Whites, women, and those with more education trust their physicians more than their counterparts; these patterns can generalize to attitudes toward the healthcare system in general (Campos-Castillo et al., 2016). The racial and ethnic differences, in particular, reflect historical and contemporary discrimination experienced by minorities, especially African Americans, in the American healthcare system (Hostetter & Klein, 2021). Moreover, as discussed in the following section, these differences have had major behavioral implications during the COVID-19 pandemic, especially in terms of willingness to seek treatment or be vaccinated.

Trust Determinants in Healthcare During the COVID-19 Pandemic: All Is Not Normal

During the COVID-19 pandemic, vulnerability has been thrust on the world in a way that obviates the "willingness to accept" clause in the classic definition of trust (described above). During the pandemic, healthcare systems shifted from consideration of individual patients' health needs to public health considerations. Elective surgeries and appointments were cancelled or postponed in order to decrease the stress on the healthcare system (i.e., to reduce the demand for personal protective equipment [PPE], decrease the potential exposure of healthcare workers to unknowingly COVID-positive patients, preserve beds for COVID-positive patients, etc.). This shift, while necessary and lifesaving for many patients who needed hospital-level care for COVID and other illnesses, represented a shift from a focus on the relationship between the healthcare system and the needs of individual patients to the needs of the population as a whole and the health of the healthcare system itself. This change in relationship dynamic was compounded further by the change in *how* patients were cared for by their healthcare teams during COVID-19: There was a shift from face-to-face care to telehealth visits (Koonin et al., 2020), such that patients no longer experienced the physical connection with their nurses, doctors, and other members of their healthcare teams; and when they were "seen" face to face, both the patients and the healthcare teams were masked, with providers sometimes in full PPE—again changing the nature of the relationship/interaction.

The shift from individual patient to population health might have contributed to the sense of vulnerability that not only patients experienced, but also healthcare workers themselves experienced—in a way that is not typical for day-to-day healthcare work. Although healthcare workers know they put themselves at risk each day by being in environments that expose them to infectious diseases, aggressive and violent behavior, and other uncertainties, these are generally well understood and to a large extent manageable and predictable (e.g., gowns, gloves, and signage outside of rooms with specific airflow parameters for patients with known infectious diseases). COVID-19 added layers of risk that were not well understood at first, and the science and understanding of the risks changed over time. Additionally, there were very real shortages and confusion over what level of PPE was needed and available for patient care, creating vulnerability for the staff providing care and the employees charged with obtaining the supplies (e.g., logistics and administrative teams). Finally, staff in some locations were overwhelmed by the sheer volume of patients and worked to the point of exhaustion.

How have the ABI (trust) factors fared during the COVID-19 pandemic? Again, there were a lot of unknowns at the beginning of COVID (and there still are). While collaboration in the scientific community has led to accelerated research and discovery, the changing understanding of diagnosis, spread, treatment, and prevention of the disease could contribute to confusion and plant seeds of doubt about the level of expertise available. For example, the question of masking, what kind, when and where was initially in question. Indeed, even though the Centers for Disease Control and Prevention and many other scientific bodies endorsed universal masking in areas with high rates of community transmission, there was uneven compliance with this recommendation, accompanied by considerable variability in regulations across states. Similarly, there were and continue to be questions about when, who, and what kind of testing should be done in what contexts. Clinical labs can detect viral genetic material (via polymerase chain reaction [PCR] testing) using nasal or oral samples (or even in wastewater) as well as the antibodies directed against viral particles in a patient's blood. However, the variety of tests and their inherent sensitivity and specificity metrics have led to disagreements and confusion even within the medical field about when to use the tests—that is, for diagnosis and treatment of individuals or for epidemiological assessments and public health planning. Testing was further complicated by the scarcity of tests and supplies to conduct them early in the pandemic. And now that vaccines are available, the public has additional data to consider in their estimates of healthcare's ability to prevent COVID-19.

Vaccine hesitancy is neither a new nor an insignificant phenomenon, and it speaks directly to the population's trust of healthcare systems, especially the extent to which they are seen as benevolent and having integrity. The 2015 U.S. National Vaccine Advisory Committee ("Assessing the State of Vaccine Confidence,"

2015) indicated that, while childhood vaccine acceptance remained high (80%–90%), the perception of providers was that families were requesting vaccination schedules different from those recommended at higher rates than in the past. Americans displayed substantial COVID-19 vaccine hesitancy, though it varied as a function of race and ethnicity. For example, when COVID vaccines were first rolled out in late 2020, over 60% of Whites and Hispanics and 83% of Asian Americans said they intended to be vaccinated, compared to only 42% of African Americans (Funk & Tyson, 2020; see also Latkin et al., 2021). As vaccinations overall became more widespread in early 2021, these racial/ethnic differences narrowed yet persisted (Funk & Tyson, 2021). These data point to significant levels of vaccine distrust engendered by a number of factors, including speed of vaccine testing and approval, with insufficient communication about the development, testing, and distribution process (including the "warp speed" process); long-standing distrust of both government in general and the healthcare profession in particular (from, e.g., the Tuskegee syphilis study; see Chapters 23–25 for more on systemic bias related to COVID-19); and the politicization and polarization of regulatory and public health bodies.

A *British Medical Journal* editorial published in the fall of 2020 suggested that a perceived lack of benevolence, due to politicization of science, is not just an American problem. According to Kamran Abbasi (2020), executive editor of the journal, membership in the Scientific Advisory Group for Emergencies underrepresented minorities, women, and clinicians. Additionally, the government suppressed scientific reports on COVID-19 and ethnic-based inequalities—and authors were instructed not to speak to the media. The consequences of politicization of science are dire: "Suppressing science, whether by delaying publication, cherry picking favourable research, or gagging scientists, is a danger to public health, causing deaths by exposing people to unsafe or ineffective interventions and preventing them from benefitting from better ones" (Abbasi, 2020, p. 2). This dynamic was seen in our country as well. (For example, the controversies surrounding hydroxychloroquine [Berlivet & Löwry, 2020], and a senator involved in sales of stocks whose worth would subsequently drop while coauthoring an opinion piece about coronavirus response [Mak, 2020]) see Chapter 3 for more on the politicization of COVID-19.)

Concerns about the equitable distribution of resources speak to the integrity component of trust. Studies have shown that Black and Hispanic communities have suffered more from COVID-19 than their White counterparts. This is aggravated by lack of access to healthcare in these communities (Douglas & Subica, 2020). For some, disparities were reinforced by the public display of the high-level care President Trump received during his bout with COVID-19, compared to the care available to many other Americans—further highlighting the need for greater integrity in our healthcare system as a whole (Baker, 2020; see Chapter 4 for more on COVID-19 ethics, Chapter 3 for COVID-19 healthcare policies, and Chapters 23–25 for systemic biases related to COVID-19).

The dissolution of trust occurs when expectations are violated. COVID-19 created a world where healthcare institutions shifted their focus from individual people to populations, where everyone was vulnerable, where changing science contributed to questioning of ability, politicization of science led to concerns about benevolence, and health inequities cast a shadow on the integrity of the system. The upside of these challenges is that they provided fertile ground for learning lessons, as discussed in the following section.

LESSONS LEARNED DURING THE PANDEMIC

One of the authors of this chapter has had the distinct privilege to work with a high-functioning healthcare system and has seen firsthand some things that worked well and some things that were less successful in achieving our aims of improving and preserving the health and well-being of our patients.

Early in the pandemic, leadership quickly shifted to an emergency management/incident command format in which administrators deferred to the expertise of experts in infectious diseases, cleaning, vaccines, and health promotion. Communication is always an essential part of leadership, and very often it is the biggest challenge for leadership and one of the largest dissatisfiers for staff in any organization. Add a pandemic in which many staff members were sent home to telework, and the challenges of communication triple. At our facility, and likely many others, we wanted to share what we knew, even though that was a moving target. Early in the pandemic, the facility's executive director started hosting a daily hour-long virtual town hall, produced by our public affairs team. He invited an infectious disease expert (who became the chief of the newly created Office of Public Health and Epidemiology) to share information about COVID-19. Other experts spoke, and as staff became weary from the work, local celebrities were invited to share their gratitude for the staff and all of our essential workers. We also found a need to bolster our abilities as healthcare providers to tackle this new disease. We set up a weekly hour-long COVID continuing medical education conference (COVID-19 Clinical Concepts for Provider Optimization—C3PO) with physician scientists and other experts that was open to all. The topics were all on the emerging literature and experience of treating COVID-19.

Demonstrating benevolence to staff and patients throughout COVID was an important and deliberate step in maintaining and even building trust. For staff, many of whom were suddenly faced with homeschooling their children while trying to maintain full-time jobs, we offered flexibility with telework, providing laptops and phones whenever possible. We also allowed, whenever possible, for shifts in tours of duty to support family challenges. Procuring masks and other PPE was a priority, and a reprocessing system was purchased early on when it was not clear that there would be sufficient N95 masks for staff providing bedside care. For our patients, we shifted services and had a several hundred-fold increase in our use of telemedicine, via both phone call and video visits.

The "digital divide" that increases health disparities exists for our patients as well. We worked to identify patients who could benefit from access to devices and expanded mechanisms to send patients modified handheld tablets to allow patients to connect with their healthcare teams. Which member of the team shares messages regarding health information may also be important. "Trusted messengers" can help allay concerns (Fadulu, 2020). Examples of this include town halls funded by the National Institutes of Health; Black scientists spoke in these town halls about vaccination to predominantly Black audiences (Fadulu, 2020); Black and other minority physicians have engaged in similar efforts (Kolata, 2020). At our facility, healthcare providers of color volunteered to reach out to populations and clinics where vaccine acceptance lagged. This behavior was not confined to physicians, nurses, pharmacists, and other professionals. Indeed, one provider (White) was having a conversation with a patient and his wife (Black) about the importance of getting vaccinated. The patient and his wife were on the fence. An environmental management worker (Black) happened to be in the room at the time and asked if he could share his story. He spoke about his hesitancy about vaccination and then what led him to choose to be vaccinated. The patient and his wife chose to be vaccinated.

In the end, it is not the amorphous organization or institution that displays trust-worthiness, but the members of the organization "through interaction and event cycles sanctioned by, and embedded in, the organization's system components" (Gillespie & Dietz, 2009). That is to say, trust is relational, and relationships are personal. During the pandemic, teams at healthcare facilities reached out to foster personal connection through events like drive-through baby showers and holiday parades in the parking lots of nursing homes. More calls were made to patients at home and more efforts to reach them via novel methods (postcards, letters, texts, social media). Additionally, healthcare systems recognized and acknowl-edged the increased vulnerability that their staff was experiencing by deploying and bolstering employee wellness teams, whole-health messaging and learning opportunities, daily devotionals and weekly support calls, and mindfulness exercises. Memberships to virtual fitness and yoga classes were offered free to healthcare workers. These are just a few of the many examples of ways that health-care institutions worked to build healthier relationships with their staff; much of that work will continue, and continue to yield benefits, even after the pandemic eases in the months and years to come.

NEXT STEPS: PRACTICAL AND EMPIRICAL

These "lessons learned" speak directly to how to build trust in the healthcare system, as well as to gaps in knowledge. Trust takes a while to establish; this is perhaps even truer when it must be restored after being diminished. Compared to other scientists, healthcare professionals differ in that they also provide services directly to consumers. Because people's response to the pandemic, and their behaviors during as well as after the pandemic, are partly driven by their trust in both the individual healthcare providers and healthcare institutions, the work of building/rebuilding trust is vital. Thus, our practical recommendations pertain both to scientists in ge-neral and to healthcare providers interacting directly with patients.

Scientists work on myriad problems relevant to people's health and well-being: nutrition (is cholesterol bad for you?), environmental risks (is lead-contaminated water harmful?), and behavior (does exercise protect against dementia?), to mention only a few. Surprisingly, however, scientists are not always very good at communicating their findings, or the findings' relevance, to the populace (Jamieson et al., 2017). Thus, medical researchers need to improve the public's familiarity with their work. An emerging "science of science communication" offers strategies for conveying scientific information to laypeople effectively (Jamieson et al., 2017).

Providers can do a number of things to raise patients' level of trust: increase transparency, open and honest communication; broaden the level of patients' involvement and teamwork in key activities; engage in public outreach (e.g., relying on public-facing resources like public affairs offices, social media, and town halls); and emphasize commonalities and shared interests (i.e., a sense that "we're all in this together" (Ghoshal & Bartlett, 1994; Hostetter & Klein, 2021; Hurley, 2006).

Secondarily, the trust relationship would benefit from increasing the overall level of personal competence at all levels, via such mechanisms as cross-training, broad membership in moving forward committee/activities, open access to data, and independent committee reviews. Relatedly, consumers will view the healthcare system as more competent to the extent that it avoids conflicts of interest, seeks to minimize mistakes and misconduct, and when those negative outcomes occur (which they inevitably will) accepts responsibility and takes appropriate remedial or disciplinary measures.

Many of these notions, especially that of patients' active engagement, are embodied in what MacCoun (2015) called an "epistemic contract" (epistemic in the sense that "it pertains to the validity of some claim of knowledge"; p. 207). According to this model of the ideal relationship between experts and consumers, experts "should strive to be calibrated, clearly delineating the strengths and limitations of his or her knowledge," and consumers "should be constrained by, and susceptible to revision in light of, available expert opinions" (p. 208). MacCoun's model exemplifies how achieving trust requires effort from both sides. Building, or rebuilding, trust requires focus on existing (and in some cases, creating new) behaviors. Within the context of COVID-19, healthcare professionals—whether wearing their scientist or their provider hat—would commit to sharing information about things like infection risk, treatment regimens, and vaccine effectiveness while acknowledging uncertainty and avoiding over- (or under-) confidence; patients, for their part, would commit to seeking information from healthcare professionals, processing it rationally, and (if warranted) modifying their beliefs and behaviors accordingly.

In addition to these practical recommendations, there are a number of empirical needs. First and perhaps foremost, trust in science and healthcare needs to be assessed on an ongoing, longitudinal basis. It is pointless to devise policies for increasing trust unless the current level of trust is known, as well as how it changes over time and responds to interventions. The Pew data, discussed above, are a step in the right direction, but such surveys need to be repeated regularly. In addition, samples must be sufficiently large to examine differences as a function of key demographic variables, such as race/ethnicity, gender, age, political affiliation, and so forth. For example, political affiliation is one of the most striking predictors of attitudes toward both science in general and various aspects of the pandemic (e.g., infection risk, vaccination, and behavioral restrictions such as social distancing, masking, and quarantine), among both citizens and political leaders (see, e.g., Funk et al., 2019).

Additional questions that research could answer include:

Does trust change depending on who is paying for the healthcare (i.e., single payer, health insurance, or patients themselves)? A unique characteristic of the COVID-19 pandemic is that the government footed the bill for most of the costs associated with testing and vaccination; it stands to reason that if patients had to pay these costs themselves—even a modest copay—compliance would be lower.

What strategies can effectively repair trust? A complicating factor is that the institution responsible for the breach (e.g., government health agencies) could be the very same institution attempting to implement reform. Consumers might ask themselves: If I don't trust you because your performance was so poor in the first place, why should I trust you to improve matters? This is where highly trusted spokespersons (e.g., Dr. Anthony Fauci at the national level or persons with high standing in local communities) and bipartisan cooperation are called for.

What works as far as combatting vaccine hesitancy and communicating complex scientific information to the public? Different communities and employers have offered various vaccination inducements and incentives, such as entertainment at vaccination sites, paid time off from work, or cash payments (the legality of some employer incentives is uncertain).

How can efforts across the myriad systems be coordinated (e.g., public vs. private) that operate in the United States/world? It is essential to acknowledge that, at least in the United States, the "system" is not actually one system. Therefore, what might work in one setting might not work in others, and healthcare leaders should refrain from mandating solutions that could create more problems than they solve.

How can profiteering and wealth/power grabs be prevented during healthcare crises? Despite the great many inspiring stories of people who acted altruistically during the pandemic (e.g., most metrics showed that charitable giving increased), other stories portrayed persons who sought to exploit the pandemic for personal gain (e.g., buying and reselling PPE; selling fake vaccination cards). Data should be collected to determine how widespread such behavior was, and what policies can combat it effectively.

CONCLUSION

As the other chapters in this volume illustrate, the COVID-19 pandemic has had, and will continue to have, far-reaching social and behavioral consequences, as well as the more obvious effects in terms of the economy and public health. Some of these consequences have to do with the public's attitudes toward the healthcare system and healthcare providers. The pandemic exposed health inequalities as a function of race and ethnicity, as well as a degree of distrust having profound behavioral and public health implications (e.g., vaccine hesitancy). However, with challenges come opportunities. Healthcare providers and researchers now have the chance to take the lessons learned during the COVID-19 pandemic and use those lessons not only to mitigate the lingering effects of the current pandemic, but also to prevent and respond more effectively to public health emergencies in the future.

NOTES

1. Although we use the term "system" as convenient shorthand, in the absence of nationalized healthcare in the United States, healthcare "systems" would be more accurate.
2. Notably, gun violence has been referred to as an "epidemic," and health departments are increasingly becoming involved in combating it, suggesting parallels with infectious epidemics/pandemics like COVID-19.

REFERENCES

Abbasi, K. (2020). Covid-19: Politicisation, "corruption," and suppression of science. *British Medical Journal, 371*(November), m4425. htpps://doi.org/10.1136/bmj.m4425

Assessing the State of Vaccine Confidence in the United States: Recommendations from the National Vaccine Advisory Committee. (2015). *Public Health Reports, 130*(6), 573–595. htpps://doi.org/10.1177/003335491513000606

Baker, V. (2020, Oct. 6). Covid and Trump: The president's healthcare v the average American's. *BBC News.* https://www.bbc.com/news/world-us-canada-54441263

Berlivet L., & Löwy I. (2020). Hydroxychloroquine controversies: Clinical trials, epistemology, and the democratization of science. *Medical Anthropology Quarterly, 34*(4), 525–541.https://doi.org/10.1111/maq.12622.

Bornstein, B. H., & Tomkins, A. J. (2015). Institutional trust: An introduction. In B. H. Bornstein & A. J. Tomkins (Eds.), *Motivating cooperation and compliance with authority: The role of institutional trust* (pp. 1–12). Springer.

Campos-Castillo, C., Woodson, B., W., Theiss-Morse, E., Sacks, T., Fleig-Palmer, M. M., & Peek, M. E. (2016). Examining the relationship between interpersonal and institutional trust in political and health care contexts. In E. Shockley, T. M. S. Neal, L. M. PytlikZillig, & B. H. Bornstein (Eds.), *Interdisciplinary perspectives on trust: Towards theoretical and methodological integration* (pp. 99–115). Springer. https://doi.org/10.1007/978-3-319-22261-5_6

Douglas, J. A., & Subica, A. M. (2020). COVID-19 treatment resource disparities and social disadvantage in New York City. *Preventive Medicine, 141*(December), 106282. https://doi.org/10.1016/j.ypmed.2020.106282

244 THE SOCIAL SCIENCE OF THE COVID-19 PANDEMIC

Fadulu, L. (2020, Dec. 7). Amid history of mistreatment, doctors struggle to sell Black Americans on coronavirus vaccine. *The Washington Post*. https://www.washingtonp ost.com/local/social-issues/black-vaccine-trust/2020/12/07/9245e82e-34c2-11eb-b59c-adb7153d10c2_story.html

Funk, C., Hefferon, M., Kennedy, B., & Johnson, C. (2019). Trust and mistrust in Americans' views of scientific experts. Pew Research Center. https://www.pewresea rch.org/science/2019/08/02/trust-and-mistrust-in-americans-views-of-scientific-experts/

Funk, C., & Tyson, A. (2020, Dec. 3). Intent to get a COVID-19 vaccine rises to 60% as confidence in research and development process increases. Pew Research Center. https://www.pewresearch.org/science/2020/12/03/intent-to-get-a-covid-19-vacc ine-rises-to-60-as-confidence-in-research-and-development-process-increases/

Funk, C., & Tyson, A. (2021, March 5). Growing share of Americans say they plan to get a COVID-19 vaccine—or already have. Pew Research Center. https://www.pewresea rch.org/science/2021/03/05/growing-share-of-americans-say-they-plan-to-get-a-covid-19-vaccine-or-already-have/

Ghoshal, S., & Bartlett, C. A. (1994). Linking organizational context and managerial action: The dimensions of quality management. *Strategic Management Journal*, *15*(S2), 91–112.

Gillespie, N., & Dietz, G. (2009). Trust repair after an organization-level failure. *The Academy of Management Review*, *34*(1), 127–145.

Hostetter, M., & Klein, S. (2021, January 14). Transforming care: Understanding and ameliorating medical mistrust among Black Americans. Advancing Health Equity. The Commonwealth Fund. https://www.commonwealthfund.org/publications/new sletter-article/2021/jan/medical-mistrust-among-black-americans

Hurley, R. F. (2006, September). The decision to trust. *Harvard Business Review*, *84*(9), 55–62, 156.

Jamieson, K. H., Kahan, D. M., & Scheufele, D. A. (2017). *The Oxford handbook of the science of science communication*. Oxford University Press.

Kolata, G. (2020, December 31). In minority communities, doctors are changing minds about vaccination. *New York Times*. https://www.nytimes.com/2020/12/31/health/ coronavirus-black-hispanic-vaccination.html

Koonin, L. M., Hoots, B., Tsang, C. A., Leroy, Z., Farris, K., Tillman Jolly, B., Antall, P., McCabe, B., Zellis, C. B. R., Tong, I., & Harris, A. M. (2020, October 30). Trends in the use of telehealth during the emergence of the COVID-19 pandemic—United States, January–March 2020. *MMWR. Morbidity and Mortality Weekly Report*, *69*(43), 1595–1599.

Kurlander, C. (2020, April 2). The deadly polio epidemic and why it matters for coronavirus. *Discover*. https://www.discovermagazine.com/health/the-deadly-polio-epide mic-and-why-it-matters-for-coronavirus

Latkin, C. A., Dayton, L., Yi, G., Konstantopoulos, A., & Boodram, B. (2021). Trust in a COVID-19 vaccine in the U.S.: A social-ecological perspective. *Social Science & Medicine*, *270*(February), 113684. https://doi.org/10.1016/j.socscimed.2021.113684

MacCoun, R. J. (2015). The epistemic contract: Fostering an appropriate level of public trust in experts. In B. H. Bornstein & A. J. Tomkins (Eds.), *Motivating cooperation and compliance with authority: The role of institutional trust* (pp. 191–214). Springer. https://doi.org/10.1007/978-3-319-16151-8_9

Mak, T. (2020, April 16). Sen. Richard Burr's pre-pandemic stock sell-offs highly unusual, analysis shows. *National Public Radio.* https://www.npr.org/2020/03/19/818192535/burr-recording-sparks-questions-about-private-comments-on-covid-19

Mayer, R. C, Davis, J. H., & Schoorman, F. D. (1995). An integrative model of organizational trust. *Academy of Management Review, 20*(3), 709–734.

McEvily, B., & Tortoriello, M. (2011). Measuring trust in organisational research: Review and recommendations. *Journal of Trust Research, 1*(1), 23–63.

Nazione, S., Perrault, E. K., & Keating, D. M. (2019). Finding common ground: Can provider-patient race concordance and self-disclosure bolster patient trust, perceptions, and intentions? *Journal of Racial and Ethnic Health Disparities, 6*(5), 962–972. https://doi.org/10.1007/s40615-019-00597-6

PytlikZillig, L. M., Hamm, J. A., Shockley, E., Herian, M. N., Neal, T. M. S., Kimbrough, C. D., Tomkins, A. J., & Bornstein, B. H. (2016). The dimensionality of trust-relevant constructs in four institutional domains: Results from confirmatory factor analyses. *Journal of Trust Research, 6*(2), 111–150. https://doi.org/10.1080/21515581.2016.1151359

Rousseau, D. M., Sitkin, S. B., Burt, R. S., & Camerer, C. (1998). Not so different after all: A cross-discipline view of trust. *Academy of Management Review, 23*(3), 393–404.

Schoenthaler, A., Montague, E., Manwell, L. B., Brown, R., Schswartz, M. D., & Linzer, M. (2014). Patient-physician racial/ethnic concordance and blood pressure control: The role of trust and medication adherence. *Ethnicity and Health, 19*(5), 565–578. https://doi.org/10.1080/13557858.2013.857764

Schoorman, F., Wood, M., & Breuer, D. (2015). Would trust by any other name smell as sweet? Reflections on the meetings and uses of trust across disciplines and context. In B. H. Bornstein & A. J. Tomkins (Eds.), *Motivating cooperation and compliance with authority: The role of institutional trust* (pp. 13–36). Springer. https://doi.org/10.1007/978-3-319-16151-8_2

Shockley, E., Neal, T. M. S., PytlikZillig, L. M., & Bornstein, B. H. (2016). *Interdisciplinary perspectives on trust: Towards theoretical and methodological integration.* Springer.

Twenge, J. M., Campbell, W. K., & Carter, N. T. (2014). Declines in trust in others and confidence in institutions among American adults and late adolescents, 1972–2012. *Psychological Science, 25*(10), 1914–1923. https://doi.org/10.1177/0956797614545133

19

Social Networks and COVID-19

Contagion and the Pandemic's Impact on Behavior

CLAYTON D. PEOPLES AND KAYLA FURLANO ■

The COVID-19 pandemic and social networks are intertwined. As a communicable illness, the virus spreads from person to person through pathways created by social networks. Consequently, some governments have instituted measures that seek to limit in-person contact, such as stay-home orders. These measures, however, change networks and alter modes of exchange. The purpose of this chapter is twofold: to use social network theory to explain COVID-19 contagion and to explore the pandemic's impact on behavior.

CHAPTER LAYOUT

As discussed shortly, social networks are central to the transmission of communicable illnesses such as COVID-19. But there are four factors related to social networks that greatly affect this process: network size, tie degree, timing of contact, and the nature of contact. Each of these is in sections below.

As much as networks are central to better understanding the spread of COVID-19, the policy response to the pandemic in turn affects social networks. For instance, things like contact tracing and mandatory quarantines are linked with social networks. Meanwhile, stay-home orders, social distancing, and mask mandates all impact social networks and the ways in which people interact with one another. These themes also are discussed in sections below.

Before concluding, the chapter expounds on "lessons learned" from the pandemic; it also proposes some future research ideas that scholars should focus on in the coming years. But before delving into these themes, it is important to introduce social network theory as well as its central concepts.

Clayton D. Peoples and Kayla Furlano, *Social Networks and COVID-19* In: *The Social Science of the COVID-19 Pandemic*. Edited by: Monica K. Miller, Oxford University Press. © Oxford University Press 2024.
DOI: 10.1093/oso/9780197615133.003.0019

SOCIAL NETWORK THEORY

The crux of social network theory is a simple—yet profound—argument that connections to others influence attitudes and behaviors. Consequently, a social network approach focuses explicitly on those connections and seeks to measure their impact on a range of social phenomena. Like other theories, social network theory is expressed in terms of relationships between concepts. Consequently, in the following paragraphs many core concepts in social network theory are introduced and defined.

Network Concepts

A social network is a set of the social entities, called actors, and the ties among the actors. Actors can be a variety of social entities, such as individual people, groups, or countries. Ties, or the relationship between the actors, can represent friendships, enemies, exchanges, work ties, communication, and more.

Ties can be categorized by both their strength and their directness. The strength of a tie is measured through the degree of connectedness. Strong ties have many mutual connections or interactions between two actors (i.e., family members), while weak ties have only one or a few mutual connections between actors (i.e., coworkers). In addition to strength, ties can be direct or indirect. A direct tie represents an actual contact relationship between actors, while an indirect tie is due to a joint affiliation, such as two students who attended the same college but have no direct contact. Strength and directness/indirectness are just two of many ways to describe and measure network ties.

Within a social network, actors are connected to both a direct and a broader network. Centrality is a term used in social network theory to describe how tied and how closely tied an actor is within a network. A central actor has many ties with other actors and/or is closely linked via short paths to many other actors. One way centrality can be measured is by degree, or number of ties. The number of ties an actor has within a social network can range from zero (no ties with any others in the network) to the total population of the network minus one (ties with every other actor in the network). Centrality and degree can each help describe an actor's position within a social network.

Social network theory can also study the structure of networks through size and density. Network size is the number of actors in a network. Network size can become more complicated when the boundaries of a network are not specified or are not clear. Networks can be studied at the microlevel through dyads and triads (relationships among two and three actors, respectively) or at the macrolevel of looking at networks as a whole. Further, the structure of a network can be studied through its density. The density of a network describes the proportion of ties present out of all possible ties within a network.

Finally, network formation is guided by proximity and homophily. Proximity refers to geographical nearness, while homophily is a tie that is from a similarity in some way (e.g., a trait, attribute, or characteristic). Both proximity and homophily help explain patterns for relationship formation and continuation within social networks. Overall, research demonstrates that networks influence and can shape behaviors, and that the behaviors of individuals are interdependent. As such, social network theory has numerous applications to pandemic-related behavior and the spread of disease.

APPLICATION TO COMMUNICABLE ILLNESSES

Social network theory has great applicability to understanding of pandemics and how diseases spread. Communicable diseases, like COVID-19, are spread through contact with others—often in the context of social networks. When thinking about how networks can apply to the question of how diseases spread, there are four elements that are especially relevant—two of which are related to networks and ties, two of which are connected to actual contact. The two related to networks and ties are network size and tie "degree"; the two connected to actual contact are timing of contact and the nature of contact. Each of these four elements is discussed below.

Network Size

Surprisingly, there is no consensus on how many people are in a typical person's social network—largely due to differences in how connections are defined. When defined very broadly—for instance, how many people a single person knows— estimates are as high as 600 or more (Gelman, 2013). When narrowed, however, to those known well enough to send a holiday card, the number drops to approximately 150 (Hill & Dunbar, 2003). Finally, if social networks are limited to close relationships—for instance, trusted others—it is closer to 25 (DiPrete et al., 2011). In short, depending on how connections are defined, networks typically range from 25 to 600 or more people.

Network size has implications for disease transmission because it represents the total number of people a contagious individual could potentially infect (note: here, this does not include the threat of spreading to strangers in public spaces). Granted, it would be very unusual for someone to infect everyone in their social network. But even infecting one other person means that the disease is spreading; infecting more than one person means that it is spreading and expanding to a larger number of people. Notice that the focus here is on "first-degree" connections—in other words, those with whom people have a personal connection. If extended to "second-degree" ties (people connected to first-degree ties) or beyond, numbers start to expand exponentially, and disease spread really ramps up.

Tie Degree

Take the most conservative estimate of network size above: 25. Roughly speaking, if extended to the second degree, that number expands to approximately 625 (25 times 25). Expanding from there to the third degree, it balloons to 15,625 (625 times 25). If further extending to the fourth degree, it shoots up to 390,625 (15,625 times 25). At the fifth degree, estimates reach nearly 10 million people (9,765,625, to be exact: 390,625 times 25). Granted, as above, it is not expected that a person carrying an illness would infect all 25 of the contacts in their network, but the above does illustrate how a disease, once transmitted beyond first-degree ties to the second degree onward, can spread exponentially.

Timing of Contact

As important as network size and tie degree are to disease transmission, they are certainly not the only factors that are relevant. One of the most important factors is timing of contact. Simply being in the same social network as someone who has a communicable illness does not put one at risk of catching the disease. First, there would need to be direct contact with the person; second, said contact would have to occur while the person is contagious. Contact prior to, or after, the person is contagious would pose no risk. Contact while the person is contagious, however, could lead to transmission, which could lead the virus to spread through the social network. This, then, segues into the nature of contact.

Nature of Contact

Although communicable diseases, by definition, spread through person-to-person contact, each disease uses a different form of contact as its primary mode of transmission. Take, for instance, sexually transmitted infections (STIs). As the name implies, STIs are spread through sexual intimacy. Gastrointestinal (GI) illnesses—colloquially known as "stomach flus"—are transmitted in a different way—through contact with someone's digestive waste. Put differently, STIs and GI illnesses cannot be spread by simply being in the presence of someone who is carrying the disease; specific forms of closer contact are required. This is not true, however, of COVID-19 and other upper respiratory infections (URIs).

As the name suggests, URIs affect the respiratory tract, including the nose, throat, and so on. URIs spread through contact with droplets expelled from the nose or mouth of an infected/contagious person. For example, URIs can spread through contact with doorknobs, TV remotes, and other frequently touched items that were handled by an infected person. Even more concerning, URIs can spread through aerosolized droplets expelled into the air by an infected person. Studies have shown that COVID-19, in particular, is spread very efficiently in this manner—especially the more contagious strains such as the "Delta variant" (Roberts, 2021).

The fact that COVID-19 transmits easily through the air implies that it can be spread by simply being in the proximity of an infected person—and there are some situations that increase the risk of transmission even further. For instance, being in the presence of an infected person who is coughing, sneezing, or otherwise expelling large numbers of droplets greatly increases the risk of transmission; likewise, spending an extended period of time with an infected person in an enclosed, poorly ventilated setting increases the risk of transmission. Regardless, the fact that COVID-19 spreads easily through the air means that people's social lives have changed dramatically in response to the virus.

APPLICATION TO THE COVID-19 PANDEMIC

In addition to its applicability to communicable illnesses in general, social network theory has great applicability to the COVID-19 pandemic specifically. This is arguably most evident in the policies and practices that have emerged during the pandemic to try to slow its spread and keep people safe. Contact tracing and mandatory quarantines, stay-home orders, social distancing guidelines, and mask mandates are among the many examples of such policies and practices (see Chapter 3 for summary of pandemic-related policies). The following paragraphs cover each of these in turn and discuss the linkages between these policies and social network theory—as well as the broader implications of these for peoples' social lives.

Contact Tracing and Mandatory Quarantines

In some countries, when a person has tested positive for COVID-19, they are asked who they have spent time with during recent days. This process is referred to as "contact tracing." Social network theory is quite important in this process—particularly some of the elements discussed in the previous section. For instance, timing of contact and nature of contact are of paramount importance when it comes to contact tracing.

Timing of contact is relevant for the reasons mentioned previously. It only matters if a person has had contact with the COVID-19 patient during a time in which the patient was likely contagious. Having contact with the person before that period of likely contagiousness would have no consequence; having contact during the period of contagiousness would be far more consequential. But this is where the nature of contact also comes into play. Brief encounters—especially outdoors and/or masked (see section on Mask Mandates below)—would likely pose little risk of transmission. Lengthier encounters—particularly those occurring indoors and/or without mask wearing—would pose a much greater risk.

If it is determined via contact tracing that someone has had contact with a confirmed-positive COVID-19 patient—and said contact is such that the timing and nature present risk of transmission—said person might be asked to self-quarantine for a period of time (e.g., 10 or 14 days). Some countries go even further and request that *anyone* entering their country quarantine for a similar period of time (10 or 14 days). Such mandatory quarantines are meant to help stop the spread of COVID-19, as are stay-home orders.

Stay-Home Orders

Stay-home orders are similar in intent to mandatory quarantines—to stop the spread of COVID-19. But unlike mandatory quarantines, which apply to specific individuals (e.g., contacts of a confirmed-positive COVID-19 individual or those traveling across national boundaries), stay-home orders apply more generally. Stay-home orders typically ask—or require—that people stay in their homes and avoid going out for any reason other than for necessities (e.g., food, medicine). But there are also other variants of stay-home orders that effectively serve the same purpose, such as converting work or schooling to an entirely online format.

Again, the intended purpose of stay-home orders is to stop the spread of COVID-19. If followed properly, they do, indeed, serve that purpose. But they do carry some unintended consequences. For instance, stay-home orders might force people to stay in close quarters with people—family members, others— who are abusive or otherwise difficult to be around (see Chapter 26 for more on relationships). In a similar vein, it might reduce the amount of quality time people can spend with those they love and trust outside their homes.

Stay-home orders also relegate contact with those outside the home to online/ virtual contact, which is arguably less rewarding than face-to-face interactions (see Chapter 22 for more on communication types during the pandemic). In a related vein, online work or schooling can exacerbate inequalities. There are undoubtedly social class issues that arise with respect to access—with those in lower class positions less likely to have access to technologies that would allow them to successfully work and/or learn remotely (see Chapters 24 and 25 for social inequalities during the pandemic).

Social Distancing

Social distancing guidelines suggest that when people are in the vicinity of others, they should maintain a distance of 6 feet (approximately 2 meters) to reduce the risk of COVID-19 transmission; they should also wear masks (more on that in the next section). Although arguably better in some respects than online interactions, social distancing—especially in combination with mask wearing (to be described next)—can alter the way in which people communicate.

Mask Mandates

Another practice that has been adopted in varying degrees across different countries is wearing masks when in public and around others outside the home. When enforced by the government, it is often referred to as a "mask mandate." In some societies, it was already a norm to wear a mask when ill (e.g., countries in Asia), so mask mandates were met with little resistance; in other societies, however, mask mandates stirred a great amount of controversy (e.g., the United States; see

Chapter 16 for more on culture and the pandemic). But as with the other measures mentioned above, the intent is to reduce the spread of COVID-19. Given that COVID-19 spreads quite efficiently through aerosolized droplets, mask wearing can allow people to interact in relatively close quarters while still reducing the spread of COVID-19. But it is not without its problems. As noted above, it can alter the way in which people communicate. Moreover, it can present challenges for those who communicate best when no masks are involved (e.g., the hard of hearing).

LESSONS LEARNED

There are a number of "lessons learned" from the COVID-19 pandemic. Some of these lessons concern the pandemic itself (e.g., its spread.); other lessons are related to social network theory. Each category of lesson learned is addressed on its own below.

Lessons Related to the COVID-19 Pandemic

One lesson learned is that unclear, nonuniform, or poorly implemented policies might have less impact on social network connections and interactions, but can increase the risk of disease spread. For example, social distancing policies implemented in airports but not on the flights themselves introduce lengthy encounters with others that could lead to the spread of disease. Further, company policies such as wearing masks and social distancing only in the public eye but not during other phases of operation can expose workers and potentially consumers to disease.

In a related vein, policy responses that restrict personal network interaction but do not restrict work interactions (e.g., office workers working from the office rather than from home) when possible also lead to greater spread of communicable diseases, particularly for workers in poorly ventilated areas for extended periods of time with others who could potentially be infected. For jobs in which in-person work is required, extra precautions should be put into place to reduce the amount of in-person contact with others, especially unmasked contact or contact with those potentially infected. This is especially relevant for people and communities that are systemically disadvantaged and might not have access or quality access to healthcare.

Lessons Related to Social Networks

A third lesson learned is that policies that reduce social network connections through isolation have the potential to decrease social support via social networks, which can adversely influence some kinds of health outcomes (Uchino et al., 2012; Usher et al., 2020). Further, isolation and limited social support can increase the risk for domestic abuse and neglect. Countries have already documented increased risks and cases of domestic abuse and neglect in response to the COVID-19 pandemic (Sserwanja et al., 2021; Usher et al., 2020). This introduces the proverbial "between a rock and a hard place" scenario: Policies intended to curb the spread of COVID-19 might keep people healthy with respect to the virus but can make them less healthy in other respects.

A fourth lesson learned is that the principles that guide social network theory still apply during the COVID-19 pandemic, but the pandemic and related behavior might change the structure and nature of social networks and interactions. For example, restricted in-person interactions can lead to greater online connections, but for some, such as those who have limited access to technology or are not "tech savvy," they might find their network connections diminishing (Nguyen et al., 2020; see also Chapter 22). Changes to in-person social networks during the pandemic, in some cases, has led to fewer casual or weak ties as well as less choice in one's social network.

FUTURE RESEARCH

A number of future research ideas can be derived from the principles and assumptions discussed in this chapter. The research questions provided in this section can be used to guide future studies as related to social networks and pandemic-related behavior. Specifically, research questions related to dyads, triads, and weak ties; network size; timing of contact; peer and social influence; and social support can be used to guide future research.

What Are the Implications of Changes in Network Size?

Network size, particularly face-to-face network size, has been altered during the COVID-19 pandemic. Future research can address how network size influenced the transmission of disease during the pandemic. Policy impacts on network size can also be studied, for both the effectiveness of policies at limiting transmission of disease through reducing network sizes and the social and psychological implications of limiting networks. The concepts of weak ties, dyadic relations, and triadic relationships can also be incorporated into these and other research ideas.

How Have Dyads, Triads, and Weak Ties Changed?

The COVID-19 pandemic has influenced various aspects of social networks, including dyadic, triadic, and weak ties relations. Dyadic and triadic network interactions can be studies as related to changes in the nature of these relationships as a result of the pandemic, as well as the frequency and strength of these network connections. Further, changes in the nature and frequency of weak ties can be studied. What are the functions of weak ties during a pandemic? Do people rely on the weak ties that remain more so than when networks are not as limited? These can be addressed in future research.

How Can Timing of Contact Influence Disease Spread?

Future research should also examine how the timing of contact can influence the spread of disease as related to social networks. Policies and practices such as stay-home orders, mask mandates, contact tracing, and more can be studied through a social network approach for their effectiveness at restricting the spread of disease by limiting (or not limiting) contact within networks. Future research can also examine if these policies and practices are about equally effective at limiting contact for all groups of people or if specific groups and networks are/were systematically excluded or influenced by their implementation.

What Are the Implications of Changes in Peer and Social Influence?

The nature of peer influence, and social influence more generally, has changed in response to the COVID-19 pandemic. For example, what are the implications of increased technology use on peer and social influence? What are the implications of decreased face-to-face social networks for peer and social influence? What are the long-term consequences of these changes? These questions can be addressed in future research.

How Have Changes in Social Support Influenced Behavior?

Finally, the influence of changes in social support on behavior can be studied through a social network approach. First, how has negative social support influenced behavior within social networks during the pandemic? What are the longer term impacts of such support? What sources of support and amount of support do people seek when their face-to-face networks are limited? Questions related to inequality (e.g., economic, gender, or racial inequality) and social support can also be addressed through a social network approach, as can ways that negative social support can be buffered. Overall, these and other research questions related to social networks in response to the pandemic can be addressed to investigate how and why disease is spread and what the most effective measures are that can be taken to decrease the spread of disease while considering other social and psychological factors.

CONCLUSION

In conclusion, social networks are critical to better understanding the COVID-19 pandemic. Networks are central to the spread of communicable illnesses such as COVID-19, but networks are themselves impacted by policies that seek to curb the spread of COVID-19. This implies that lessons learned from the application of network theory to the pandemic include lessons for better understanding COVID-19 and other communicable diseases *plus* lessons for scholarship on social networks. In that respect, there are a number of possible research ideas presented here for future research. The hope is that these ideas represent a "call for action" for researchers to explore these topics and study how networks have impacted the COVID-19 pandemic and vice versa.

REFERENCES

DiPrete. T. A., Gelman, A., McCormick, T., Teitler, J., & Zheng, T. (2011). Segregation in social networks based on acquaintanceship and trust. *American Journal of Sociology, 116*, 234–283. https://doi.org/10.1086/659100

Gelman, A. (2013, February 18). The average American knows how many people? *The New York Times.* https://www.nytimes.com/2013/02/19/science/the-average-american-knows-how-many-people.html

Hill, R. A., & Dunbar, R. I. M. (2003). Social network size in humans. *Human Nature, 14*, 53–72. https://doi.org/10.1007/s12110-003-1016-y

Nguyen, M. H., Gruber, J., Fuchs, J., Marler, W., Hunsaker, A., & Hargittai, E. (2020). Changes in digital communication during the COVID-19 global pandemic: Implications for digital inequality and future research. *Social Media + Society, 6*(3), 2056305120948255. https://doi.org/10.1177/2056305120948255

Roberts, M. (2021, July 1). What are the India, Brazil, South Africa and UK variants? *BBC News.* https://www.bbc.com/news/health-55659820

Sserwanja, Q., Kawuki, J., & Kim, J. H. (2021). Increased child abuse in Uganda amidst COVID-19 pandemic. *Journal of Paediatrics and Child Health, 57*(2), 188–191. https://doi.org/10.1111/jpc.15289

Uchino, B. N., Bowen, K., Carlisle, M., & Birmingham, W. (2012). Psychological pathways linking social support to health outcomes: A visit with the "ghosts" of research past, present, and future. *Social Science & Medicine, 74*, 949–957. https://doi.org/10.1016/j.socscimed.2011.11.023

Usher, K., Bhullar, N., Durkin, J., Gyamfi, N., & Jackson, D. (2020). Family violence and COVID-19: Increased vulnerability and reduced options for support. *International Journal of Mental Health Nursing, 29*(4), 549–552. https://doi.org/10.1111/inm.12735

FURTHER READING

Christakis, N. A., & Fowler, J. H. (2007). The spread of obesity in a large social network over 32 years. *New England Journal of Medicine, 357*(4), 370–379. https://doi.org/10.1056/NEJMsa066082

Felmlee, D. H., & Faris, R. (2013). Interactions in social networks. In J. Delamater & A. Ward (Ed.), *Handbook of social psychology* (2nd ed., pp. 439–464). Springer.

Hanneman, R., & Riddle, M. (n.d.). *Introduction to social network methods.* http://www.faculty.ucr.edu/~hanneman/nettext

Experiences During the Pandemic

20

The Collective Trauma and Chronic Stress of COVID-19

Risk and Resilience

DANA ROSE GARFIN AND KAYLEY D. ESTES ■

Collective traumas are large-scale, negative life events that impact the populace broadly, by both proximal exposure and media coverage. No prior collective trauma has impacted so many for such a long duration than the COVID-19 pandemic. The pandemic shares many characteristics with other collective traumas (e.g., terrorism, hurricanes, shootings) in that it was a catastrophic event that shattered assumptions of safety and security, occurred without warning, and involved a crisis of meaning with respect to our experience of continuity, community, and self (Hirschberger, 2018). Yet unlike many other collective traumas, there was no clear demarcation of the "end" of the public health emergency, when the crisis ended, and healing began. Thus, the pandemic shared many features of chronic stressors—ongoing events that influence a person's physical and mental health through disruption of daily life. COVID-19 and the associated dramatic social disruption, staggering loss of life, and cascade of stressful events created a mental health crisis for many. Yet resilience was also common. Type of exposure (e.g., direct exposure, media-based exposure, secondary stressors) as well as demographic indicators explained variability in responses.

In sum, people's experiences of the COVID-19 pandemic varied greatly due to differential exposures; individual-level indicators (e.g., demographics, prior mental health); and contextual factors associated with resilience compared to distress. Opportunities for capitalizing on individual and social resilience can inform strategies to facilitate coping during the recovery process and beyond. This chapter reviews the current state of COVID-19 mental health research and provide an overview of methodological and empirical limitations to inspire rigorous research moving forward.

Dana Rose Garfin and Kayley D. Estes, *The Collective Trauma and Chronic Stress of COVID-19* In: *The Social Science of the COVID-19 Pandemic*. Edited by: Monica K. Miller, Oxford University Press. © Oxford University Press 2024. DOI: 10.1093/oso/9780197615133.003.0020

CONCEPTUALIZING EXPOSURE TO COVID-19

Exposure to the COVID-19 pandemic, like many other collective traumas, occurred from multiple imputes. Yet the COVID-19 pandemic was distinct from most other events in that many people experienced so many different types of exposures concurrently. The following section reviews key types of exposures associated with the COVID-19 pandemic: direct exposure (e.g., proximal exposure); secondary stressors (e.g., events that stem from direct exposure to the trauma); media-based exposure; cascading traumas (e.g., associated collective trauma that occurs as part of the disaster cascade); and chronic stress. The confluence of these exposures portended increased distress in many individuals. However, understanding the interrelationships between these exposures and psychological outcomes could yield information for targeted intervention efforts that guide recovery efforts and healing.

Direct Exposure

Traumatic events involve direct threat to the life of the individual or their loved one or by hearing of a trauma through professional work (American Psychiatric Association, 2013). In the collective trauma literature, direct exposure is being geographically at or near the physical location of the traumatic event or having someone close to you (i.e., friend or family) at or near the event (Holman et al., 2014). During COVID-19, direct exposure included personal illness (i.e., self or close friend or family member diagnosed with COVID-19) and loss of life (i.e., death of a close friend or family member due to COVID-19), with such exposures linked with increased psychological maladies in the general populace (Holman et al., 2020). Witnessing patient death was a particularly potent predictor of post-traumatic stress in healthcare workers treating patients with COVID-19, highlighting the relationship between direct exposure and mental health outcomes, especially for those at high risk of such exposures (Mosheva et al., 2021; see Chapters 27 and 31 of this volume for more on post-traumatic stress disorder (PTSD) associated with COVID-19).

Secondary Stressors

Secondary stressors are individual-level events associated with the disaster cascade (Garfin et al., 2014). Prior disaster research demonstrated that number of secondary stressors experienced in the aftermath of earthquakes (Garfin et al., 2014) and hurricanes (Kessler et al., 2012) was positively associated with mental health maladies. During the early phase of the COVID-19 outbreak, secondary stressors included job loss, decreased wages, canceled travel plans, waiting in long lines, and inability to obtain necessary supplies; these experiences were in turn associated with incremental increases in acute stress and depressive symptoms

(Holman et al., 2020). As the pandemic continued, stressors shifted to include missed events such as graduations, inability to attend religious services, school closures, and separation from friends and family (see Chapter 2 of this volume for more on how COVID-19 affected daily life). Indeed, between March 11, 2020, and February 2, 2021, schools averaged 95 closure days globally (UNICEF, 2021), highlighting the severe and ongoing duration of secondary stressors globally.

Cascading Traumas

Collective traumas rarely occur in isolation; rather, the occurrence of one event frequently triggers a series of interconnected disasters that create a compounding crisis (Silver et al., 2021). The COVID-19 outbreak was associated with restrictions leading to business closures and an economic crisis. The first few months of lockdowns resulted in the highest U.S. unemployment rate on record (since 1948), peaking at 14.8% in April 2020 (Falk et al., 2021). A year later, the unemployment rate was still 6.1%, which was 2.6% higher than February 2020, the month preceding widespread lockdown measures. As the economy reopened, inflation spiked, with rising costs in nearly all sectors of consumer goods, including food, transportation, and housing (Bureau of Labor Statistics, 2021). The COVID-19 pandemic also begot increased political polarization and a social justice reckoning in the United States and elsewhere, occurring concurrently with seasonal natural hazards (e.g., hurricanes, wildfires, tornados). These events created the "perfect storm" of compounding crises, the mental health effects of which are still largely unknown (Silver et al., 2021). Prior research regarding responses to terrorist attacks (Garfin et al., 2015) and natural disasters (Garfin et al., 2014) suggested that exposure to COVID-19-related compounding crises that occurred in both rapid succession and over time will likely be linked with increased distress; longitudinal research with nuanced assessments of event exposure is necessary to confirm.

Media-Based Exposure to COVID-19

Early in the crisis, the likely deleterious mental health effects of COVID-19-related media exposure were evident (Garfin et al., 2020). A robust body of prospective research on prior collective trauma, including terrorist attacks, shootings, natural disasters, and previous viral epidemics (e.g., Ebola and H1N1 outbreaks), demonstrated the striking association between increased event-related media exposure and mental health maladies. During COVID-19, the problem was exacerbated by the increased time people spent engaging with media. Stay-at-home orders eliminated commute times and socialization opportunities for many, with global online content consumption substantially increasing (Garfin, 2020). Indeed, average daily hours spent consuming media content on the Internet increased in 2020 from just over 3 hours to 6 hours and 59 minutes (Koetsier,

2020). This was compounded by people's reliance on the media for critical updates. As COVID-19 emerged, scientific information was rapidly evolving, risks were amplifying, and government mandates changing by the months, weeks, and even days (Garfin et al., 2021), necessitating people stay informed as information emerged. Media exposure and distress can form a reciprocal, amplification relationship and a cycle of distress over time; that is, those who are distressed seek out more media and in turn become more distressed (Thompson et al., 2019). Longitudinal research should explore this in the COVID-19 context.

As expected, early findings from nationally representative samples documented the association between COVID-19 media exposure and psychological distress. Data from a representative sample of U.S. adults ($N = 6,329$) assessed in March 2020 found time spent on social media and number of traditional media sources consulted were independently associated with increased mental distress (Riehm et al., 2020). However, differential conceptualization of media exposure (e.g., type vs. number of sources) makes cross-medium comparisons tenuous. A distinct nationally representative sample of U.S. adults assessed between March 18, 2020 and April 18, 2020, found hours of COVID-19-related media exposure (including both traditional and new media) were positively associated with acute stress and depressive symptoms (Holman et al., 2020). Importantly, during the COVID-19 pandemic, there was also an "infodemic" of misinformation and contradictory communications (see Chapter 36 of this volume for more in misinformation related to COVID-19). Exposure to this conflicting news coverage was independently associated with increased psychological distress, even after accounting for total amount of media exposure, demographic indicators, and prepandemic mental health ailments (Holman et al., 2020). Taken together, these early findings suggest future research should account for content, amount, type, and source of media consumption during COVID-19 and future crises.

Chronic Stress

Stress theorists have long struggled to precisely define the concept of stress, in part because it is contingent on one's perception of the event and their resources (including support, ability, prior experiences) to meet its demands (Baum, 1990). A classic definition of chronic stress is "demands, threats, perceived harm or loss, or responses that persist for long periods of time" (p. 662). By that definition, the COVID-19 pandemic would clearly be considered a chronic stressor in addition to an acute and compounding trauma. A classic example of the effect of chronic stressors is the Three Mile Island (TMI) disaster in the late 1970s, when a nuclear reactor accident caused radiation exposure to nearby communities. Like COVID-19, the radiation was an invisible threat and covered widely by the media, with conflicting and confusing information and a high degree of uncertainty. Longitudinal research found those living near TMI experienced elevated psychological distress and physiological stress responses that persisted years postevent (Baum, 1990). Given this and the likely prolonged social and economic recovery of the COVID-19 pandemic, longitudinal research is essential to document the long-term effects of COVID-19 and the persistence of the stress response—using multiple metrics—over time.

COVID-19 AND MENTAL HEALTH OUTCOMES

Research on the mental health effects of the COVID-19 pandemic has exploded since the crisis began. Early research suggested that, as COVID-19 spread in the United States, psychological distress increased (Holingue et al., 2020; Holman et al., 2020). Hundreds of articles were published on mental health and COVID-19, in conjunction with a national conversation about the potential rise in mental health ailments as a result of the virus, lockdowns, and other public health mitigation efforts (e.g., social distancing policies). Key ailments of concern included depression, anxiety, PTSD, general distress, and suicide (Pfefferbaum & North, 2020). Research on prior epidemics requiring substantial quarantines noted irritability, insomnia, emotional exhaustion, and substance abuse, and long-term avoidance behavior could also be problematic (Brooks et al., 2020).

A few key studies utilized prepandemic mental health data to examine change associated with the emergence of COVID-19. Early research from an ongoing nationally representative sample (N = 1,470) compared prevalence rates of depression from 2017 to 2018 to those collected during March–April 2020, demonstrating a threefold increase in depression (Ettman et al., 2020). Similarly, a longitudinal, nationally representative sample in the United Kingdom found a significant increase in mental health ailments during the beginning of the pandemic (April, May, and June) compared to assessments taken in 2017–2019 (Daly et al., 2021), yet a large attrition rate cautions strong inferences. Using a sequential cohort design, epidemiological findings from a nationally representative sample of 6,514 Americans found that both acute stress and depressive symptoms increased between March 18 and April 18, 2020 (Holman et al., 2020). That study found that psychological distress increased along with case counts, deaths, and restrictions. Importantly, that research accounted for prepandemic mental and physical health ailments, potent predictors of COVID-19-related mental-health maladies. Further follow-up on that sample demonstrated that individual-level and media-based exposures were more potent predictors of psychological distress than statewise restrictions (Thompson et al., 2022). Such data facilitate inferences regarding increases in symptoms attributable to the pandemic and its associated morbidities, mortalities, and social disruptions.

Relatedly, data from the Centers for Disease Control and Prevention found changes in several types of emergency department visits, including mental health conditions and suicide attempts; results illustrated both increased during mid-March to October 2020 compared to March–October 2019 (Holland et al., 2021). In contrast, other research indicated suicide rates did not uniformly increase during 2020 and sometimes decreased (John et al., 2020). Such findings may have been due to less access to self-harm modalities during the lockdowns, an early "pulling together" period, or differential presentation by age or other sociodemographic factors. Indeed, national data on deaths in Japan during the later months in 2020 found suicides increased (Sakamoto et al., 2021). Such findings demonstrate the value of longitudinal, population-based research to track the pandemic's impact on mental health over time and for interventions that target those with prior mental health ailments, who are particularly vulnerable.

GRIEF

Uniquely, this public health crisis involved protracted quarantines and lockdowns at regional and national levels. As a result, pandemic-associated grief likely occurred from a variety of losses: the loss of loved ones from the virus itself and the loss of life-cycle events (e.g., graduations, weddings) and daily routines resulting from social distancing and other mitigation efforts (Bertuccio & Runion, 2020). Experiencing multiple losses in a constricted time frame can lead to bereavement overload, with negative consequences for physical and mental health (Zhai & Du, 2020). Other concerns included unexpected death circumstances (e.g., for people who believed the virus was not deadly) or perceiving the death as preventable. Moreover, travel restrictions and limited ability to gather in groups hindered common rituals surrounding death (e.g., funerals); lack of formal social and cultural recognition of grief may reduce availability and/or perception of resources (e.g., social support) that typically aid the grieving process (Zhai & Du, 2020).

Preliminary empirical evidence supports these initial concerns. Greater functional impairment from COVID-19 losses was associated with risk factors, including not being present when the death occurred, distress about the memorial service, and postloss loneliness (Neimeyer & Lee, 2021). Dysfunctional grief symptoms were associated with several of those same risk factors (e.g., distress about the deceased dying alone, distress about the memorial service, loneliness from isolation policies) and a unique risk factor (e.g., worry about losing others to COVID-19). A cross-sectional survey of 1,600 bereaved adults found COVID-19-related deaths were a potent predictor of grief when compared to natural causes, perhaps due to COVID-19 deaths operating like an unexpected and shocking loss (Eisma et al., 2021). Given that acute grief severity is a strong predictor of persistent complex grief disorder, these phenomena suggest COVID-19-related losses could be associated with more long-term problems. Longitudinal research is critical to examine if the intensity of this acute grief translates into protracted problems.

DEMOGRAPHIC RISK FACTORS FOR MENTAL HEALTH AILMENTS

Most research suggests that key demographic factors help predict who is at risk for mental health problems following exposure to collective trauma (see Silver

& Garfin, 2016). During the COVID-19 pandemic, social and contextual factors exacerbated some common risk factors (e.g., low socioeconomic status [SES]) for poor outcomes. Of critical importance to the recovery efforts, COVID-19 deepened some health disparities, calling to action research, services, and policies that can help address these inequities.

Age

Although everyone was susceptible to contracting COVID-19, older adults, especially those above 65 years old, were at higher risk of severe illness. Yet COVID-19-related psychological distress has not followed the same pattern as the risk for illness severity. In a nationally representative sample, age was negatively associated with acute stress symptoms in the first month of the lockdown (Holman et al., 2020). Several plausible explanations exist. Younger workers were more susceptible to COVID-19-related unemployment compared to older workers (Dua et al., 2021). The daily life of older adults might have been less affected, and they might have felt it easier to avoid infections and crowds through greater availability of social support (e.g., younger friends or neighbors willing to grocery shop or cook). Younger adults in the United Kingdom reported more mental health symptoms, including depression and anxiety symptoms; retired individuals reported the least mental health symptoms (Pieh et al., 2021). This bolsters the theory that older adults might not have had to suddenly shift to working-from-home situations, continue working in a high-risk, in-person environment as an essential worker, or balance the demands of work with child care and homeschooling (see Chapters 29 and 44 of this volume for more on these experiences).

Ethnicity/Race

Generally, being an underrepresented minority is associated with physical and mental health disparities; during COVID-19, this relationship was especially pronounced (Hooper et al., 2020). Mental health disparities are common after collective trauma; early in the pandemic it became clear that risk factors for mental health problems were not equitably distributed (Hooper et al., 2020; Purtle, 2020). There were disparities in the risks of COVID-19 susceptibility and severity, which in turn could lead to increased trauma exposure, experiences of secondary stressors, and associated grief. Preexisting financial inequities were likely exacerbated; indeed, the ability to isolate in a safe home, work from home with stable Internet access, and maintain income during the pandemic was not equitable across ethnic and racial populations (see Chapters 23–25 for more on racial disparities during the pandemic) (Yancy, 2020). Moreover, perceptions of COVID-19-related discrimination increased over time during the early phase of the pandemic, which was in turn associated with increased psychological distress (Liu et al., 2020). However, most literature on such health disparities was conducted early on in the pandemic, with neither longitudinal follow-ups nor an incorporation of the history effects of the Black Lives Matter protests, the international reckoning on racism, and the highly publicized murder of George Floyd by a Minneapolis, Minnesota, police officer.

Sex/Gender

Generally, women report greater distress following collective trauma exposure. During COVID-19, although women tended to die from COVID-19 at a lower rate than men, they may have endured higher social, psychological, and economic costs associated with the pandemic (see Chapters 11 and 12 of this volume for more on gender differences) (Gausman & Langer, 2020). They were more likely to be front-line workers and to be the primary caregiver for children and other family members. Consequently, during COVID-19, women reported more anxiety, depression, and loneliness compared to men (McQuaid et al., 2021). There was early speculation that women might suffer more economically, which bore out in economic projections regarding the pandemic's impact on women (see Chapter 29 of this volume for more on the experiences of women and families). Indeed, estimates suggested that 56% of workforce departures were women, despite the fact women make up 48% of the workforce (Dua et al., 2021). As estimates suggest these trends will persist in the short and medium term, it is critical that future research account for these phenomena in longitudinal inquiry.

Socioeconomic Status

Lower income has been associated with greater risk for mental health problems during the COVID-19 pandemic, including depression (Holman et al., 2020) and loneliness, which is associated with a variety of negative downstream effects on physical and mental health (McQuaid et al., 2021). It has been robustly established that those with lower SES typically experience worse physical and mental health, with COVID-19 exacerbating these inequities (Purtle, 2020). Not only do those with lower SES typically have less access to high-quality healthcare, they often have jobs that require in-person interaction, putting them at higher risk for COVID-19 exposure (see Chapter 25 of this volume for more on SES inequities). Moreover, low SES households faced nearly a twofold rate of unemployment compared to higher income households, with projections indicating a much slower economic recovery for such households (Dua et al., 2021).

BUILDING RESILIENCE

Despite the confluence of risk factors and the importance of addressing mental health during the pandemic and throughout the recovery efforts, there is reason for hope. Indeed, as the myriad research projects on responses to disasters suggest, resilience is common (see Chapters 20 and 21 for more on resilience). While many people experience elevated psychological distress during and in the immediate aftermath of a traumatic event, humans have a marked capacity for resilience, even during times of great difficulty. Although early research from COVID-19 suggested somewhat elevated symptoms of acute stress and depression, taken at a population level, distress was relatively low (Holman et al., 2020) and was associated with identifiable risk factors (e.g., prior mental health ailments) that could facilitate targeted psychological interventions.

Despite the inherent challenges of COVID-19, new opportunities for more equitable distribution of mental health and self-care resources flourished during the pandemic. Telehealth services expanded, providing greater access and affordability to a larger segment of the populace (Garfin, 2020). Online opportunities to explore and develop healthy interests that reduce stress and facilitate healthy coping also increased dramatically (Garfin, 2020). Options included mediation, yoga, exercise, cooking, reading clubs, art classes, dancing, and so on. During the COVID-19 pandemic, the availability of these activities increased globally, while barriers to access (e.g., cost, transportation, geographic availability) reduced dramatically. Opportunities for social connection also increased as people turned to technology to engage with others. Findings regarding loneliness during COVID-19 have therefore been mixed, with sociodemographic groups at risk for loneliness before the pandemic similarly at risk during COVID-19, with several caveats (e.g., students were more at risk during the pandemic than before) (Bu et al., 2020). Such a finding could be due to the ingenuity of people transitioning to family functions, coworker happy hours, and other social functions via videoconferencing. As the world transitions to a post-COVID-19 reality, individual people, organizations, and providers might reflect on which innovations and opportunities that expanded during COVID-19 might be helpful moving forward.

CONCLUSION AND FUTURE DIRECTIONS

Resiliency and recovery from COVID-19 will likely be heterogeneous. Many will return to prepandemic levels of functioning relatively quickly with few lasting negative mental health consequences. Others will need a period of readjustment before fully returning to life and a mental health state that mirrors their pre-COVID-19 world. Yet, based on prior research on disasters and trauma, a substantial minority of the populace will continue to experience the residual mental health effects of this collective trauma in the years to come. As such, people's exposure to trauma and capacity for resilience shape people's experiences of the pandemic and can inform efforts to bolster resilience and recovery in those with protracted distress responses.

Previous longitudinal research on chronic stressors (Baum, 1990) and collective trauma like the September 11, 2001, terrorist attacks indicated measurable impacts on mental health many years after the event (Garfin et al., 2018). Given the global reach and pervasive disruption of COVID-19 on nearly every aspect of daily life, it could be expected that for many, the mental health crisis may continue long after the vaccine rollout.

The research on the mental health effects of COVID-19 provided key insights into the acute response. Longitudinal research that follows participants over time and throughout the recovery process is necessary to clarify the potential long-term effects. While many studies in the early phase of the outbreak used opt-in online surveys and other forms of convenience samples that provided time-sensitive information, such data should be validated using representative, probability-based samples that integrate prepandemic metrics and follow participants over time. Future research on COVID-19 should take a nuanced approach to measuring exposure and take the perspective that for many—and particularly those groups at risk for high health disparities—many secondary stressors (e.g., job loss) will likely turn into chronic stress with resulting long-term psychological strain. Scholars should also assess what positive outcomes people experienced as a result of the pandemic, and which coping strategies and intervention were effective at mitigating and managing this multifaceted collective trauma. With that perspective, researchers, clinicians, and public health officials can glean information that will clarify the experience of COVID-19 on the populace and learn what might be helpful in preparing for future events.

ACKNOWLEDGMENTS

This work was funded by the National Institute on Minority Health and Health Disparities (K01 MD013910) and National Science Foundation Grant/Award Numbers 2026337 and 2030139.

REFERENCES

American Psychiatric Association. (2013). *Diagnostic and statistical manual of mental disorders* (5th ed.). American Psychiatric Publishing. https://doi.org/10.1176/appi. books.9780890425596.744053

Baum, A. (1990). Stress, intrusive imagery, and chronic distress. *Health Psychology, 9*(6), 653–675. https://doi.org/10.1037/0278-6133.9.6.653

Bertuccio, R. F., & Runion, M. C. (2020). Considering grief in mental health outcomes of COVID-19. *Psychological Trauma: Theory, Research, Practice, and Policy, 12*, 87–89. https://doi.org/10.1037/tra0000723

Brooks, S. K., Webster, R. K., Smith, L. E., Woodland, L., Wessely, S., Greenberg, N., & Rubin, G. J. (2020). The psychological impact of quarantine and how to reduce it: Rapid review of the evidence. *The Lancet, 395*(10227), 912–920. https://doi.org/ 10.1016/S0140-6736(20)30460-8

Bu, F., Steptoe, A., & Fancourt, D. (2020). Who is lonely in lockdown? Cross-cohort analyses of predictors of loneliness before and during the COVID-19 pandemic. *Public Health, 186*, 31–34. https://doi.org/10.1016/j.puhe.2020.06.036

Bureau of Labor Statistics, U.S. Department of Labor. (2021). Consumer price index up 4.2 percent from April 2020 to April 2021. *The Economics Daily.* Consumer price index up 4.2 percent from April 2020 to April 2021 at https://www.bls.gov/opub/ted/2021/consumer-price-index-up-4-2-percent-from-april-2020-to-april-2021.htm

Daly, M., Sutin, A. R., & Robinson, E. (2021). Longitudinal changes in mental health and the COVID-19 pandemic: Evidence from the U.K. Household Longitudinal Study. *Psychological Medicine*, 1–10. https://doi.org/10.1017/S0033291720004432

Dua, A., Ellingrud, K., Lazar, M., Luby, R., Srinivasan, S., & Van Aken, T. (2021, February 3). Achieving an inclusive U.S. economic recovery. *McKinsey & Company.* https://www.mckinsey.com/industries/public-and-social-sector/our-insights/achieving-an-inclusive-us-economic-recovery

Eisma, M. C., Tamminga, A., Smid, G. E., & Boelen, P. A. (2021). Acute grief after deaths due to COVID-19, natural causes and unnatural causes: An empirical comparison. *Journal of Affective Disorders Journal*, *278*, 54–56. https://doi.org/10.1016/j.jad.2020.09.049

Ettman, C. K., Abdalla, S. M., Cohen, G. H., Sampson, L., Vivier, P. M., & Galea, S. (2020). Prevalence of depression symptoms in U.S. adults before and during the COVID-19 pandemic. *JAMA Network Open*, *3*(9), 1–12. https://doi.org/10.1001/jamanetworkopen.2020.19686

Falk, G., Carter, J., Nicchitta, I., Nyhof, E., & Romero, P. (2021). Unemployment rates during the COVID-19 Pandemic. Congressional Research Service, R46554, 1–25. https://crsreports.congress.gov/product/pdf/R/R46554

Garfin, D. R. (2020). Technology as a coping tool during the coronavirus disease 2019 (COVID-19) pandemic: Implications and recommendations. *Stress and Health*, *36*(4), 555–559. https://doi.org/10.1002/smi.2975

Garfin, D. R., Fischhoff, B., Holman, E. A., & Silver, R. C. (2021). Risk perceptions and health behaviors as COVID-19 emerged in the United States: Results from a probability-based nationally representative sample. *Journal of Experimental Psychology: Applied*, *27*(4), 584–598. https://doi.org/https://doi.org/10.1037/xap0000374

Garfin, D. R., Holman, E. A., & Silver, R. C. (2015). Cumulative exposure to prior collective trauma and acute stress responses to the Boston marathon bombings. *Psychological Science*, *26*(6), 675–683. https://doi.org/10.1177/0956797614561043

Garfin, D. R., Poulin, M. J., Blum, S., & Silver, R. C. (2018). Aftermath of terror: A nationwide longitudinal study of posttraumatic stress and worry across the decade following the September 11, 2001 terrorist attacks. *Journal of Traumatic Stress*, *31*(1), 146–156. https://doi.org/10.1002/jts.22262

Garfin, D. R., Silver, R. C., & Holman, E. A. (2020). The novel coronavirus (COVID-2019) outbreak: Amplification of public health consequences by media exposure. *Health Psychology*, *39*(5), 355–357. https://doi.org/10.1037/hea0000875

Garfin, D. R., Silver, R. C., Ulgade, F., Linn, H., & Inostroza, M. (2014). Exposure to rapid succession disasters: A study of residents at the epicenter of the Chilean Bio-Bio earthquake. *Journal of Abnormal Psychology*, *123*, 545–556.

Gausman, J., & Langer, A. (2020). Sex and gender disparities in the COVID-19 pandemic. *Journal of Women's Health*, *29*(4), 465–466. https://doi.org/10.1089/jwh.2020.8472

Hirschberger, G. (2018). Collective trauma and the social construction of meaning. *Frontiers in Psychology*, *9*(August), 1–14. https://doi.org/10.3389/fpsyg.2018.01441

Holland, K. M., Jones, C., Vivolo-Kantor, A. M., Idaikkadar, N., Zwald, M., Hoots, B., . . . & Houry, D. (2021). Trends in US emergency department visits for mental health, overdose, and violence outcomes before and during the COVID-19 pandemic. *JAMA Psychiatry*, *78*(4), 372–379. https://www.doi.org/10.1001/jamapsychia try.2020.4402

Holingue, C., Kalb, L. G., Riehm, K. E., Bennett, D., Kapteyn, A., Veldhuis, C. B., Johnson, R. M., Fallin, M. D., Kreuter, F., Stuart, E. A., & Thrul, J. (2020). Mental distress in the United States at the beginning of the COVID-19 pandemic. *American Journal of Public Health*, *110*(11), 1628–1634. https://doi.org/10.2105/AJPH.2020.305857

Holman, E. A., Garfin, D. R., & Silver, R. C. (2014). Media's role in broadcasting acute stress following the Boston Marathon bombings. *Proceedings of the National Academy of Sciences of the United States of America*, *111*(1), 93–98. https://doi.org/ 10.1073/pnas.1316265110

Holman, E. A., Thompson, R. R., Garfin, D. R., & Silver, R. C. (2020). The unfolding COVID-19 pandemic: A probability-based, nationally representative study of mental health in the U.S. *Science Advances*, *5390*, eabd5390. https://doi.org/10.1126/ sciadv.abd5390

Hooper, M. W., Napoles, A. M., & Perez-Stable, E. J. (2020). COVID-19 and racial/ethnic disparities. *JAMA*, *323*(24), 2466–2467. https://doi.org/10.1002/jclp.20757

John, A., Pirkis, J., Gunnell, D., Appleby, L., & Morrissey, J. (2020). Trends in suicide during the COVID-19 pandemic. *BMJ*, *371*, m4352. https://doi.org/10.1136/ bmj.m4352

Kessler, R. C., McLaughlin, K. A., Koenen, K. C., Petukhova, M., & Hill, E. D. (2012). The importance of secondary trauma exposure for post-disaster mental disorder. *Epidemiology and Psychiatric Sciences*, *21*(1), 35–45. https://www.doi.org/10.1017/ S2045796011000758

Koetsier, J. (2020, September 26). Global online content consumption doubled in 2020. *Forbes*. https://www.forbes.com/sites/johnkoetsier/2020/09/26/global-online-cont ent-consumption-doubled-in-2020/?sh=4583b6b52fde

Liu, Y., Finch, B. K., Brenneke, S. G., Thomas, K., Le, P. D., & Tag, M. P. H. (2020). Perceived discrimination and mental distress amid the COVID-19 pandemic: Evidence from the Understanding America Study. *American Journal of Preventive Medicine*, *59*(4), 481–492. https://doi.org/10.1016/j.amepre.2020.06.007

McQuaid, R. J., Cox, S. M. L., Ogunlana, A., & Jaworska, N. (2021). The burden of loneliness: Implications of the social determinants of health during COVID-19. *Psychiatry Research*, *296*, 113648. https://doi.org/10.1016/j.psychres.2020.113648

Mosheva, M., Gross, R., Hertz-Palmor, N., Hasson-Ohayon, I., Kaplan, R., Cleper, R., Kreiss, Y., Gothelf, D., & Pessach, I. M. (2021). The association between witnessing patient death and mental health outcomes in frontline COVID-19 healthcare workers. *Depression and Anxiety*, *38*(4), 468–479. https://doi.org/10.1002/da.23140

Neimeyer, R. A., & Lee, S. A. (2022). Circumstances of the death and associated risk factors for severity and impairment of COVID-19 grief. *Death Studies*, *46*(1), 34–42. https://www.doi.org/ 10.1080/07481187.2021.1896459

Pfefferbaum, B., & North, C. S. (2020). Mental health and the COVID-19 pandemic. *JAMA*, *383*(6), 510–512. https://www.doi.org/10.1056/NEJMp2008017

Pieh, C., Budimir, S., Delgadillo, J., Barkham, M., Fontaine, J. R. J., & Probst, T. (2021). Mental health during COVID-19 lockdown in the United Kingdom. *Psychosomatic Medicine*, *83*(4), 328–337. https://doi.org/10.1097/PSY.0000000000000871

Purtle, J. (2020). COVID-19 and mental health equity in the United States. *Social Psychiatry and Psychiatric Epidemiology, 55*(8), 969–971. https://doi.org/10.1007/s00127-020-01896-8

Riehm, K. E., Holingue, C., Kalb, L. G., Bennett, D., Kapteyn, A., Jiang, Q., Veldhuis, C. B., Johnson, R. M., Fallin, M. D., Kreuter, F., Stuart, E. A., & Thrul, J. (2020). Associations between media exposure and mental distress among U.S. adults at the beginning of the COVID-19 pandemic. *American Journal of Preventive Medicine, 59*(5), 630–638. https://doi.org/10.1016/j.amepre.2020.06.008

Sakamoto, H., Ishikane, M., Ghaznavi, C., & Ueda, P. (2021). Assessment of suicide in Japan during the COVID-19 pandemic vs previous years. *JAMA Network Open, 4*(2), 1–10. https://doi.org/10.1001/jamanetworkopen.2020.37378

Silver, R. C., & Garfin, D. R. (2016). Coping with disasters. In J. C. Norcross, G. R. VandenBos, & D. K. Freedheim (Editors-in-Chief), *APA handbook of clinical psychology: Psychopathology and health* (Vol. 4, pp. 597–611). Washington, DC: American Psychological Association.

Silver, R. C., Holman, E. A., & Garfin, D. R. (2021). Coping with cascading collective traumas in the United States. *Nature Human Behaviour, 5*(1), 4–6. https://doi.org/10.1038/s41562-020-00981-x

Thompson, R. R., Jones, N. M., Holman, E. A., Garfin, D. R., & Silver, R. C. (2022). COVID-19 community restrictions and mental health in the United States. *Health Psychology, 41*(11), 817–825. https://doi.org/10.1037/hea0001233 [IF: 5.56]

Thompson, R. R., Jones, N. M., Holman, E. A., & Silver, R. C. (2019). Media exposure to mass violence events can fuel a cycle of distress. *Science Advances, 5*, eaav3502. https://doi.org/10.1126/sciadv.aav3502

UNICEF. (2021). COVID-19 and school closures one year of education disruption. https://data.unicef.org/resources/one-year-of-covid-19-and-school-closures/

Yancy, C. W. (2020). COVID-19 and African Americans. *JAMA, 60611*, 2020–2021. https://doi.org/10.1001/jama.2020.6548

Zhai, Y., & Du, X. (2020). Loss and grief amidst COVID-19: A path to adaptation and resilience. *Brain, Behavior, and Immunity, 87*, 80–81.

FURTHER READING

Garfin, D. R., & Silver, R. C. (2016). Responses to natural disasters. In H. S. Friedman (Ed.), *Encyclopedia of mental health* (2nd ed., Vol. 4, pp. 35–46). Academic Press.

Silver, R. C., & Garfin, D. R. (2016). Coping with disasters. In J. C. Norcross, G. R. VandenBos, & D. K. Freedheim (Eds.-in-Chief), *APA handbook of clinical psychology: Vol. 4. Psychopathology and health* (pp. 597–611). American Psychological Association.

Stroebe, M., & Schut, H. (2020). Bereavement in times of COVID-19: A review and theoretical framework. *OMEGA-Journal of Death and Dying, 82*(3), 500–522. https://doi.org/10.1177/0030222820966928.

21

Collective Resilience and the COVID-19 Experience

CHRIS COCKING, EVANGELOS NTONTIS, SARA VESTERGREN,
AND KATARZYNA LUZYNSKA ■

This chapter explores how social psychological theories of collective resilience from the social identity tradition have been applied to understanding people's experiences during the COVID-19 pandemic. The social identity tradition originates from the work of Tajfel and Turner (1979) and Turner (1982), who proposed that as well as having personal identities (i.e., categories that emphasize individual uniqueness vis-à-vis other individuals), people can also derive a sense of self from membership in the various social groups that they identify with (e.g., local neighborhood, nation, etc.). The social norms associated with these multiple identities can influence both individual and collective behavior, and such identities become more or less salient depending on the social context. Social identities and the meaning derived from their group memberships are central for health and well-being. Thus, the social identity approach has been applied to a range of health-related areas (Haslam et al., 2018), including the impact of and public responses to mass emergencies and disasters (e.g., Drury, 2018; Drury et al., 2019). Considering the widespread impact of COVID-19 on psychological well-being, exploring the psychology that underpins public responses to COVID-19 is vital to understanding people's experiences during the pandemic. Therefore, we explore mutual aid and solidarity during the pandemic in this chapter, as well as how having a greater understanding of these concepts can help guide responses to future pandemics.

PUBLIC BEHAVIOR IN EXTREME EVENTS

Public emergency responses are traditionally seen as potentially problematic. Until relatively recently, emergency planning and response guidelines were based on the idea that people cannot be trusted to behave rationally and are prone to "panic." This often resulted in paternalistic or even coercive emergency planning models to prevent and/or control "mass panic." However, research of mass emergencies, going back to World War II and beyond (Fritz & Williams 1957; Quarantelli, 1999; Solnit, 2009), has found that civilian populations can behave much more resiliently than is often expected, and assumptions of panic and/or irrational behavior are rarely supported by empirical evidence. Evidence from emergencies such as bombings, sinking ships, fires, and crowd crushes shows that in times of crisis, people often come together and provide each other with social support (Drury et al., 2009a, 2009b). Pathologizing narratives of individual irrationality such as "panic buying" that are common in public discourse are not supported by empirical evidence. Rather, stockpiling behavior is often attributed to people's perceptions of shortages by observing other people's behavior in person or through media reports (Sterman & Dogan, 2015; Zheng et al., 2020). Crucially, during mass emergencies people might try to minimize trips to supermarkets and thus engage in slightly increased and less frequent purchases, which can cause problems to fragile supply chains that are designed for immediate demands and do not stock additional products (Kantar World Panel, 2020; Lewis, 2020). Thus, the expectations that people will panic is not the reality of the overall experience of the pandemic.

Rather than being too shocked or panicked to help others during the acute phase of emergencies, evidence shows that public intervention before the arrival of emergency first responders is common, and such members of the public are known as "zero responders" (Cocking, 2013). Social psychologists from the social identity tradition have developed the social identity model of collective psychosocial resilience (SIMCPR) to explain how such spontaneous collective resilience occurs (Drury, 2018; Ntontis et al., 2019). The SIMCPR argues that disasters can create a sense of shared fate ("we're all in this together") that enables a shared social identity to emerge among those affected, which becomes the basis of various emotional, relational, and behavioral changes. For example, people start to consider themselves less in terms of individual characteristics and more as members of the same group. This shift to a shared identity leads them to expect support from and provide support to other fellow group members and facilitates collective coordination. This common identity can emerge from survivors' experiences of the incident itself, and such social bonds might not have been present (or at least not as strong) before the start of the emergency. Therefore, collective resilience can occur not only *despite* an emergency, but also *because of it*.

Apart from emergent groups in the absence of preexisting bonds, people's responses to extreme events can also be influenced by the existence of social capital, which is defined as "the aggregate of the actual or potential resources which are linked to possession of a durable network of more or less institutionalized relationships of mutual acquaintance and recognition" (Bourdieu, 1986, p. 21). This refers to how dense social networks can facilitate norms of reciprocity, trust, and social bonds (Helliwell & Putnam, 2004; see also Chapter 19 for more on social networks and the pandemic). Communities with dense social capital are characterized by a sense of continuity and creativity during disasters (Dynes, 2006).

Such bonds provide social support and assistance toward those in need, mobilize resources more effectively, and improve recovery from extreme events (Aldrich, 2017; Chamlee-Wright & Storr, 2011; Elliott et al., 2010). The SIMCPR has been applied to promoting greater crowd resilience and safety during emergencies, with recent recommendations (e.g., Drury et al., 2019) calling for emergency planners and responders to better understand crowd psychology and to work more collaboratively with the public to encourage greater collective resilience.

UNDERSTANDING PANDEMIC BEHAVIOR

This section explores human behavior in pandemics and the social support and mutual aid that can occur during them. Before the COVID-19 pandemic, the SIMCPR drew evidence mainly from acute, short-term "big-bang" incidents—such as terrorist attacks or fires (see Drury et al., 2009a, 2009b)—or more medium-term, "rising-tide" events, such as flooding (Ntontis et al., 2018). The "Spanish influenza" from 1918 to 1920[1] was the last long-term global pandemic previous to COVID-19 and pre-dated most modern research into emergencies. However, it quickly become apparent that social identity models of human behavior were also relevant to COVID-19, and that application of the SIMCPR could help with responses to mitigate the effects of the pandemic. Therefore, in early 2020, psychologists began to explore psychosocial responses to the pandemic and encourage greater collective resilience in public behavior, highlighting the crucial role of group processes (Van Bavel et al., 2020). Encouraging collectively resilient behaviors was especially important when countries around the world introduced national lockdowns from February 2020 onward, and populations were expected to conform to far-reaching behavioral restrictions to break the transmission cycle of COVID-19. Lockdowns had a major impact on people's daily lives, affecting travel, working practices, and social interactions on a global scale. Social identity psychologists argued that to respond effectively to these required changes it was necessary to move beyond the pathologizing narratives prevalent in public discourses in relation to behavior in emergencies (Drury et al., 2020). Furthermore, shortly before the first U.K. lockdown began in March 2020, Reicher and Drury (2020)[2] argued that individualized responses ("Will I survive?") to the pandemic were less likely to be effective, and that it would be better to encourage more collective responses ("How do we all get through this?") as a tactic to promote the mass behavioral changes that were necessary to combat the spread of COVID-19 infection.

Unfortunately, appeals from social psychologists to trust the public's collective resilience in the face of the pandemic were not heeded by policymakers in the United Kingdom, and the notion of "behavioral fatigue" (that people would quickly tire of lockdown measures and cease complying with them) was used as a reason to delay the national U.K. lockdown in March 2020 (BBC, 2020). The decision to delay lockdown was challenged by clinicians, with some arguing that it may have cost thousands more lives compared to initiating it earlier (Mahase,

2020). Additionally, a subsequent media investigation found that there was no evidence from either psychology or from the broader social sciences to substantiate the notion of behavioral fatigue (BBC, 2020), with behavioral experts advising the U.K. Scientific Advisory Group on Emergencies (SAGE)[3] disputing the very existence of the term.

SOCIAL SUPPORT AND MUTUAL AID

Rather than the selfish and/or "irrational" behavior during the COVID-19 pandemic that was widely predicted beforehand, there were mass outpourings of social support and spontaneous volunteering as lockdown restrictions were imposed in the United Kingdom (Alakeson & Brett, 2020; Greenaway, 2020; Tiratelli & Kaye, 2020). By May 2020, it was estimated that there were over 4,300 mutual aid groups comprising approximately 3 million people in the United Kingdom—more than the total number of civilians that volunteered for the U.K. Civilian Defense Service throughout the duration of World War II.[4] Over 750,000 people also volunteered to help the U.K. National Health Service's call for volunteers, but it was estimated that only one in three of these volunteers was used, as it was not possible for the system to accommodate all offers. Therefore, many of these volunteers gravitated toward involvement in mutual aid schemes within their local communities instead (Butler, 2020). Such cooperation was often manifested on a reciprocal level within people's local communities, and a survey by the U.K. Office for National Statistics (ONS) found that two thirds of respondents believed their local community would provide them with social support if they needed it, one third had done shopping for others in their local community, and two thirds had checked on their neighbors' well-being in the previous week (ONS, 2020).

The cooperation seen during the pandemic supports social identity models, with Goldberg et al. (2020) finding that disease prevention behavior was linked to positive social influence from friends and family. Furthermore, interviews with members of mutual aid groups during the first U.K. COVID-19 lockdown (Cocking et al., 2023; Mao et al., 2021) found that the reciprocal nature of the mutual aid relationship was important for participants not only from helping others, but also because they felt they could draw on such support themselves if they ever needed it. The perceived reciprocal support echoes previous work by Sani (2012) showing that belonging to valued social groups can be beneficial for physical and mental well-being, independently of whether support from the groups in question was accessed by its members. Furthermore, Mao et al. (2021) also found that participation offered members of mutual aid groups positive emotional experiences, increased engagement in life, increased a sense of control, and improved social relationships. Additionally, participation in mutual aid facilitated the creation of new social identities and, when seen through a political lens, created a sense of empowerment among participants and enhanced their willingness to address the structural roots of inequality.

Therefore, by supporting others within their local community, participants stressed the importance of neighborhood action as beneficial for both community cohesion and individual mental well-being. Identification with one's local neighborhood was recognized as an important source of social support in work pre-dating the COVID-19 pandemic (Fong et al., 2019; Stevenson et al., 2019). Furthermore, identification with one's local community may also be easier to maintain psychologically than broader regional or national identities. Consequently, members of local COVID-19 mutual aid groups may have found it easier to empathize with, and so help other ingroup members. Such community resilience can also become a source of positive feedback that encourages other related prosocial behaviors. For instance, Stevenson et al. (2021) found that community identification not only predicted the giving and receiving of pandemic-related support, but also positively predicted adherence to lockdown restrictions. The increased sense of shared collective identity that emerges from providing social support for others can also promote an enhanced sense of mental well-being. For example, Röselet al. (2022) found that social support was positively linked to ability to cope with the negative mental health impacts of the pandemic. With regard to involvement in mutual aid groups, Cocking et al. (2023) found that participants reported positive personal benefits from their involvement in community groups. For instance, some reported that their involvement in local community groups helped them deal with the pandemic better, and that these benefits were also realized through the creation of new personal relationships with others in their community that outlasted the initial lockdown. Furthermore, some participants who offered to do dog walking for those self-isolating under COVID-19 restrictions reported that they continued this activity after the end of the self-isolation period to maintain the connection with the person they had been supporting (and perhaps also with their dog!). Therefore, involvement in mutual aid groups during the COVID-19 lockdown provided participants with a reciprocal sense of social support and, consequently, an enhanced sense of individual and collective well-being (see also Chapter 20 for more in individual resilience and well-being).

ENDURING RESILIENCE?

While there is a wide body of evidence to support the notion of collective resilience developing from a shared experience of adversity during emergencies, such resilience can decline as the emergency becomes less acute. This decline in resilience can be an issue in ongoing incidents, such as a global pandemic that requires repeated lockdowns to prevent infection spread. There is some evidence that the solidarity seen during the early stages of disasters later declines (Fritz & Williams, 1957; Kaniasty & Norris, 1999). This reduction in solidarity can result from the shared experience of adverse events dissipating over time due to a shift in people's self-perception away from social identities related to the disaster (Ntontis et al., 2020). Cocking et al.'s (2023) study of mutual aid involvement during the first U.K. COVID-19 lockdown in March 2020 found that involvement in mutual cooperation can decrease over time, but that this was more likely a result of structural factors impacting participants' ability to continue supporting others (e.g., a need to return to work, child care commitments, etc.) and not because of any reduced personal motivation. Existing societal inequalities can also hinder enduring collective resilience. For instance, Templeton al. (2020) argued that while the shared sense of common fate that emerges in response to adversity should underpin community responses to COVID-19, some aspects of the pandemic could also exacerbate existing economic, ethnic, and gender-based inequalities, which could in turn undermine such community action. This is consistent with previous work by Ntontis et al. (2020), who found that participants' perceptions of inequitable treatment by the authorities could diminish the collective identity that had originally emerged from their community being flooded. Perceived inconsistencies in messaging and/or behavior from those in authority can also erode public confidence in and adherence to lockdown restrictions. This is because if people believe that those in authority are not leading by example, then the sense of shared adversity ("We're all in this together") can decline. Such discrepancy in messaging and action happened in May 2020 after the U.K. prime minister's aide Dominic Cummings broke lockdown regulations while potentially infectious with COVID-19 (Cocking, 2020). However, Jackson et al. (2020) argued that such behavior could have served as an anti–role model and may have even encouraged some to maintain their own compliance with lockdown regulations, as those who were already likely to adhere to lockdown restrictions could believe that it became even less acceptable to do so after this story emerged.

IMPLICATIONS AND FUTURE DIRECTIONS

The COVID-19 pandemic is likely to have an impact for the foreseeable future; hence, it is vital to consider the implications of taking more collective perspectives in such crises and the possible directions that future research should take. The field of social psychology is ideally placed to take up this challenge, and relevant perspectives from within this discipline (especially the social identity approach) can be applied to explore how we respond to global emergencies such as the COVID-19 pandemic. For example, among possible priorities for further research, O'Connor et al. (2020) suggested that making collective identities more salient (and hence developing a greater concern for the well-being of others) could also encourage greater compliance with COVID-19 lockdown restrictions. Collectivizing the response to the pandemic was evident in the speeches of New Zealand Prime Minister Jacinda Ardern, who (in contrast to the UK Prime Minister Boris Johnson; see Chapter 14 for more on pandemic related messages and Chapter 32 for discussion of leadership during the pandemic) framed governmental decisions as moral imperatives for the nation's health, positioned herself and the government as parts of the people (rather than as outgroups), invoked the capacity of the nation to overcome the pandemic collectively, and constructed norms of social support and mutual aid as core aspects of New Zealand's national identity (Vignoles et al., 2021).

The nature of COVID-19 transmission means that mass adherence to restrictions to prevent infection (e.g., self-isolation after possible exposure) is necessary, and feeling a sense of social support can be crucial for encouraging such adherence. However, reported adherence to self-isolation after possible exposure to COVID-19 in the United Kingdom varied during the pandemic, and up to 75% of symptomatic respondents reported leaving their home within the previous 24 hours (Smith et al., 2021). Nevertheless, coercive measures are unlikely to be effective in ensuring compliance, and in any case, local and national authorities would rarely have the resources to enforce such mass compliance.

Therefore, getting the public to identify with, and thereby comply with, more facilitative approaches to necessary behavioral changes is likely to be more effective. Indeed, earlier work by Smith et al. (2020) found that those in receipt of social support from others in their local community were more likely to adhere to self-isolation lockdown restrictions. Finally, more research on how to best encourage enduring collective resilience in the long term is necessary, as the nature of the COVID-19 outbreak (and any future pandemics) means that long-term behavior change may be necessary to combat such emergencies more effectively. In short, those in authority should see the public as a partner in pandemic responses (rather than as a potential problem), and more collaborative approaches that encourage a collective sense of identity would be more effective in responding to similar future global emergencies.

CONCLUSION AND "TAKE-HOME" MESSAGES

It is undeniable that the COVID-19 pandemic brought great deprivation and hardship across the globe. However, the mass displays of mutual cooperation and social support that emerged as the scale of the pandemic became apparent illustrates how such dark times can also bring about the best in human nature. Such collective resilience displayed by the public is not guaranteed though, and it needs to be enabled and facilitated by those in authority who are responsible for mass emergency planning and response. Therefore, we finish this chapter with the following take-home messages on how to encourage such collective resilience in future pandemics:

- Those in authority must stop assuming that the public cannot behave resiliently in mass emergencies and/or pandemics and should not adopt "panic" models in their planning responses.
- Mass emergencies can create a shared sense of adversity that creates a common identity and cooperative behavior among those affected ("We're all in this together").
- Emergency planning guidelines need to recognize the potential for collective resilience and help facilitate the potential for the collective resilience that can emerge during global pandemics.

- Such collective resilience can be manifested via spontaneous volunteering and/or involvement in local mutual aid groups outside of traditional governmental structures and/or nongovernmental organizations, and this should be recognized in emergency planning guidelines.
- More collective and collaborative approaches would encourage more effective responses to future emergencies and/or pandemics.

In conclusion, therefore, we would argue that while much needs to be learned from negative experiences during the COVID-19 pandemic, more attention needs to be paid to the overall resilient nature of public responses, and to learning more about these positive collective experiences will improve responses to future pandemics.

NOTES

1. https://www.cdc.gov/flu/pandemic-resources/1918-pandemic-h1n1.html
2. See Drury and Reicher (2020).
3. BBC Newsnight on Twitter: "There's no science behind the term behavioural fatigue."—Professor Robert West, member of the government's scientific pandemic influenza group on behaviours. Watch @lewis_goodall's report into why the United Kingdom didn't lockdown sooner. https://t.co/1HNCCQ3DP7 #Newsnight https://t.co/gem3gb4b2Y
4. https://en.wikipedia.org/wiki/Civil_Defence_Service#:~:text=The%20Civil%20Defence%20Service%20was,Service%20(CD)%20in%201941

REFERENCES

Alakeson, V., & Brett, W. (2020). Local heroes. How to sustain community spirit beyond Covid-19. Power to Change, National Lottery Community Fund. https://www.powertochange.org.uk/blog/local-heroes-sustain-community-spirit-beyond-covid-19/

Aldrich, D. P. (2017). The importance of social capital in building community resilience. In W. Yan & W. Galloway. (Eds.), *Rethinking resilience, adaptation and transformation in a time of change* (pp. 357–364). Springerhttps://doi.org/10.1007/978-3-319-50171-0_23

BBC. (2020, July 20). Behavioural science and the pandemic. https://www.bbc.co.uk/sounds/play/m0001207

Bourdieu, P. (1986). Pierre Bourdieu 1986—The forms of capital. In J. Richardson (Ed.), *Handbook of theory and research for the sociology of education* (pp. 241–258). The Guardian.

Butler, P. (2020, March 8). NHS coronavirus crisis volunteers frustrated at lack of tasks. *The Guardian.* https://www.theguardian.com/world/2020/may/03/nhs-coronavirus-crisis-volunteers-frustrated-at-lack-of-tasks

Chamlee-Wright, E., & Storr, V. (2011). Social capital as collective narratives and post-disaster community recovery. *Sociological Review, 59*(2), 266–282. https://doi.org/10.1111/j.1467-954X.2011.02008.x

Cocking, C. (2013). The role of "zero-responders" during 7/7: Implications for the emergency services. *International Journal of the Emergency Services, 2*(2), 79–93.

Cocking, C. (2020, May 25). Resilience requires those in authority to be honest, open and consistent. *The Psychologist.* https://www.bps.org.uk/psychologist/resilience-requires-those-authority-be-honest-open-and-consistent

Cocking, C., Vestergren, S., Ntontis, E., & Luzynska, K. (2023). "All together now": Facilitators and barriers to engagement in mutual aid during the first UK COVID-19 lockdown. *Plos One, 18*(4), e0283080. https://doi.org/10.1371/journal.pone.0283080

Drury, J. (2018). The role of social identity processes in mass emergency behaviour: An integrative review. *European Review of Social Psychology, 29*(1), 38–81.

Drury, J., Carter, H., Cocking, C., Ntontis, E., Guven, S. T., & Amlot, R. (2019). Facilitating collective resilience in the public in emergencies: Twelve recommendations based on the social identity approach. *Frontiers in Public Health, 7,* 1–21. https://doi.org/10.3389/fpubh.2019.00141

Drury, J., Cocking, C., & Reicher, S. (2009a). Everyone for themselves? Understanding how crowd solidarity can arise in an emergency: An interview study of disaster survivors. *British Journal of Social Psychology, 48,* 487–506. https://doi.org/10.1348/014466608X357893

Drury, J., Cocking, C., & Reicher, S. (2009b). The nature of collective "resilience": Survivor reactions to the July 7th (2005) London bombings. *International Journal of Mass Emergencies and Disasters, 27*(1), 66–95.

Drury, J., & Reicher, S. (2020). Don't personalise, collectivise! The Psychologist. https://thepsychologist.bps.org.uk/dont-personalise-collectivise

Drury, J., Reicher, S., & Stott, C. (2020). COVID-19 in context: Why do people die in emergencies? It's probably not because of collective psychology. *British Journal of Social Psychology, 59*(3), 689–693. https://doi.org/10.1111/bjso.12393

Dynes, R. (2006). Social capital: Dealing with community emergencies. *Homeland Security Affairs, 2*(2), 1–26.

Elliott, J. R., Haney, T. J., & Sams-Abiodun, P. (2010). Limits to social capital: Comparing network assistance in two New Orleans neighborhoods devastated by Hurricane Katrina. *The Sociological Quarterly, 51*(4), 624–648.

Fong, P., Cruwys, T., Haslam, C., & Haslam, S. A. (2019). Neighbourhood identification and mental health: How social identification moderates the relationship between socioeconomic disadvantage and health. *Journal of Environmental Psychology, 61,* 101–114.https://doi.org/10.1016/j.jenvp.2018.12.006

Fritz, C., & Williams, H. (1957). The human being in disasters: A research perspective. *Annals of the American Academy of Political & Social Science, 309*(1), 42–51. https://doi.org/10.1177/000271625730900107

Goldberg, M., Maibach, E. W., Van der Linden, S., & Kotcher, J. (2020). Social norms motivate COVID-19 preventive behaviors. PsyArXiv. https://doi.org/10. 31234/osf.io/9whp4

Greenaway, K., (2020). Group threat. In J. Jetten, S. Reicher, S. Haslam, & T. Cruwys (Eds.), *Together apart: The psychology of COVID-19* (pp. 61–67). Sage.

Haslam, C., Jetten, J., Cruwys, T., Dingle, G., & Haslam, S. A. (2018). *The new psychology of health: Unlocking the social cure*. Routledge.

Helliwell, J. F., & Putnam, R. D. (2004). The social context of well-being. *Philosophical Transactions of the Royal Society B: Biological Sciences, 359*(1449), 1435–1446. https://doi.org/10.1098/rstb.2004.1522

Jackson, J., Bradford, B., Yesberg, J., Hobson, Z., Kyprianides, A., Pósch, K., & Solymosi, R. (2020, June 15). Public compliance and COVID-19: Did Cummings damage the fight against the virus, or become a useful anti-role model? *LSE BPP.* https://blogs.lse.ac.uk/politicsandpolicy/public-compliance-covid19-june/

Kaniasty, K., & Norris, F. (1999). The experience of disaster: Individuals and communities sharing trauma. In R. Gist & B. Lubin (Eds.), *Response to disaster: Psychosocial, community, and ecological Approaches* (pp. 25–62). Bruner/Mazel. http://dx.doi.org/10.1016/S0022-3999%2802%2900418-X

Kantar World Panel. (2020). Accidental stockpilers driving shelf shortages in the U.K. Kantar World Panel. *https://www.kantar.com/inspiration/fmcg/accidental-stockpilers-driving-shelf-shortages-in-the-uk*

Lewis, H. (2020). How panic-buying revealed the problem with the modern world. *The Atlantic.* https://www.theatlantic.com/international/archive/2020/03/coronavirus-panic-buying-britain-us-shopping/608731/

Mao, G., Drury, J., Fernandes-Jesus, M., & Ntontis, E. (2021). How participation in Covid-19 mutual aid groups affects subjective wellbeing and how political identity moderates these effects. *Analyses of Social Issues and Public Policy, 21*(1), 1082–1112. https://doi.org/10.1111/asap.12275

Mahase, E. (2020). Covid-19: Was the decision to delay the U.K.'s lockdown over fears of "behavioural fatigue" based on evidence? *BMJ, 370,* m3166. http://dx.doi.org/10.1136/bmj.m3166

Ntontis, E., Drury, J., Amlôt, R., Rubin, J. G., & Williams, R. (2018). Emergent social identities in a flood: Implications for community psychosocial resilience. *Journal of Community and Applied Social Psychology, 28*(1), 3–14. https://doi.org/10.1002/casp.2329

Ntontis, E., Drury, J., Amlôt, R., Rubin, J. G., & Williams, R. (2019). What lies beyond social capital? The role of social psychology in building community resilience to climate change. *Traumatology, 26*(3), 253–265. http://dx.doi.org/10.1037/trm0000221

Ntontis, E., Drury, J., Amlôt, R., Rubin, G., & Williams R. (2020). Endurance or decline of emergent groups following a flood disaster: Implications for community resilience. *International Journal of Disaster Risk Reduction, 45.* https://doi.org/10.1016/j.ijdrr.2020.101493

O'Connor, D., Aggleton, J., & Chakrabarti, B. (2020). Research priorities for the COVID-19 pandemic and beyond: A call to action for psychological science. *British Journal of Psychology, 111*(4), 609–623. https://onlinelibrary.wiley.com/doi/full/10.1111/bjop.12468

Office for National Statistics (ONS). (2020). Coronavirus and the social impacts on Great Britain: 16 April 2020. https://www.ons.gov.uk/peoplepopulationandcommunity/healthandsocialcare/healthandwellbeing/bulletins/coronavirusandthesocialimpactsongreatbritain/16april2020

Quarantelli, E. L. (1999). Disaster related social behavior: Summary of 50 years of research findings. https://udspace.udel.edu/items/57c4515d-7714-4154-9dce-1a167334aa3b

Rösel, I., Bauer, L. L., Seiffer, B., Deinhart, C., Atrott, B., Sudeck, G., . . . Wolf, S. (2022). The effect of exercise and affect regulation skills on mental health during the COVID-19 pandemic: A cross-sectional survey. *Psychiatry Research*, *312*, 114559. https://doi.org/10.1016/j.psychres.2022.114559

Sani, F. (2012). Group identity, social relationships and health. In J. Jetten, C. Haslam, & S. A. Haslam. (Eds.), *The social cure: Identity, health and well-being* (pp. 21–37). Taylor & Francis.

Smith, L. E., Amlôt, R., Lambert, H., Oliver, I., Robin, C., Yardley, L., & Rubin, G. J. (2020). Factors associated with adherence to self-isolation and lockdown measures in the UK: A cross-sectional survey. *Public Health*, *187*, 41–52. https://doi.org/10.1016/j.puhe.2020.07.024

Smith, L. E., Potts, H., Amlôt, R., Fear, N., Michie, S., Rubin, G. J. (2021). Adherence to the test, trace, and isolate system in the U.K.: Results from 37 nationally representative surveys. *BMJ*, *372*, n608. https://doi.org/10.1136/bmj.n608

Solnit, R. (2009). *A paradise built in hell: The extraordinary communities that arise in disaster*. Penguin Books.

Sterman, J. D., & Dogan, G. (2015). "I'm not hoarding, I'm just stocking up before the hoarders get here": Behavioral causes of phantom ordering in supply chains. *Journal of Operations Management*, *39–40*, 6–22. https://doi.org/10.1016/j.jom.2015.07.002

Stevenson, C., Easterbrook, M., Harkin, L., McNamara, N., Kellezi, B., & Shuttleworth, I. (2019). Neighbourhood identity helps residents cope with residential diversification: Contact in increasingly mixed neighbourhoods of Northern Ireland. *Political Psychology*, *40*, 227–295. https://doi.org/10.1111/pops.12510

Stevenson, C., Wakefield, J., Felsner, I., Drury, J., & Costa, S. (2021). Collectively coping with coronavirus: Local community identification predicts giving support and lockdown adherence during the COVID-19 pandemic. *British Journal of Social Psychology*, *60*(4), 1403–1418. https://doi.org/10.1111/bjso.12457

Tajfel, H., & Turner, J. C. (1979). An integrative theory of intergroup conflict. In W. Austin & S. Worchel (Eds.), *The social psychology of intergroup relations* (pp. 33–37). Brooks/Cole.

Templeton, A., Guven, S. T., Hoerst, C., Vestergren, S., Davidson, L., Ballentyne, S., & Choudhury, S. (2020). Inequalities and identity processes in crises: Recommendations for facilitating safe response to the COVID-19 pandemic. *British Journal of Social Psychology*, *59*(3), 674–685. https://doi.org/10.1111/bjso.12400

Tiratelli, L., & Kaye, S. (2020). *Communities vs coronavirus: The rise of mutual aid*. New Local Government Network.

Turner, J. C. (1982). Towards a cognitive redefinition of the social group. In H. Tajfel (Ed.), *Social identity and intergroup relations* (pp. 15–40). Cambridge University Press.

Van Bavel, J., Baicker, K., Boggio, P. S., Capraro, V., Cichocka, A., Cikara, M., Crockett, M., Crum, A., Douglas, K., Druckman, J., Drury, J., Dube, O., Ellemers, N., Finkel, E., Fowler, J., Gelfand, M., Han, S., Haslam, A., Jetten, J., . . . Willer, R. (2020). Using social and behavioural science to support COVID-19 pandemic response. *Nature Human Behaviour*, *4*, 460–471. https://doi.org/10.1038/s41562-020-0884-z

Vignoles, V., Jaser, Z., Taylor, F., & Ntontis, E. (2021). Harnessing shared identities to mobilize resilient responses to the COVID-19 pandemic. *Political Psychology*, *42*(5), 817–826. https://doi.org/10.1111/pops.12726

Zheng, R., Shou, B., & Yang, J. (2020). Supply disruption management under consumer panic buying and social learning effects. *Omega*, *101*, 102238. https://doi.org/10.1016/j.omega.2020.102238

FURTHER READING/USEFUL RESOURCES

British Psychological Society. (2020). COVID resources. https://www.bps.org.uk/coro navirus-resources

UK Health Security Agency (UKHSA). (2020). COVID-19 pages. https://www.gov.uk/ government/organisations/uk-health-security-agency

U.K. Scientific Advisory Group (SAGE) Pandemic Influenza Behavioural group (SPI-B). (2020). Home page. https://www.gov.uk/government/groups/independent-scienti fic-pandemic-influenza-group-on-behaviours-spi-b

University of Sussex. Groups and COVID. (2020). Research web pages. https://www.sus sex.ac.uk/research/projects/groups-and-covid/

22

Staying Together While Apart

How Digital Media Both Helped and Harmed Our Sense of Connection During the COVID-19 Pandemic

ANDREA BAYER, SARA V. WHITE, AND
SAMUEL E. EHRENREICH ∎

Over the past decade, social media and digital communication have become increasingly important platforms people use to interact and connect with their peers and peer networks. Digital communication platforms have established themselves as the preferred method for adolescents and young adults to interact with their peers (Nesi et al., 2018a; Rideout & Robb, 2018) and have become increasingly common among older adults as well (Greenwood et al., 2016). Although this trend toward digital peer interactions has been unfolding for years, the COVID-19 pandemic—and the associated social distancing—amplified this transition and forced many individuals to rely almost exclusively on these digital platforms for peer interaction. Whereas digital forms of interaction had been consistently increasing in popularity over the past decade (Ehrenreich et al., 2021), the COVID-19 pandemic forced many people across the world to rely on digital platforms exclusively for social interaction. This abrupt and categorical shift to digital interactions provides a unique opportunity to examine how interactions in these digital spaces shape and define peer relationships. This chapter applies the transformation framework to understand how social media facilitated (and at times hindered) efforts to stay connected with peers during COVID-19 social distancing procedures. The chapter examines how individuals' pandemic experiences can offer insight into future research on peer relationships. The lessons that can be learned for policymakers, educators, and parents are also discussed.

Andrea Bayer, Sara V. White, and Samuel E. Ehrenreich, *Staying Together While Apart* In: *The Social Science of the COVID-19 Pandemic*. Edited by: Monica K. Miller, Oxford University Press. © Oxford University Press 2024.
DOI: 10.1093/oso/9780197615133.003.0022

THE TRANSFORMATIONAL FRAMEWORK

The transformation framework proposes that adolescents and adults do not simply transition their existing peer interactions into digital spaces, but that these digital platforms can fundamentally transform the ways in which we interact with our peers. For purposes of this chapter, social media are broadly defined, and the description used by Nesi et al. (2018a) is adopted. Social media constitutes any "media used for social interaction, including digital applications or tools where users share content and communicate with others" (Nesi et al., 2018a, p. 270). This definition includes, but is not limited to, websites and apps such as Facebook, Snapchat, Instagram, Tiktok, YouTube, Twitter, and Tumblr and more dyadic communication tools such as text messaging.

This framework proposes five conceptual ways that social media can transform peer experiences (Nesi et al., 2018a). First, social media has the potential to transform peer experiences "by changing the *frequency or immediacy* those interactions," permitting nearly constant access to the entire peer network regardless of physical location (Nesi et al., 2018b, p. 296). Next (and building on the increased *immediacy*): "Social media may *amplify* peer experiences and demands by increasing their intensity and scale" (Nesi et al., 2018b, p. 296). The ability to contact peers immediately and continuously could create the expectation that an individual be responsive. Third, social media could "*alter the qualitative nature* of peer experiences," for example by changing or eliminating a variety of social cues, such as tone of voice, physical touch, or eye contact (Nesi et al., 2018b, pp. 296–298). Social media may also "transform peer experiences by creating *new opportunities for compensatory behaviors*—i.e., behaviors that would have been less likely or more challenging offline" (Nesi et al., 2018b, p. 298). Last, social media has the potential to "create opportunities for *entirely novel behaviors*, or behaviors that would have been impossible offline" (Nesi et al., 2018b, p. 298).

This chapter applies the five categories of transformation to the ways in which social media impacted people's ability to stay connected during the COVID-19 pandemic. Nesi et al. (2018a) used the transformation framework to understand adolescents' peer experiences; however, this chapter employs a more expansive interpretation of the framework and uses it to examine the large-scale impact of social media during the social distancing practices of the COVID-19 pandemic.

TRANSFORMED PEER EXPERIENCES DURING THE COVID-19 PANDEMIC

In an effort to minimize the spread of the COVID-19 virus, many of the primary sources of peer interaction were restricted, including the closing of many offices, schools and universities, and public recreation sites. Face-to-face interactions were limited through social distancing mandates. Given the restrictions on in-person contact, it is not surprising that social media became a primary way for people to cope with social distancing and provided opportunities for people to remain connected. The five categories of transformation discussed by Nesi et al. (2018a) provide a framework for understanding how the nearly complete transition to digital social interaction experienced by many people shaped their relationships and sense of connection during this period.

Frequency and Immediacy of Peer Experiences

The first way that social media transforms peer relationships is by altering the *frequency or immediacy* of interactions (Nesi et al., 2018b, p. 296). Social media allows "peer interactions and communication to occur rapidly and often" (Nesi et al., 2018a, p. 278). Because peers are constantly available via social media, and these interactions are often public and stored permanently, this may increase the potential for frequent and immediate social support during COVID-19 (Nesi et al., 2018a, p. 284). During a time when face-to-face contact was discouraged with individuals outside the household, social media ensured that social interactions could occur any time of day from any location. People could consistently and instantaneously develop and maintain relationships with social networks. This allowed individuals to find a source of connection during a time of isolation 24 hours a day and 7 days a week. Several media sources confirmed that, since the beginning of the pandemic, the number of hours individuals are exposed to screen time has increased dramatically for both children[1] and adults.[2] For example, between 2019 and March 2020, adult screen time increased more than 3 hours per day.[3] Similarly, since the lockdowns of March 2020, children's screen time was up 50%.[4] The pandemic dominated virtual school and work discussions, after-hours remote happy hours, and late-night Facebook messaging. The frequency and immediacy of social media also meant that individuals were less likely to find a "sanctuary" to escape information related to COVID-19. This may have heightened negative feelings associated with the pandemic.

Amplification of Peer Experiences and Demands

Social media can also transform peer interactions through an *amplification* of peer experiences and demands (Nesi et al., 2018a). The availability of social media increases the expectations associated with maintaining peer networks (Nesi et al., 2018a). For example, the capacity to be in contact with peers at any point often comes with an implicit expectation that an individual should be responsive at a moment's notice. For example, one of the ways that social media use can negatively impact adolescents' sleep is an unwillingness to "sign off" as one gets tired due to the perception that peers expect teens to be constantly available to respond to messages, posts, or comments (Scott et al., 2019).

One interesting way that social media has amplified peer experiences is through passive social media use (scrolling through peers' social media feeds without directly interacting), which increases social comparison and social influence.

Adolescents and young adults who spend significant amounts of time passively viewing peers' posts are at risk for negative social comparison, often feeling like their own lives do not compare to the highly curated content of peers' posts (Fardouly & Vartanian, 2016). On the flip side of this, the perception that peers are constantly viewing and evaluating one's own posts often creates pressure to present an idealized image (Yau & Reich, 2019). Indeed, passive social media use amplifies social comparison, envy, and anxiety about missing out on fun activities and has been one of the most consistent predictors of maladjustment (Frison & Eggermont, 2020; Vogel et al., 2015).

The amplification of peer experiences on social media likely remained during the pandemic, as people may have devoted considerably more time and energy to social media in an effort to stay connected. This may have resulted in an increased perception of obligation to be accessible. Additionally, the ability of social media to amplify experiences and demands may have led individuals to feel even more isolated during the pandemic. Scrolling through social media and seeing repeated posts about a lack of in-person connection and separation may have led to rumination. Interestingly, in our own examination of young adults' social media usage during social distancing procedures, we did not find the expected correlations between passive social media use and loneliness or depression (White & Ehrenreich, 2021). It is possible that, although many used social media as a platform to gripe and express negativity, the risk of negative social comparison and anxiety about missing out on social events was diminished since the lack of fun social events was a shared experience.

Altered Qualitative Nature of Peer Experiences

Peer interactions that occur in digital spaces are in many ways fundamentally distinct from face-to-face social interactions. Nesi and colleagues (2018a) highlighted the loss of social cues that may make digital peer experiences less rich. The inability to provide physical touch, eye contact, and supportive body language may undermine efforts to support and console a friend. Similarly, the asynchronicity of many social media platforms may disrupt social connection. If an individual is seeking support and help from a peer, the delay between messages may impair a feeling of connection. The absence of body language and tone of voice may also lead to miscommunication and misunderstanding (Madell & Muncer 2007). For example, a sardonic statement made as a joke might instead be interpreted as an actual attack directed at the partner.

As socially distanced individuals were increasingly forced to interact with peers exclusively via social media, the distinct qualitative feel of these digital interactions became increasingly salient. As teenagers' education and social relationships moved exclusively online, many found themselves feeling increasingly lonely and isolated.[5] Perhaps most disturbingly, as hospitals attempted to curtail the spread of COVID-19, many families were unable to be with quarantined relatives during their final moments. There were heart-wrenching stories of healthcare workers using FaceTime to allow families to be "present" as loved ones passed away. Although the opportunity to connect with loved ones in their final moments was a powerful affordance of digital communication, the inability to be physically present, holding a hand at the end, also served as a stark reminder of how these media lack much of the interpersonal richness of being face to face.[6]

New Opportunities for Peer Experiences: Compensatory Behaviors and Novel Experiences

The final two proposed mechanisms for how social media can transform peer relationships emphasize how these technologies can facilitate new opportunities for behaviors (Nesi et al., 2018a). First, social media creates *new opportunities for compensatory behaviors* (Nesi et al., 2018a). Although certain behaviors could have been possible without social media, the online experience may make people more likely to engage in these activities (Nesi et al., 2018a). The COVID-19 pandemic intensified the importance of social media in compensating for the loss of face-to-face interactions. Nesi et al. (2018a) proposed that social media could support peer relationships that would be difficult to maintain in person, perhaps due to geographic distance. However, during the COVID-19 pandemic, nearly all relationships had to rely on social media to compensate for the loss of face-to-face interactions that were discouraged or explicitly prohibited. For example, online dating is not a new phenomenon, but after the start of the pandemic, the number of daily messages on dating sites such as Tinder, Bumble, and Plenty of Fish substantially increased.[7] During the pandemic, people had more time and were starving for human connection. More people gravitated to online dating to find companionship. A virtual coffee date became a common occurrence in the online dating scene and provided a platform that allowed individuals to take time to get to know each other before meeting up in person. Online dating may have increased people's willingness to message strangers and increased the perception of safety associated with dating during a pandemic.

Social media helped people form romantic connections during the pandemic; however, it also forced individuals to compensate for all social interaction using online platforms. Virtual happy hours, coffee breaks, or lunches were an attempt for families, friends, and coworkers to foster a sense of togetherness and camaraderie. Even sites like that of Martha Stewart (https://www.marthstewart.com) offered tips on how to host a virtual happy hour with the appropriate guest list, dress code, snacks, and party games.[8] Meeting up at a favorite bar or restaurant with a group of people was impossible throughout most of the pandemic. Social media facilitated the sense of community for isolated individuals. However, it provided the only sense of community and forced people to rely on social media for all community interactions. One interesting outcome of the COVID-19 pandemic has been the realization that, although social media can compensate for social interaction that is otherwise unavailable, it does a poor job of completely *replacing* in-person social interactions. Although Zoom happy hours provided some semblance of connection, many people quickly tired of them.[9] The rapid decline in adolescent mental health and well-being while engaging in remote schooling was perhaps most telling (see Chapter 20 for more on mental health related to the pandemic). Although adolescents are among the most enthusiastic users of social media for peer connection (Rideout & Robb, 2018), the pandemic has highlighted that these platforms do not adequately replace all in-person interaction.

In addition to compensating for social connection that was otherwise not possible in person, the transformation framework also proposes that social media provides the potential for entirely novel experiences and interactions (Nesi et al., 2018a), truly redefining how we interact with or peers and coworkers. When we think of the social experiences that defined the COVID-19 pandemic, many of them represent transitioning our offline relationships into these digital spaces. Zoom happy hours and remote game nights may best be conceptualized as leveraging social media to facilitate the existing social interactions that were lost during social distancing. But as we begin to emerge from COVID-induced isolation, we are beginning to embark on a discussion of how this period of remote interaction may have permanently shifted how we work and socialize.[10] Many companies are now grappling with employees' desires for the continued option for remote work.[11] Although many jobs cannot be done remotely, this experience has forced companies and educators to reevaluate how we can coordinate with colleagues and peers on a more permanent basis* (see also Chapter 2 for more on work related to the pandemic).

Lessons Learned: How Social Distancing Has Redefined Digital Peer Interaction

Perhaps the most significant "lesson learned" about social media usage during the pandemic is that, although social media served was a critically important compensatory outlet during periods of restricted access to peers, it was generally inadequate in completely replacing in-person interaction. Although social media have become an increasingly important outlet for socializing over the past decade (Ehrenreich et al., 2021), there was a dramatic increase in loneliness and isolation while individuals were sheltering in place and were prevented from face-to-face interaction with others (Killgore et al., 2020). As we transition back to "normal" peer interactions, this period of largely exclusively digital socialization can serve as a guide, cautioning against moving too far away from in-person interactions. Nonetheless, it is also important to note that, while social media did not adequately replace in-person interaction, it does not mean it was unimportant during

---

* Related to this, the second and third authors of this chapter collaborated on a research project during the pandemic period: developing a study, collecting data, and coauthoring a manuscript entirely remotely. Since Sara then transitioned to a doctoral program on graduation, their entire collaboration occurred without ever meeting in person.

the pandemic. As difficult as it was for individuals to be limited to FaceTime to say their goodbyes as loved ones died in isolated hospital rooms, this was nonetheless preferable to having no opportunity at all. Moving forward, parents, educators, and individuals themselves can use this period as informative of both the values *and* the limitations of peer interaction in digital spaces.

A second lesson learned from this pandemic experience (or more appropriately, "*relearned*") is that the driving force behind social media is not the technology itself, but the people and relationships. A great deal of concern and consternation has surrounded if people—particularly teens—are eschewing "real" relationships in favor of digital social networks (see Twenge et al., 2018). However, COVID-19's forced isolation has reiterated the importance of in-person relationships and interactions. The dramatic increases in isolation and loneliness reiterate an important point made by danah boyd: "Most teens aren't addicted to social media; if anything, they're addicted to each other" (boyd, 2014, p. 80). Although individuals are drawn to social media because of the immediate, frequent, and convenient interactions they afford (Nesi et al., 2018a), they nonetheless represent attempts to connect with people.

Relating to this, a final important lesson that is hoped will be learned by individuals as we emerge from the COVID-19 pandemic is the importance of introspecting about how we use social media, what our motivations are for using these platforms, and how social media may undermine our own social goals and well-being. Although the association between social media use and well-being have been mixed (George et al., 2018), there is growing consensus that there are indeed specific behaviors that are likely especially problematic, such as spending a significant amount of time passively viewing peers' social media feeds. The challenge is that many of these problematic behaviors are appealing in the short term (e.g., passively viewing peers posts initially makes us feel more connected with them, but over time actually leads to problematic social comparisons, fear of missing out, and loneliness; Burnell et al., 2021). Preliminary evidence suggests that individuals are beginning to recognize that social media comes with challenges in addition to benefits (Yau & Reich, 2019); being more mindful of these issues with social media might facilitate healthier (and more moderated) usage patterns. Perhaps one silver lining of the pandemic-induced increase in screen time and social media use will be a greater recognition of the toll these platforms can have on our well-being when overused.[12]

FUTURE DIRECTIONS

One important direction for future research is to understand how the dramatic transition to interacting almost exclusively in digital spaces shapes people's perceptions and use of these platforms going forward. There has already been discussion about how the COVID-19 pandemic will reshape our social contexts, ranging from establishing a renewed appreciation for casual human interactions[13] to the ushering in of the end of office work altogether.[14] And indeed, individual's social experiences during the pandemic will likely ultimately define these changes. Many adolescents found remote schooling to be largely devoid of the in-person socialization they were accustomed to (even if they reported preferring text messaging to face-to-face interaction; Rideout & Robb, 2018) and reported feeling lonely and isolated from their friends. Alternatively, many adults reported appreciating the flexibility and reduced social expectations while working from home.[15] A critical next step for researchers is assessing individuals' perceptions of how they would like their social lives to look after COVID restrictions are lifted as this will likely guide what "returning to normal" looks like.

Younger generations, particularly those defined as "digital natives" have generally been more comfortable navigating relationships in social media compared to older generations (Bowe & Wohn, 2015; Fietkiewicz et al., 2016). However, older adults were nonetheless active participants on a variety of social media platforms before the pandemic, and adults of all ages saw dramatic increases in the amount of time spent online while social distancing.[16] Given that older individuals were at greater risk of suffering significantly adverse reactions to COVID-19, older adults were at significant risk of feeling isolated, anxious, and depressed as a result of social distancing (Sepúlveda-Loyola et al., 2020). As a result of this, many older adults found themselves engaging with a variety of social media technologies that were previously viewed as overly technical or undesirable outlets for social connection.[17] Although it is hoped we will not be forced into social distancing again within older adults' lifetime, the increased comfort that digital platforms provides may translate into more digitally literate older generations, who can translate these skills into opportunities for continued social connection going forward.

Finally, additional research should continue to examine the experiences of individuals navigating social distancing through the transformational framework. This theoretical lens is relatively new and has only begun to gain empirical inquiry and support (e.g., Choukas-Bradley et al., 2019). The transformational framework provides a blueprint for understanding how digital social interactions are shaped by the features of the context. The COVID-19 pandemic provides a unique window in time when nearly all relationships were diverted into these digital contexts. Empirically testing the transformational framework in the context of COVID-19 will allow researchers to test the limits of interactions occurring in social media, understanding how the framework holds up when face-to-face interactions are abruptly and rapidly transitioned into digital spaces.

CONCLUSION

The COVID-19 pandemic was a uniquely challenging moment in history. In the midst of extraordinary medical and economic challenges, people were forced to socially distance from one of their most important coping mechanisms: family and peer relationships. In this context, social media became a critically important resource, allowing individuals to maintain a sense of connection and social support. Although social media platforms have been an increasingly important form of peer interaction over the past decade for both adolescents and adults, this abrupt transition to nearly exclusive digital interaction with family and friends provides insight into both benefits and challenges of interacting with peers via social media. The transformational framework (Nesi et al., 2018a) provides a useful tool in understanding how the frequency, immediacy, and intensity of social media shaped people's experiences during the pandemic and became an important way to compensate for the challenges of social distancing.

NOTES

1. https://www.axios.com/kids-screen-time-pandemic-112650a6-743c-4c15-b84a-7d86103262bb.html
2. https://eyesafe.com/covid-19-screen-time-spike-to-over-13-hours-per-day/
3. See Note 2.
4. See Note 1.
5. https://www.washingtonpost.com/lifestyle/style/teenagers-covid-pandemic-mental-health/2021/02/10/3389983a-39d6-11eb-9276-ae0ca72729be_story.html; also see Note 1.
6. https://www.charlotteobserver.com/news/coronavirus/article241678926.html
7. https://www.dw.com/en/love-in-the-time-of-coronavirus-covid-19-changes-the-game-for-online-dating/a-52933001
8. https://web.archive.org/web/20200409144914/https://www.marthastewart.com/7781469/how-host-virtual-happy-hour-coronavirus-pandemic
9. https://www.thecut.com/article/i-hate-my-mandatory-zoom-happy-hours.html
10. https://www.forbes.com/sites/forbestechcouncil/2021/05/20/the-future-of-work-isnt-about-technology---its-about-people/?sh=34fa74c22e74
11. https://www.bbc.com/worklife/article/20201023-coronavirus-how-will-the-pandemic-change-the-way-we-work
12. https://www.nytimes.com/2021/01/28/learning/what-students-are-saying-about-excessive-screen-time-presidential-priorities-and-fashion-statements.html
13. https://qz.com/work/1941620/covid-19-and-the-surprising-effects-of-casual-human-interactions/
14. https://www.forbes.com/sites/zengernews/2020/12/11/covid-and-the-end-of-the-office-as-you-knew-it/?sh=16827b1b2c2f
15. https://www.nytimes.com/2020/05/05/business/pandemic-work-from-home-coronavirus.html
16. See Note 2.
17. https://www.bloomberg.com/news/features/2020-05-06/in-lockdown-seniors-are-becoming-more-tech-savvy

REFERENCES

Bowe, B. J., & Wohn, D. Y. (2015, July). Are there generational differences? Social media use and perceived shared reality. In *Proceedings of the 2015 International Conference on Social Media & Society* (pp. 1–5). https://doi.org/10.1145/2789187.2789200

boyd, d. (2014). *It's complicated: The social lives of networked teens*. Yale University Press

Burnell, K., George, M. J., & Underwood, M. K. (2021). New media and solitude: Implications for peer relations. In R. J. Coplan, J. C. Bowker, & L. J. Nelson (Eds.), The *handbook of solitude*: Psychological *perspectives on social isolation, social withdrawal, and being alone* (pp. 254–267). Wiley. https://doi.org/10.1002/978111 9576457.ch18

Choukas-Bradley, S., Nesi, J., Widman, L., & Higgins, M. K. (2019). Camera-ready: Young women's appearance-related social media consciousness. *Psychology of Popular Media Culture*, 8(4), 473. https://doi.org/10.1037/ppm0000196

Ehrenreich, S. E., George, M. J., Burnell, K., & Underwood, M. K. (2021). Importance of digital communication in adolescents' development: Theoretical and empirical advancements in the last decade. *Journal of Research on Adolescents*, 31(4), 928–943.

Fardouly, J., & Vartanian, L. R. (2016). Social media and body image concerns: Current research and future directions. *Current Opinion in Psychology*, 9, 1–5. https://doi.org/10.1016/j.copsyc.2015.09.005

Fietkiewicz, K. J., Lins, E., Baran, K. S., & Stock, W. G. (2016, January). Inter-generational comparison of social media use: Investigating the online behavior of different generational cohorts. In 2016 49th Hawaii International Conference on System Sciences (HICSS) (pp. 3829–3838). IEEE. https://doi.org/10.1109/HICSS.2016.477

Frison, E., & Eggermont, S. (2020). Toward an integrated and differential approach to the relationships between loneliness, different types of Facebook use, and adolescents' depressed mood. *Communication Research*, 47, 701–728. https://doi.org/10.1177/0093650215617506

George, M. J., Russell, M. A., Piontak, J. R., & Odgers, C. L. (2018). Concurrent and subsequent associations between daily digital technology use and high-risk adolescents' mental health symptoms. *Child Development*, 89(1), 78–88. https://doi.org/10.1111/cdev.12819

Greenwood, S., Perrin, A., & Duggan, M. (2016, November 10). Social media update 2016. Pew Research Center. https://www.pewresearch.org/internet/2016/11/11/social-media-update-2016/

Killgore, W. D., Cloonan, S. A., Taylor, E. C., Miller, M. A., & Dailey, N. S. (2020). Three months of loneliness during the COVID-19 lockdown. *Psychiatry Research*, 293, 113392. https://doi.org/10.1016/j.psychres.2020.113392

Madell, D. E., & Muncer, S. J. (2007). Control over social interactions: An important reason for young people's use of the internet and mobile phones for communication? *Cyber Psychology and Behavior*, 10(1), 137–140. https://doi.org/10.1089/cpb.2006.9980

Moreno, M., & Kota, R. (2013). Social media. In V. C. Strasburger, B. Wilson, & A. B. (Beth) Jordan (Eds.), *Children, Adolescents, and the Media* (3rd ed.). SAGE Publications, Inc. https://us.sagepub.com/en-us/nam/children-adolescents-and-the-media/book235807

Nesi, J., Choukas-Bradley, S., & Prinstein, M. J. (2018a). Transformation of adolescent peer relations in the social media context: Part 1—A theoretical framework and application to dyadic peer relationships. *Clinical Child and Family Psychology Review*, 21(3), 267–294. https://doi.org/10.1007/s10567-018-0261-x

Nesi, J., Choukas-Bradley, S., & Prinstein, M. J. (2018b). Transformation of adolescent peer relations in the social media context: Part 2—Application to peer group processes and future directions for research. *Clinical Child and Family Psychology Review*, *21*, 295–319. https://doi.org/10.1007/s10567-018-0262-9

Rideout, V., & Robb, M. B. (2018). Social media, social life: Teens reveal their experiences. Common Sense Media.https://www.commonsensemedia.org/research/social-media-social-life-2018

Scott, H., Biello, S. M., & Woods, H. C. (2019). Identifying drivers for bedtime social media use despite sleep costs: the adolescent perspective. *Sleep Health*, *5*(6), 539–545. https://doi.org/10.1016/j.sleh.2019.07.006

Sepúlveda-Loyola, W., Rodríguez-Sánchez, I., Pérez-Rodríguez, P., Ganz, F., Torralba, R., Oliveira, D. V., & Rodríguez-Mañas, L. (2020). Impact of social isolation due to COVID-19 on health in older people: Mental and physical effects and recommendations. *The Journal of Nutrition, Health & Aging*, *24*, 938–947. https://doi.org/10.1007/s12603-020-1469-2

Twenge, J. M., Joiner, T. E., Rogers, M. L., & Martin, G. N. (2018). Increases in depressive symptoms, suicide-related outcomes, and suicide rates among U.S. adolescents after 2010 and links to increased new media screen time. *Clinical Psychological Science*, *6*(1), 3–17. https://doi.org/10.1177/2167702617723376

Vogel, E. A., Rose, J. P., Okdie, B. M., Eckles, K., & Franz, B. (2015). Who compares and despairs? The effect of social comparison orientation on social media use and its outcomes. *Personality and Individual Differences*, *86*, 249–256. https://doi.org/10.1016/j.paid.2015.06.026

White, S. V., & Ehrenreich, S. E. (2021). Social media use and psychological well-being during the COVID-19 pandemic [Manuscript in preparation]. University of Nevada, Reno.

Yau, J. C., & Reich, S. M. (2019). "It's just a lot of work": Adolescents' self-presentation norms and practices on Facebook and Instagram. *Journal of Research on Adolescence*, *29*(1), 196–209. https://doi.org/10.1111/jora.12376

FURTHER READING

Allington, D., Duffy, B., Wessely, S., Dhavan, N., & Rubin, J. (2021). Health-protective behaviour, social media usage and conspiracy belief during the COVID-19 public health emergency. *Psychological Medicine*, *51*(10), 1763–1769. Advance online publication. https://doi.org/10.1017/S003329172000224X

Bendau, A., Petzold, M. B., Pyrkosch, L., Mascarell Maricic, L., Betzler, F., Rogoll, J., Große, J., Ströhle, A., & Plag, J. (2021). Associations between COVID-19 related media consumption and symptoms of anxiety, depression and COVID-19 related fear in the general population in Germany. *European Archives of Psychiatry and Clinical Neuroscience*, *271*(2), 283–291. https://doi.org/10.1007/s00406-020-01171-6

boyd, d. (2014). *It's complicated: The social lives of networked teens*. Yale University Press.

Killgore, W. D., Cloonan, S. A., Taylor, E. C., Miller, M. A., & Dailey, N. S. (2020). Three months of loneliness during the COVID-19 lockdown. *Psychiatry Research*, *293*, 113392. https://doi.org/10.1016/j.psychres.2020.113392

Nesi, J., Choukas-Bradley, S., & Prinstein, M. J. (2018). Transformation of adolescent peer relations in the social media context: Part 1—A theoretical framework and application to dyadic peer relationships. *Clinical Child and Family Psychology Review*, *21*(3), 267–294. https://doi.org/10.1007/s10567-018-0261-x

23

Xenophobia, Prejudice, Stigma, and the COVID-19 Pandemic

VICTORIA ESTRADA-REYNOLDS AND CYNTHIA WILLIS-ESQUEDA ■

The COVID-19 pandemic upended lives everywhere as the world struggled with containment. Some COVID-19 costs are apparent, such as the global death toll, increased unemployment, strained healthcare systems, and ongoing health problems of those who recovered from the virus. However, the pandemic also affected the way people feel, think, and act toward others, particularly those seen as "different." During the pandemic, numerous examples of prejudice and discrimination in the United States were reported across media outlets. People hurled anti-Asian slurs and avoided those who appeared to be of East Asian descent, even resorting to physical attacks.[1] Then-President Donald Trump tweeted: "I always treated the *Chinese Virus* very seriously, and have done a very good job from the beginning, including my very early decision to close the 'borders' from China." (emphasis added)[2]; he defended his use of the term "Chinese Virus," stating: "It's not racist at all. No, not at all. It comes from China."[3] Further, the Centers for Disease Control and Prevention (CDC) added a "Reducing Stigma" webpage outlining how certain groups (e.g., racial/ethnic minorities, those who have or are suspected of having COVID-19) could be subject to prejudice during the pandemic.[4] As these examples suggest, prejudice, discrimination, and stigma dramatically altered the pandemic experiences of some people.

The purpose of this chapter is to highlight how the COVID-19 pandemic potentially increased prejudice and discrimination toward others, affecting the pandemic experiences of some (e.g., Asian Americans). In doing so, we use psychological concepts and theories to explain why this occurs. First, we examine how people naturally categorize other people and how this can produce prejudice and discrimination under certain conditions (i.e., feeling threatened). Next, we examine how emotions can drive prejudice toward others. For example, fear

Victoria Estrada- and Cynthia Willis-Esqueda, *Xenophobia, Prejudice, Stigma, and the COVID-19 Pandemic* In: *The Social Science of the COVID-19 Pandemic*. Edited by: Monica K. Miller, Oxford University Press. © Oxford University Press 2024.
DOI: 10.1093/oso/9780197615133.003.0023

may trigger prejudice and discrimination to reduce terror experienced due to the deadly and unknown nature of COVID-19. For instance, disgust can lead to prejudice against those suspected of harboring disease. Throughout the chapter, we apply these psychological concepts to the COVID-19 pandemic, discuss applications of these concepts to past epidemics, and provide suggestions for policy and future research to help reduce stigma and prejudice during times of pandemic. We hope that this chapter will bring attention to the destructive nature of prejudice during pandemics and inspire new policy and research to help reduce stigma and hate toward others.

"US VERSUS THEM": CATEGORIZATION AND PREJUDICE

It is understood that a person's ability to categorize is central to simplifying and understanding the world. For instance, a person has knowledge of what defines a gas station (e.g., the positions of pumps outside a building), so they might drive on unfamiliar roads but are still able to identify a gas station when they pass one by. This gas station knowledge provides the ability to categorize and act in one's environment. This knowledge gained through categorization is helpful; drivers can refuel their cars before running out of gas. From these basic, nonsocial processes, research on social intergroup relations has extended categorization principles to help understand how categorization can lead to prejudice toward dissimilar others.

In social interactions, the categorization process leads to the formation of social categories or groups. Tajfel and colleagues (1971) demonstrated that simply assigning a person an arbitrary group label (e.g., randomly telling someone they underestimated or overestimated the number of dots presented to them) can predict treatment toward the new ingroup (e.g., awarding more money to ingroup versus outgroup members). This consistent ingroup favoritism is explained through social identity theory (SIT; Tajfel & Turner, 1979).

Social identity theory proposes that people categorize individuals into groups, and from their notions of group membership and our place within a group, they ascribe group characteristics to the self and develop a social identity. Social categorization theory (SCT; Turner et al., 1987) further explains that people possess multiple identities (i.e., human, social, and personal identities), and shifting to a social group identity increases ingroup favoritism. Identifying with a group is likely to occur when group identity is made salient or when feeling uncertain. Building from SIT and SCT, uncertainty-categorization theory (Hogg, 2012) suggests that when faced with uncertainty, people are motivated to reduce this feeling with group identification. This helps people feel a sense of purpose, as groups offer information on how to think, feel, and behave.

COVID-19 was a novel disease that spread quickly, forced large behavioral changes, and left the world uncertain of the future. At the beginning of the pandemic, much was unknown about the virus and how best to contain it or avoid infection. The U.S. government often contradicted CDC and World Health Organization recommendations on containing the virus's spread, minimized virus seriousness, and politicized the pandemic, further adding to uncertainty for how to behave in response. Further, Americans perceive the COVID-19 virus as coming from China, and this potentially increased perceived nationality differences. As a result, people might have sought to reaffirm memberships to ingroups to reduce uncertainty, resulting in more positive ingroup favoritism, but at the expense of outgroups.

In addition, people are motivated to belong to an ingroup and for it to be viewed positively, as this positivity halo extends to ingroup members. As a result, people will engage in behavior that preserves or increases positive perceptions of the group. For example, people give valuable resources to the ingroup, are more willing to trust and cooperate with ingroup members, and make more positive and less negative attributions for the ingroup's behavior (Dietz-Uhler & Murrell, 1998; Wit & Kerr, 2002).

The social identity account provides an explanation for why people cling to social categories in times of uncertainty and how this affects interaction with outgroup members. This framework has been applied to past epidemics and prejudice. For instance, HIV infection risk was associated with stigmatized social groups (e.g., homosexual men, those who injected drugs), which increased perceived differences between the stigmatized outgroup and the ingroup (i.e., those *not* infected with HIV; Devine et al., 1999). Further categorizations are made between ourselves and those perceived as responsible for contracting HIV (e.g., unprotected sex, sharing needles), which acts to protect the ingroup's status (e.g., nonpromiscuous, non–drug user; Devine et al., 1999).

The result of social categorization is typically ingroup favoritism (e.g., cooperating more with ingroup members) and less so outgroup derogation (e.g., cooperating less with outgroup members; Balliet et al., 2014). Therefore, social categorization alone does not explain outgroup derogation in the pandemic, such as healthcare workers being denied services in Nepal[5] or physical attacks on Asian people.[6] What then might account for this type of discrimination? Threat, prejudice, and discrimination also have explanatory contributions.

THREAT AND PREJUDICE

Intergroup threat occurs if the outgroup's characteristics, beliefs, or behaviors jeopardize the goals or well-being of the ingroup. If a person feels threatened by another group, they are likely to express prejudice toward that group (Riek et al., 2006). Intergroup threat predicts outgroup prejudice, and several theories provide insight regarding why this occurs. Realistic group conflict theory (LeVine & Campbell, 1972) suggests that people may become threatened if groups are in competition for power or tangible and limited resources, which threatens their existence. Integrated threat theory (Stephan & Stephan, 2000) extended the types of threats. For example, when people perceive outgroups as threatening their actual existence (realistic), belief systems (symbolic), future interactions (i.e., unfamiliarity with interactions toward outgroup members; intergroup), or hold negative beliefs about those groups (negative stereotypes), then outgroup threat produces prejudice.

The COVID-19 virus posed a realistic threat. At times, the pandemic resulted in increased prejudice toward people who were sick; those showing signs of illness/infection (e.g., coughing, sneezing); or those who did not comply with preventative measures (e.g., wearing a mask, maintaining proper distance). Further, scientists proposed the virus potentially originated in China, and this could have increased perceived ingroup-outgroup differences and notions of a virus threat to the ingroup (i.e., for those not of Chinese descent). As a result, individuals of East Asian descent experienced increased incidents of prejudice and discrimination.[7]

Implementation of social distancing and increased isolation created a symbolic threat, as connections to social ingroups decreased. People may interpret the consequences of social distancing and lockdowns as threatening their group's culture and identity because group members cannot meet and maintain their identity (Kachanoff et al., 2020). In response to this symbolic threat, people will act in discriminatory ways toward those who are threatening. This behavior has been observed related to the pandemic.[8]

Integrated threat theory has been applied to perceptions of people with HIV/AIDS. Berrenberg et al. (2002) found those who perceived high realistic threats (e.g., economic and/or emotional strains), high symbolic threats (e.g., beliefs that those with AIDS have different values/beliefs), and high intergroup anxiety (e.g., how they felt when interacting with someone diagnosed with AIDS) toward people diagnosed with AIDS had more negative attitudes toward people with AIDS.

Those who perceive intergroup threat are also likely to experience negative emotions (e.g., fear, disgust, and anger), and intergroup threat could reduce empathy for outgroup members (Stephan et al., 2009), dividing people and increasing prejudice. Emotions are known to predict prejudice against outgroup members. Next, we focus on anger, fear, and disgust as possible sources of prejudice during the COVID-19 pandemic.

EMOTIONS AND PREJUDICE

Several emotions are thought to be universally experienced across cultures because they are evolutionarily beneficial (e.g., anger, fear, and disgust; Tracy & Randles, 2011). For example, fear and disgust can warn of potential threats (Cottrell & Neuberg, 2005). However, emotions may be attached to certain appraisals and action tendencies (e.g., approach/avoidance), and we act according to the emotion elicited (e.g., fear produces flight), so experiencing emotions could lead to negative responses toward others.

Anger and Approach Tendencies

Generally, less positive and more negative emotions toward an outgroup are predictive of negative outgroup attitudes (Stangor et al., 1991). That is, if people experience less positive and more negative emotions toward Asian Americans, those with COVID-19 symptoms, or those viewed as "outsiders," they may show increased prejudice and discrimination. However, specific emotions can result in specific actions toward others. For example, anger is typically described as having an approach action tendency. Those who experience anger might "approach" the targets of their anger by attacking or confronting them (Smith & Mackie, 2008). Further, when the individual person or ingroup is perceived as stronger than the "outside" individual person or outgroup, then anger is more likely expressed toward the outgroup compared to fear (Mackie et al., 2000).

Thus, if one perceives their status as greater than another's (or their ingroup as more powerful than the outgroup), they are more likely to experience anger and approach the target of anger. Regarding the COVID-19 pandemic, Americans might blame Asian Americans for the COVID-19 pandemic, experience anger, and actively attack Asians by yelling racial slurs or even physically assaulting them.[9] For example, in the AIDS epidemic when diseases were perceived to be contracted through avoidable behaviors, anger and blame increased (Weiner, 1993).

Fear, Avoidance, and Terror Management Theory

Fear is also related to prejudice and discrimination. Experiencing threat (as when faced with a global virus) could lead to fear. The behavioral reaction associated with fear is different from anger; a fearful person is likely to avoid the threatening person or outgroup (Smith & Mackie, 2008). Again, this may have served an evolutionary purpose, as experiencing fear helped trigger an avoidance or flee response and provided protection from danger. However, this fear response might also lead to a prejudiced response toward those who are feared, such as people with signs of illness, those not following COVID-19 pandemic safety guidelines, or those seen as the source of illness.

Terror management theory (TMT; Greenberg et al., 1986) effectively explains the connection between fear and prejudice (see Chapter 33 in this book for an in-depth discussion of TMT and the pandemic). TMT states that humans, like all living creatures, are motivated toward self-preservation, but humans can think of the past and future and contemplate their own mortality. As a result, awareness of one's inevitable death (i.e., mortality salience) leads to feelings of terror and a motivation to manage that terror. One way to decrease the fear of death is to develop a cultural worldview, which is a group's belief system that helps provide structure and a sense of purpose or self-esteem for an individual (e.g., instructs people on how to behave and outlines what will occur after death). When fear arises from mortality salience, people seek to reduce fear by protecting their cultural worldview. Others who threaten the worldview are met with prejudice (e.g., acting or thinking negatively about another person with different beliefs helps to decrease the threat they pose to their worldview), attempts to convert others to conform to our beliefs or, in extreme cases, extermination of the outgroup (Greenberg & Kosloff, 2008). Previous TMT research has found that increased mortality salience results in more negative attitudes toward outgroup members (Burke et al., 2010). The COVID-19 pandemic has likely increased fears of death, which could lead to negative attitudes toward those who are "different" or threaten one's cultural worldview.

In previous epidemics, Arrowood et al. (2017) found that those who were asked to think about Ebola (e.g., describing thoughts of contracting the disease), increased mortality salience, and belief adherence. Based on previous findings of TMT, disease that threatens our survival can go beyond belief adherence and increase negative attitudes and behaviors toward threatening others.

Disgust and the Behavioral Immune System

Experiencing disgust can result in avoidance behavior and lead to negative outgroup attitudes. For example, disgust has predicted increased prejudice toward homosexual (Terrizzi et al., 2010) and obese (Vartanian et al., 2016) people and a range of other perceived deviant or low-status groups (e.g., immigrants or "foreigners," ethnic minorities, Jewish individuals, Aboriginals, AIDS patients, low socioeconomic status groups; Hodson et al., 2013). One explanation for the connection between disgust and prejudice is provided by the behavioral immune system (BIS) framework (Schaller, 2011).

According to the BIS, the physiological immune system activates when it detects pathogens, but this response costs energy that could be used for other bodily functions. As a result, humans evolved a BIS that activates emotions, cognitions, and behaviors that help us avoid perceived pathogen threats and avoid activation of the physiological immune system. For instance, smelling rotting food may trigger feelings of disgust and avoidance of potentially harmful food (Schaller, 2011). Thus, people who are perceived to be sick, at risk for illness, or a health risk will be viewed more negatively and avoided, particularly when the threatened person feels they are at increased infection risk (Schaller, 2011).

One outcome of the BIS is that people might think and act negatively toward people who pose no immune threat (i.e., older people) because they are associated with disease (Duncan & Schaller, 2009) or perceived as "foreign" people who might bring foreign pathogens (Kusche & Barker, 2019). Thus, people desire less contact with unfamiliar immigrant groups when feeling susceptible to disease (Navarrete et al., 2007) and express more negative attitudes toward those groups (Hodson et al., 2013).

The BIS provides yet another explanation for why prejudice occurred during the COVID-19 pandemic. Oversensitivity to threats associated with the COVID-19 virus or feared groups that could carry communicable disease can result in prejudice and discrimination. For example, people might show prejudice to people not wearing masks, showing symptoms of COVID-19 or general illness (e.g., sneezing), or those perceived as "different." Additionally, travel bans could increase threat perceptions of immigrant groups, thus increasing xenophobia and ethnocentrism. In particular, Asian Americans increasingly became targets of prejudice during the COVID-19 pandemic. The Center for the Study of Hate and Extremism reported a 145% increase in Asian American hate crimes among 16 largest cities in the United States from 2019 to 2020 despite the fact that overall hate crimes decreased across those same cities.[10] The first COVID-19 case was reported in Wuhan, Hubei Province, China, and use of the term "Chinese virus" and other derogatory terms for the COVID-19 virus by public figures (e.g., former President Donald Trump, former Secretary of State Mike Pompeo[11]) could have increased disgust against Asian Americans. Finally, as the virus can be passed by asymptomatic people, this could increase reliance on nonsymptom cues associated with disease or potential pathogen threat. Chinese and Asian stereotypes in the United States have focused on perceived unsanitary habits and "unusual" food choices (Roberto et al., 2020), which could increase disgust against these groups and, in turn, increase prejudice and discrimination.

Research on past epidemics clarifies the connection between risk of disease and increased prejudice during the COVID-19 pandemic. For instance, Prati and Pietrantoni (2016) found that increased risk perception and fear of contracting Ebola by Italian people were related to increased prejudice against African immigrants. Further, people who have high general intergroup disgust have more negative attitudes toward those associated with disease (e.g., people diagnosed with AIDS; Hodson et al., 2013).

As these examples illustrate, people's experiences of the pandemic can be shaped by prejudice, discrimination, and stigma. This was particularly true for people, including Asians, because of the nature of COVID-19. The theories discussed above offer explanations for not only prejudice and resulting behavior but also lessons learned.

LESSONS LEARNED

There are several strategies for reducing prejudice and discrimination. First, changing a person's group identity to a more inclusive group could help reduce prejudice in a pandemic, as proposed by the common ingroup identity model (Gaertner & Dovidio, 2008). For example, virus mitigation and vaccine campaigns could promote cooperation as a community and reduce language that increases nationality and racial/ethnic categorizations. The hope is that people will stop viewing the targets of prejudice as outgroup members and instead include them as part of their community identity.

Second, reducing uncertainty at multiple stages of the pandemic can help reduce prejudice against outgroup members. For example, in the United States, political officials across states could agree to communicate the same clear messages regarding virus explanations, how it is transmitted, guidelines and rules for reducing community spread, and vaccination information. This would reduce uncertainty about how to defend against COVID-19. However, early in the pandemic, there was a large emphasis on COVID-19 novelty and how much was not (and still is not) known about the virus. This might be necessary to avoid drawing precipitous conclusions, but it is still important to emphasize what *is* known and to have a unified message to avoid threats and negative emotions. The extent to which one can reduce uncertainty and threat in a pandemic is challenging. For instance, it may not be possible to know when the pandemic will "end" or when a return to "normalcy" might occur. Further complicating these efforts are multiple sources of information via social media and the Internet, which can transmit misinformation and cause uncertainty (see Chapter 36 for more about media messages during the COVID-19 pandemic).

Third, principles of intergroup contact theory (Allport, 1954; Pettigrew et al., 2011) could be applied to reduce prejudice during pandemics. This theory proposes that increased positive contact with outgroups will reduce prejudice. This contact can contain equal status among those seeking contact, common goals, cooperation to fulfill those goals, and authority support, but not all are required to reduce prejudice. Although physical contact is restricted during a pandemic, authorities and respected community members can promote messages that promote notions of equal status, common goals, cooperation, and support (e.g., get vaccinated, wear a mask) to achieve a common goal (e.g., reduce spread of the virus, return to "normal" life sooner).

Last, alongside these pandemic messages to promote intergroup contact goals, one could attempt to insert strategies for long-term prejudice reduction (Devine et al., 2012). For example, asking people to take the perspective of those experiencing prejudice and discrimination and/or sharing stories of people who experience prejudice during the pandemic can help to increase empathy and reduce prejudice. Sharing stories also serves to individuate the stereotyped person, which can decrease prejudice.

DIRECTIONS FOR FUTURE RESEARCH

Future research could examine which groups experienced prejudice/discrimination during the pandemic and to what degree. For example, there was an increase in Asian American hate crimes in large cities in the United States. Were there also increases in hate crimes and/or prejudice against other, typically denigrated, groups (e.g., Jewish individuals[12])? Further, what types of groups were the target of prejudice outside the United States? Depending on the circumstances in different countries or regions across the world, groups other than East Asians might have been scapegoats and experienced increases in prejudice and discrimination. In addition, people attach specific traits to groups, such as perceiving Asians as competent but cold and untrustworthy (Fiske et al., 2007). To what extent do preexisting stereotypes and attitudes affect whether outgroups are perceived to be a threat during a pandemic?

Last, some lessons can be learned from previous epidemics (e.g., HIV/AIDS), but the way people communicate and consume information has changed drastically with increased access to the Internet and social media. Future research should examine the connection between misinformation regarding the pandemic (causing uncertainty, fear, or anger) and increases in prejudice. Conversely, authorities' and public figures' messages could serve to mitigate those messages thought to increase prejudice.

CONCLUSIONS

Heightened prejudice during a pandemic has many causes. People categorize and favor people who are part of their own social ingroup. However, real and symbolic threats to our existence can increase prejudice and discrimination toward outgroups and their members. Emotions, such as fear, anger, and disgust, can drive negative thoughts and actions toward those perceived as carrying disease. These theories suggest that some groups (e.g., Asians) likely had pandemic experiences that were quite different from the experiences of other groups. The creation of clear, unified messages during the pandemic, promoted by those in authority and trusted positions, could potentially reduce prejudice and increase empathy and individuation for targets of prejudice. Future research should take care to specifically examine prejudice in the wake of the COVID-19 pandemic, applying old theory and examining new approaches to understand pandemic-related prejudice and discrimination.

NOTES

1. https://www.npr.org/local/309/2020/03/31/824397216/asian-americans-feel-the-bite-of-prejudice-during-the-c-o-v-i-d-19-pandemic
2. https://twitter.com/realDonaldTrump/status/1240243188708839424
3. https://trumpwhitehouse.archives.gov/briefings-statements/remarks-president-trump-vice-president-pence-members-coronavirus-task-force-press-briefing-5/
4. https://stacks.cdc.gov/view/cdc/89490/
5. https://kathmandupost.com/national/2020/05/01/stigma-against-health-workers-patients-and-area-locals-continues-in-covid-19-hotspots
6. https://time.com/5797836/coronavirus-racism-stereotypes-attacks/
7. https://www.nbcnews.com/news/asian-america/there-were-3-800-anti-asian-racist-incidents-mostly-against-n1261257
8. https://www.today.com/health/mask-protest-t186064
9. https://www.nytimes.com/2021/02/12/us/asian-american-racism.html
10. https://www.csusb.edu/sites/default/files/FACT%20SHEET-%20Anti-Asian%20Hate%202020%20rev%203.21.21.pdf
11. https://www.nytimes.com/2020/03/10/us/politics/wuhan-virus.html
12. https://apnews.com/article/health-bombings-race-and-ethnicity-religion-coronavirus-0ba3503646bbb707a37685a2e23d5cd8

REFERENCES

Allport, G. W. (1954). *The nature of prejudice*. Perseus Books Publishing.

Arrowood, R. B., Cox, C. R., Kersten, M., Routledge, C., Shelton, J. T., & Hood, R. W. (2017). Ebola salience, death-thought accessibility, and worldview defense: A terror management theory perspective. *Death Studies, 41*(9), 585–591. https://doi.org/ 10.1080/07481187.2017.1322644

Balliet, D., Wu, J., & De Dreu, C. K. W. (2014). Ingroup favoritism in cooperation: A meta-analysis. *Psychological Bulletin, 140*(6), 1556–1581. https://doi.org/10.1037/ a0037737

Berrenberg, J. L., Finlay, K. A., Stephan, W. G., & Stephan, C. (2002). Prejudice toward people with cancer or AIDS: Applying the integrated threat model. *Journal of Applied Biobehavioral Research, 7*(2), 75–86. https://doi.org/10.1111/j.1751-9861.2002.tb00078.x

Burke, B. L., Martens, A., & Faucher, E. H. (2010). Two decades of terror management theory: A meta-analysis of mortality salience research. *Personality and Social Psychology Review, 14*(2), 155–195. https://doi.org/10.1177/1088868309352321

Cottrell, C. A., & Neuberg, S. L. (2005). Different emotional reactions to different groups: A sociofunctional threat-based approach to "prejudice." *Journal of Personality and Social Psychology, 88*(5), 770–789. https://doi.org/10.1037/0022-3514.88.5.770

Devine, P. G., Forscher, P. S., Austin, A. J., & Cox, W. T. L. (2012). Long-term reduction in implicit race bias: A prejudice habit-breaking technique. *Journal of Experimental Psychology, 48*(6), 1267–1278. https://doi.org/10.1016/j.jesp.2012.06.003

Devine, P. G., Plant, E. A., & Harrison, K. (1999). The problem of "us" versus "them" and AIDS stigma. *American Behavioral Scientist, 42*(7), 1212–1228. https://doi.org/ 10.1177/00027649921954732

Dietz-Uhler, B., & Murrell, A. (1998). Effects of social identity and threat on self-esteem and group attributions. *Group Dynamics: Theory, Research, and Practice, 2*(1), 24–35. https://doi.org/10.1037/1089-2699.2.1.24

Duncan, L. A., & Schaller, M. (2009). Prejudicial attitudes toward older adults may be exaggerated when people feel vulnerable to infectious disease: Evidence and implications. *Analyses of Social Issues and Public Policy, 9*(1), 97–115. https://doi.org/10.1111/j.1530-2415.2009.01188.x

Fiske, S. T., Cuddy, A. J., & Glick, P. (2007). Universal dimensions of social cognition: Warmth and competence. *Trends in Cognitive Sciences, 11*(2), 77–83. https:// doi.org/10.1016/j.tics.2006.11.005

Gaertner, S. L., & Dovidio, J. F. (2008). Addressing contemporary racism: The common ingroup identity model. In C. Willis-Esqueda (Ed.), *Motivational aspects of prejudice and racism* (pp. 111–133). Springer.

Greenberg, J., & Kosloff, S. (2008). Terror management theory: Implications for understanding prejudice, stereotyping, intergroup conflict, and political attitudes. *Social and Personality Psychology Compass, 2*(5), 1881–1894. https://doi.org/10.1111/ j.1751-9004.2008.00144.x

Greenberg, J., Pyszczynski, T., & Solomon, S. (1986). The causes and consequences of a need for self-esteem: A terror management theory. In R. F. Baumeister (Ed.), *Public self and private self* (pp. 189–212). Springer. https://doi.org/10.1007/978-1-4613-9564-5_10

Hodson, G., Choma, B. L., Boisvert, J., Hafer, C. L., MacInnis, C. C., & Costello, K. (2013). The role of intergroup disgust in predicting negative outgroup evaluations.

Journal of Experimental Social Psychology, 49(2), 195–205. https://doi.org/10.1016/j.jesp.2012.11.002

Hogg, M. A. (2012). Uncertainty-identity theory. In P. A. M. Van Lange, A. W. Kruglanski, & E. T. Higgins (Eds.), *Handbook of theories of social psychology* (Vol. 2. pp. 62–80). Sage. https://doi.org/10.4135/9781446249222.n29

Kachanoff, F. J., Bigman, Y. E., Kapsaskis, K., & Gray, K. (2020). Measuring realistic and symbolic threats of COVID-19 and their unique impacts on well-being and adherence to public health behaviors. *Social Psychological and Personality Science, 12*(5), 603–616. https://doi.org/10.1177/1948550620931634

Kusche, I., & Barker, J. L. (2019). Pathogens and immigrants: A critical appraisal of the behavioral immune system as an explanation of prejudice against ethnic outgroups. *Frontiers in Psychology, 10*, 1–9. https://doi.org/10.3389/fpsyg.2019.02412

LeVine, R. A., & Campbell, D. T. (1972). *Ethnocentrism: Theories of conflict, ethnic attitudes, and group behavior.* John Wiley & Sons.

Mackie, D. M., Devos, T., & Smith, E. R. (2000). Intergroup emotions: Explaining offensive action tendencies in an intergroup context. *Journal of Personality and Social Psychology, 79*(4), 602–616. https://doi.org/10.1037/0022-3514.79.4.602

Navarrete, C. D., Fessler, D. M., & Eng, S. J. (2007). Elevated ethnocentrism in the first trimester of pregnancy. *Evolution and Human Behavior, 28*(1), 60–65. https://doi.org/10.1016/j.evolhumbehav.2006.06.002

Pettigrew, T. F., Tropp, L. R., Wagner, U., & Christ, O. (2011). Recent advances in intergroup contact theory. *International Journal of Intercultural Relations, 35*(3), 271–280. https://doi.org/10.1016/j.ijintrel.2011.03.001

Prati, G., & Pietrantoni, L. (2016). Knowledge, risk perceptions, and xenophobic attitudes: Evidence from Italy during the Ebola outbreak. *Risk Analysis, 36*(10), 2000–2010. https://doi.org/10.1111/risa.12537

Riek, B. M., Mania, E. W., & Gaertner, S. L. (2006). Intergroup threat and outgroup attitudes: A meta-analytic review. *Personality and Social Psychology Review, 10*(4), 336–353. https://doi.org/10.1207/s15327957pspr1004_4

Roberto, K. J., Johnson, A. F., & Rauhaus, B. M. (2020). Stigmatization and prejudice during the COVID-19 pandemic. *Administrative Theory & Praxis, 42*(3), 364–378. https://doi.org/10.1080/10841806.2020.1782128

Schaller, M. (2011). The behavioural immune system and the psychology of human sociality. *Philosophical Transactions of the Royal Society B: Biological Sciences, 366*(1583), 3418–3426. https://doi.org/10.1098/rstb.2011.0029

Smith, E. R., & Mackie, D. M. (2008). Intergroup emotions. In M. Lewis, J. M. Haviland-Jones, & L. F. Barrett (Eds.), *Handbook of emotions* (3rd ed., pp. 428–439). Guilford Press.

Stangor, C., Sullivan, L. A., & Ford, T. E. (1991). Affective and cognitive determinants of prejudice. *Social Cognition, 9*(4), 359–380. https://doi.org/10.1521/soco.1991.9.4.359

Stephan, W. G., & Stephan, C. W. (2000). An integrated threat theory of prejudice. In S. Oskamp (Ed.), *Reducing prejudice and discrimination* (pp. 23–45). Lawrence Erlbaum Associates Publishers.

Stephan, W. G., Ybarra, O., & Rios Morrison, K. (2009). Intergroup threat theory. In T. D. Nelson (Ed.), *Handbook of prejudice, stereotyping, and discrimination* (pp. 43–59). Psychology Press. https://psycnet.apa.org/record/2008-09974-000

Tajfel, H., Billig, M. G., & Bundy, R. P. (1971). Social categorization and intergroup behaviour. *European Journal of Social Psychology, 1*(2), 149–178. https://doi.org/10.1002/ejsp.2420010202

Tajfel, H., & Turner, J. C. (1979). An integrative theory of intergroup conflict. In W. G. Austin & S. Worchel (Eds.), *The social psychology of intergroup relations* (pp. 33–47). Brooks/Cole.

Terrizzi, J. A., Jr., Shook, N. J., & Ventis, W. L. (2010). Disgust: A predictor of social conservatism and prejudicial attitudes toward homosexuals. *Personality and Individual Differences, 49*(6), 587–592. https://doi.org/10.1016/j.paid.2010.05.024

Tracy, J. L., & Randles, D. (2011). Four models of basic emotions: A review of Ekman and Cordaro, Izard, Levenson, and Panksepp and Watt. *Emotion Review, 3*(4), 397–405. https://doi.org/10.1177/1754073911410747

Turner, J. C., Hogg, M. A., Oakes, P. J., Reicher, S. D., & Wetherell, M. S. (1987). *Rediscovering the social group: A self-categorization theory.* Basil Blackwell.

Vartanian, L. R., Trewartha, T., & Vanman, E. J. (2016). Disgust predicts prejudice and discrimination toward individuals with obesity. *Journal of Applied Social Psychology, 46*(6), 369–375. https://doi.org/10.1111/jasp.12370

Weiner, B. (1993). AIDS from an attributional perspective. In J. B. Pryor & G. D. Reeder (Eds.), *The social psychology of HIV infection* (pp. 287–302). Lawrence Erlbaum Associates. https://psycnet.apa.org/record/1995-98031-010

Wit, A. P., & Kerr N. L. (2002). "Me versus just us versus us all." Categorization and cooperation in nested social dilemmas. *Journal of Personality and Social Psychology, 83*(3), 616–637. https://psycnet.apa.org/doi/10.1037/0022-3514.83.3.616

FURTHER READING

Demirtaş-Madran, H. A. (2020). Exploring the motivation behind discrimination and stigmatization related to COVID-19: A social psychological discussion based on the main theoretical explanations. *Frontiers in Psychology, 11*, 1–17. https://doi.org/10.3389/fpsyg.2020.569528

Forscher, P. S., Mitamura, C., Dix, E. L., Cox, W. T. L., & Devine, P. G. (2017). Breaking the prejudice habit: Mechanisms, timecourse, and longevity. *Journal of Experimental Psychology, 72*, 133–146. https://doi.org/10.1016/j.jesp.2017.04.009

Schaller, M., & Neuberg, S. L. (2012). Danger, disease, and the nature of prejudice. In J. M. Olson & M. P. Zanna (Eds.), *Advances in experimental social psychology* (Vol. 46, pp. 1–54). Academic Press. https://doi.org/10.1016/B978-0-12-394281-4.00001-5

Van Bavel, J. J., Baicker, K., Boggio, P. S., Capraro, V., Cichocka, A., Cikara, M., Crockett, M. J., Crum, A. J., Douglas, K. M., Druckman, J. N., Drury, J., Dube, O., Ellemers, N., Finkel, E. J., Fowlser, J. H., Gelfand, M., Han, S., Haslam, S. A., Jetten, J., . . . Willer, R. (2020). Using social and behavioural science to support COVID-19 pandemic response. *Nature Human Behavior, 4*(5), 460–471. https://doi.org/10.1038/s41562-020-0884-z

24

Inequality and the COVID-19 Experience

CYNTHIA WILLIS-ESQUEDA AND
VICTORIA ESTRADA-REYNOLDS ■

This chapter addresses the structural and systemic disadvantages that race/ethnic minorities face in life in general and especially during the pandemic. Every society has a structure, including hierarchies, governments, and institutions, that serves to organize efforts, distribute resources (Murdock, 1949), and provide goals and norms (Merton, 1938). However, not all people within a society will benefit from the structure. Consequently, the study of structural inequality has a long history within the social sciences. In 1905, Tonnies noted the shift from studying biological approaches to studying the impact of social structures and contextual factors in order to understand social behaviors and outcomes. Tonnies challenged the social sciences to examine how social structures define "collective entities," composed of individual people. Moreover, there can be conflict between these collective entities (e.g., state governments vs. federal governments, workers vs. business enterprises, individual people vs. governments).

Social structures define what cultural goals are possible and accepted (e.g., amassing wealth, gaining an education, racial/ethnic groupings, maintaining health) and the means to achieve one's goals (e.g., legal business practices, medically prescribed treatments, responses to conflict, racial/ethnic segregation; Merton, 1938). They also demonstrate where a group is positioned within a society's hierarchy and determine the material and nonmaterial resources a group and its members possess, along with attitudes toward the group (Bobo, 1999). Social structure and consensual attitudes about groups can explain underlying race bias and inequalities.

Racism refers to biased behavior (often negative) based on perceived race/ethnicity (Dovidio & Gaertner, 1986). Systemic racism refers to the biased policies

Cynthia Willis-Esqueda and Victoria Estrada-Reynolds, *Inequality and the COVID-19 Experience* In: *The Social Science of the COVID-19 Pandemic.* Edited by: Monica K. Miller, Oxford University Press. © Oxford University Press 2024.
DOI: 10.1093/oso/9780197615133.003.0024

and practices imbedded in societal institutions (Zambrana, 2020). Thus, structural and systemic race biases influence quality of life and disparities within health that are present for Black, Indigenous, and people of color (BIPOC; Smedley et al., 2003).

There are two means by which societal structures at the international level can produce inequality. The first focuses on internal social structures for various countries and inequality. For example, Allen (2019) noted industrial developments within England produced changes in the social classes for income and social power. Research in Australia has demonstrated that subjective well-being is tied to objective social structural issues (M. Western & Tomaszewski, 2016). The second means focuses on the ways in which global social structures impact nations and their people (Finn & Kobayashi, 2020). Finn and Kobayashi noted structural inequalities from colonization at the global level lent themselves to increased health risks for over 100 years for sub-Saharan African countries, with a lack of infrastructure, medical personnel, and poor living standards. Prior pandemic events (e.g., bubonic plague, Spanish influenza) and their aftermath for sub-Sharan Africa were related to the global social structures that created inequalities between nations (i.e., colonization and domination over resources).

SOCIAL STRUCTURES AND INEQUITY IN THE UNITED STATES

While global perspectives are important, the purpose here is to focus on the implications of structural inequality in the United States. Disparities exist between social categories in the social structure of the United States, and such disparities are present in social indicators (e.g., income, employment, education, health). For example, due to the U.S. social structure and categories, disparities exist by gender (Carian & Johnson, 2022); sexual orientation (lesbian, gay, bisexual, transgender, queer/questioning [LGBTQ]; American Psychological Association, 2010); and socioeconomic status (SES; Sorenson, 1996). Moreover, immigrants to the United States are perceived as an outgroup in the social structure (Lee & Fiske, 2006), and myriad factors coalesce to impact immigrant health (Viruell-Fuentes et al., 2012).

Race discrimination has been examined as a function of social structures. "Structural racism is a complex, dynamic system of conferring social benefits on some groups and imposing burdens on others that results in segregation, poverty, and denial of opportunity for millions of people of color" (Wiecek, 2011, p. 5). Some of the reasoning for structural and systemic race/ethnic inequalities is outlined in this book (see Chapters 23 and 25). Structural racism can entail psychological acceptance of a social structure and even acceptance of actual physical structures that highlight group boundaries, enforcing the social structural and cultural norms. For example, in Kansas City, Missouri, a city street marks the traditional boundaries for White and Black segregation (Xu, 2021).

In Detroit, Michigan, a wall was erected to mark the race boundaries (Einhorn & Lewis, 2021).

As part of a social structure, Bobo (1999) characterized group membership and the position of a group in the social structure as predictors of outcomes— possession of both material and nonmaterial recourses. Thus, groups (and their members) are in conflict over resources, with some groups possessing an unfair share. Structural racism then is a means to explain inequalities that BIPOC face and how those inequalities impact quality-of-life outcomes.

By 1946, Kurt Lewin acknowledged the necessity of examining social structures and individual attitudes to explain race discrimination as part of "action research" and to improve the social condition (Lewin, 1946). Research on the impact of social structures and systemic racism has been historically recent, but extensive in the social sciences (Bonilla-Silva, 1997). For example, scholars have investigated the impact of unequal social structural issues on biological functioning for BIPOC. Dougherty et al. (2020) examined the influence of disparities in structural factors (e.g., housing, schools, incarceration rates, poverty) between Blacks and Whites, and if structural factors would impact body mass index (BMI) scores. White adults had the lowest obesity rates (29.9%), followed by Hispanics (33.8%) and non-Hispanic Blacks (39.8%; Centers for Disease Control and Prevention, 2021). With a national sample, results indicated that a county structural racism (CSR) measure was predictive of BMI. However, for Blacks, higher CSR indicated higher BMI, but for Whites higher CSR meant lower BMI.

Lukachko et al. (2014) focused on connections between structural racism and myocardial infarction. With a national sample, state-level measures of structural racism were obtained (e.g., political participation, employment and job status, educational attainment, and judicial treatment). Results indicated higher disparities in political participation, employment, and judicial treatment meant higher myocardial infarction rates for Blacks. However, Whites from states with high structural racism against Blacks had lower myocardial infarction rates. Thus, structural racism produces differences at the biological level for BIPOC.

In addition to the impact of structural racism on biological functioning, several other issues highlight the ramifications of social structure for BIPOC. For example, Burrell et al. (2021) examined how structural racism can create a confluence of issues (e.g., oppressive civil authorities, community strain, internalization of tension) that produce increased violence among Black males in urban communities. Powell (2008) has noted: "At the level of societal organization, the structural model helps us analyze how housing, education, employment, transportation, health care, and other systems interact to produce racialized outcomes" (p. 793).

Several issues highlight structural and systemic inequality that contribute to increased vulnerability in times of pandemic. Consequently, structural disparities in employment, poverty, education, and the criminal justice system (CJS) are examined for the potential to increase the vulnerability of BIPOC in times of pandemic.

EMPLOYMENT DISPARITIES: HISTORICALLY AND DURING THE PANDEMIC

In the American colonies, an economic structure that contained slavery defined the type of employment one could engage in. On Europeans' first arrival, race categorizations occurred within the Spanish (Resendez, 2016) and British (Lloyd, 1951; Sharfstein, 2007) colonies. Within the British colonies, differences in ethnic experiences gave shape to social structures and systems. Indigenous people were enslaved within the Spanish (Resendez, 2016) and British (Newell, 2009) colonies and later the Southwest (Resendez, 2016). The majority of those of African descent became slaves for life in the 1640s (Nagayama Hall, 2010), eliminating employment choices. Reliance on race categories for social structure meant differences in worthiness (S. J. Gould, 1994) and the dehumanization of those enslaved (*Dred Scott v. Sandford*, 1857; Geotting, 2008). Dehumanization is the denial of human qualities or emphasis on animal-like tendencies of a group and its members (Haslam, 2006). For example, the *Scott* decision proclaimed those of African descent were of an inferior race, incapable of citizenship, and the law upheld this understanding. Mexican Americans (Willis-Esqueda, 2020) and American Indians (Freng & Willis Esqueda, 2011) were also deemed lacking human qualities. Thus, race beliefs, reliance on race categories, and slavery set up a social structure that dictated employment opportunities, with ongoing disparities seen today.

Employment disparities, with BIPOC experiencing higher unemployment than Whites, are a long-standing concern. Since the beginnings of employment tracking in 1972 and through 2019, Blacks have been twice as likely to be unemployed compared to Whites (Ajilore, 2020). In 2019, Blacks (6.1%), American Indians and Alaska Natives (6.1%), and Hispanics (4.3%) held higher unemployment rates compared to Whites (3.3%) or Asians (2.7%; Bureau of Labor Statistics, 2020). In April 2021, the unemployment rate for all ethnic groups (e.g., Whites, Asians, Hispanics, and Blacks) indicated Hispanics and Blacks had higher unemployment risk and the problems that accompany sustained lack of income (food instability, healthcare access, loss of health insurance; Bureau of Labor Statistics, 2021). Between 1970 and 2010, and taking employee sex into account, occupations where BIPOC are more likely employed had low wages, low status, and more instability compared to Asians and Whites, who had higher wages and more stable, professional jobs (Byars-Winston et al., 2015).

This means BIPOC are less likely to be able to work from home (E. Gould & Shierholz, 2020) and are more likely to have high COVID-19 risk occupations (i.e., fast food workers, farmworkers, and those working in warehouses, factories, and food processing; Velasco-Mondragon et al., 2016). While BIPOC lost more jobs than Whites during the pandemic (Benfer et al., 2021), women of color, particularly Latinas, have been most affected by job loss (Galvan, 2021; Kurtz, 2021). Consequently, with downturns in business, BIPOC were more likely to lose employment during COVID-19 restrictions (Coats et al., 2022).

BIPOC POVERTY: FOOD INSECURITY, HOUSING, AND HEALTH IN THE PANDEMIC

With employment disparities, poverty of BIPOC is the outcome. For example, in 1863, Black Americans held less than 1% of the national wealth, and as of 2019 Black Americans held only 1.5% of the national wealth (Schermerhorn, 2019). This means that in over 150 years, Blacks have made virtually no progress in wealth accumulation. While there has been improvement in poverty rates for Blacks and Hispanics over time, Asians and Whites still maintain the lowest poverty rates, with little variation. As of 2019, Asians and Whites were tied for the lowest poverty rate (Creamer, 2020). Asians had the highest median household income, followed by Whites, Hispanics, and Blacks (Wilson, 2020). Income disparities are so pervasive that poverty has become equated with being a BIPOC (Hunt, 2016).

While most Americans still believe in unending opportunity, individual effort, and hard work and perseverance producing wealth (Royce, 2019), the truth is: "The historical data also reveal that no progress has been made in reducing income and wealth inequalities between black and white households over the past 70 years" (Kuhn et al., 2018, p. 1). Thus, misperceptions about wealth accumulation, race disparities in poverty, and structural barriers that hinder income increases indicate the need to understand the history of race-based poverty as an additional risk factor of the social structural system (Schermerhorn, 2019). These structural issues vary by ethnic group, with different historical and current issues that hinder wealth improvement.

For example, food insecurity is the limited or indeterminate means to obtain adequate food for a household (Anderson, 1990), and approximately 12.3% of American households are food insecure (Odoms-Young, 2018). Racial and ethnic minority groups are disproportionately likely to have food insecurity (Morales et al., 2020), particularly Blacks and Hispanics (Hernandez et al., 2017). In fact, for over 20 years the U.S. government has tracked racial disparities in food security, with Whites having higher security than BIPOC (Odoms-Young, 2018). Structural racism predicts food insecurity (Odoms-Young, 2018), and it has been advocated that elimination of racial disparities in a variety of areas (e.g., housing, education, employment, food access) could reduce the risk.

In addition to food insecurity, poverty creates housing instability. Across SES categories, Blacks and Latinx are less likely to afford rent, compared to Whites and Asian Americans, and this was exacerbated during a pandemic (Ong et al., 2020). During a pandemic, minorities are more likely to live in overcrowded living environments or be homeless, largely because of evictions and housing instability among BIPOC (Benfer et al., 2021). "Further, when families are unable to pay their bills, they face difficult trade-offs, including skipping meals, delaying or avoiding medical treatment, and risking eviction" (Ong et al., 2021, p. 4). Further, poverty and precarious living conditions make healthcare more difficult to achieve (see Chapter 25 for more on health-related disparities during COVID-19).

Outcomes from poverty had a profound effect on BIPOC during the COVID-19 pandemic. For example, sheltering in place is more difficult for impoverished families due to unpaid rent and food insecurity (Wright et al., 2020). Inability to pay utility bills is a major concern for BIPOC (Ong et al., 2021). The effects of poverty on major life events could become the largest barrier to overcoming risk factors in times of pandemic and dooms BIPOC to increased risk for negative life outcomes. The seriousness of poverty becomes even more salient when one considers: "If average black family wealth continues to grow at the same pace it has over the past three decades, it would take black families 228 years to amass the same amount of wealth white families have today" (Collins et al., 2016).

In terms of COVID-19, the United States relies on a private healthcare system, and people are responsible for paying for healthcare services. Better and more frequent access to care and a healthier lifestyle (e.g., food, gyms) are related to income (Mouzon & Brock, 2021). Unfortunately, because poverty is higher among BIPOC, health and healthcare are influenced by structural racism, which impacts BIPOC disproportionately.

EDUCATIONAL OPPORTUNITIES AND DISPARITIES: HISTORICALLY AND DURING THE PANDEMIC

Employment and poverty disparities are tied with the structural racism embedded in educational opportunities. Historically, there have been structural and even legal barriers for BIPOC's education. Education was legally forbidden for most slaves (Williams, 2005). BIPOC were denied equal education with Whites through a variety of means (e.g., unequal facilities, separate but equal facilities, denial of access). Various legal cases highlighted Blacks and Mexican Americans efforts to obtain education, including the famous *Brown v. Topeka Board of Education* case (Aguirre, 2005; Valencia, 2005). In early history, eastern American Indian nations' children attended church-sponsored schools (e.g., Moravians and the Cherokee Nation) (Giunca, 2009), but by 1880 the United States forcibly put children in boarding schools for assimilation into White culture (Lomawaima, 1993), leaving generations of traumatized children and adults with mental health issues. Asian Americans faced race segregation into separate schools as well (Kuo, 1998). Thus, there have been race disparities in educational access and quality from the beginning of the republic.

This has meant a lasting disparity in educational achievement for BIPOC (Soblich, 2016), and it has been estimated that, between 2009 and 2020, little changed to close race disparities in educational attainment (Dorn et al., 2020). BIPOC students at all ages are at a disadvantage compared to White and Asian students (Lips, 2019; Soblich, 2016), with school infrastructure, quality of teachers, bias in interpretation of student behaviors, food security, and fund allocations as issues. Race differences in educational attainment are significant because Black and Hispanic students are less likely to graduate from high school or college compared to White and Asian students (Soblich, 2016), and education level predicts employment status and type of occupation (Bureau of Labor Statistics, 2020).

The education system was not designed for pandemics such as COVID-19. Thus, educational race disparities become exacerbated. Although school personnel and parents worked to organize a meaningful learning experience, remote learning posed additional problems. Black and Hispanic students had less access to computers and technology prior to COVID-19, compared to White and Asian students, and this disparity did not subside (McDonald, 2020). Without school lunches, BIPOC students face food insecurities (Wright et al., 2020) and hunger. With remote learning the alternative to in-person learning, minority students are at a disadvantage.

In addition, BIPOC parents, if employed, are less likely to be able to work from home (E. Gould & Shierholz, 2020) and provide homework assistance. BIPOC parents work longer hours and are more likely to have multiple jobs (Bureau of Labor Statistics, 2014). They are more likely to be less educated compared to White and Asian parents (Soblich, 2016). Hispanic parents are more likely to be educated outside the United States (Krogstad & Radford, 2018) and less able to assist with education.

As Merolla and Jackson (2019) noted, structural racism is the overarching cause of educational achievement disparities, and the unequal education components are exacerbated during times of system stress, such as COVID-19. The consistent racial disparities in the educational social structure highlights additional barriers that students of color must overcome. Unfortunately, during times of pandemics such as COVID-19, these barriers could have resulted in higher dropout rates for BIPOC (Dorn et al., 2020), which then impacted employment and income during challenging national crises.

BIPOC AND INCARCERATION: HISTORICALLY AND DURING THE PANDEMIC

Finally, the structure of the CJS produces biased outcomes for BIPOC. Structural racism for criminal issues has existed since the 18th century (Gross, 2008; Rocque, 2011), with race categories determining defendant rights. Race bias within the CJS produces the most devastating outcomes for BIPOC in the United States, including stigma, persistent poverty, family dysfunction, and mental health issues (B. Western & Pettit, 2005).

The United States incarcerates more people than any other country, with $185 billion spent on the incarceration system (Prison Policy Initiative, 2021). BIPOC are overrepresented at all levels (local, state, and federal) compared to Whites (Prison Policy Initiative, 2021). For example, Black and Hispanic males are more likely to go to prison than White males (Alexander, 2010; Bonczar, 2003) at state and federal systems (Carson, 2015; Nellis, 2022). One of three Black males and one of six Hispanic males will be incarcerated at some point in their life (Bonczar, 2003).

In addition to social structural race issues (e.g., unemployment, housing insta-bility, poor quality education), poverty is a central feature of CJS treatment (Cole, 1999). Those who face poverty are overrepresented in the CJS, and they are at a disadvantage at each step of the process (Cole, 1999). Once incarcerated, Black males never reach income parity with those not incarcerated or with Whites (B. Western & Petit, 2005).

Similar to incarcerated adults, Black, Latinx, and American Indian youth are all overrepresented in correctional detention compared to White youth (The Sentencing Project, 2021b), and youth of color have negative perceptions of the CJS (Hagan, et al, 2005). In addition to race as a juvenile incarceration risk factor, being male, raised in poverty, experiencing substance abuse issues, and having an incarcerated parent are additional predictive factors (Ng et al., 2013).

Ramifications of pandemics are not well researched for prison populations, but there are indications that incarcerated persons face the worst possible conditions for spread of a disease like COVID-19. With significant deficits in the medical care offered incarcerated populations (Massoglia & Remster, 2019) and overcrowding of jails (Mortaji et al., 2021), incarcerated adults and staff faced an unusually high risk for diseases like COVD-19 (Denney & Valdez, 2021). In addition, youth in adult prisons and in youth detention centers faced high risk for contracting COVID-19 (Barnert, 2020). These pandemic risks fell mostly on BIPOC, and there is a growing demand for governments to implement protocols to protect those incarcerated and to address the structural racism that left BIPOC so over-whelmingly present in the CJS.

LESSONS LEARNED AND FUTURE RESEARCH

Macrolevel structural and systemic issues dramatically affect life experiences, and during times of social upheaval and hardship, vulnerable populations experi-ence heightened risk for negative effects (Egede & Walker, 2020). Inequalities left BIPOC with vulnerabilities within systems that would normally provide support during pandemics, such as COVID-19. Employment disparities, unemployment rates, housing shortages, food insecurities, educational disparities, and techno-logical absences left BIPOC with less ability to survive and thrive when any/all of these systems are challenged.

The findings on disparities signal a need for a concerted effort to bolster the employment, housing, food, education, and health systems that provide for a high quality of life. There have been attempts to improve the quality of life of vulner-able groups, such as BIPOC (e.g., war on poverty; Santiago, 2015). The unique structural and psychological issues for BIPOC need a renewed focus in a holistic system that considers how the social structures work individually and in unison to impede the quality of life for BIPOC and ensure adequate supports to with-stand pandemics or other national emergencies.

As Boulware et al. (2003) noted, BIPOC often have a distrust of authority due to historical and contemporary experiences (see Chapter 18 for a review).

Addressing and improving the structures and systems that have failed BIPOC will do much to overcome distrust and be a major step toward improving BIPOC's responses to pandemics, such as COVID-19 protocols, now and in the future.

CONCLUSIONS

Structural and systemic racism for BIPOC is not new, but we know the consequences are far reaching, impacting daily life as well as future prospects. This sets up a context where BIPOC experience barriers to overcoming poverty and to access quality employment, housing, education, and more. The CJS also contributes to the disparities by leaving the formerly incarcerated, the majority of whom are BIPOC, with lifelong barriers to equity. During times of pandemic, like COVID-19, the disparities pose an increased burden for BIPOC when trying to navigate through a national crisis. Elimination of the overcoming, persistent structural racism should be the foremost goal to ensure the most vulnerable are not left to negotiate the ravages of disease with no support system to promote survival.

REFERENCES

Aguirre, F. P. (2005). *Mendez v. Westminster School District*: How it affected *Brown v. Board of Education. Journal of Hispanic Higher Education*, 4(4), 321–332. https://doi.org/10.1177/1538192705279406

Ajilore, O. (2020, February 14). On the persistence of the Black-White unemployment gap. Center for American Progress. https://www.americanprogress.org/issues/economy/reports/2020/02/24/480743/persistence-black-white-unemployment-gap/

Alexander, M. (2010). *The New Jim Crow: Mass Incarceration in the Age of Colorblindness*. The New Press.

Allen, R. C. (2019). Class structure and inequality during the industrial revolution: Lessons from England's social tables, 1688–1867. *Economic History Review*, 72(1), 88–125. https://doi.org/10.1111/ehr.12661

American Psychological Association. (2010). Lesbian, gay, bisexual and transgender persons and socioeconomic status. https://www.apa.org/pi/ses/resources/publications/lgbt

Anderson, S. A. (1990). Core indicators of nutritional state for difficult-to-sample populations. *Journal of Nutrition, 120*, 1555–600. https://www.sciencedirect.com/science/article/abs/pii/S0022316622176613?via%3Dihub

Barnert, E. S. (2020, August). COVID-19 and youth impacted by juvenile and adult criminal justice systems. *Pediatrics, 146*(2). E20201299. https://doi.org/10.1542/peds.2020-1299

Benfer, E. A., Vlahov, D., Long, M. Y, Walker-Wells, E., Pottenger, J. L., Jr., Gonsalves, G., & Keene, D. E. (2021). Eviction, health inequity, and the spread of COVID-19: Housing policy as a primary pandemic mitigation strategy. *Journal of Urban Health, 98*, 1–12. https://doi.org/10.1007/s11524-020-00502-1

Bobo, L. D. (1999). Prejudice as group position: Microfoundations to a sociological approach to race and racism. *Journal of Social Issues, 55*(3), 445–472. https://doi.org/10.1111/0022-4537.00127

Bonczar, T. P. (2003). Prevalence of Imprisonment in the U.S. Population, 1974–2001 (NCJ-197976). U.S. Department of Justice. https://bjs.ojp.gov/content/pub/pdf/piusp01.pdf

Bonilla-Silva, E. (1997). Rethinking racism: Toward a structural interpretation. *American Sociological Review, 62*(3), 465–480. https://www.jstor.org/stable/2657316

Boulware, L. E., Cooper, L. A., Ratner, L. E., LaVeist, T. A., & Powe, N. R. (2003). Race and trust in the health care system. *Public Health Reports, 118*, 358–365. https://doi.org/10.1093/phr/118.4.358

Bureau of Labor Statistics (2014, May). *Job characteristics among working parents: differences by race, ethnicity, and nativity.* Retrieved from https://www.bls.gov/opub/mlr/2014/article/job-characteristics-among-working-parents.htm

Bureau of Labor Statistics. (2020). Labor force characteristics by race and ethnicity, 2019. https://www.bls.gov/opub/reports/race-and-ethnicity/2019/pdf/home.pdf

Bureau of Labor Statistics. (2021). Labor force statistics from the current population survey. https://www.bls.gov/web/empsit/cpseea04.htm

Burrell, M., White, A. M., Frerichs, L., Funchess, M., Cerulli, C., DiGiovanni, L., & Hassmiller Lich, K. (2021). Depicting "the system": How structural racism and disenfranchisement in the United States can cause dynamics in community violence among males in urban Black communities. *Social Science & Medicine, 272*, 113469. https://doi.org/10.1016/j.socscimed.2020.113469

Byars-Winston, A., Fouad, N., & Wen, Y. (2015). Race/ethnicity and sex in U.S. occupations, 1970–2010: Implications for research, practice, and policy. *Journal of Vocational Behavior, 87*, 54–70. https://doi.org/10.1016/j.jvb.2014.12.003

Carian, E. K., & Johnson, A. L. (2022). The agency myth: Persistence in individual explanations for gender inequality. *Social Problems, 69*(1), 123–142. https://10.1093/socpro/spaa072

Carson, E. A. (2015, September). Prisoners in 2014 (NCJ 248955). Bureau of Justice Statistics, U.S. Department of Justice. https://bjs.ojp.gov/content/pub/pdf/p14.pdf

Centers for Disease Control and Prevention. (2021). Adult obesity maps. https://www.cdc.gov/obesity/data/prevalence-maps.html#race

Coats, J. V., Humble, S., Johnson, K. J., Pedamallu, H., Drake, B. F., Geng, E., Goss, C. W., & Davis, K. L. (2022, August 18). Employment Loss and Food Insecurity — Race and Sex Disparities in the Context of COVID-19. Preventing Chronic Disease. *Centers for Disease Control.* Retrieved from https://www.cdc.gov/pcd/issues/2022/22_0024.htm

Cole, E. (1999). *No equal justice: Race and class in the American criminal justice system.* The New Press.

Collins, C., Asante-Muhammad, D., Hoxie, J., & Nieves, E. (2016, August 8). The ever-growing gap. Institute for Policy Studies, Racial Wealth Divide Initiative. https://ips-dc.org/report-ever-growing-gap/

Creamer, J. (2020, September 15). Inequalities persist despite decline in poverty for all major race and Hispanic origin groups. United State Census Bureau. https://www.census.gov/library/stories/2020/09/poverty-rates-for-blacks-and-hispanics-reached-historic-lows-in-2019.html

Denney, M. G. T., & Valdez, R. G. (2021). Compounding racialized vulnerability: COVID-19 in prisons, jails, and migrant detention centers. *Journal of Health, Political Policy and Law, 46*(5), 861–887. https://doi.org/10.1215/03616878-9156019

Dorn, E., Hancock, B., Sarakatsannis, J., & Viruleg, E. (2020). COVID-19 and student learning in the United States: The hurt could last a lifetime. https://www.mckinsey.com/industries/education/our-insights/covid-19-and-student-learning-in-the-united-states-the-hurt-could-last-a-lifetime

Dougherty, G. B., Golden, S. H., Gross, A. L., Colantuonia, E., & Dean, L. T. (2020). Measuring structural racism and its association with BMI *American Journal of Preventive Medicine, 59*(4), 530–537. https://doi.org/10.1016/j.amepre.2020.05.019

Dovidio, J. F., & Gaertner, S. L. (1986). Prejudice, discrimination, and racism: Historical trends and contemporary approaches. In J. F. Dovidio & S. L. Gaertner (Eds.). *Prejudice, discrimination, and racism* (pp. 1–34). Academic Press.

Dred Scott v. John F. A. Sandford. (1857). 60 U.S. 393.

Egede, L. E., & Walker, R. J. (2020, September 17). Structural racism, social risk factors, and Covid-19—A dangerous convergence for Black Americans. *New England Journal of Medicine, 383*, E77.https://doi.org/10.1056/NEJMp2023616

Einhorn, E., & Lewis, O. (2021, July 19). Built to keep Black from White. *NBC News.* https://www.nbcnews.com/specials/detroit-segregation-wall/index.html

Finn, B. M., & Kobayashi, L. C. (2020). Structural inequality in the time of COVID-19: Urbanization, segregation, and pandemic control in sub-Saharan Africa. Dialogues in *Human Geography, 10*(2), 217–220. https://10.1177/2043820620934310

Freng, S., & Willis Esqueda, C. (2011). A question of honor: Chief Wahoo and American Indian stereotype activation among a university-based sample. *The Journal of Social Psychology, 151*, 577–591. https://doi.org/10.1080/00224545.2010.507265

Galvan, A. (2021, June 16). Latinas left workforce at highest rate, see slow recovery. Associated Press. https://apnews.com/article/coronavirus-pandemic-technology-race-and-ethnicity-health-lifestyle-e21f94341735cc2c59042edcb09fb345

Geotting, N. (2008). The Marshall Trilogy and the constitutional dehumanization of American Indians. *Guild Practitioner, 65*, 207–226.

Giunca, M. (2009, September 8). https://journalnow.com/news/local/cherokee-revealed---translated-moravian-records-disclose-a-forgotten-history/article_7ab2e4dc-e315-5a72-ad4d-d9d99a15db1a.html

Gould, E., & Shierholz, H. (2020, March 19). Not everybody can work from home: Black and Hispanic workers are much less likely to be able to telework. Economic Policy Institute. https://www.epi.org/blog/black-and-hispanic-workers-are-much-less-likely-to-be-able-to-work-from-home/

Gould, S. J. (1994, November). The geometer of race. *Discover*, 65–69.

Gross, A. J. (2008). *What blood won't tell: A history of race on trial in America.* Harvard University Press.

Hagan, J., Shedd, C., & Payne, M. R. (2005). Race, ethnicity, and youth perceptions of criminal injustice. *American Sociological Review, 70*, 381–407. https://doi.org/10.1177/000312240507000302

Haslam, N. (2006). Dehumanization: An integrative review. *Personality and Social Psychology Review, 10*(3), 252–264. https://doi.org/10.1207/s15327957pspr1003_4

Hernandez, D. C., Reesor, L. M., & Murillo, R. (2017). Food insecurity and adult over-weight/obesity: Gender and race/ethnic disparities. *Appetite, 117*, 373–378. https://doi.org/10.1016/j.appet.2017.07.010

Hunt, M. O. (2016). Race, ethnicity, and lay explanations of poverty in the United States: Review and recommendations for stratification beliefs research. *Sociology of Race and Ethnicity, 2*(4) 393–401. https://doi.org/10.1177/2332649216666544

Krogstad, J. M., & Radford, J. (2018, September 14). Education levels of U.S. immigrants are on the rise. Pew Research Center. https://www.pewresearch.org/fact-tank/2018/09/14/education-levels-of-u-s-immigrants-are-on-the-rise/

Kuhn, M., Schularick, M., Steins, U. I. (2018). Income and wealth inequality in America, 1949–2016 (Institute Working Paper 9). Federal Reserve Bank of Minneapolis. https://doi.org/10.21034/iwp.9

Kuo, J. (1998). Excluded, segregated and forgotten: Historical view of the discrimination of Chinese Americans in public schools. *Asian Law Journal, 5*, 181–212.

Kurtz, A. (2021, January 8). The U.S. economy lost 140,000 jobs in December. All of them were held by women. https://www.cnn.com/2021/01/08/economy/women-job-losses-pandemic/index.html

Lee, T. L., & Fiske, S. T. (2006). Not an outgroup, not yet an ingroup: Immigrants in the stereotype content model. *International Journal of Intercultural Relations, 30*(6), 751–768. https://doi.org/10.1016/j.ijintrel.2006.06.005

Lewin, K. (1946). Action research and minority problems. *Journal of Social Issues, 2*(4), 34–46.

Lips, D. (2019). The state of equal opportunity in American K–12 education. Freeopp. https://freopp.org/the-state-of-equal-opportunity-in-american-k-12-education-42c78f5b67d2

Lloyd, R. G. (1951). The first great battle regarding life servitude in America. *The Negro Educational Review, 2*, 8–13.

Lomawaima, K. T. (1993). Domesticity in the federal Indian schools: The power of authority over mind and body. *American Ethnologist, 20*(2), 227–240. https://doi.org/10.1525/ae.1993.20.2.02a00010

Lukachko, A., Hatzenbuehler, M. L., & Keyes, K. M. (2014). Structural racism and myocardial infarction in the United States. *Social Science & Medicine, 103*, 42–50. https://doi.org/10.1016/j.socscimed.2013.07.021

Massoglia, M., & Remster, B. (2019). Linkages between incarceration and health. *Public Health Reports, 134*, 8S–14S. https://doi.org/10.1177/0033354919826563

McDonald, J. (2020, December 8). Despite improved access, digital divide persists for minority, low-income students. *UCLA Newsroom*. https://newsroom.ucla.edu/releases/digital-divide-persists-for-minority-low-income-students

Merolla, D. M., & Jackson, O. (2019). Structural racism as the fundamental cause of the academic achievement gap. *Sociological Compass, 13*, 1–13. https://doi.org/10.1111/soc4.12696

Merton, R. K. (1938). Social structure and anomie. *American Sociological Review, 3*(5), 672–682.

Morales, D. X., Morales, S. A., & Beltran, T. F. (2020). Racial/ethnic disparities in household food insecurity during the COVID-19 pandemic: A nationally representative study. *Journal of Racial and Ethnic Health Disparities, 8*, 1300–1314. https://doi.org/10.1007/s40615-020-00892-7

Mortaji, P., Corbisiero, M. F., Vrolijk, M. A., Henao-Martinez, A. F., & Franco-Paredes, C. (2021, June 01). Chronicle of jails and prisons COVID-19 deaths foretold. *American Journal of Medical Sciences, 361*(6), 801–802. https://doi.org/10.1016/j.amjms.2021.01.002

Mouzon, D. M., & Brock, B. D. (2021). If only they would make better choices: Confronting myths about ethnoracial health disparities. In S. M. McClure & C. A. Harris (Eds.), *Getting real about race* (pp. 1–21). Sage.

Murdock, G. P. (1949). *Social structure.* Macmillan.

Nagayama Hall, G. C. (2010). *Multicultural psychology.* Prentice Hall.

Nellis, A. (2022, September). Racial impact statements can help address disparities. *Lincoln Journal Star.* Lincoln, NE. Retrieved from https://journalstar.com/opin ion/columnists/guest-column-racial-impact-statements-can-help-address-disp arities/article_c667cb13-0bce-570c-935c-b0d5f631f89c.html#tracking-source= home-top-story

Newell, M. S. (2009). Indian slavery in colonial New England. In A. Gallay (Ed.), *Indian slavery in early America* (pp. 33–66). University of Georgia Press.

Ng, I. Y. H., Sarri, R. C., & Stoffregen, E. (2013). Intergenerational incarceration: Risk factors and social exclusion. *Journal of Poverty, 17*(4), 437–459. https://doi.org/10.1080/10875549.2013.833161

Odoms-Young, A. M. (2018). Examining the impact of structural racism on food insecurity: Implications for addressing racial/Ethnic disparities. *Family and Community Health, 41*, S3–S6. https://doi.org/10.1097/FCH.0000000000000183

Ong, P., Gonzalez, S., Trumbull, K., & Pierce, G. (2021). *Keeping the lights and heat on: COVID-19 utility debt.* UCLA: Center for Neighborhood Knowledge. https:// escholarship.org/uc/item/47h4b7s6

Ong, P., Wong, K., & Gonzalez, S. R. (2020). Systemic racial inequality and the COVID-19 homeowner crisis. https://escholarship.org/uc/item/2z99b26v

Powell, J. A. (2008). Structural racism: Building upon the insights of John Calmore. *North Carolina Law Review, 86*(3), 791–816.

Prison Policy Initiative. (2021). United States profile. https://www.prisonpolicy.org/profi les/US.html

Resendez, A. (2016). *The other slavery.* Houghton Mifflin Harcourt.

Rocque, M. (2011). Racial disparities in the criminal justice system and perceptions of legitimacy: A theoretical linkage. *Race and Justice, 3*, 292–315. https://doi.org/10.1177/2153368711409758

Royce, E. (2019). *Poverty and power: The problem of structural inequality.* Rowman and Littlefield.

Santiago, A. M. (2015). Fifty years later: From a war on poverty to a war on the poor. *Social Problems, 62*(1), 2–14. https://doi.org/10.1093/socpro/spu009

Schermerhorn, C. (2019, June 19). Why the racial wealth gap persists, more than 150 years after emancipation. *Washington Post.* https://www.washingtonpost.com/ outlook/2019/06/19/why-racial-wealth-gap-persists-more-than-years-after-emanc ipation/

Sharfstein, D. J. (2007). Crossing the color line: Racial migration and the one drop rule, 1600–1860. *Minnesota Law Review, 91*, 592–656.

Smedley, B. D., Stith, A. Y., & Nelson, A. R. (2003). Unequal treatment: Confronting racial and ethnic disparities in health care. National Academies Press. http://www. nap.edu/catalog/12875.html

Soblich, L. (2016, June 6). 7 findings that illustrate racial disparities in education. Brookings Institute. https://www.brookings.edu/blog/brown-center-chalkboard/2016/06/06/7-findings-that-illustrate-racial-disparities-in-education/

Sorenson, A. (1996). The structural basis of social inequality. *American Journal of Sociology, 101*(5), 1333–1365. https://www.jstor.org/stable/2782357

The Sentencing Project. (2021a). Racial justice.https://www.sentencingproject.org/issues/racial-disparity/

The Sentencing Project. (2021b). Youth justice. https://www.sentencingproject.org/issues/juvenile-justice/

Tonnies, F. (1905). The present problems of social structure. *American Journal of Sociology, 10*(5), 569–588.

Valencia, R. R. (2005). The Mexican American struggle for equal educational opportunity in *Mendez v. Westminster*: Helping to pave the way for *Brown v. Board of Education*. *Teachers College Record, 107*(3), 389–423.

Velasco-Mondragon, E., Jimenez, A., Palladino-Davis, A. G., Davis, D., & Escamilla-Cejudo, J. A. (2016). Hispanic health in the USA: A scoping review of the literature. *Public Health Review, 37*, 31. https://doi.org/10.1186/s40985-016-0043-2

Viruell-Fuentes, E. A., Miranda, P. Y., & Abudulrahim, S. (2012). More than culture: Structural racism, intersectionality theory, and immigrant health. *Social Science & Medicine, 75*, 2099–2106. https://doi.org/10.1016/j.socscimed.2011.12.037

Western, B., & Pettit, B. (2005). Black-White wage inequality, employment rates, and incarceration. *American Journal of Sociology, 111*(2), 553–578.

Western, M., & Tomaszewski, W. (2016). Subjective wellbeing, objective wellbeing and inequality in Australia. *PLoS One, 11*(10). https://doi.org/10.1371/journal.pone.0163345

Wiecek, W. M. (2011). Structural racism and the law in America today: An introduction. *Kentucky Law Journal, 100*(1), 1–22.

Williams, H. A. (2005). *Self-Taught: African American education in slavery and freedom*. University of North Carolina, Chapel Hill Press.

Willis-Esqueda, C. (2020). Bad characters and desperados: Latinxs and causal explanations for legal system bias. *UCLA Law Review, 67*(5), 1204–1223.

Wilson, V. (2020, September 16). Racial disparities in income and poverty remain largely unchanged amid strong income growth in 2019. Economics Policy Institute. https://www.epi.org/blog/racial-disparities-in-income-and-poverty-remain-largely-unchanged-amid-strong-income-growth-in-2019/

Wright, A. L., Sonin, K., Driscoll, J., & Wilson, J. (2020). Poverty and economic dislocation reduce compliance with COVID-19 shelter-in-place protocols. *Journal of Economic Behavior and Organization, 180*, 544–554. https://doi.org/10.1016/j.jebo.2020.10.008

Xu, C. (2021, July 17). Hundreds walk on Troost to promote unity along Kansas City's historic racial divide. *Kansas City Star*. https://www.kansascity.com/news/local/

Zambrana, R. E. (2020, October 15). Prioritizing equity: Structural racism and the Latinx community. American Medical Association. https://www.ama-assn.org/delivering-care/population-care/prioritizing-equity-video-series-structural-racism-and-latinx

FURTHER READING

Blumer, H. (1958). Race prejudice as a sense of group position. *The Pacific Sociological Review, 1*(3), 3–7.

Harris, A. P., & Pamukcu, A. (2020). The civil rights of health: New approach to challenging structural inequality. *UCLA Law Review, 67*(4), 758–833.

Norton, M. I., & Ariely, D. (2011). Building a better America—One wealth quintile at a time. *Perspectives on Psychological Science, 6*(1) 9–12. https://doi:10.1177/1745691610393524

Riley, A. R. (2008). Neighborhood disadvantage, residential segregation, and beyond—Lessons for studying structural racism and health. *Racial and Ethnic Health Disparities, 5*(2), 357–365. https://doi.org/10.1007/s40615-017-0378-5

25

Inequality in Healthcare

Theoretical Explanations for Disparities in COVID-19 Experience

EMILY R. BERTHELOT AND SUSAN G. BORNSTEIN ■

This chapter describes social and structural theories for inequality in general, in the healthcare system, and applied to COVID-19 (coronavirus severe acute respiratory syndrome coronavirus 2 [SARS-CoV-2]). The effects of such inequality are discussed, highlighting the resulting disadvantages to people of color (POC), older adults, and those of low socioeconomic status (SES).

INEQUALITIES IN HEALTHCARE AND HEALTH OUTCOMES

Inequalities in healthcare and health outcomes have been well documented in the literature. The COVID-19 pandemic exacerbated hardships for already vulnerable populations. A marked disparity occurred in the number of COVID-19 infections and deaths based on race,[1] ethnicity, age, and SES, with some of these categories overlapping, producing additive harm. The purpose of this chapter is to elucidate inequalities in healthcare, with respect to COVID-19, associated with race/ethnicity, age, and SES and to apply social psychological theories to explain these inequalities.

Inequality, Race, and Ethnicity

As of August 5, 2022, Blacks and Hispanics in the United States had experienced one and a half greater risk of infection, twice the risk of death, and large disparities in hospitalizations compared to non-Hispanic Whites.[2] The numbers of Blacks

Emily R. Berthelot and Susan G. Bornstein, *Inequality in Healthcare* In: *The Social Science of the COVID-19 Pandemic.* Edited by: Monica K. Miller, Oxford University Press. © Oxford University Press 2024. DOI: 10.1093/oso/9780197615133.003.0025 and Hispanics who died from COVID-19 exceeded their percentage makeup of the population.[3]

There are many explanations for these disparities in infection rates and deaths. Given that 11.5% of Blacks and 19% of Hispanics are uninsured, compared to only 7.5% uninsured Caucasians,[4] it is reasonable to infer that concern regarding costs, and inability to pay, may have diminished healthcare access and use, resulting in poorer outcomes. In addition, factors such as discrimination, occupation (particularly essential workers), educational/income/wealth gaps, and housing circumstances (e.g., living in crowded conditions) affected health equity and were associated with the unequal risk of COVID-19 infections, hospitalizations, and death in racial and ethnic minority groups compared to Whites.[5]

Inequality and Age

Of those who contracted COVID-19, older adults experienced the highest risk of severe illness and death. This population was more likely to have underlying medical conditions, such as heart disease, diabetes, kidney disease, and respiratory illness, which increased their risk of severe illness. By May 12, 2021, of COVID-19 deaths 30% had occurred in those aged 85 and older, and 95.5% occurred in people aged 50 and older.[6] Between February 1, 2020, and May 22, 2021, the United States experienced between 580,751 and 713,873 more deaths than predicted.[7]

Many COVID-19 deaths occurred among long-term care facility (LTCF) residents and staff, as these facilities housed concentrated populations of older adults and those with chronic medical conditions, who were inherently susceptible to infectious illness and less resilient to disease. In the United States as of June 1, 2021, while LTCFs accounted for 4% of COVID-19 cases, they were the source of 32% of U.S. COVID-19 deaths overall, ranging from 9% of deaths in Hawaii to 66% of COVID-19 deaths in New Hampshire.[8] Elaine Ryan, American Association of Retired Persons vice president of government affairs for state advocacy, described the disastrous response as a failure of accountability. The federal government passed responsibility to the states, and the states left the LTCFs in charge.[9] There was also a failure to make LTCFs a priority early in the pandemic, with inadequate testing supplies resulting in the rapid spread of infections throughout their facilities. Federal recognition of the need for widespread testing in LTCFs did not occur until May 2020.[9]

Disturbingly, while the average U.S. case fatality rate was 2%, in LTCFs the median case fatality rate was 10%.[10] Furthermore, with its staff itself comprising a COVID-19 high-risk population (minority workers, low wages); frequent personnel shift changes; and shortages of adequate personal protective equipment (PPE), the vulnerable LTCF population was even more likely to be exposed to the virus.

Inequality and SES

People with low SES are disproportionately likely to contract and die from COVID-19. SES is determined by income, education level, and occupational status. Research has proven that there is a clear relationship between SES and health outcomes (Brooks-Gunn & Duncan, 1997; Singh & Siahpush, 2006; Wagstaff et al., 2003). Low SES has been linked to increased risk of both mental (Belle & Doucet, 2003) and physical health problems (Braveman et al., 2010), higher mortality, and lower life expectancy (Singh & Siahpush, 2006).

Some people of low SES are at greater risk of poor health outcomes. Although many factors (e.g., income, education, occupation, marital status, geographic location) can influence one's SES, age and race/ethnicity are among the strongest predictors of deleterious health outcomes among the low-SES population. For example, aging low-SES people are more likely to be disabled and are at greater risk for death (Minkler et al., 2006), and racial and ethnic minorities are disproportionately likely to be of low SES relative to their White counterparts (Mode et al., 2016). The aging population is not the only low-SES group, however, that experiences increased risk of adverse health outcomes. Children are at greater risk for negative health outcomes, and this is more prevalent in children of color and is often due to the costs associated with care and the lack of health literacy among parents (Edelstein & Chinn, 2009).

INEQUALITY RELATED TO THE COVID-19 VACCINE

In the absence of curative treatment for COVID-19 and the morbidity and mortality that would ensue from pursuit of a herd immunity strategy, the most effective method identified to combat the COVID-19 pandemic was widespread uptake of vaccines. The Pfizer-BioNTech and Moderna vaccines were found to prevent 94%–95% of symptomatic infections and the Johnson & Johnson vaccine 72%.[11] However, there was significant racial disparity in access to the vaccine and willingness to undergo vaccination. As of May 24, 2021, in the 40 states for which data were available, 43% of Whites had received at least one COVID vaccine dose, compared to 29% of Blacks and 32% of Hispanics, with a White–Black discrepancy of as much as minus 25 percentage points (Iowa).[12]

Another source of COVID-19 disparity was related to vaccine distribution. Allocation to states was based on population size[13] rather than the number of high-risk individuals who were more susceptible to COVID-19 complications and death. States were then tasked with formulating their own injection disbursement plans.[14] Many initially adhered, with some modifications, to the Advisory Committee on Immunization guidelines. The guidelines prioritized vaccination of LTCF residents and staff, as well as hospital personnel, followed by those persons 75 years of age and older.[15] Initially, vaccine demand exceeded supply. However, over time, the focus shifted to reach low-information, vaccine-hesitant, and transportation-challenged persons.

THE SCIENCE AND THEORY
OF STRUCTURAL INEQUALITY

This section discusses theory and statistics illustrating that structural inequality exists, along with possible explanations. Specifically, COVID-19 experiences of POC, older adults, and those with low SES are examined through the lens of social-ecological models of health and critical race theory to identify areas of research needed to effect social change. This section focuses on social-ecological models of inequality and critical race theory to explain discriminatory attitudes and behaviors such as racism and ageism (see Chapters 23 and 24 for more on discrimination and COVID-19).

Within most societies (although to varying degrees), power and inequality are not evenly distributed. Some groups are historically oppressed, typically based on demographic categories (e.g., race, ethnicity, religion, SES, gender, immigrant status, age). Intersectionality refers to the intersection of numerous bases of inequality (including race, class, gender, and dis/ability), (Gillborn, 2015) and provides a theoretical framework for identifying who is most at risk for experiencing discrimination and disadvantage. Experiencing more than one of these characteristics (e.g., an aging Native American woman) compounds the disadvantage. These groups are less likely to live in areas that have quality schools, employment opportunities, or healthcare; to earn as much money as those in advantaged groups; or to be technologically savvy (See Chapter 24 for more on structural inequality in areas outside of healthcare). In addition, they may mistrust groups that have historically oppressed them, making interactions with such groups (e.g., law enforcement, healthcare providers) less productive, with suboptimal outcomes (see Chapter 18 for more on trust in healthcare).

Social-Ecological Models of Inequality

Social-ecological models posit that there are multiple levels of influence on behavior. These models allow researchers, using population-wide approaches, to consider the impacts of several levels of influence on behavioral (in this case health) outcomes simultaneously. These influences are found at individual, interpersonal, community, and societal levels. Biological and historical factors (individual level); family and peer factors (interpersonal level); neighborhood, school, and work factors (community level); and social, cultural, and policy factors (social level) can all impact health behaviors and outcomes. Research (Braveman & Gottlieb, 2014; McAllister et al., 2018; McCormack et al., 2017) focused on social-ecological models has long shown negative implications of structural inequality on physical and mental health outcomes.

Individual-level factors impacting health outcomes include age, race, education, income, and health history (Hu et al., 2021; Shorey & Ng, 2020). Conflict resolution, life skills training, literacy efforts, and violence prevention strategies are the most effective techniques found to prevent negative health outcomes at this level. Interpersonal-level factors impacting health outcomes include the influence of an individual's closest friends, family, and partners. Interpersonal skills development techniques are the most effective prevention strategies at this level. Community-level factors include school, work, neighborhood, and other social settings that may lead to disproportionate levels of disadvantage in health outcomes. Prevention strategies here include limiting disorder in the physical and social environment and addressing socioeconomic issues such as poverty and residential segregation. At the social level, broader social matters, such as social and cultural norms, work to perpetuate inequalities in health outcomes between groups in society, including health, economic, educational, and social policies. Promotion of societal norms that prevent inequalities is the most effective prevention strategy.

Social-ecological models allow researchers to better understand how these influences impact health outcomes and behaviors. These models focus on the influence of individual, interpersonal, community, and societal factors. Research that emerges from social-ecological models provides a foundation through which intervention strategies can be developed to implement change at specific levels of influence (Glanz et al., 2008).

Critical Race Theory

Research focused on critical race theory examines how certain beliefs, policies, and practices allow for racism to occur and persist, along with attempts to eliminate structural racism and systemic racism (Riley, 2018). Structural racism is the system that privileges certain racial/ethnic groups over others through policies, practices, representations, and social norms leading to racial inequities. Systemic racism, or institutionalized racism, refers to the laws, policies, and procedures (either current or historical) throughout all systems in society that have presented a public image of equality, but are either not racially neutral or have been applied inconsistently across races and ethnicities. The effects of these laws, policies, and procedures have led to racial inequalities that are long standing and pervasive. Examples of racist policies and practices that perpetuate structural racism include redlining in housing, laws that disproportionately restrict voting rights of POC, and school segregation laws (see Chapter 24 for more on structural inequality).

Critical race theory goes beyond identifying race and racism, however, by attempting to uncover how race and racism are understood and experienced, while also examining societal and cultural responses to race and racism (Ford & Airhihenbuwa, 2010). Further, critical race theory provides a lens through which racism leads to inequality and prejudice across several spheres of society, including health inequalities.

IMPORTANT DEFINITIONS RELATED TO CRITICAL RACE THEORY
- Privilege consists of five major components: "First, privilege is a special advantage; it is neither common nor universal. Second, it is granted, not

earned or brought into being by one's individual effort or talent. Third, privilege is a right or entitlement that is related to a preferred status or rank. Fourth, privilege is exercised for the benefit of the recipient and to the exclusion or detriment of others. Finally, a privileged status is often outside of the awareness of the person possessing it" (Black & Stone, 2005, p. 244).

- Microaggressions "are defined as the everyday, subtle, intentional—and oftentimes unintentional—interactions or behaviors that communicate some sort of bias toward historically marginalized groups. . . . They would deny it because they don't recognize that their behaviors communicate their racial biases" (Torino et al., 2018).

- The social construction of race is a multifaceted concept: "First, humans rather than abstract social forces produce races. Second, as human constructs, races constitute an integral part of a whole social fabric that includes gender and class relations. Third, the meaning-systems surrounding race change quickly rather than slowly. Finally, races are constructed relationally, against one another, rather than in isolation" (Lopez, 1994).

Racial inequality disproportionately impacts Black individuals and leads to several disadvantages, including socioeconomic, environmental, and adverse health outcomes. Many health policies fail to address how racism influences health outcomes. Additionally, the intersectionality between SES and systemic racism is often the cause of poor health.

STRUCTURAL INEQUALITY AND THE HEALTHCARE SYSTEM

This section provides examples of structural inequality in healthcare. Examples include both historical and more modern examples of structural inequality.

Historical Examples of Inequality in Healthcare

Medical history has been rife with examples of mistreatment of, or disregard for, the lives and dignity of patients of color. In medical studies, patients of color have been used as nonconsensual research subjects who did not receive proper treatment. For example, in the notorious Tuskegee study, for 40 years, from 1932 to 1972, Black men with syphilis were told that they were receiving free care from the federal government but were intentionally left untreated so that the researchers could assess their progression of disease.

Another example is the 1951 harvesting of Henrietta Lack's cervical cancer cells, known as HELA cells, for research without her consent or attribution (Skloot, 2017). Sixty-five years later, a study by Hoffman et al. (2016) demonstrated that

50% of medical students and residents surveyed endorsed false beliefs pertaining to biologic differences between Blacks and Whites (e.g., Black people having thicker skin or less sensitive nerve endings than White people), which translated into lower pain ratings for Black versus White patients and thus less accurate treatment recommendations.

Current Example of Inequality in Healthcare

In their review of communication and race in a medical setting, Cooper and Roter (2003) found that negative stereotypes of minority and disadvantaged groups had a negative effect on both the elicitation and conveyance of information by the provider. Although assertive behavior by Black and low-SES patients made it more likely that their providers would order more comprehensive testing (Krupat et al., 1999), another factor is that most outgoing communication is delivered by White, educated physicians and epidemiologists. Perhaps patients' inability to communicate in similar language influenced their ability to get appropriate care. Effectiveness of communication may also be hampered by the environment in which communication is taking place, messaging style, and/or cultural tone-deafness.

STRUCTURAL INEQUALITY AND COVID-19

This section gives COVID-19-related examples of the structural inequality described in the theory section above. Both social-ecological models of inequality and critical race theory provide frameworks for the disparities seen in health outcomes related to race, age, and SES.

Social-Ecological Models of Inequality and COVID-19 Health Disparities

The COVID-19 pandemic highlighted inequalities in behavioral (i.e., health) outcomes at all four levels of the socioecological model of inequality and magnified disparities in housing; educational, income, and wealth gaps; occupation; and healthcare access and utilization.

INDIVIDUAL-LEVEL HEALTH OUTCOMES
Racial/ethnic minorities have disproportionate representation among essential workers, which may lead to some of the disparate rates of infection and death of COVID-19 in these populations. Based on data compiled by the Economic Policy Institute, 10% of essential workers had a high school education or less; only 11% had an advanced degree; 49% were female, 51% male; 15% were Black, and 21% were Hispanic, while 55% were White. Only 12% were covered by a

union contract, which confers greater likelihood of employer-provided health insurance.[16] Of Hispanic adults aged 18–64, 69% had noncitizens in the family, and 49% of adults whose families contained no noncitizens lost jobs or income because of the pandemic, as opposed to 41% of non-Hispanic Blacks and 38% of non-Hispanic Whites.[17] Uninsured people are more likely to have poor health status, less likely to receive medical care, more likely to be diagnosed later in their course of illness, and more likely to die early.[18] These individual-level characteristics are associated with increased risk of COVID-19 infection death and perpetuate COVID-19 inequality across SES, race, and age.

INTERPERSONAL-LEVEL HEALTH OUTCOMES

Social determinants of health that may influence risk of exposure to COVID-19 include neighborhood and physical environment, housing, occupation, education, and economic stability. Specifically, the SES of those who contracted COVID-19 had important implications on the quality of healthcare they received. For example, Rudy Giuliani, former President Trump's personal attorney, bragged about receipt of treatment not available to most Americans: "If it wasn't me, I wouldn't have been put in a hospital frankly," Mr. Giuliani told WABC radio in New York. "Sometimes when you're a celebrity, they're worried if something happens to you, they're going to examine it more carefully, and do everything right."[19]

Giuliani, Mr. Trump, former N.J. Governor Chris Christie, and U.S. Department of Housing and Urban Development (HUD) Secretary Ben Carson all received special treatment for COVID-19, including the use of monoclonal antibodies, not widely available to the general public at the time.[20] There is no question that the morbidity and mortality of COVID-19 infections would be much different nationally if everyone had the same access, quality of care, and attention as Mr. Trump and those in his inner circle.

Because Medicare does not provide for home services such as assistance with daily living, delivered meals, or 24/7 care,[21] aging or disabled persons are more likely to reside in congregant care facilities, where they have exposure to far more people than they would in an independent home setting. Not only might they have a roommate, with whom they are in near-continuous close contact, but with the rotation of staffing and visitors (albeit with the latter being eliminated or severely restricted at various points during the pandemic), there was an ever-changing stream of people coming and going, any of whom conferred risk of viral transmission. Furthermore, by the very definition of their need to reside in a LTCF, the referenced population is far more likely to be aging, debilitated, acutely ill, or have underlying health comorbidities, all of which make it more difficult to recover from an acquired COVID-19 infection.

Regarding interpersonal-level factors and COVID-19's disproportionately deleterious effect on older adults, a key factor was inadequate supply of PPE for use in nursing homes, despite housing a particularly vulnerable population. In addition, hospitals sent infected patients back to the nursing homes despite the risk that they posed to the other residents. Paradoxically, with shortages of PPE and rapid spread of COVID-19 within LTCFs, the Centers for Medicaid and Medicare

Services suspended routine inspection of nursing homes, making it possible for an unfortunate situation to become worse. Meanwhile, LTCFs lobbied to be absolved of liability.[22] In a fitting example of intersectionality: "nursing homes with significant Black and Latino populations, no matter their location, size, government rating or infection history—(were) twice as likely to get hit by the coronavirus as their mostly White counterparts."[16]

COMMUNITY-LEVEL HEALTH OUTCOMES

Community-level factors that may lead to disproportionate levels of disadvantage in COVID-19 health outcomes include school, work, neighborhood, and other social settings. Rural and public hospitals struggle with staffing and revenue. Patients may not have Internet access or the digital skills to participate in telemedicine visits,[23] limiting access to providers. "Access to testing was lower in rural areas, and rural Black Americans were 70% more likely to be in a testing desert than the general rural population."[24] A testing desert is an area with limited access to COVID-19 tests. Living in pharmacy deserts also makes it difficult for many minorities or low-SES people to have access to the vaccine. A pharmacy desert is an area within which a person cannot fill a prescription within a short distance from their home. The distance varies between half a mile for low-income people without cars and a mile or more.

In addition, lack of health literacy and limited exposure to healthcare personnel due to workforce shortages may contribute to inequalities in healthcare in rural and disadvantaged communities. Health literacy is defined as "the degree to which individuals have the capacity to obtain, process, and understand basic health information needed to make appropriate health decisions"[25] and is most common among older adults, minority populations, those who have low SES, and medically underserved people.[26]

Low health literacy and limited exposure to healthcare personnel have direct implications for COVID-19 infections because knowledge helps people understand how the infection is spread and the importance of using masks and social distancing as a social responsibility. Patients of color and older adults in disadvantaged communities might feel intimidated in medical settings due to lack of familiarity and lower health literacy, limiting their ability to effectively communicate with their providers. In turn, these individuals may be less likely to ask questions, challenge their doctors' diagnoses, and/or admit they do not understand. The result of these inequalities is delayed care, failure to follow treatment recommendations, greater severity of disease, and increased likelihood of death.

Community-level influences on COVID-19 in the older adult population have also been a topic of political discourse. Some officials went so far as to offer to sacrifice the "senior" population to keep the economy rolling and avoid personal inconveniences. For example, Lt. Governor Dan Patrick of Texas indicated that he and others who were 70 years of age or older would rather risk death than compromise the economy by adopting public health measures, which at that time involved shutting down businesses and wearing masks when away from home and indoors. "You know, Tucker, no one reached out to me and said, 'As a senior citizen, are you willing to take a chance on your survival in exchange for keeping the America that all America loves for your children and grandchildren?'" Patrick said. "And if that's the exchange, I'm all in." Despite being at increased risk for complications from COVID-19, he stated that the aging adults could take care of themselves.[27]

SOCIAL-LEVEL HEALTH OUTCOMES

There are also substantial social-level contributions to COVID-19-induced inequalities. County-level income inequality has consistently been one of the strongest predictors of higher rates of COVID-19 infection and death rates (Tan et al., 2021). According to the National Institute for Health Care Management Foundation, there was bias in allocation of federal resources and funding, with initial relief based on hospital revenue.[28] Therefore, smaller hospitals with larger numbers of Black patients received less funding. In addition: "Patients at some community hospitals in NYC were three times more likely to die than patients at medical centers in the wealthiest parts of the city."[28]

Structural racism, according to researchers at the Harvard T. H. Chan School of Public Health, is making COVID-19 deadlier for Black Americans. "Environmental inequities" in Black communities make residents more likely to be exposed to pollution, have limited access to healthy food and medical care, live in crowded homes due to poverty (making social distancing difficult or impossible), and higher likelihood of being low-wage, low-skill, essential workers. Further, this population is also more likely to have underlying health conditions, like diabetes, heart failure, kidney disease, obesity, and respiratory and cardiac conditions. These environmental and medical conditions, coupled together, put them at higher risk for COVID-19 infection and make them more susceptible to severe symptoms and death.[29]

Critical Race Theory and COVID-19 Health Disparities

Critical race theory also provides a strong theoretical foundation to explain some of the inequalities in healthcare associated with COVID-19. The experience and tragic outcome of Dr. Monica Brown is exemplary of the effects of systemic racism within the healthcare delivery system and provide a strong example of the divergent experiences of people of color (even educated and affluent ones) compared to Whites as highlighted by the tenets of critical race theory. Dr. Brown's experience with healthcare for her COVID-19 diagnosis included microaggressions in response to her healthcare needs and accusations of drug-seeking behaviors, which are consistent with structural and systemic racism critical race theory outlines.

Dr. Brown was a Black, female family physician who presented with symptomatic COVID-19. As she described in posts and a video posted to Facebook,[30] her request for pain medication for severe neck pain was rebuffed by the White physician treating her, who made her feel as if she were considered a drug addict. In fact, Dr. Brown only received analgesia once an emergent computed tomographic scan showed new pulmonary infiltrates. The doctor also refused her pleas for additional doses of remdesivir. "This is how Black people get killed, when you send them home and they don't know how to fight for themselves," Moore said. "I put forth and I maintain if I was White, I wouldn't have to go through that." She died from the complications of COVID-19 3 weeks after falling ill.[30,31] Dr. Brown's experience, especially as a medical doctor of color, provides strong evidence that systematic racism is a pervasive problem in healthcare settings.

LESSONS LEARNED

Drawing from the information provide in this chapter, this section offers thoughts on how public health officials and policymakers might address structural inequality through a theoretical lens. This chapter provides several examples of discrimination against Black Americans and older adults throughout history and within the context of the COVID-19 pandemic. Inequalities in healthcare and society at large were highlighted and magnified by the COVID-19 pandemic. Early in the pandemic, it became abundantly clear that there were significant racial and age-related differences among those who became severely ill and those who died from COVID-19. Rates of infection, hospitalization, and death were significantly greater among low-SES, minority, and older populations.

It is crucial for national, state, and local governments to address social determinants of health, especially in older, impoverished, and minority populations. Public policy responses should include making healthcare and insurance universally accessible and affordable, improving housing assistance programs, and improving accountability in nursing homes and LTCFs. Additionally, given the proximity of impoverished communities to industrial plants, increasing residents' risk for adverse health conditions, including COVID-19 (Terrell & James, 2022), environmental strategies should be established to reduce toxic emissions.

Although vaccines were widely distributed among older adult populations, Black communities often had limited access and longer travel times to obtain vaccines, which likely deterred some Black Americans from getting vaccinated.[32] Special care must be taken to ensure equitable distribution of the COVID-19 vaccine (and any future vaccines). Broad and equal access to vaccinations and other medical advancements is one of the best ways to limit the spread of disease.

Additionally, health literacy efforts should be expanded to ensure that older adults, minorities, those of low SES, and other medically underserved individuals have greater understanding of their health, the ability to communicate effectively with their providers, and the confidence to demand better healthcare. At least equity with regard to COVID-19 appears to be underway as part of President Biden's National Strategy for the COVID-19 Response and Pandemic Preparedness by investing $250 million to encourage COVID-19 safety and vaccination among underserved populations.[33] Health literacy should also be fostered beyond the COVID-19 response to improve overall knowledge of health and healthcare access.

Relatedly, medical professionals should also advance their knowledge of the presence and consequences of structural racism and biases in healthcare, which disproportionately impact minority and impoverished populations. Research has revealed significant biases based on false beliefs toward several marginalized groups, including minorities (Hoffman et al., 2016). Innovative training strategies should be widely adopted to eliminate racial (and other) disparities in healthcare access, communication, and treatment.

FUTURE RESEARCH

Future research should focus on how systemic racism and the numerous other risk factors experienced by minorities, older adults, and those with low SES negatively impact the health outcomes of these individuals. Specifically, scholars should examine understudied factors that were amplified by the COVID-19 pandemic, such as the impact of being an essential worker, joblessness, and extended use of unemployment benefits on health outcomes and the relationship between environmental inequalities and the COVID-19 pandemic on community level health. Additionally, future research should study how increasing health literacy among patients and developing and implementing effective training programs for medical professionals focused on the consequences of structural racism and biases in healthcare can improve health outcomes in marginalized populations.

CONCLUSION

Health outcomes are not random. Rather, they are predominantly products of interactions, systems, and beliefs that can be altered to the benefit of individuals and society. The COVID-19 pandemic exacerbated hardships for already vulnerable populations. A marked disparity occurred in the number of COVID-19 infections and deaths based on race, ethnicity, age, and SES. This chapter examined the COVID-19 experiences of people of color, older adults, and low-SES people through the lens of social-ecological models of health and critical race theory to identify areas of research needed to effect social change. Prior to the COVID-19 pandemic, American history was already marked with several examples of disadvantaged people being mistreated in the name of public health. The COVID-19 pandemic shed light on these inequalities and highlighted the need for medical and social research to inform decisions of practice and policy to identify critical points of intervention in healthcare.

NOTES

1. Although race is an artificially constructed concept, we refer to skin color as race throughout this chapter.

2. https://www.kff.org/racial-equity-and-health-policy/issue-brief/covid-19-cases-and-deaths-by-race-ethnicity-current-data-and-changes-over-time/
3. https://covid.cdc.gov/covid-data-tracker/#demographics
4. https://www.kff.org/racial-equity-and-health-policy/issue-brief/changes-in-health-coverage-by-race-and-ethnicity-since-the-aca-2010-2018/
5. https://www.cdc.gov/coronavirus/2019-ncov/community/health-equity/race-ethnicity.html
6. https://www.statista.com/statistics/1191568/reported-deaths-from-covid-by-age-us/
7. https://www.cdc.gov/nchs/nvss/vsrr/covid19/excess_deaths.htm
8. https://www.nytimes.com/interactive/2020/us/coronavirus-nursing-homes.html
9. https://www.aarp.org/caregiving/health/info-2020/covid-19-nursing-homes-who-is-to-blame.html
10. https://www.nytimes.com/interactive/2020/us/coronavirus-nursing-homes.html
11. https://www.yalemedicine.org/news/covid-19-vaccine-comparison
12. https://www.kff.org/coronavirus-covid-19/issue-brief/latest-data-on-covid-19-vaccinations-race-ethnicity/
13. https://www.defense.gov/Explore/News/Article/Article/2441698/pro-rata-vaccine-distribution-is-fair-equitable/
14. https://www.hhs.gov/coronavirus/covid-19-vaccines/distribution/index.html
15. https://www.cdc.gov/mmwr/volumes/69/wr/mm695152e2.htm
16. https://www.epi.org/blog/who-are-essential-workers-a-comprehensive-look-at-their-wages-demographics-and-unionization-rates/
17. https://www.urban.org/urban-wire/immigrant-families-hit-hard-pandemic-may-be-afraid-receive-help-they-need
18. https://www.healthypeople.gov/2020/topics-objectives/topic/Access-to-Health-Services
19. https://www.nytimes.com/2020/12/09/us/politics/trump-coronavirus-treatments.html
20. https://www.usatoday.com/story/news/health/2020/12/21/monoclonal-antibodies-covid-19-donald-trump-regeneron-lilly/3895201001/
21. https://www.medicare.gov/coverage/home-health-services
22. https://www.aarp.org/caregiving/health/info-2020/covid-19-nursing-homes-an-american-tragedy.html
23. https://www.nytimes.com/2020/12/16/upshot/biden-trump-health-pandemic.html
24. https://nihcm.org/publications/systemic-racism-health-care-covid-treatment
25. https://health.gov/our-work/healthy-people/healthy-people-2030/health-literacy-healthy-people-2030
26. https://www.hrsa.gov/about/organization/bureaus/ohe/health-literacy/index.html
27. https://www.theguardian.com/world/2020/mar/24/older-people-would-rather-die-than-let-covid-19-lockdown-harm-us-economy-texas-official-dan-patrick
28. https://nihcm.org/publications/systemic-racism-health-care-covid-treatment
29. https://news.harvard.edu/gazette/story/2021/04/with-covid-spread-racism-not-race-is-the-risk-factor/
30. https://www.facebook.com/susan.moore.33671748/posts/3459157600869878
31. https://www.nytimes.com/2020/12/23/us/susan-moore-black-doctor-indiana.html

32. https://www.inquirer.com/health/coronavirus/mapping-vaccine-sites-study-coro
navirus-racial-disparities-20210204.html?utm_campaign=KHN%3A%20Da
ily%20Health%20Policy%20Report&utm_medium=email&_hsmi=109671949&_
hsenc=p2ANqtz--xiRyf7JjF2w3UFM98DnNhLLGBHwxNhaZanaaSdueBAcV6r
ORr__AUCvN2-DYzD4Qbsn_U_moRh69LW5WoYxRroxdWVg&utm_content=
109671949&utm_source=hs_email
33. https://minorityhealth.hhs.gov/omh/Content.aspx?ID=21533&lvl=2&lvlid=8

REFERENCES

Belle, D., & Doucet, J. (2003). Poverty, inequality, and discrimination as sources of depression among US women. *Psychology of Women Quarterly, 27*(2), 101–113. https://doi.org/10.1111/1471-6402.00090

Black, L. L., & Stone, D. (2005). Expanding the definition of privilege: The concept of social privilege. *Journal of Multicultural Counseling and Development, 33*(4), 243–255. https://doi.org/10.1002/j.2161-1912.2005.tb00020.x

Braveman, P. A., Cubbin, C., Egerter, S., Williams, D. R., & Pamuk, E. (2010). Socioeconomic disparities in health in the United States: What the patterns tell us. *American Journal of Public Health, 100*(S1), S186–S196. https://doi.org/10.2105/AJPH.2009.166082

Braveman, P., & Gottlieb, L. (2014). The social determinants of health: It's time to consider the causes of the causes. *Public Health Reports, 129*(1, Suppl. 2), 19–31. https://doi.org/10.1177/00333549141291S206

Brooks-Gunn, J., & Duncan, G. J. (1997). The effects of poverty on children. *The Future of Children, 7*(2), 55–71. https://doi.org/10.2307/1602387

Cooper, L. A., & Roter, D. L. (2003). Patient-provider communication: The effect of race and ethnicity on process and outcomes of healthcare. In B. D. Smedley, A. Y. Stith, & A. R. Nelson (Eds.), *Unequal treatment: Confronting racial and ethnic disparities in health care* (pp. 552–593). National Academies Press.

Edelstein, B. L., & Chinn, C. H. (2009). Update on disparities in oral health and access to dental care for America's children. *Academic Pediatrics, 9*(6), 415–419. https://doi.org/10.1016/j.acap.2009.09.010

Ford, C. L., & Airhihenbuwa, C. O. (2010). Critical race theory, race equity, and public health: Toward antiracism praxis. *American Journal of Public Health, 100*(S1), S30–S35. https://doi.org/10.2105/AJPH.2009.171058

Gillborn, D. (2015). Intersectionality, critical race theory, and the primacy of racism: Race, class, gender, and disability in education. *Qualitative Inquiry, 21*(3), 277–287. https://doi.org/10.1177/1077800414557827

Glanz, K., Rimer, B. K., & Viswanath, K. (Eds.). (2008). *Health behavior and health education: Theory, research, and practice.* John Wiley & Sons.

Hoffman, K. M., Trawalter, S., Axt, J. R., & Oliver, M. N. (2016). Racial bias in pain assessment and treatment recommendations, and false beliefs about biological differences between Blacks and Whites. *Proceedings of the National Academy of Sciences of the United States of America, 113*(16), 4296–4301. https://doi.org/10.1073/pnas.1516047113

Hu, D., Zhou, S., Crowley-McHattan, Z. J., & Liu, Z. (2021). Factors that influence participation in physical activity in school-aged children and adolescents: A systematic review from the social ecological model perspective. *International Journal of Environmental Research and Public Health*, *18*(6), 3147–3168. https://doi.org/10.3390/ijerph18063147

Krupat, E., Irish, J. T., Kasten, L. E., Freund, K. M., Burns, R. B., Moskowitz, M. A., & McKinlay, J. B. (1999). Patient assertiveness and physician decision-making among older breast cancer patients. *Social Science & Medicine*, *49*(4), 449–457. https://doi.org/10.1016/S0277-9536(99)00106-9

Lopez, I. F. H. (1994). The social construction of race: Some observations on illusion, fabrication, and choice. *Harvard Civil Rights-Civil Liberties Law Review*, *29*, 1–62.

McAllister, A., Fritzell, S., Almroth, M., Harber-Aschan, L., Larsson, S., & Burström, B. (2018). How do macro-level structural determinants affect inequalities in mental health? A systematic review of the literature. *International Journal for Equity in Health*, *17*(1), 1–14. https://doi.org/10.1186/s12939-018-0879-9

McCormack, L., Thomas, V., Lewis, M. A., & Rudd, R. (2017). Improving low health literacy and patient engagement: A social ecological approach. *Patient Education and Counseling*, *100*(1), 8–13. https://doi.org/10.1016/j.pec.2016.07.007

Minkler, M., Fuller-Thomson, E., & Guralnik, J. M. (2006). Gradient of disability across the socioeconomic spectrum in the United States. *New England Journal of Medicine*, *355*(7), 695–703. https://doi.org/10.1056/NEJMsa044316

Mode, N. A., Evans, M. K., & Zonderman, A. B. (2016). Race, neighborhood economic status, income inequality and mortality. *PloS One*, *11*(5), e0154535.

Riley, A. R. (2018). Neighborhood disadvantage, residential segregation, and beyond—Lessons for studying structural racism and health. *Journal of Racial and Ethnic Health Disparities*, *5*(2), 357–365. https://doi.org/10.1007/s40615-017-0378-5

Shorey, S., & Ng, E. D. (2022). A social–ecological model of grandparenting experiences: A systematic review. *The Gerontologist*, *62*(3), e193–e205. https://academic.oup.com/gerontologist/article/62/3/e193/5955961

Singh, G. K., & Siahpush, M. (2006). Widening socioeconomic inequalities in U.S. life expectancy, 1980–2000. *International Journal of Epidemiology*, *35*(4), 969–979. https://doi.org/10.1093/ije/dyl083

Skloot, R. (2017). *The immortal life of Henrietta Lacks*. Broadway Paperbacks.

Tan, A. X., Hinman, J. A., Magid, H. S. A., Nelson, L. M., & Odden, M. C. (2021). Association between income inequality and county-level COVID-19 cases and deaths in the U.S. *JAMA Network Open*, *4*(5), e218799. https://doi.org/10.1001/jamanetworkopen.2021.8799

Terrell, K. A., & James, W. (2022). Racial disparities in air pollution burden and COVID-19 deaths in Louisiana, USA, in the context of long-term changes in fine particulate pollution. *Environmental Justice*, *15*(5), 286–207. https://doi.org/10.1089/env.2020.0021

Torino, G. C., Rivera, D. P., Capodilupo, C. M., Nadal, K. L., & Sue, D. W. (Eds.). (2018). *Microaggression theory: Influence and implications*. John Wiley & Sons.

Wagstaff, A., Van Doorslaer, E., & Watanabe, N. (2003). On decomposing the causes of health sector inequalities with an application to malnutrition inequalities in Vietnam. *Journal of Econometrics*, *112*(1), 207–223. https://doi.org/10.1016/S0304-4076(02)00161-6

FURTHER READING

Chotiner, I. (2020, April 14). The interwoven threads of inequality and health. *The New Yorker.* https://www.newyorker.com/news/q-and-a/the-coronavirus-and-the-interwoven-threads-of-inequality-and-health

Lopez, L., Hart, L. H., & Katz, M. H. (2021). Racial and ethnic health disparities related to COVID-19. *JAMA,* 325(8), 719–720. https://doi.org/10.1001/jama.2020.26443

Ndugga, N., & Artiga, S. (2021, May 11). Disparities in health and health care: 5 key questions and answers. Kaiser Family Foundation. https://www.kff.org/racial-equity-and-health-policy/issue-brief/disparities-in-health-and-health-care-5-key-question-and-answers/

Patel, J. A., Nielsen, F. B. H., Badiani, A. A., Assi, S., Unadkat, V. A., Patel, B., Ravindrane, R., & Wardle, H. (2020). Poverty, inequality, and COVID-19: the forgotten vulnerable. *Public Health,* 183, 110–111. https://doi.org/10.1016/j.puhe.2020.05.006

26

How Will Couples Adapt to Stress From the COVID-19 Pandemic?

A Relationship Science Perspective

PAULA R. PIETROMONACO AND NICKOLA C. OVERALL ∎

The COVID-19 pandemic has produced widespread challenges, including those in financial, economic, and social spheres. Close relationships, in particular, have been disrupted (see also Chapters 19, 22, and 29 for how COVID-19 interacts with relationships). Quarantines and social distance mandates have separated people from their broader social networks (friends, family, neighbors, coworkers) and restricted key resources for navigating daily life (child care, elder care, health-care), increasing risks for social isolation and feelings of loss. These challenges can create stress that puts at risk the quality and stability of couples' relationships (Neff & Karney, 2017) and, as a result, health and well-being (Pietromonaco & Collins, 2017). This chapter draws on a key framework from relationship science—the vulnerability-stress-adaptation (VSA) model (Karney & Bradbury, 1995)—which suggests that the extent to which the pandemic disrupts couples' ability to adapt to the challenges of the pandemic will depend on the amount and severity of their pandemic-related stress along with their enduring personal vulnerabilities (Pietromonaco & Overall, 2021). The chapter presents findings from new, emerging research examining relationship functioning prior to and during the pandemic that support this framework and applies these findings as well as the broader literature to identify pathways through which individuals, couples, and societal policies could mitigate adverse effects of the pandemic on relationships and promote resilience.

Paula R. Pietromonaco and Nickola C. Overall, *How Will Couples Adapt to Stress From the COVID-19 Pandemic?* In: *The Social Science of the COVID-19 Pandemic.* Edited by: Monica K. Miller, Oxford University Press. © Oxford University Press 2024.
DOI: 10.1093/oso/9780197615133.003.0026

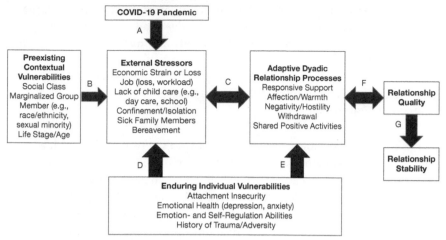

Figure 26.1 How the COVID-19 pandemic may shape relationship processes and outcomes. The framework (adapted from Karney & Bradbury, 1995) suggests that the COVID-19 pandemic will create a variety of external stressors, such as economic strain or job loss, that may interfere with adaptive dyadic relationship processes, which in turn can intensify the impact of external stressors as well as lower relationship quality and threaten relationship stability. The impact of pandemic-related stressors can be exacerbated by preexisting stressors, such as having a low income or being a member of a marginalized group. Couples in which one or both members have enduring vulnerabilities (e.g., attachment insecurity, depression) will be more likely to experience greater negative and fewer positive interactions, and the impact of external stressors may be heightened. (Figure from "Applying Relationship Science to Evaluate How the COVID-19 Pandemic May Impact Couples' Relationships" by P. R. Pietromonaco and N. C. Overall, 2020, *American Psychologist*, p. 3 [http://dx.doi.org/10.1037/amp0000 714]. Copyright © 2020 by the American Psychological Association. Reproduced with permission.)

THE VULNERABILITY-STRESS-ADAPTION MODEL APPLIED TO THE COVID-19 PANDEMIC

Figure 26.1 depicts Karney and Bradbury's VSA model adapted to focus on stress from the COVID-19 pandemic (Pietromonaco & Overall, 2021). The model suggests that the pandemic will create myriad stressors (Path A; e.g., economic loss, job/career loss or disruption, isolation and separation, lack of child care) that can undermine adaptive relationship processes, such as couples' ability to be supportive versus hostile during stressful relationship interactions (Path C). Preexisting contextual stressors (lower social class, marginalized group member) as well as enduring personal vulnerabilities (attachment insecurity, poor emotion regulation, depression) can exacerbate pandemic-related stress (Paths B and D), amplifying the strain on dyadic functioning. Enduring vulnerabilities also can interfere with adaptive relationship processes by increasing maladaptive patterns, such as hostility, criticism and withdrawal, poor support giving, and less affection and warmth, at a time when having a reliable, supportive, and caring partner is critical (Path E). Finally, the impairment of adaptive dyadic relationship processes adversely impacts longer term relationship quality and stability (Paths F and G).

External Stress and Relationship Processes and Outcomes (Paths C, F, G)

A large literature has shown that stress external to the relationship, such as from economic hardship or job loss, harms relationships. People confronted with stress are more likely to be critical or hostile, blame the partner for negative behavior, or provide little or ineffective support (Neff & Karney, 2017), and these patterns lead to greater relationship dissatisfaction over time (Nguyen et al., 2020). One reason that stress disrupts adaptive relationship processes is that coping with stress requires considerable attention and effort, thereby reducing a person's capacity to marshal additional resources to effectively engage with and support their partner (Buck & Neff, 2012). For example, experiencing the pressure of a hectic, conflict-filled day while working remotely can exhaust the energy and resources required to respond constructively during couples' discussions about child care or financial difficulties. Instead, when resources are depleted, people are more likely to become irritated or hostile or blame their partner for the problem, all behaviors that are apt to make the situation worse.

The COVID-19 pandemic has created a variety of stressors, placing demands on people to socially distance, remain at home while fulfilling job responsibilities, supervise children, and attempt to cope with diminished control and disruptions across many life domains (financial, relational). These combined sources of stress are likely to strain cognitive and emotional resources, hindering the ability to be a responsive, supportive partner and effectively negotiate when problems arise. Moreover, people are confronting this array of stressors within a context in which they view family as more important and conflict as more likely during the pandemic than before (Funder et al., 2021). Combined, this unique situation could amplify the pressure for couples to support one another and resolve relational problems, but depletion arising from increased stress likely means couples will struggle to do so.

Research in the early stages of the pandemic has provided evidence that the stress of this major disruptive event has negatively impacted relationship functioning. We review work that provided strong tests of the impact of pandemic-related stress by assessing relationship functioning prior to and during the pandemic. Drawing on an existing longitudinal panel study in Germany, analyses of 781 respondents illustrated that relationship satisfaction within marital/cohabiting relationships declined from before to during the pandemic (Schmid et al., 2021). In another study of 157 couples with children, people who experienced greater quarantine-related stress (living conditions, parenting, health) or had difficulty equitably distributing the increased household labor (housework, parenting) showed increased relationship problem severity and dissatisfaction (Overall,

Chang, Pietromonaco, et al., 2021; Waddell et al., 2021). Parents (N = 365) who experienced greater stress during mandatory quarantine also evidenced greater verbal aggression toward their intimate partners and children, poorer responsiveness to their children, and poorer family functioning (e.g., increased home chaos, decreased family cohesion; McRae et al., in press; Overall, Chang, Cross, et al., 2021).

Although the pandemic is accompanied by a variety of stressors, it also has initiated changes in daily lives that could open opportunities for couples to strengthen their relationships, such as by spending more quality time together or tackling the common threat together as a team (Pietromonaco & Overall, 2021). Consistent with this idea, people (N = 654) in married, cohabiting, or dating relationships who reported better coping, or lower relationship conflict, during the early months of the pandemic showed greater relationship satisfaction and less partner blaming compared to before the pandemic (Williamson, 2020). These findings suggest that couples who are able to engage in adaptive processes, such as reducing partner blame and sustaining affection/warmth during a stressful time, could reap relationship benefits. This idea is further supported by the decline observed in the divorce rate in 2020, compared to two prior prepandemic years (2018 and 2019) in four of five U.S. states (Florida, Missouri, New Hampshire, and Oregon), remaining about the same in the fifth state (Arizona) included in this study (Manning & Payne, 2020).

Whether stress from the pandemic disrupts relationships, or couples are able to maintain adaptive functioning, will vary depending on many factors. Many couples who are trying to manage the challenges of the pandemic while being confined at home with their children, for example, must negotiate the balance among work, child care, and household demands, which are likely to produce greater stress (Twenge & Joiner, 2020) and tax the cognitive and emotional resources needed to engage in adaptive dyadic processes. Accordingly, the studies reviewed above focusing on couples with children showed more negative outcomes (Overall, Chang, Cross, et al., 2021; Overall, Chang, Pietromonaco, et al., 2021; Schmid et al., 2021). Similarly, couples who already experienced economic (e.g., low income) or social challenges (e.g., discrimination based on race/ethnicity) prior to the pandemic are likely faced with greater stress over the course of the pandemic, placing them at greater risk for relationship problems (see Chapters 24 and 25, for more on inequality related to the pandemic). Moreover, these risks could be greater as the stress continues past the early months of the pandemic, as examined in the studies reviewed above, and could be magnified by other preexisting personal vulnerabilities shown to undermine adaptive dyadic relationship processes.

Enduring Personal Vulnerabilities (Paths D and E)

The VSA model (Karney & Bradbury, 1995) and its application to the COVID-19 pandemic (Pietromonaco & Overall, 2021) specifies that the impact of the

COVID-19 pandemic on couples' relationships also will vary depending on preexisting vulnerabilities (or strengths), which can influence how people perceive, react to, and behave within stressful situations (see Figure 26.1). For example, research examining individual vulnerabilities has indicated that maladaptive emotion regulation strategies (expressive suppression, rumination) and greater neuroticism were associated with poorer psychological, social and physical well-being during the pandemic (Kroencke et al., 2020; Low et al., 2020). Vulnerabilities that create greater distress and defensiveness within stressful situations also disrupt constructive dyadic exchanges and undermine relationship quality for both partners. Furthermore, enduring vulnerabilities will more adversely impact relationship outcomes when people confront more severe or more numerous stressors. This proposition was supported by research evaluating the effects of preexisting vulnerabilities on relationship functioning prior to and during the pandemic.

Attachment insecurity is a vulnerability that could be particularly significant in the context of the pandemic. The pandemic could trigger attachment insecurities by raising a variety of threats, including fears related to mortality (see Chapter 33 for more), uncertainty about the future, and isolation/separation from wider social networks. As a result, people are likely to turn to close others for comfort and security, but the affect regulation strategies of those who are insecurely attached could undermine their ability to effectively seek comfort from others or provide comfort to others (Mikulincer & Shaver, 2017; Simpson & Rholes, 2017). People high in attachment anxiety typically show more intense distress when faced with threat, and their attempts to cope often include overly relying on their partner for support and reassurance. These strategies can lead to relationship difficulties, including destructive communication and poor support provision, especially in the face of ongoing stress. Findings from a recent study illustrated how these processes affect relationship functioning during the pandemic. More anxiously attached people (assessed prepandemic) showed an increase in relationship problem severity during a COVID-19 quarantine, controlling for prepandemic problem severity, but only if they also reported a high level of quarantine-related stress (Overall, Chang, Pietromonaco, et al., 2021). Furthermore, partners of anxiously attached people—who likely were dealing with repeated requests for reassurance and support along with destructive communication—also showed a decrease in relationship satisfaction and commitment, an increase in relationship problem severity, and lower family cohesion if they reported a high level of quarantine-related stress.

Attachment avoidance is another form of attachment insecurity that is characterized by downplaying distress and distancing from the partner in the face of threat. These strategies also undermine relationship well-being for individuals and their partners because they restrict closeness and responsiveness and lead to damaging behaviors, such as hostility and withdrawal (Simpson & Rholes, 2017). In the same study described above, people with partners high in attachment avoidance (assessed prepandemic) showed decreased problem-solving efficacy and family cohesion whether or not they experienced high pandemic-related stress. This pattern of decreased relationship functioning likely reflects that their avoidant partners' strategies of distancing and disengaging made it difficult to negotiate conflicts and to sustain intimacy and closeness. The key point is that relationship functioning depends on both partners and is shaped by not only a person's own vulnerabilities but also those of their partner.

Preexisting vulnerabilities also can come in the form of broad societal attitudes that can impact how romantic partners negotiate power in their relationship. One such factor is men's hostile sexism, which includes beliefs sanctioning men's (and not women's) greater power and authority in the family (Glick & Fiske, 1996). Men's hostile sexism is linked to greater risk of aggression in intimate relationships (see Chapter 12 for more), especially when men believe that they have low control or low power (Cross et al., 2019). This situation is highly likely during quarantines in which couples are isolated together at home and have a hard time soliciting outside sources of support. The risk of hostile sexism is illustrated in a recent study showing that men higher in hostile sexism (assessed prepandemic) showed greater aggression toward their partner, especially if they experienced less power when interacting with their partner during a COVID-19 quarantine (Overall, Chang, Cross, et al., 2021).

Other personal vulnerabilities (e.g., depression, childhood adversity) that shape couples' functioning in general also are likely to interfere with adaptive relationship processes during the pandemic (see Figure 26.1), but research examining these factors in relation to the pandemic has not yet emerged. Depression, for example, leads people to focus more heavily on negative aspects of their situation (Wilde & Dozois, 2019), a pattern that is likely to amplify negative aspects of the pandemic (Path C). Furthermore, the negative views, hostility, and defensiveness of people with depressive symptoms also can lead to destructive interactions (hostility, defensiveness) with relationship partners (Barry et al., 2019; Pietromonaco et al., 2022) and heighten pandemic-related stress (Path B).

LESSONS LEARNED: MITIGATING RELATIONSHIP DISRUPTIONS, PROMOTING RESILIENCE

Although the COVID-19 pandemic has created widespread disruptions that are likely to present challenges for couples, how couples respond and manage their relationships under stress will vary considerably depending on couples' contexts and vulnerabilities. This key lesson can be applied to consider diversity in the long-term impact of the pandemic on relationship quality and stability, as well as the factors that predict when the pandemic will likely have a differential impact. For example, research on how people respond to major losses and trauma suggested that responses range from trajectories of chronic distress and long-term disruption to stable well-being and resilience (Bonanno, 2004). Similarly, couples will likely vary in their responses to pandemic-related stress, showing a range of trajectories from chronic, long-term relationship distress to a stable pattern of resilience (Pietromonaco & Overall, 2021). Figure 26.1 highlights that differences in couples' trajectories will be determined by a combination of their situational contexts, enduring vulnerabilities, and subsequent adaptive relationship processes.

Couples who face relatively low levels of loss and disruption (economic, job/career) from the pandemic, who can minimize isolation by connecting with others using methods that allow for social distancing (e.g., via video calls), and who have few enduring vulnerabilities are likely to be able to maintain a satisfying relationship and be resilient, especially if they already were able to skillfully and effectively negotiate conflict and provide support. Greater time together also could offer these couples the chance to share enjoyable activities (taking walks together, playing a new game or learning a new skill together, sharing happy memories), which can enhance closeness and strengthen their bond (see Pietromonaco & Overall, 2021). Moreover, working as a team to overcome obstacles arising from the pandemic could lead to a greater appreciation of their partner and relationship.

The majority of couples, however, will face relatively more significant challenges, and their relationship trajectories will be shaped by the extent to which they can engage in adaptive relationship processes over the course of the pandemic. Similar to the protective effect of vaccines against COVID-19, adaptive relationship processes will help to protect couples against the detrimental effects of stress from the pandemic (Neff & Karney, 2017). Relationship science points to two sets of behaviors that are especially important for safeguarding relationships: providing responsive support and effective communication. Responsive support entails listening to and trying to understand one's partner's concerns along with being willing to offer support that matches the particular needs of one's partner and reduces the potential negative consequences of stress and personal vulnerabilities on relationship well-being (Pietromonaco et al., 2022). Effective communication that helps resolve problems involves both avoiding certain responses, such as expressing hostility, being critical, or withdrawing from one's partner, as well as more active, positive engagement, involving both partners being motivated to work as a team to address the issue (Overall & McNulty, 2017). Applied to the pandemic, couples with partners who are both supportive and work as a team to tackle the parenting challenges of COVID-19 quarantines reduce the risk of poor relationship and family functioning (McRae et al., in press). Moreover, although the pandemic still might create short-term distress, couples who provide responsive support and engage in effective communication could recover more quickly and even develop a stronger defense that will help to protect them from future challenges.

Some couples will face extreme stress, loss, and disruption from the pandemic, such as those who entered the pandemic with greater socioeconomic disadvantage, members of racial/ethnic minority groups who have been hit particularly hard by the pandemic, as well as those struggling to care for children or elderly family members (see Pietromonaco & Overall, 2021). For these couples, adapting to the stress and challenges raised by the pandemic could take a toll on their relationships and increase their risk for relationship dissatisfaction and breakup. Sustaining adaptive relationship processes will be much more difficult under these adverse circumstances, which are likely to be exacerbated by the pandemic, and mitigating disruptions and promoting resilience could require efforts by policymakers and advocates that originate outside of the couple. Social policies that alleviate some of the economic burden, provide jobs or education and training, offer child care assistance, and healthcare (Karney et al., 2018) would allow couples some relief from intractable problems and open opportunities for further enhancing their relationships by engaging in adaptive relationship processes.

The overarching lessons learned emphasize that couples are not all the same, and thus the most effective pathways for mitigating disruptions and promoting resilience will depend on contextual and enduring vulnerabilities, stress, and adaptive relationship processes. Researchers, practitioners, policymakers, and couples will need to take into account variations in these factors in order to address the impact of the pandemic. The most effective strategies for supporting couples will need to be responsive to couples' contexts and vulnerabilities when they entered the pandemic as well as the extent to which the pandemic disrupted key aspects of their lives.

FUTURE RESEARCH DIRECTIONS

The theoretical framework presented in Figure 26.1 highlights the importance of taking into account multiple factors—life contexts, enduring individual vulnerabilities, and couples' adaptive relationship processes—in investigating how disruptions from the COVID-19 pandemic could shape couples' continued relationship functioning as well as relationship stability. These factors will shape not only how couples navigate throughout the crisis but also how they fare after the crisis has ended. Yet, only a few studies have provided evidence for these processes. For example, the initial work we reviewed has examined how key components of the model jointly influenced couples' functioning during the early months of the pandemic, but further work is needed to evaluate how stress and enduring individual vulnerabilities combine to impact adaptive relationship processes such as communication and responsive support. In addition, the current research on the impact of COVID-19 on couples' relationships has (necessarily) focused on short-term changes within the early months of the pandemic, but continued work is needed to determine how relationships evolve over the course of the pandemic as well as whether couples are able to recover once the strains of the pandemic begin to ease.

Our multifaceted theoretical framework also identifies several pressing questions for the development of future theory and research. First, to what extent will the current crisis produce different long-term trajectories for couples who entered the pandemic with different contexts and vulnerabilities, and will the crisis widen or exaggerate differences among these couples? Second, what kinds of interventions and policies will be most effective in mitigating risks and promoting resilience among couples who either entered the pandemic with greater risks and/or accrued greater risks over the course of the crisis? To adequately address these questions, future work will need to incorporate diverse samples, including diversity in socioeconomic status, race/ethnicity, parental status, culture, and country, which will allow for comparisons between different contexts and external stressors. In addition, longitudinal research that assesses both contextual and individual vulnerabilities prior to the pandemic and follows couples both throughout the pandemic and after the intensity of the crisis has ended will be important to pinpoint the extent to which the factors in Figure 26.1 shape couples' long-term functioning. Finally, research on interventions and policies will help to identify the best avenues for alleviating detrimental effects of the pandemic and fostering resilience among couples with different entry points, vulnerabilities, relationship skills, and trajectories.

Finally, just as the unique challenges of the pandemic put to the test couples' adaptability, the pandemic also puts to the test whether psychological science provides insight into risk, resilience, and recovery within a real-world crisis. The emerging evidence reviewed above supported the utility of relationship science theory and research for explaining the relative risks versus resilience of poor relationship functioning in the unprecedented context of a global pandemic. However, our recommendations for future research provide not only valuable targets for intervention to help couples effectively navigate such crises, but also persuasive tests of the relative importance of the contextual, personal, and relationship vulnerabilities (and strengths) identified in Figure 26.1 and, in turn, the central theories that identify these processes as essential for understanding relationship functioning.

CONCLUSION

Our analysis draws on the VSA model to illustrate the importance of couples' life contexts, their vulnerabilities, and their adaptive (or maladaptive) relationship processes for understanding how the COVID-19 pandemic could shape couples' relationship functioning and stability. Couples who entered the pandemic with different life contexts, vulnerabilities, and relationship skills might vary considerably in how the pandemic impacts their relationships. Furthermore, this variability means that the interventions and social policies that will be most successful for reducing relationship stress and promoting resilience will likely differ across couples. Future research investigating the multiple and interacting factors in the theoretical model will help to determine how the pandemic shapes couples' responses over time, whether couples who enter the pandemic from different contexts and with different vulnerabilities show distinct relationship trajectories, and which interventions and policies will be the most effective in supporting couples with different trajectories. Pandemic-related research also offers powerful tests of the utility of relationship science in accounting for relationship risk and resilience within real-world crises.

REFERENCES

Barry, R. A., Barden, E. P., & Dubac, C. (2019). Pulling away: Links among disengaged couple communication, relationship distress, and depressive symptoms. *Journal of Family Psychology*, *33*(3), 280–293. https://doi.org/10.1037/fam0000507

Bonanno, G. A. (2004). Loss, trauma, and human resilience: Have we underestimated the human capacity to thrive after extremely aversive events? *American Psychologist*, *59*(1), 20–28. https://doi.org/10.1037/0003-066X.59.1.20

Buck, A. A., & Neff, L. A. (2012). Stress spillover in early marriage: The role of self-regulatory depletion. *Journal of Family Psychology*, *26*(5), 698–708. https://doi.org/10.1037/a0029260

Cross, E. J., Overall, N. C., Low, R. S. T., & McNulty, J. K. (2019). An interdependence account of sexism and power: Men's hostile sexism, biased perceptions of low power, and relationship aggression. *Journal of Personality and Social Psychology*, *117*(2), 338–363. https://doi.org/10.1037/pspi0000167

Funder, D. C., Lee, D. I., Baranski, E., & Baranski, G. G. (2021). The experience of situations before and during a COVID-19 shelter-at-home period. *Social Psychological and Personality Science*, *112*(8), 1499–1504. https://doi.org/10.1177/1948550620985388

Glick, P., & Fiske, S. T. (1996). The Ambivalent Sexism Inventory: Differentiating hostile and benevolent sexism. *Journal of Personality and Social Psychology*, *70*(3), 491–512. https://doi.org/10.1037/0022-3514.70.3.491

Karney, B. R., & Bradbury, T. N. (1995). The longitudinal course of marital quality and stability: A review of theory, methods, and research. *Psychological Bulletin*, *118*(1), 3–34. https://doi.org/10.1037/0033-2909.118.1.3

Karney, B. R., Bradbury, T. N., & Lavner, J. A. (2018). Supporting healthy relationships in low-income couples: Lessons learned and policy implications. *Policy Insights From the Behavioral and Brain Sciences*, *5*(1), 33–39. https://doi.org/10.1177/2372732217747890

Kroencke, L., Geukes, K., Utesch, T., Kuper, N., & Back, M. D. (2020). Neuroticism and emotional risk during the COVID-19 pandemic. *Journal of Research in Personality*, *89*, 104038. https://doi.org/10.1016/j.jrp.2020.104038

Low, R. S. T., Overall, N. C., Chang, V. T., & Henderson, A. M. E. (2020). Emotion regulation and psychological and physical health during a nationwide COVID-19 lockdown. Manuscript submitted for Publication. https://doi.org/10.31234/osf.io/pkncy

Manning, W. D., & Payne, K. K. (2020). Marriage and divorce decline during the COVID-19 pandemic: A case study of five states. Unpublished manuscript, Bowling Green State University. https://doi.org/10.31235/osf.io/tdfvc

McRae, C. S., Overall, N. C., Low, R. S. T., & Chang, V. T. (2021). Parents' distress and poor parenting during COVID-19: The buffering effects of partner support and co-operative coparenting. *Developmental Psychology*, *57*(10), 1623–1632. https://doi.org/10.1037/dev0001207

Mikulincer, M., & Shaver, P. R. (2017). *Attachment in adulthood: Structure, dynamics, and change (Second)*. Guilford Press.

Neff, L. A., & Karney, B. R. (2017). Acknowledging the elephant in the room: How stressful environmental contexts shape relationship dynamics. *Current Opinion in Psychology*, *13*, 107–110. https://doi.org/10.1016/j.copsyc.2016.05.013

Nguyen, T. P., Karney, B. R., & Bradbury, T. N. (2020). When poor communication does and does not matter: The moderating role of stress. *Journal of Family Psychology*, *34*(6), 676–686. https://doi.org/10.1037/fam0000643

Overall, N. C. (2020). Behavioral variability reduces the harmful longitudinal effects of partners' negative-direct behavior on relationship problems. *Journal of Personality and Social Psychology*, *119*(5), 1057–1085. https://doi.org/10.1037/pspi0000231

Overall, N. C., Chang, V. T., Cross, E. J., Low, R. S. T., & Henderson, A. M. E. (2021). Sexist attitudes predict family-based aggression during a COVID-19 lockdown. *Journal of Family Psychology*, *35*(8), 1043–1052. https://doi.org/10.1037/fam0000834

Overall, N. C., Chang, V. T., Pietromonaco, P. R., Low, R. S. T., & Henderson, A. M. E. (2021). Partners' attachment insecurity and stress predict poorer relationship functioning during COVID-19 quarantines. *Social Psychological and Personality Science*, *13*(1), 285–298. https://doi.org/10.1177/1948550621992973

Overall, N. C., & McNulty, J. K. (2017). What type of communication during conflict is beneficial for intimate relationships? *Current Opinion in Psychology*, *13*, 1–5. https://doi.org/10.1016/j.copsyc.2016.03.002

Pietromonaco, P. R., & Collins, N. L. (2017). Interpersonal mechanisms linking close relationships to health. *American Psychologist*, *72*(6), 531–542. https://doi.org/10.1037/amp0000129

Pietromonaco, P. R., & Overall, N. C. (2021). Applying relationship science to evaluate how the COVID-19 pandemic may impact couples' relationships. *American Psychologist*, *76*(3), 438–450. https://doi.org/10.1037/amp0000714

Pietromonaco, P. R., Overall, N. C., & Powers, S. I. (2022). Depressive symptoms, external stress, and marital adjustment: The buffering effect of partner's responsive behavior. *Social Psychological and Personality Science*, *13*(1), 22-0–232. https://doi.org/10.1177/19485506211001687

Schmid, L., Wörn, J., Hank, K., Sawatzki, B., & Walper, S. (2021). Changes in employment and relationship satisfaction in times of the COVID-19 pandemic: Evidence from the German family panel. *European Societies*, *23*(Supp. 1), S743–S758. https://doi.org/10.1080/14616696.2020.1836385

Simpson, J. A., & Rholes, W. S. (2017). Adult attachment, stress, and romantic relationships. *Current Opinion in Psychology*, *13*, 19–24. https://doi.org/10.1016/j.copsyc.2016.04.006

Twenge, J. M., & Joiner, T. E. (2020). Mental distress among U.S. adults during the COVID-19 pandemic. *Journal of Clinical Psychology*, *76*(12), 2170–2182. https://doi.org/10.1002/jclp.23064

Waddell, N., Overall, N. C., Chang, V. T., & Hammond, M. D. (2021). Gendered division of labor during a nationwide COVID-19 lockdown: Implications for relationship problems and satisfaction. *Journal of Social & Personal Relationships*, *38*(6), 1759–1781. https://doi.org/10.1177/0265407521996476

Wilde, J. L., & Dozois, D. J. A. (2019). A dyadic partner-schema model of relationship distress and depression: Conceptual integration of interpersonal theory and cognitive-behavioral models. *Clinical Psychology Review*, *70*, 13–25. https://doi.org/10.1016/j.cpr.2019.03.003

Williamson, H. C. (2020). Early effects of the COVID-19 pandemic on relationship satisfaction and attributions. *Psychological Science*, *31*(12), 1479–1487. https://doi.org/10.1177/0956797620972688

FOR FURTHER READING

Chen, S., & Bonanno, G. A. (2020). Psychological adjustment during the global outbreak of COVID-19: A resilience perspective. *Psychological Trauma: Theory, Research, Practice, and Policy,12*(S1), S51–S54. https://doi.org/10.1037/tra0000685

Overall, N. C., & McNulty, J. K. (2017). What type of communication during conflict is beneficial for intimate relationships? *Current Opinion in Psychology, 13*, 1–5. https://doi.org/10.1016/j.copsyc.2016.03.002

Prime, H., Wade, M., & Browne, D. T. (2020). Risk and resilience in family well-being during the COVID-19 pandemic. *American Psychologist, 75*(5), 631–643. https://doi.org/10.1037/amp0000660

Randall, A. K., & Bodenmann, G. (2009). The role of stress on close relationships and marital satisfaction. *Clinical Psychology Review, 29*(2), 105–115. https://doi.org/10.1016/j.cpr.2008.10.004

27

The COVID-19 Pandemic as a Trauma Trigger

Lessons From Bosnia and Herzegovina

ALMA JEFTIĆ AND TOSHIAKI SASAO ∎

INTRODUCTION

Even though it seems that stress and post-traumatic stress disorder (PTSD) are possible outcomes for many people during the COVID-19 pandemic, it is still unexplored what happens to those who are already stressed and/or suffering from PTSD, such as war survivors. During the pandemic, measures imposed by governments in the form of isolation or quarantine have the potential to act as powerful stimuli of war reminders that can trigger memories related to the traumatic event. In addition, media coverage similar to what had been experienced during the war and a fear of the invisible enemy (the virus) can further provoke traumatic memories. Such events could dramatically affect the experiences of war survivors during the COVID-19 pandemic.

The empirical research conducted in Bosnia-Herzegovina as a part of the large COVIDiSTRESS Global Survey is used as a background for the explanation regarding how government measures of quarantine and lockdown influenced people who survived the 1992–1995 war in Bosnia-Herzegovina and to analyze if the COVID-19 pandemic acted as a trauma reminder. However, the purpose of this chapter is not to further discuss the results of the empirical research, but to compare different aspects of the pandemic (lockdown, restrictions to travel, media coverage, lack of food in the supermarkets) in terms of their role in provoking the post-traumatic stress symptoms and traumatic memories. Therefore, the major aims are to analyze and discuss the social-psychological theories of war trauma and PTSD, the social aspects of the lockdown in specific situations such as a postwar

Alma Jeftić and Toshiaki Sasao, *The COVID-19 Pandemic as a Trauma Trigger* In: *The Social Science of the COVID-19 Pandemic*. Edited by: Monica K. Miller, Oxford University Press. © Oxford University Press 2024.
DOI: 10.1093/oso/9780197615133.003.0027

developing country together with the challenges social scientists (psychologists and sociologists particularly) may face, and the potential of the global health crisis (COVID-19) to act as a war trauma trigger. The chapter discusses the lessons about how previous trauma and PTSD can impact experiences of the COVID-19 pandemics and will provide lessons learned from the Bosnian example together with the recommendations for researchers in the area of social science.

WAR TRAUMA REMINDERS AND PTSD

The connection between war trauma reminders and PTSD has been widely explored in literature (Duraković-Belko et al., 2003; Howell et al., 2015). This section reviews the theories and studies relevant to the explanation of trauma triggers and their impact on our experiences during crisis situations such as the COVID-19 pandemic. First described is the relationship between trauma reminders and PTSD, and second is a brief discussion of how media coverage might act as a trauma trigger during the pandemic.

War Trauma Reminders and PTSD: A Brief Overview

One of the major challenges in trauma research is the analysis of its transgenerational transmission as well as behavior of the first generation of survivors over time (see Chapter 44 for more on historical experiences that can affect COVID-19 experiences). The development of traumatic memories at the time of stress exposure represents a major vulnerability through repeated environmental triggering of the increasing dysregulation of a person's neurobiology (McFarlane, 2010). That is especially true for survivors of war trauma, who keep coping with their traumatic memories over the course of their lives. Different crisis situations (including pandemics) involve preventive measures that to a certain extent resemble the state of emergency proclaimed during the war (quarantine, isolation, curfew) and as such have the power to act as a trauma trigger. Besides curfew, quarantine, and lockdown, some behaviors, such as food hoarding, can have a similar impact.

Trauma reminders either symbolize or resemble aspects of previous traumatic experiences and have the potential to reactivate post-traumatic stress reactions (Layne et al., 2006). Hence, such reminders have the power to provoke memories of the past traumatic events and can be used to predict the onset of post-traumatic stress symptoms (Howell et al., 2015).

From the clinical point of view, the major characteristics of PTSD include reexperiencing symptoms of the traumatic event (i.e., intrusive memories and recurrent nightmares); protective reactions, such as avoidance of the stimuli associated with the trauma; and arousal symptoms, such as the startled response and hypervigilance (Ducrocq et al., 2001). However, PTSD is much more complex and includes a combination of the most frequent symptoms with not very common ones. However, Ai et al. (2002) stated physical reactivity to trauma provides reminders of one of the most common PTSD symptoms. Although it is expected that trauma reminders can lose their strength over time, Glad et al. (2017) discovered that the connection between trauma reminders and PTSD can even be stronger over time.

Media Coverage as a Trauma Reminder

In the context of pandemics, the media coverage that uses historical analogy while describing the situation can act as a trauma reminder. Historical analogy is defined as the process of drawing parallels between a past event and a current situation (Ghilani et al., 2017) and as such is applied "when a person or group draws upon parts of their personal and/or collective memories, and/or parts of 'history', to deal with current situations and problems'" (Brändström et al., 2004, p. 193). According to Ghilani et al. (2017), such analogies have two functions: They act as cognitive devices that people use to make sense of unfamiliar events, and they have instrumental purposes (i.e., helping policymakers establish their political agendas).

Although historical analogies have been used in the past by different media outlets and for various reasons, when used in a postwar environment they can act as a trauma reminder for the subset of the population that survived the war. It is well explored that memory for traumatic events lies at the core of PTSD (Kevers et al., 2016); hence, the exposure to war analogies in media during crisis situations such as pandemics can trigger higher stress levels. As such, media coverage of crisis situations may serve as a strong trauma trigger when reports include analogies to the previous war and/or language that corresponds to the war vocabulary (battlefield, enemy, fight, survival, isolation, etc.). However, recent studies showed that media can strengthen social support and provide important content and resources during pandemics (Galea et al., 2020).

BOSNIA-HERZEGOVINA 26 YEARS AFTER THE WAR

The war experience leaves lasting consequences on the survivors and as such significantly affects the way they react in not only everyday life but also crisis situations. This section provides a brief overview of the 1992–1995 war in Bosnia-Herzegovina and its consequences with special emphasis on mental health.

Brief Overview of the 1992–1995 War in Bosnia-Herzegovina

The war in Bosnia-Herzegovina started in 1992 and lasted 3 years. During that time, many people lost their lives or suffered from life-threatening injuries. Concentration camps, siege, and destruction are just some of the characteristics of that period that left lasting consequences on the citizens of Bosnia-Herzegovina, including those who managed to leave the country but suffered from the indirect consequences of war.

The war ended in 1995 after the ratification of the Dayton Peace Agreement on November 21, 1995, which kept the country as a single state made up of two parts, the Federation Bosnia-Herzegovina (Bosniak-Croat majority) and the Republic of Srpska (Serb majority) (Jeftić, 2019). Although the agreement brought some sense of relief at the beginning, very soon signs of despair appeared as the country remained deeply divided across ethnic lines (Maček, 2009). Besides poverty, unemployment, and destroyed buildings, the symptoms of war trauma were present, but there was no adequate psychological and psychiatric assistance in that period (Jeftić, 2019).

Mental Health in Bosnia-Herzegovina After the 1992–1995 War

Health and psychosocial well-being were affected in a number of ways during the 1992–1995 war in Bosnia-Herzegovina, particularly due to the forced displacement, disruption, and loss of life, relatives, and property (Carballo et al., 2004). Studies have shown signs of psychological maladjustment and PTSD in war survivors (e.g., Comtesse et al., 2019; Duraković-Belko et al., 2003; Hasanović et al., 2006). Both displaced and nondisplaced people experienced feelings of depression, fatigue, anxiety, and lack of sense of worth (Carballo et al., 2004).

Although citizens of Bosnia-Herzegovina had to cope with various stressors during and after the war, lack of awareness about mental health problems and stigma and labeling due to psychiatric hospitalization have had a powerful influence on their willingness to seek support, which has resulted in lower quality of life (Hasanović et al., 2006). Subjective perception of stigmatization and discrimination is an underexplored phenomenon; however, postwar stressors have led to an increase in the intensity and prevalence of PTSD symptoms (Klaric et al., 2007). In their study conducted 8 years after the war, Ringdal et al. (2008) found that about 13% of respondents had war-related distress symptoms above the threshold. A recent longitudinal study in three samples of Bosnian war survivors showed high levels of general psychological distress with current stressful living conditions, including health problems, debts, separation from loved ones, and similar acting as important predictors (Comtesse et al., 2019). The described conditions were further influenced by the COVID-19 pandemics.

COVID-19 PANDEMICS IN BOSNIA-HERZEGOVINA: PREVALENCE, RESPONSES, AND EXPERIENCES

This section discusses the main aspects of the COVID-19 pandemics in Bosnia-Herzegovina and current studies that explore the connection between war trauma reminders, PTSD, and the experiences of pandemics.

Basic Facts About the COVID-19 Pandemic in Bosnia-Herzegovina

The first registered case of COVID-19 in Bosnia-Herzegovina was reported on March 5, 2020, while a state of emergency was declared on March 17, 2020.[1] The curfew and the preventive measures (physical distancing, use of masks and disinfectant) were introduced almost immediately (Turjačanin et al., 2020). Lockdown was not imposed; however, feelings of anxiety were intensified by contradictory media reports and official statements (Turjačanin et al., 2020) that included historical analogies and collective memories of the last war (Banjeglav& Moll, 2021). Hence, citizens of Bosnia-Herzegovina had to cope with different war trauma reminders, including controversial media reports, lockdowns and border restrictions, and restriction and/or closure of business that provoked feelings of economic instability they went through during the 1992–1995 war.

War Trauma Reminders and PTSD Explain Some Experiences of the COVID-19 Pandemic in Bosnia-Herzegovina

Previous studies of the psychological impact of COVID-19 on citizens of Bosnia-Herzegovina were mostly concerned with the stress levels, behaviors, and quality of life. Janković et al. (2020) have shown that citizens' stress levels during the COVID-19 pandemic were low to moderate, but overthinking, change in sleep patterns, and nervousness were very frequent. Gobbi et al. (2020) reported signs of worsening of preexisting psychiatric conditions that led to the deterioration of life quality. However, not many studies explored the relationship between war trauma reminders, PTSD, and the COVID-19 pandemic. It is interesting to notice that such a connection was not explored during previous pandemics and epidemics. Reasons for this could include the complexity of such a study, the difficulty of conducting research with a vulnerable population, and the difficulty of separating the impact of a pandemic on previously diagnosed PTSD and PTSD developing under the influence of the pandemic itself. However, the connection between these variables was explored in two studies conducted at two different geographic areas during the COVID-19 pandemics.

Ellis and Rawicki (2020) discussed the possible link between the COVID-19 pandemic and experiences of war, hunger, and a concentration camp (Ellis & Rawicki, 2020). Based on the personal recollections of a 93-year-old Holocaust survivor, their article provides some insights into his struggles during lockdown while positioning the virus as an invisible enemy and a war trauma trigger. Although Ellis and Rawicki (2020) conducted an in-depth interview and discussed the meaning of trauma for war survivors during pandemics, it is hard to generalize their conclusions to the wider population. Hence, empirical study that would connect war trauma reminders, PTSD, and the COVID-19 pandemic was needed to fill that gap.

Jeftić et al. (2023) conducted an empirical study to test the relationship between war trauma reminders, PTSD, and the COVID-19 pandemic. They explored perceived stress and severity of PTSD symptoms during the COVID-19 pandemic in people who experienced the 1992–1995 war in Bosnia-Herzegovina, as well as how reminders of past trauma and loneliness related to current stress and PTSD symptoms. However, due to the restrictions caused by the COVID-19 pandemic, this study was conducted online as a part of the large COVIDiSTRESS Global Survey, and participants responded to the assessments of exposure to COVID-related information, concerns over disease, severity of exposure to war, frequency and intensity of war trauma reminders, loneliness, stress, and PTSD symptoms (Jeftić et al., 2020). The sample consisted of 123 participants (81.3% experienced war as a civilian), and the results confirmed that those who scored high on PTSD symptoms experienced higher levels of stress during the pandemic, which was especially present in those who reported feelings of loneliness. The intensity of exposure to war trauma reminders was positively associated with higher levels of PTSD symptom severity (Jeftić et al., 2023). However, the amount of consumption of COVID-related news coverage was not significantly associated with severity of PTSD symptoms and stress. This variable was assessed using items about seeking information from the government, news outlets, social media, and friends and family more frequently than usual, which suggests further that participants found this information helpful but not traumatizing (Jeftić et al., 2023). That is in line with previous research on social/news media as a risk factor for psychological distress during the COVID-19 pandemic, according to which media can also strengthen social support and provide valuable content and resources to the consumers (Galea et al., 2020). This underlies the importance of providing relevant content and support through local media during crisis/pandemics.

Much higher stress and PTSD levels were reported by those who were forcibly displaced, while firsthand experience of war and loss of family members was associated with more frequent and intense reminders during the pandemic. It was also shown that those who reported higher levels of perceived loneliness (living alone, being separated from family members, lack of friends/relatives/partner) experienced higher levels of stress and PTSD symptoms, all of which opens up a larger debate on the importance of examining negative experiences during pandemic.

Although the above described study explains some of the experiences during a pandemic, much deeper exploration of PTSD and the pandemic is needed in order to differentiate between war trauma-related PTSD and PTSD symptoms resulting from a pandemic itself. Also, studies like this would benefit from in-depth interviews with war survivors and a larger sample size. However, this is at the moment the first and only empirical study of this type; therefore, it provides a valuable starting point for future research. The results obtained through this study are supported by previous studies, such as that of Besser et al. (2009), who confirmed the coexistence of post-traumatic and perceived stress; the 2015 study of Howell et al. in which the authors indicated that the exposure to trauma reminders could predict PTSD symptoms; the work of Dekel et al. (2013), who discovered that PTSD symptoms predicted negative cognition of the self and the world in a sample exposed to war trauma; and the exploration by Mitchell et al. (2011) of the alleviating effects of social support on perceived stress in people who had experienced active combat. Besides that, several lessons can be drawn from the described study.

LESSONS LEARNED: HOW TO PROVIDE ASSISTANCE TO THE MOST VULNERABLE GROUPS (WAR SURVIVORS AND THEIR FAMILIES)

The first lesson learned is that PTSD and perceived stress appear together; there-fore, the negative appraisals during the pandemic can worsen the existing PTSD symptoms and further increase stress levels (Jeftić et al., 2023). The COVID-19 pandemic is perceived as a very stressful event, and it is expected that people who suffer from PTSD need social support and (in severe cases) psychological assis-tance to help them handle the crisis effectively.

The second lesson is that repeated exposure to content related to war trauma content and situations can trigger PTSD symptoms and increase stress levels. During the COVID-19 pandemic, the preventive measures of lockdown and curfew resembled measures introduced during the 1992–1995 war in Bosnia-Herzegovina regarding food and supply hoarding and COVID-19 media coverage. However, the latter was related to neither the higher levels of stress nor PTSD, which could be due to several facts: either such news provided beneficial information to citizens, hence they preferred to follow it or the level of trust in media was low, so people decided not to believe and react to what was presented to them. Hence, preventive measures should be designed in a way that does not trigger war trauma and PTSD symptoms in vulnerable populations, while media should display relevant, trustworthy infor-mation and avoid fake news and historical analogies.

The third lesson is that forced displacement and total time spent during the war highly influenced perceived stress levels and severity of PTSD symptoms. Also, direct experience of war and loss of close ones impacted how someone reacts to war trauma reminders.

The fourth lesson is that feelings of loneliness (being isolated, being abandoned, without company) can mediate the link between preexisting PTSD and increased stress levels during the pandemic. Hence, the importance of social support to vul-nerable groups should be emphasized during the pandemic as maintaining social interactions and preserving close attachments enables coping with war-related stressors. Lack of social support impacts how someone reacts to the war trauma reminders and can be an important factor in planning prevention programs.

FUTURE RESEARCH ON WAR TRAUMA, PTSD, AND EXPERIENCES DURING THE PANDEMIC

The future research ideas are supposed to examine further the topics discussed above. Although only one empirical study has been conducted in

Bosnia-Herzegovina with the aim to test the impact of the COVID-19 pandemic and its preventive measures on people who suffered from war trauma and PTSD, additional studies are needed. Hence, a few research questions can be formulated in future studies.

Why Do People Differ in the Way They React to Trauma Reminders?

While the authors (Jeftić et al., 2023) of the empirical study presented above focused on war-related stressors and perceived loneliness as factors that could determine why people differ in the way they react to the war trauma reminders, it remains unknown if some other factors, such as personality traits, general intelligence, moral values, and trust in government, can influence someone's reaction to trauma reminders. It will be important to test these assumptions in the future while including both vulnerable groups (war survivors, people who suffer from PTSD or other mental illnesses) and nonvulnerable groups.

Are the Children of War Survivors Impacted by Trauma Reminders During Crisis?

Trauma has been transmitted through generations, and such mechanisms have been widely explored. However, current studies of people suffering from PTSD and struggling during the COVID-19 pandemic did not explore the behavior of their children. Considering how trauma (especially war-related trauma) can be transmitted from parents to children (and from grandparents to their grandchildren), it is important to examine their behaviors during a pandemic. While applying similar methodology, (grand)children of war survivors should be considered a vulnerable group, and their susceptibility to develop PTSD (or similar symptoms) during crises such as the COVID-19 pandemic should be further analyzed.

What Type of Preventive Measures Should Be Provided to People Who Suffer From PTSD During the Pandemic or Similar Crisis?

Although psychotherapy is recommended to those who suffer from PTSD, including hospitalization for more severe cases, there has not been much evidence of treatment and measures to be applied during a pandemic. Puspitasari et al. (2021) recommended their approach to quickly adapt to a teletherapy technology platform for an intensive outpatient program guided by cognitive and behavioral modular principles for adults with serious mental illness, while Fina et al. (2021) discussed the prolonged exposure therapy as a highly effective treatment for PTSD across trauma-exposed populations and that has been implemented effectively via telehealth. However, specific adaptations during the COVID-19 pandemic should be required due to the physical distancing (Fina et al., 2021). Hence, new studies should investigate further how to implement standard and novel psychotherapies in the time of a pandemic while taking into consideration that people might need more time to adapt to the new methodologies while still coping with the crisis. Knowing how people who survived trauma react to new crises is important as it informs the wider audience how to act and behave (i.e., how to prepare the news for local media; how to prepare mental health professionals to better assist the most vulnerable groups). Providing regular psychotherapy and assistance to nonhospitalized people during lockdown and quarantine is a challenge that requires an integrative approach and cooperation of mental health professionals, government, and families of those in need.

Is the COVID-19 Pandemic Going to Cause PTSD or Other Mental Health Problems, and What Type of Psychological Assistance Should Be Provided in Such a Case?

Previous studies have indicated that the COVID-19 pandemic caused PTSD symptomatology in young adults (Liu et al., 2020) and in the general population (Fekih-Romdhane et al., 2020), as well as in health workers (Blekas et al., 2020; Johnson et al., 2020). Future studies should provide more insights on methods and treatments for preventing the onset of PTSD symptoms in a crisis. A longitudinal study of patients who were diagnosed with the PTSD before the pandemic would provide more insights on how the symptoms develop over time during the pandemic (under the special measures of lockdown and/or quarantine and afterward). Such studies would help differentiate symptoms of trauma-related PTSD and PTSD symptoms as a consequence of pandemics solely.

CONCLUSION

Experiences of the COVID-19 pandemic are largely impacted by the historical and psychological state of both the environment and people affected by it. Societies affected by war are more vulnerable to the new crisis, and previously traumatized people can experience worsening of PTSD symptoms and higher levels of perceived stress. Future studies should explore the connection between reminders of trauma and its connection to PTSD symptoms during a pandemic and similar crisis situations in order to develop functional preventive programs for vulnerable groups.

NOTE

1. Radio Slobodna Evropa (2020). *Prvi slučaj virusa korona u Bosni i Hercegovini, zaraženi otac i dijete.* https://www.slobodnaevropa.org/a/30469735.html

REFERENCES

Ai, A. L., Peterson, C., & Ubelhor, D. (2002). War-related trauma and symptoms of posttraumatic stress disorder among adult Kosovar refugees. *Journal of Traumatic Stress, 15*(2), 157–160. https://doi.org/10.1023/A:1014864225889

Banjeglav, T., & Moll, N. (2021.) Outbreak of war memories? Historical analogies of the 1990s wars in discourses about the coronavirus pandemic in Bosnia and Herzegovina and Croatia. *Southeast European and Black Sea Studies, 21*(3), 353–372. https://doi.org/10.1080/14683857.2021.1942656

Besser, A., Neria, Y., & Haynes, M. (2009). Adult attachment, perceived stress, and PTSD among civilians exposed to ongoing terrorist attacks in Southern Israel. *Personality and Individual Differences, 47*(8), 851–857. https://doi.org/10.1016/j.paid.2009.07.003

Blekas, A., Voitsidis, P., Athanasiadou, M., Parlapani, E., Chatzigeorgiou, A. F., Skoupra, M., Syngelakis, M., Holeva, V., & Diakogiannis, I. (2020). COVID-19: PTSD symptoms in Greek health care professionals. *Psychological Trauma: Theory, Research, Practice, and Policy, 12*(7), 812–819. https://doi.org/10.1037/tra0000914

Brändström, A., F. Bynander, & P. t'Hart. 2004. Governing by looking back: Historical analogies and crisis management. *Public Administration, 82*(1), 191–210. https://doi.org/10.1111/j.0033-3298.2004.00390.x

Carballo, M., Smajkic, A., Zeric, D., Dzidowska, M., Gebre-Medhin, J., & Van Halem, J. (2004). Mental health and coping in a war situation: The case of Bosnia and Herzegovina. *Journal of Biosocial Science, 36*(4), 463–477. https://doi.org/10.1017/s0021932004006753

Comtesse, H., Powell, S., Soldo, A., Hagl, M., & Rosner, R. (2019). Long-term psychological distress of Bosnian war survivors: An 11-year follow-up of former displaced persons, returnees, and stayers. *BMC Psychiatry, 19*(1), 1. https://doi.org/10.1186/s12888-018-1996-0

Dekel, S., Peleg, T., & Solomon, Z. (2013). The relationship of PTSD to negative cognitions: A 17-year longitudinal study. *Psychiatry, 76*(3), 241–255. https://doi.org/10.1521/psyc.2013.76.3.241

Ducrocq, F., Vaiva, G., Cottencin, O., Molenda, S., & Bailly, D. (2001). Etat de stress post-traumatique, dépression post-traumatique et episode dépressif majeur: la littérature [Post-traumatic stress, post-traumatic depression and major depressive episode: literature]. *L'Encephale, 27*(2), 159–168.

Duraković-Belko, E., Kulenović, A., & Đapic, R. (2003). Determinants of posttraumatic adjustment in adolescents from Sarajevo who experienced war. *Journal of Clinical Psychology, 59*(1), 27–40. https://doi.org/10.1002/jclp.10115

Ellis, C., & Rawicki, J. (2020). A researcher and survivor of the Holocaust connect and make meaning during the COVID-19 pandemic. *Journal of Loss and Trauma, 25*(8), 605–622. https://doi.org/10.1080/15325024.2020.1765099

Fekih-Romdhane, F., Ghrissi, F., Abbassi, B., Cherif, W., & Cheour, M. (2020). Prevalence and predictors of PTSD during the COVID-19 pandemic: Findings from a Tunisian community sample. *Psychiatry Research, 290*, 113131. https://doi.org/10.1016/j.psychres.2020.113131

Fina, B. A., Wright, E. C., Rauch, S. A. M., Norman, S. B., Acierno, R., Cuccurullo, L.-A. J., Dondanville, K. A., Moring, J. C., Brown, L. A., & Foa, E. B. (2021). Conducting prolonged exposure for PTSD during the COVID-19 pandemic: Considerations for treatment. *Cognitive and Behavioral Practice, 28*(4), 532–542. https://doi.org/10.1016/j.cbpra.2020.09.003

Galea, S., Merchant, R. M., & Lurie, N. (2020). The mental health consequences of COVID-19 and physical distancing: The need for prevention and early intervention. *JAMA Internal Medicine, 180*(6), 817–818. https://doi.org/10.1001/jamaintern med.2020.1562

Ghilani, D., Luminet, O., Erb, H.-P., Flassbeck, C., Rosoux, V., Tames, I., & Klein, O. (2017). Looking forward to the past: An interdisciplinary discussion on the use of historical analogies and their effects. *Memory Studies, 10*(3), 274–285. https://doi.org/10.1177/1750698017701609

Glad, K. A., Hafstad, G. S., Jensen, T. K., & Dyb, G. (2017). A longitudinal study of psychological distress and exposure to trauma reminders after terrorism. *Psychological Trauma: Theory, Research, Practice, and Policy, 9*(Suppl. 1), 145–152. https://doi.org/10.1037/tra0000224

Gobbi, S., Płomecka, M. B., Ashraf, Z., Radziński, P., Neckels, R., Lazzeri, S., Dedić, A., Bakalović, A., Hrustić, L., Skórko, B., Eshaghi, S., Almazidou, K., Rodríguez-Pino, L., Alp, A. B., Jabeen, H., Waller, V., Shibli, D., Behnam, M. A., Arshad, A. H., . . . & Jawaid, A. (2020). Worsening of preexisting psychiatric conditions during the COVID-19 pandemic. *Frontiers in Psychiatry, 11*, 581426. https://doi.org/10.3389/fpsyt.2020.581426

Hasanović, M., Sinanović, O., Pajević, I., Avdibegović, E., & Sutović, A. (2006). Postwar mental health promotion in Bosnia-Herzegovina. *Psychiatria Danubina, 18*(1–2), 74–78.

Howell, K. H., Kaplow, J. B., Layne, C. M., Benson, M. A., Compas, B. E., Katalinski, R., Pasalic, H., Bosankic, N., & Pynoos, R. (2015). Predicting adolescent posttraumatic stress in the aftermath of war: Differential effects of coping strategies across trauma reminder, loss reminder, and family conflict domains. *Anxiety, Stress & Coping, 28*(1), 88–104. https://doi.org/10.1080/10615806.2014.910596

Janković, A., Bakal, M., Hadžiahmetović, A., Kovačević, L., Omić, N., & Čehajić-Clancy, S. (2020). Social and behavioural responses during the COVID-19 pandemic in Bosnia and Herzegovina. *Sarajevo Social Science Review, 9*(2), 123–142.

Jeftić, A. (2019). *Social aspects of memory. Stories of victims and perpetrators from Bosnia and Herzegovina*. Routledge.

Jeftić, A., Ikizer, G., Tuominen, J., Chrona, S., Kumaga, R., & Yamada, Y. (2020). "Stay at home": Connection between the coronavirus pandemic, prevention measures and war trauma in Bosnia and Herzegovina. Open Science Framework. https://doi.org/10.17605/OSF.IO/R4VT9

Jeftić, A., Ikizer, G., Tuominen, J., Chrona, S., & Kumaga, R. (2023). Connection between the COVID-19 pandemic, war trauma reminders, perceived stress, loneliness, and PTSD in Bosnia-Herzegovina. *Current Psychology, 42*, 8582–8594. https://doi.org/10.1007/s12144-021-02407-x

Johnson, S. U., Ebrahimi, O. V., & Hoffart, A. (2020). PTSD symptoms among health workers and public service providers during the COVID-19 outbreak. *PLoS One, 15*(10), e0241032. https://doi.org/10.1371/journal.pone.0241032

Kevers, R., Rober, P., Derluyn, I., & Haene, L. D. (2016). Remembering collective violence: Broadening the notion of traumatic memory in post-conflict rehabilitation.

Culture, Medicine, and Psychiatry, *40*, 620–640. https://doi.org/10.1007/s11 013-016-9490-y

Klaric, M., Klarić, B., Stevanović, A., Grković, J., & Jonovska, S. (2007). Psychological consequences of war trauma and postwar social stressors in women in Bosnia and Herzegovina. *Croatian Medical Journal*, *48*(2), 167–176.

Layne, C. M., Warren, J. S., Saltzman, W. R., Fulton, J. B., Steinberg, A. M., &Pynoos, R. S. (2006). Contextual influences on posttraumatic adjustment: Retraumatization and the roles of revictimization, posttraumatic adversities, and distressing reminders. In L. A. Schein, H. I. Spitz, G. M. Burlingame, P. R. Muskin (Eds.) & S. Vargo (Collaborator), *Psychological effects of catastrophic disasters: Group approaches to treatment* (pp. 235–286). Haworth Press.

Liu, C. H., Zhang, E., Wong, G. T. F., & Hyun, S. (2020). Factors associated with depression, anxiety, and PTSD symptomatology during the COVID-19 pandemic: Clinical implications for U.S. young adult mental health. *Psychiatry Research*, *290*, 113172. https://doi.org/10.1016/j.psychres.2020.113172

Maček, I. (2009). *Sarajevo under siege: Anthropology in wartime.* University of Pennsylvania Press.McFarlane A. C. (2010). The long-term costs of traumatic stress: Intertwined physical and psychological consequences. *World Psychiatry: Official journal of the World Psychiatric Association (WPA)*, *9*(1), 3–10. https://doi.org/10.1002/j.2051-5545.2010.tb00254.x

Mitchell, M. M., Gallaway, M. S., Millikan, A., & Bell, M. R. (2011). Combat stressors predicting perceived stress among previously deployed soldiers. *Military Psychology*, *23*(6), 573–586. https://doi.org/10.1080/08995605.2011.616478

Puspitasari, A. J., Heredia, D., Gentry, M., Sawchuk, C., Theobald, B., Moore, W., Tiede, M., Galardy, C., & Schak, K. (2021). Rapid adoption and implementation of telehealth group psychotherapy during COVID 19: Practical strategies and recommendations. *Cognitive and Behavioral Practice*, *28*(4), 492–506. https://doi. org/10.1016/j.cbpra.2021.05.002

Ringdal, G. I., Ringdal, K., &Simkus, A. (2008). War experiences and war-related distress in Bosnia and Herzegovina eight years after war. *Croatian Medical Journal*, *49*, 75–86. https://doi.org/10.3325/cmj.2008.1.75

Turjačanin, V., Puhalo, S., Damnjanović, K., &Pralica, M. (2020). The new normal: Perception, attitudes and behavior of the citizens of Bosnia and Herzegovina at the beginning of the COVID-19 pandemic. *Friedrich Ebert Stiftun BiH*.

FURTHER READING

Okorn, I., Jahović, S., Dobranić-Posavec, M., Mladenović, J., & Glasnović, A. (2020). Isolation in the COVID-19 pandemic as re-traumatization of war experiences. *Croatian Medical Journal*, *61*(4), 371–376. https://doi.org/10.3325/cmj.2020.61.371

Van Der Kolk, B. (2015). *The body keeps the score. Brain, mind and body in the healing of trauma*. Penguin Books.

28

Nostalgia and Protection of Psychological Well-Being During the COVID-19 Pandemic

TIM WILDSCHUT AND CONSTANTINE SEDIKIDES ∎

The COVID-19 pandemic has triggered a wave of nostalgia ("a sentimental longing or wistful affection for the past"; *The New Oxford Dictionary*). A Nielsen/Media Rating Council (MRC) survey among 945 members of the U.S. general public (ages 13+) during the initial stage of the pandemic (March 25–29, 2020) revealed that the majorities of respondents had recently rewatched episodes of an old favorite television show (54%) and listened to music they used to listen to but had not heard in a while (55%).[1] Nostalgic trends have also emerged on social media. The subreddit r/Nostalgia has enjoyed growing popularity since the start of the pandemic, and tweets with the phrase "I Miss" have surged on Twitter.[2] New nostalgic social media challenges have sprung up; these invite users to post pictures of their younger selves (#MeAt20), recreate childhood photographs (#ImJustAKid), or describe favorite pastimes and products from their past (#DistractA90sKid).[3] Old-fashioned board games have come back in vogue, and sepia-tinted broadcasts of classic sporting events have attracted captivated audiences.[4]

Why does pandemic-induced malaise trigger nostalgia? In turn, what does nostalgia do for the beleaguered person? We address these questions from the perspective of the regulatory model of nostalgia (Wildschut & Sedikides, 2021). This model proposes that nostalgia shapes people's experiences of the COVID-19 pandemic by acting as a homeostatic corrective: Negative states trigger nostalgia, which in turn restores balance by counteracting these negative states. To set the stage, the first part of our chapter outlines the model by means of illustrative studies. We present evidence that aversive psychological states, such as those created by the pandemic, trigger nostalgia. We next show how, in turn, nostalgia serves a number of

Tim Wildschut and Constantine Sedikides, *Nostalgia and Protection of Psychological Well-Being During the COVID-19 Pandemic* In: *The Social Science of the COVID-19 Pandemic*. Edited by: Monica K. Miller, Oxford University Press.
© Oxford University Press 2024. DOI: 10.1093/oso/9780197615133.003.0028

important psychological functions. We then combine these threads by reviewing studies that tested the complete model, demonstrating the positive downstream effects of adversity-induced nostalgia. In the second part of our chapter, we present the findings from six studies conducted during the COVID-19 pandemic. Based on the regulatory model, these studies demonstrated how loneliness (an aversive state) during the pandemic not only undermined well-being, but also animated nostalgia. Nostalgia, in turn, was positively associated with well-being, counteracting the adversity of loneliness (see Chapter 28 for more on well-being). In concluding the chapter, we consider lessons learned and future opportunities. We begin, however, by briefly addressing the definitional question: What is nostalgia?

WHAT IS NOSTALGIA?

Studies in which laypersons were asked to identify which features or attributes they considered most characteristic (or prototypical) of the construct "nostalgia" revealed that they conceptualized nostalgia as a predominantly positive, social, and past-oriented emotion (Hepper et al., 2012). In nostalgic reverie, one brings to mind a fond and personally meaningful event, typically involving one's childhood or a close relationship. The person often sees the event through rose-colored glasses, misses that time or relationship, and might even long to return to the past. As a result, they feel sentimental, mostly happy but with a tinge of sadness. These lay conceptions of nostalgia dovetail with contemporary dictionary definitions, as do the findings of content analyses and automated text analyses of nostalgic narratives (Wildschut et al., 2018). This prototypic view of nostalgia transcends cultural boundaries (Hepper et al., 2014).

TRIGGERS OF NOSTALGIA

The first tenet of the regulatory model proposes that aversive states, such as those induced by the COVID-19 pandemic, trigger nostalgia. Boredom is a case in point. The pandemic has imposed constraints on people that have eroded their sense of agency and induced aversive feelings of boredom (Boylan et al., 2020). Van Tilburg and colleagues (2013, Study 2) hypothesized that boredom would increase nostalgia. To test this, they experimentally manipulated boredom by randomly assigning participants to trace a line through either three (low-boredom condition) or nine (high-boredom condition) large spirals. The manipulation successfully induced boredom. The researchers then instructed participants to retrieve an unspecified autobiographical memory (i.e., a past event) and to indicate how nostalgic they felt after recalling the event. Participants rated two items (i.e., "Right now, I am feeling quite nostalgic," "Right now, I'm having nostalgic feelings"), which were averaged to create an index. Participants in the high-boredom condition felt more nostalgic than those in the low-boredom condition. Boredom increased nostalgia.

Loneliness serves as another example. A longitudinal survey among a nation-wide sample of U.S. adults revealed that loneliness increased significantly during the initial phase of the pandemic (April to September 2020). Respondents who reported that they were under stay-at-home, shelter-in-place, or lockdown orders evinced higher loneliness levels than those reporting no restrictions (Killgore et al., 2020; cf. Luchetti et al., 2020). Wildschut and colleagues (2006, Study 4) examined the impact of an experimental loneliness induction on momentary feelings of nostalgia. They manipulated loneliness via false feedback. U.K. undergraduates first completed 15 items measuring loneliness. In the high-loneliness condition, the researchers phrased these items to elicit agreement by prefacing them with the words "sometimes" (e.g., "I sometimes feel isolated from others"). In the low-loneliness condition, they phrased the items to elicit disagreement by prefacing them with the stem "always" (e.g., "I always feel isolated from others"). As intended, participants in the high-loneliness (compared to low-loneliness) condition were more likely to agree with the statements. The researchers then informed participants in the high-loneliness condition that they fell in the 62nd percentile of the loneliness distribution and therefore were "above average on loneliness." Those in the low-loneliness condition were told that they fell in the 12th percentile and therefore were "very low on loneliness." Participants then generated reasons for their purported loneliness level and completed a (successful) manipulation check. Next, nostalgia was assessed by instructing participants to rate how much they missed 18 aspects of their past (e.g., "my family," "music," "having someone to depend on," "holidays I went on"; Batcho, 1995). We averaged the 18 responses to create a nostalgia index. Participants in the high-loneliness condition felt more nostalgic than those in the low-loneliness condition. Loneliness increased nostalgia. These findings invite an important question: When triggered, what does nostalgia do for people who experience adversity?

FUNCTIONS OF NOSTALGIA

The second tenet of the regulatory model proposes that nostalgia serves a number of key psychological functions. These functions fall into four broad domains: social, self-oriented, existential, and future oriented. Within the social domain, nostalgia promotes perceived social connectedness and interpersonal competence, which provide the scaffolding for prosocial goals, action tendencies, and behavior (Sedikides & Wildschut, 2019). With regard to its self-oriented function, nostalgia builds, maintains, and enhances self-positivity. Specifically, it heightens the accessibility of positive self-attributes and boosts self-esteem (Vess et al., 2012). As for the existential domain, nostalgia is a source of meaning in life and fosters a sense of continuity between one's past and present self (Sedikides & Wildschut, 2018). Relating to its future-oriented function, nostalgia raises optimism, inspiration, and creativity (Sedikides & Wildschut, 2020). We zoom in on two domains that are particularly pertinent to the COVID-19 pandemic: existential and social.

Chasson and colleagues (2021) examined the presence and search for meaning in life in two samples of new mothers: one that was recruited before the pandemic and one recruited during the pandemic. New mothers reported lower presence of meaning in life and higher search for meaning in life during the pandemic than prior to it. Can nostalgia replenish meaning in life? Reid and colleagues (2015) examined the relation between scent-evoked nostalgia and meaning among U.S. undergraduates. Participants sampled, in random order, 12 pleasantly or neutrally scented oils presented in glass tubes (e.g., Chanel No. 5, baby powder, lavender). They rated each scent for nostalgia (i.e., "How nostalgic does this scent make you feel?") and responded to two meaning items (i.e., "life is meaningful," "life has a purpose"). Higher levels of scent-evoked nostalgia were positively correlated with greater meaning in life.

To test the causal impact of nostalgia on meaning in life, Routledge and colleagues (2011, Study 2) experimentally induced nostalgia with song lyrics. The study involved two sessions, approximately 1 week apart. In the initial session, participants were instructed to generate the titles and performing artists of three songs that made them feel nostalgic. During the interim period that followed, the researchers randomly allocated participants to conditions and yoked each participant in the nostalgia condition to a participant in the control condition (i.e., creating pairs of participants). They then retrieved, for each participant assigned to the nostalgia condition, the lyrics of one of the three personally nostalgic songs they listed in the initial session. In the subsequent experimental session, the researchers presented these lyrics to both participants in each yoked pair. Thus, the lyrics were constant across conditions, but only participants in the nostalgia condition viewed lyrics of a personally nostalgic song. After reading the lyrics, participants completed the Presence of Meaning in Life scale (Steger et al., 2006). Participants in the nostalgia condition reported greater presence of meaning in life than yoked controls. Nostalgia increased meaning in life.

Turning to the social domain, the COVID-19 pandemic has disrupted the provision of healthcare (e.g., cessation of in-person counseling, reduced availability of medical facilities), creating even greater obstacles to adequate professional support than usual and discouraging people from seeking help when they need it (Lueck, 2021). Juhl and colleagues (2021, Study 4) hypothesized that nostalgia, by virtue of its capacity to strengthen social bonds and interpersonal trust, can promote help seeking. To test this, they experimentally induced nostalgia with the event reflection task. Participants were randomly assigned to reflect on either a personally experienced nostalgic event (nostalgia condition) or an ordinary (e.g., everyday, regular) event (control condition). After bringing the relevant event to mind, participants listed four keywords capturing its essence and provided a brief written account. Following a (successful) manipulation check, they first rated four items assessing social connectedness ("With this event in mind, I feel connected to loved ones," ". . . protected," ". . . loved," ". . . I can trust others") and then worked on an (unsolvable) insight problem, in which they had to trace each line of a geometric figure only once, without lifting the pencil and without retracing any existing lines. They were instructed to contact the experimenter by pushing a red button on an intercom system if they wanted help solving the insight problem. Participants in the nostalgia condition sought help sooner than those in the control condition. This beneficial effect of nostalgia on help seeking was mediated by perceived social connectedness.

THE COMPLETE REGULATORY MODEL

So far, we have presented evidence for discrete paths in the regulatory model. The first path links aversive states, such as boredom and loneliness, to increased nostalgia. The second path links nostalgia to vital psychological outcomes, including increased meaning in life and help seeking. We now consider two studies by Zhou and colleagues (2008, Studies 1 and 2) that tested the complete regulatory model by examining both paths simultaneously. The researchers examined the relations among loneliness, nostalgia, and perceived social support. The regulatory model posits that loneliness affects social support in two distinct ways. The direct effect of loneliness is negative: Loneliness undermines feeling socially supported. Yet, the indirect effect of loneliness via nostalgia is positive: Loneliness increases nostalgia, which in turn boosts perceptions of social support.

The first study by Zhou's team was a survey among Chinese migrant children and teenagers, in which the researchers assessed individual differences in loneliness (UCLA Loneliness Scale; Russell, 1996; e.g., "How often do you feel completely alone?"), nostalgia (Southampton Nostalgia Scale; Barrett et al., 2010; e.g., "How often do you experience nostalgia?"), and social support (Multidimensional Scale of Perceived Social Support; Zimet et al., 1988; e.g., "I can count on my friends when things go wrong"). Participants who were high (compared to low) in loneliness perceived less social support, but they were also more nostalgic. In turn, nostalgia strengthened perceptions of social support, thereby offsetting the negative impact of loneliness. In their second study, the team experimentally manipulated loneliness in a sample of Chinese university students by giving them false feedback regarding questionnaire scores (as described previously in this chapter). Following the loneliness induction, participants' momentary nostalgia and social support were assessed with state versions of the Southampton Nostalgia Scale and Multidimensional Scale of Perceived Social Support, respectively. Participants in the high-loneliness (compared to low-loneliness) condition perceived less social support, but they also felt more nostalgic. Nostalgia, in turn, strengthened their perceptions of social support.

In summary, a rich body of empirical evidence supports the regulatory model of nostalgia across diverse domains. Nostalgia offsets adversity and maintains homeostasis.

THE REGULATORY ROLE OF NOSTALGIA DURING THE COVID-19 PANDEMIC

Having outlined the regulatory model of nostalgia, we now turn to the second part of our chapter, which sees nostalgia "in action" during the COVID-19 pandemic. The pertinent evidence stems from six studies completed at various stages of the pandemic by Zhou and colleagues (2022, Studies 1–6). Studies 1–3 were surveys conducted in China (March 8–14, 2020), the United States (April 3–12, 2020), and the United Kingdom (April 20–21, 2020), examining the cross-sectional relations among loneliness, nostalgia, and happiness. In Study 1 ($N = 1,546$), loneliness was operationalized as social isolation ("During the outbreak, have you been living alone for more than a week?"; $0 = no$, $1 = yes$). Social isolation refers to objective lack of social interactions, whereas loneliness refers to the subjective perception that one lacks meaningful social interactions. Although they are conceptually distinct, social isolation is a good proxy of loneliness (Savikko et al., 2005). Happiness was measured with two items: "For the past week, how happy has your life been?" and "For the past week, how meaningful has your life been?" ($1 = not at all$, $7 = very much$). The researchers assessed nostalgia with a validated (Hepper et al., 2012) three-item measure (e.g., "I feel nostalgic;" $1 = not at all$, $7 = very much$). Results revealed that lonely participants were less happy than nonlonely ones, but they also felt more nostalgic. Nostalgia, in turn, was positively associated with happiness. When happiness was regressed onto both loneliness and nostalgia simultaneously, loneliness negatively predicted happiness, whereas nostalgia positively predicted it. The direct effect of loneliness was negative: Loneliness was prognostic of less happiness. Yet, the indirect effect of loneliness via nostalgia was positive: Loneliness predicted higher nostalgia, which in turn was associated with more happiness.[5]

To test the robustness and generality of Study 1 findings, Zhou's team next surveyed U.S. (Study 2; $N = 1,572$) and U.K. (Study 3; $N = 571$) samples. Both surveys used identical measures. Loneliness was assessed with two items: "How isolated from the rest of the world did you feel in the past week?" ($1 = not at all$, $7 = very much$) and "How lonely did you feel in the past week?" ($1 = not at all lonely$, $7 = very lonely$). Happiness was assessed with three items: "I consider myself as ($1 = not a very happy person$; $7 = a very happy person$)"; "Compared with my peers, I consider myself ($1 = much less happy$, $7 = much more happy$)"; and "I think my life is ($1 = not meaningful at all$, $7 = very meaningful$)." Nostalgia was measured as in Study 1. Indices of loneliness, happiness, and nostalgia were created by averaging the corresponding items. Study 1 findings were replicated in both new samples. Loneliness was negatively associated with happiness, but positively associated with nostalgia. Nostalgia, in turn, was positively associated with happiness. When happiness was regressed onto both loneliness and nostalgia, loneliness was a negative predictor, whereas nostalgia was a positive one. Again, the direct effect of loneliness on happiness was negative, but its indirect effect via nostalgia was positive.

The results of these three cross-sectional studies converged in supporting the regulatory model of nostalgia across cultures. Loneliness during the pandemic was associated negatively with happiness but positively with nostalgia. Nostalgia, through its positive link with happiness, counteracted loneliness. An integrative data analysis (IDA; Curran & Hussong, 2009), which pooled the three studies and tested associations in the aggregated sample, reinforced these conclusions. Cross-sectional studies, however, cannot definitively determine direction of causation. Whereas evidence indicates that loneliness causes unhappiness (Cacioppo et al., 2006) and loneliness causes nostalgia (Wildschut et al., 2006), support for a causal path from nostalgia to increased happiness is limited. Zhou and colleagues filled this gap in their next three (experimental) studies (Studies 4–6). Additionally, they asked, for the first time, whether experimentally induced nostalgia has lasting effects—up to 2 days—on happiness.

Study 4 ($N = 209$) was conducted from April 19 to April 24, 2020, Study 5 ($N = 196$) from April 29 to April 30, 2020, and Study 6 ($N = 190$) from December 21 to December 22, 2020. Participants in all three studies were Western MTurkers. Each study involved two time points (T1 and T2). At T1, nostalgia was induced with the event reflection task. This was followed by a manipulation check and collection of the well-being measures. In Study 4, happiness was assessed with two items (e.g., "Right now, I consider myself . . ." 1 = *not a very happy person*; 7 = *a very happy person*). In Studies 5 and 6, happiness was measured with three items (e.g., "Right now, how much do you experience happiness?"). In all three studies, positive affect and negative affect were assessed with the Positive and Negative Affect Schedule (Watson et al., 1988). At T2, one or two days after the original assessment, participants completed the same measures as at T1. In Studies 4 and 5, this was preceded by a brief induction booster. Participants in the nostalgia (control) condition read: "In our previous questionnaire, you were asked to recall a nostalgic (ordinary) event and write down a few keywords. Do you still remember the event? Please write it down in the blank space below." In Study 6, this induction booster was omitted to examine whether its absence would weaken the intervention's impact at T2.

In addition to testing the effects of the nostalgia intervention on measures of well-being at each time point within each study, the researchers also pooled the data across studies in an IDA. For the sake of parsimony and to avoid repetition, we focus on the IDA results. The IDA took the form of a 2 (nostalgia vs. control) × 2 (T1 vs. T2) × 3 (Study 4 vs. Study 5 vs. Study 6) multilevel analysis, with time points nested within participants and study membership treated as a fixed characteristic of each participant in the pooled sample. Results revealed that the nostalgia induction (compared to control) significantly increased happiness and positive affect (but had no effect on negative affect). The absence of higher order interactions indicated that these beneficial effects did not decline significantly from T1 to T2 and did not vary between studies. Further, the absence of significant Nostalgia × Time × Study three-way interactions indicates that the absence of an induction booster in

Study 6 did not result in a diminution of the nostalgia effects at T2 (compared to Studies 4 and 5). It is tempting, then, to conclude that the beneficial effects of a brief nostalgia induction can endure for up to 2 days. Still, separate analyses of Study 6 showed that the nostalgia effects on T2 happiness and positive affect were in the predicted direction but nonsignificant, potentially due to participant attrition. A cautious interpretation suggests that a booster was sufficient to reinstate nostalgia's beneficial effects at T2, but more research is needed to ascertain if it is necessary.

Jointly, these six studies, conducted during the pandemic, demonstrate that nostalgia is a valuable psychological resource that is harnessed during periods of social isolation and contributes to preventing downward spirals of declining mental health. Nostalgia inductions are easy to implement and can be self-initiated, raising the prospect of cost- and time-effective interventions.

LESSON LEARNED

Nostalgia has a checkered past. The term was coined in 1688 by Johannes Hofer, a medical student, who combined the Greek words *nostos* ("home-coming") and *algos* ("suffering") to denote a collection of negative physical symptoms displayed by itinerants, in particular Swiss mercenaries. Nostalgia was thought to be the suffering caused by an incessant desire to return home, with symptoms including weeping, fainting, stomachache, fever, palpitations, and suicidal ideation. Hofer's classification of nostalgia as a medical or neurological disease remained influential through the 18th and 19th century. Views changed in the 20th century, albeit not for the better. Nostalgia was regarded a psychiatric disorder marked by anxiety, sadness, pessimism, loss of appetite, and insomnia.

Over the past 15 years, a growing body of empirical research has reversed the tide and formed the basis for a new look on nostalgia. The picture of nostalgia that has emerged is not of a medical disease, psychiatric disorder, or psychological illness, but rather of a nourishing and invigorating psychological resource. Nostalgia does not cause adverse symptoms but instead is recruited to counter those symptoms and maintain psychological equanimity. Hofer (and many contemporary or succeeding writers) made an inferential error by confusing the direction of causation between symptoms and nostalgia. We sympathize because nostalgia is enigmatic: What other emotion is positively associated with both boredom and meaning in life or with both loneliness and happiness? An important lesson, then, is that one should resist the temptation to infer that because nostalgia "occurs in the context of present fears discontents, anxieties, or uncertainties" (Davis, 1979, pp. 34–35), it must be maladaptive. The COVID-19 pandemic has vividly illustrated that adversity and nostalgia are often contiguous in time but—just as a viral infection is followed by an immune response—this association should be attributed to the emotion's functional, rather than dysfunctional, role.

CONCLUSION

Nostalgia plays an important role in shaping people's experiences of the COVID-19 pandemic. We have highlighted the utility of a regulatory model for understanding the nostalgic response to adversity. An urgent question for future research pertains to the potential therapeutic role of nostalgia. Recent studies have documented the benefits of nostalgia for vulnerable populations, including people living with dementia (Ismail et al., 2018), refugees (Wildschut et al., 2019), and bereaved people (Reid et al., 2021). We propose that there is now sufficient evidence for the efficacy of nostalgia inductions to warrant the development of therapeutic interventions and have recently completed the first steps in this direction (Layous et al., 2021).

NOTES

1. https://www.digitalmusicnews.com/wp-content/uploads/2020/04/COVID-19-Entertainment-Tracker-Release-1-1586793733.pdf
2. https://shares.pulsarplatform.com/trends/newnormal-i-miss-P8vD-3gQNQ3V
3. https://www.forbes.com/sites/mattklein/2020/04/29/our-coronavirus-security-blanket-nostalgia-for-old-music-movies-and-much-more/?sh=70acd1a1256f
4. https://www.theguardian.com/commentisfree/2020/may/03/nostalgia-for-the-beautiful-world-outside-has-made-a-collector-of-me
5. By using the terms *direct effect* and *indirect effect* in the context of correlational analyses, we are adopting the terminology of intervening-variable analyses and do not mean to imply causation.

REFERENCES

Barrett, F. S., Grimm, K. J., Robins, R. W., Wildschut, T., Sedikides, C., & Janata, P. (2010). Music-evoked nostalgia: Affect, memory, and personality. *Emotion, 10*(3), 390–403. https://doi.org/10.1037/a0019006

Batcho, K. I. (1995). Nostalgia: A psychological perspective. *Perceptual & Motor Skills, 80*(1), 131–143. https://doi.org/10.2466/pms.1995.80.1.131

Boylan, J., Seli, P., Scholer, A. A., & Danckert, J. (2020). Boredom in the COVID-19 pandemic: Trait boredom proneness, the desire to act, and rule-breaking. *Personality and Individual Differences, 171*, Article 110387. https://doi.org/10.1016/j.paid.2020.110387

Cacioppo, J. T., Hawkley, L. C., Ernst, J. M., Burleson, M., Berntson, G. G., Nouriani, B., & Spiegel, D. (2006). Loneliness within a nomological net: An evolutionary perspective. *Journal of Research in Personality, 40*(6), 1054–1085. https://doi.org/10.1016/j.jrp.2005.11.007

Chasson, M., Ben-Yaakov, O., & Taubman-Ben-Ari, O. (2021). Meaning in life among new mothers before and during the COVID-19 pandemic: The role of mothers' marital satisfaction and perception of the infant. *Journal of Happiness Studies*, *22*(8), 3499–3512. https://doi.org/10.1007/s10902-021-00378-1

Curran, P. J., & Hussong, A. M. (2009). Integrative data analysis: The simultaneous analysis of multiple data sets. *Psychological Methods*, *14*(2), 81–100. https://doi.org/10.1037/a0015914

Davis, F. (1979). *Yearning for yesterday: A sociology of nostalgia*. The Free Press.

Hepper, E. G., Ritchie, T. D., Sedikides, C., & Wildschut, T. (2012). Odyssey's end: Lay conceptions of nostalgia reflect its original Homeric meaning. *Emotion*, *12*(1), 102–119. https://doi.org/10.1037/a0025167

Hepper, E. G., Wildschut, T., Sedikides, C., Ritchie, T. D., Yung, Y.-F., Hansen, N., Abakoumkin, G., Arikan, G., Cisek, S. Z., Demassosso, D. B., Gebauer, J. E., Gerber, J. P., González, R., Kusumi, T., Misra, G., Rusu, M., Ryan, O., Stephan, E., Vingerhoets, A. J. J. M., & Zhou, X. (2014). Pancultural nostalgia: Prototypical conceptions across cultures. *Emotion*, *14*(4), 733–747. https://doi.org/10.1037/a0036790

Ismail, S., Christopher, G., Dodd, E., Wildschut, T., Sedikides, C., Ingram, T. A., Jones, R. W., Nooman, K. A., Tingley, D., & Cheston, R. (2018). Psychological and mnemonic benefits of nostalgia for people with dementia. *Journal of Alzheimer's Disease*, *65*(4), 1327–1344. https://doi.org/10.3233/JAD-180075

Juhl, J., Wildschut, T., Sedikides, C., Xiong, X., & Zhou, X. (2021). Nostalgia promotes help seeking by fostering social connectedness. *Emotion*, *21*(3), 631–643. https://doi.org/10.1037/emo0000720

Killgore, W. D. S., Cloonan, S. A., Taylor, E. C., Lucas, D. A., & Dailey, N. S. (2020). Loneliness during the first half-year of COVID-19 Lockdowns. *Psychiatry Research*, *294*, Article 113551. https://doi.org/10.1016/j.psychres.2020.113551

Layous, K., Kurtz, J. L., Wildschut, T., & Sedikides, C. (2021). The effect of a multi-week nostalgia intervention on well-being: Mechanisms and moderation. *Emotion*, *22*(8), 1952–1968. https://doi.org/10.1037/emo0000817

Luchetti, M., Lee, J. H., Aschwanden, D., Sesker, A., Strickhouser, J. E., Terracciano, A., & Sutin, A. R. (2020). The trajectory of loneliness in response to COVID-19. *American Psychologist*, *75*(7), 897–908. https://doi.org/10.1037/amp0000690

Lueck, J. A. (2021). Help-seeking intentions in the U.S. population during the COVID-19 pandemic: Examining the role of COVID-19 financial hardship, suicide risk, and stigma. *Psychiatry Research*, *303*, Article 114069. https://doi.org/10.1016/j.psychres.2021.114069

Reid, C. A., Green, J. D., Short, S. D., Willis, K. D., Moloney, J. M., Collison, E. A., Wildschut, T., Sedikides, C., & Gramling, S. (2021). The past as a resource for the bereaved: Nostalgia predicts declines in distress. *Cognition and Emotion*, *35*(2) 256–268. https://doi.org/10.1080/02699931.2020.1825339

Reid, C. A., Green, J. D., Wildschut, T., & Sedikides, C. (2015). Scent-evoked nostalgia. *Memory*, *23*(2), 157–166. https://doi.org/10.1080/09658211.2013.876048

Routledge, C., Arndt, J., Wildschut, T., Sedikides, C., Hart, C., Juhl, J., Vingerhoets, A. J., & Scholtz, W. (2011). The past makes the present meaningful: Nostalgia as an existential resource. *Journal of Personality and Social Psychology*, *101*(3), 638–652. https://doi.org/10.1037/a0024292

Russell, D. W. (1996). UCLA Loneliness Scale (Version 3): Reliability, validity, and factor structure. *Journal of Personality Assessment*, *66*(1), 20–40. https://doi.org/10.1207/s15327752jpa6601_2

Savikko, N., Routasalo, P., Tilvis, R. S., Strandbert, T. E., & Pitkala, K. H. (2005). Predictors and subjective causes of loneliness in an aged population. *Archives of Gerontology and Geriatrics, 41*(3), 223–233. https://doi.org/10.1016/j.archger.2005.03.002

Sedikides, C., & Wildschut, T. (2018). Finding meaning in nostalgia. *Review of General Psychology, 22*(1), 48–61. https://doi.org/10.1037/gpr0000109

Sedikides, C., & Wildschut, T. (2019). The sociality of personal and collective nostalgia. *European Review of Social Psychology, 30*(1), 23–173. https://doi.org/10.1080/10463 283.2019.1630098

Sedikides, C., & Wildschut, T. (2020). The motivational potency of nostalgia: The future is called yesterday. *Advances in Motivation Science, 7*, 75–111. https://doi.org/ 10.1016/bs.adms.2019.05.001

Steger, M. F., Frazier, P., Oishi, S., & Kaler, M. (2006). The meaning in life questionnaire: Assessing the presence of and search for meaning in life. *Journal of Counseling Psychology, 53*(1), 80–93. https://doi.org/10.1037/0022-0167.53.1.80

Van Tilburg, W. A. P., Igou, E. R., & Sedikides, C. (2013). In search of meaningfulness: Nostalgia as an antidote to boredom. *Emotion, 13*(3), 450–461. https://doi.org/ 10.1037/a0030442

Vess, M., Arndt, J., Routledge, C., Sedikides, C., & Wildschut, T. (2012). Nostalgia as a resource for the self. *Self and Identity, 11*(3), 273–284. https://doi.org/10.1080/15298 868.2010.521452

Watson, D., Clark, L. A., & Tellegen, A. (1988). Development and validation of brief measures of positive and negative affect: The PANAS scales. *Journal of Personality and Social Psychology, 54*(6), 1063–1070. https://doi.org/10.1037/0022-3514.54.6.1063

Wildschut, T., & Sedikides, C. (2021). Psychology and nostalgia: Toward a functional approach. In M. H. Jacobsen (Ed.), *Intimations of nostalgia* (pp. 110–128). Bristol University Press.

Wildschut, T., Sedikides, C., & Alowidy, D. (2019). *Hanin*: Nostalgia among Syrian refugees. *European Journal of Social Psychology, 49*(7), 1368–1384. https://doi.org/ 10.1002/ejsp.2590

Wildschut, T., Sedikides, C., Arndt, J., & Routledge, C. (2006). Nostalgia: Content, triggers, functions. *Journal of Personality and Social Psychology, 91*(5), 975–993. https://doi.org/10.1037/0022-3514.91.5.975

Wildschut, T., Sedikides, C., & Robertson, S. (2018). Sociality and intergenerational transfer of older adults' nostalgia. *Memory, 26*(8), 1030–1041. https://doi.org/ 10.1080/09658211.2018.1470645

Zhou, X., Sedikides, C., Mo, T., Li, W., Hong, E. K., & Wildschut, T. (2022). The restorative power of nostalgia: Thwarting loneliness by raising happiness during the COVID-19 pandemic. *Social Psychological and Personality Science, 13*(4), 803–815. https://doi.org/10.1177/19485506211041830.

Zhou, X., Sedikides, C., Wildschut, T., & Gao, D. G. (2008). Counteracting loneliness: On the restorative function of nostalgia. *Psychological Science, 19*(10), 1023–1029. https://doi.org/10.1111/j.1467-9280.2008.02194.x

Zimet, G. D., Dahlem, N. W., Zimet, S. G., & Farley, G. K. (1988). The Multidimensional Scale of Perceived Social Support. *Journal of Personality Assessment, 52*(1), 30–41. https://doi.org/10.1207/s15327752jpa5201_2

FURTHER READING

Sedikides, C., Wildschut, T., Arndt, J., & Routledge, C. (2008). Nostalgia: Past, present, and future. *Current Directions in Psychological Science, 17*(5), 304–307. https://doi. org/10.1111/j.1467-8721.2008.00595.x

Sedikides, C., Wildschut, T., Routledge, C., Arndt, J., Hepper, E. G., & Zhou, X. (2015). To nostalgize: Mixing memory with affect and desire. *Advances in Experimental Social Psychology, 51*, 189–273. https://doi.org/10.1016/bs.aesp.2014.10.001

29

The Burden of Pandemic Life for Families With Young Children

JENNIFER A. MORTENSEN, LYDIA DEFLORIO, AND MELISSA M. BURNHAM ∎

As the famous adage goes: "It takes a village." Unfortunately, COVID-19 fractured villages and isolated families from traditional means of support such as child care, school, family, and friends. In this chapter, we examine the burden of pandemic life for families with young children using the tenets of family systems theory (FST) as a lens for understanding current and future research. We focus on families with young children (ages 0–8) because of their time-intensive caregiving needs. We also emphasize the experiences of mothers, who have been disproportionately overwhelmed with child care responsibilities (Heggeness & Fields, 2020) and employment issues (Bick & Blandin, 2020). This has caused unprecedented instability within families, particularly for economically disadvantaged families and families of color—both groups disproportionately affected by COVID-19 (Gould & Wilson, 2020; Gould et al., 2020; Yavorsky et al., 2021; see Chapters 23–25 for more on the impact of the pandemic on minorities, and Chapter 44 for more on families and the pandemic). Below we examine how pandemic instability in family systems affected the pandemic experience, as well as include suggestions for future research.

THE CONTEXT OF PANDEMIC LIFE FOR FAMILIES WITH YOUNG CHILDREN

U.S. school/child care closures varied, but most parents found themselves without reliable access to school/child care at some point in 2020 (Alon et al., 2020). Closures were not only necessary for public health safety, but also catastrophic for working parents. In the United States, most two-parent families are dual earners

Jennifer A. Mortensen, Lydia DeFlorio, and Melissa M. Burnham, *The Burden of Pandemic Life for Families With Young Children* In: *The Social Science of the COVID-19 Pandemic*. Edited by: Monica K. Miller, Oxford University Press.
© Oxford University Press 2024. DOI: 10.1093/oso/9780197615133.003.0029

(U.S. Census, 2020), so one parent needed to be home full time for child care and supervising distance learning; this burden fell overwhelmingly to mothers. In comparison to men, women are simultaneously more likely to be employed in positions that can be done from home and in jobs that require close physical proximity with others (Mongey et al., 2020). Therefore, mothers in dual-earner families were two to three times more likely than fathers to reduce working hours or leave careers to manage new homeschooling responsibilities (Heggeness & Fields, 2020). Employment data show that across 2020, women's rate of employment and number of working hours dropped significantly lower than men's (Bick & Blandin, 2020). Indeed, one study found that mothers decreased their work hours four to five times more than fathers during the period of February to April 2020 alone (Collins et al., 2020). Collins et al. (2020) reported that women worked 20%–50% less than men, depending on the age of the child; mothers with children aged 1–5 were hit the hardest. U.S. Census data collected since the pandemic indicate that school closures coincided with women leaving the workforce, with no similar increase for fathers (Heggeness & Fields, 2020).

Mothers working from home were more likely to have flexible hours and a steady paycheck—but endless distractions often meant working late at the expense of sleep and mental well-being (Hertz et al., 2021; Whiley et al., 2020; see Chapter 21 for more on pandemic-related mental health). Moreover, mothers working essential jobs in the community (overwhelmingly Latina and Black women) juggled child care and low pay, inflexible leave policies, and increased risk of COVID-19 exposure (Gould & Wilson, 2020; Gould et al., 2020). Mothers are also more likely to be single parents (23% of all mothers in comparison to 6% of all fathers; U.S. Census, 2020), so many women were left to juggle child care and work alone. Single mothers reported greater work productivity decline compared to mothers in multiadult households and felt more strained by the loss of child care (Hertz et al., 2021).

Across 2020, women reported record unemployment (Alon et al., 2020). Men's employment is typically the victim of economic crises, but COVID-19's impact on service, leisure, and education industries meant that this time women suffered the worst (Alon et al., 2020). Latina women faced some of the highest unemployment rates, mostly due to overrepresentation in service industries, massive COVID-19 outbreaks in states with large Latinx populations (e.g., Arizona, California), and racist immigration policies that keep Latinx workers disempowered at work (Gould et al., 2020). Similarly, Black women also faced disproportionate unemployment fueled by long-standing racism and economic inequality (Gould & Wilson, 2020). At the time of this writing, June 2021, COVID-19 numbers were decreasing and demand for workers in certain industries was rising; however, low wages and lack of affordable child care make it hard to fill positions (Dingel et al., 2020; Shierholz, 2021), and women of color have experienced slower job recovery in recent months than men or White women (Yavorsky et al., 2021).

As this review illustrates, being a woman—and especially a minority woman—greatly affected one's experiences during the pandemic. Taken together, the loss of child care and parenting support, increase in home responsibilities, and mothers' overall reduced economic power has created a new context for families with young children. As families build back what was lost, it is critical for researchers to consider how the recent instability reverberates across the rest of the family system.

FAMILY SYSTEM THEORY

"The whole is greater than the sum of its parts" captures the main premise of FST. Systems-based thinking applies everywhere, from planetary systems and ecosystems to military systems, including families (Whitchurch & Constantine, 2004). At their core, all systems are "set(s) of elements standing in interrelation among themselves and with the environment" (von Bertalanffy, 1975, p. 159). All systems (1) are made up of interconnected components, (2) must be viewed as a whole, (3) interact with the environment (anything outside the system boundaries), and (4) are not tangible—they are simply a way of understanding how individual components are interrelated and work together (White et al., 2019). Families are systems—all individual family members are interconnected, and it is only possible to understand individual people by examining the whole system (Whitchurch & Constantine, 2004). Like all systems, families are affected by the environment, as well as act on the environment (White et al., 2019). From this perspective, we can view the COVID-19 pandemic—as well as associated disparities and oppressions for some families—as environmental forces shaping family systems (James et al., 2018).

The FST tenet of *mutual influence* speaks to the interdependent nature of family systems (Whitchurch & Constantine, 2004). Because individual family members are "held together" within the system, the actions of one reverberate across the rest of the family. In this sense, parents and children are never operating in isolation: Their behaviors and experiences affect everyone else, as well as contribute to overall system functioning. Family systems also function best with clear (but flexible) *roles and boundaries* (Cox & Paley, 1997). Each family member plays a role, whether it is parent, child, sibling, spouse, or others. Roles are prescribed meanings for who does what within the system, and systems function best when roles are clearly defined (White et al., 2019). Boundaries delineate who is in and out of the system (Whitchurch & Constantine, 2004). All family systems have "open" boundaries in that they interact with the environment, but some families are more closed off than others. Within the family, boundaries also help define subsystems (Cox & Paley, 1997). For example, parents make up a parent subsystem, while children make up a child subsystem, and there are clear boundaries demarcating the difference between these subsystems (e.g., parental authority). In two-parent households, there are also boundaries between the parental subsystem and the marital subsystem (e.g., not talking about children during a romantic evening). Family systems operate best when boundaries are clear but flexible; clear boundaries help the system function, but boundaries should not be so rigid that the system is incapable of change when necessary (Cox & Paley, 1997). Finally, like all systems, families strive for *homeostasis* (Whitchurch & Constantine, 2004). Systems are self-regulating and calibrate to maintain stability. Clear roles and boundaries help maintain homeostasis (Cox & Paley, 1997), but all families experience events that upset the status quo. When this happens, families can engage in patterns of interaction and communication that encourage either adaptation (positive feedback loops) or resistance to change (negative-feedback loops) (White et al., 2019). Both types of feedback loops help families maintain—or adapt to a different—homeostasis. It is important to note that the terms positive and negative do not denote value, simply whether or not the system is moving toward change.

Family systems theory is typically used to understand how family members establish roles, set and maintain boundaries—and also to understand processes such as communication, conflict, cohesion, and adaptation to change (Whitchurch & Constantine, 2004). FST is also useful for understanding major family transitions such as becoming parents (Holmes et al., 2013; Kluwer, 2010); marriage (Johnson, 2001; Olson, 2000); divorce (Van Gasse & Mortelmans, 2020); responses to mental and behavioral health issues (Feinberg et al., 2012); co-parenting (McHale & Lindahl, 2011; Robin & Foster, 2002); or the death of a family member (Kazak & Noll, 2004; Mehta et al., 2009). Transitions create vulnerability in the system because new roles and boundaries are established or adjusted. The system might resist the transition through negative-feedback loops or move toward systems-level change through positive-feedback loops. Recent iterations of FST also explore the role of race, ethnicity, and racism in systems, particularly in terms of how they affect the marital and parent-child subsystems, as well as shape the historical context the system is operating within (James et al., 2018). Given this, FST is a useful framework for understanding the burden of pandemic life for families with young children and offers important insights for pandemic family science research.

APPLICATION OF FAMILY SYSTEMS THEORY TO PANDEMIC LIFE

In the following sections, we explore how pandemic life threatens the stability of family systems while recognizing the importance of context (James et al., 2018). First, in comparison to similar nations, the United States has notoriously unfriendly work-family policies, as well as minimal social support services (Trask, 2017), instead relying on women's unpaid labor. The pandemic has exposed that "a system built on women's backs, and on the backs of mothers in particular, cannot be maintained when multiple competing demands are exposed" (Friedman & Satterthwaite, 2021, p. 60). Second, families of color are simultaneously operating in contexts of oppression characterized by disparate COVID-19 outcomes and high-profile instances of race-related violence. All of this sets the backdrop for family system functioning.

Maternal Mental Health

The sudden onset of quarantine and the reconfiguration of parenting, work, and school under one roof dissolved established boundaries and forced parents—primarily mothers—to assume a number of new roles, often at the same time—caretaker, employee, preschool teacher, spouse, and more (Hertz et al., 2021). The pandemic also forced isolation from family, friends, babysitters, and other parenting support (Hertz et al., 2021). Approximately 30% of the parent workforce has children under age 6 (Dingel et al., 2020), which means that loss of formal and informal child care was a major disruption to families. Given FST, boundary dissolution between work, school/child care, and home is not conducive to family functioning; homeostasis is thrown off and new roles need to be negotiated (Cox & Paley, 1997). It is no surprise, then, that mothers' mental health has suffered as a result. For example, in heterosexual two-parent households, mothers working from home because of COVID-19 have reported increased anxiety, depression, and loneliness at significantly higher levels than working-at-home fathers (Lyttelton et al., 2020). These mothers were also more likely to take on a larger share of the house and care work than fathers, despite both working from home (Lyttelton et al., 2020). In a nationally representative sample, Ruppanner and colleagues (2021) found that pandemic-related increases in housework and care work for mothers contributed to increased anxiety and poorer sleep. Interestingly, these changes did not affect fathers' mental health. The construction of roles—and the boundaries associated with those roles—is important here. In the United States, motherhood tends to be heavily romanticized with impossible standards of perfection (Whiley et al., 2020). One person managing the competing demands of multiple roles is going to experience stress and burnout.

The family system's degree of flexibility in adopting new roles and modifying boundaries should also be critical to maternal mental health. Some evidence suggests that all working mothers—no matter their economic circumstances—report that COVID-related parenting stress (specifically parental role strain) is linked to lower perceived quality of life (Limbers et al., 2020). Perceived ability to adapt to these challenges is important, but the reality is that many mothers are having to adjust roles and boundaries while also navigating structural and/or individual racism, both of which have been exacerbated by the pandemic (see Chapters 24 and 25). In the United States, COVID-19 has disproportionately impacted communities of color. Both hospitalization and mortality rates have been highest among those who identify as African American, Native American, and Latinx (Centers for Disease Control and Prevention, 2021). These disparities stem from a number of factors, including overrepresentation in "essential" occupations, dense and often racially segregated living arrangements, less access to health care, and higher rates of comorbid health conditions (Lopez et al., 2021). For many, this means higher levels of anxiety, trauma, and other pandemic-related distress as they worry about their own health and safety and that of those they love (Hibel et al., 2021; Novacek et al., 2020). Racism during the pandemic has likely impacted mothers' mental health (and family systems, by extension) in other ways as well. For example, it is too soon to know empirically how the highly publicized killings of Breonna Taylor and George Floyd by police early in the pandemic impacted African American mothers or how the rise in violence toward Asian Americans that has occurred throughout the pandemic has impacted Asian American mothers, but associations between experiencing racial trauma and mental health are well established (Shim & Starks, 2021). How exactly these issues are compounded by COVID-19 and play out within family systems is an important area of future study (James et al., 2018; Shim & Starks, 2021).

Spillover in the Family System

Given the FST tenet of mutual influence, maternal stress does not reside purely in her psychology alone. Stress, anxiety, depression, and more will spill over to other areas of the family system. For mothers with a cohabiting partner, pandemic-related stressors (and mental health sequelae) can cause maladaptive dyadic processes in the marital/romantic relationship subsystem, such as negativity, hostility, and withdrawal (Pietromonaco & Overall, 2021; see Chapter 26). Pandemic research from the United States and around the globe has found decreased relationship and sexual satisfaction (Luetke et al., 2020; Mousavi, 2020; Turliuc & Candel, 2021; see also Chapter 26 for more on the relationships during the pandemic), including increased rates of intimate partner violence toward women (Piquero et al., 2021). For families of color, James and colleagues (2018) also stressed the importance of accounting for one's history of discrimination as it exacerbates strain in the marital subsystem. It will be important to consider the intersecting effects of the pandemic and oppressions when studying the marital/romantic relationship subsystem.

For families with young children, the co-parental and parent-child subsystems are also vulnerable to spillover. Co-parenting is the joint childrearing aspect of an adult relationship (McHale & LIndahl, 2011). In heterosexual families, the pandemic forced many fathers to play a larger role in child care (Ruppanner et al., 2021), but there is some evidence that the pandemic has resulted in a shift away from egalitarian toward more conventional gender roles with fathers as financial providers and mothers as caretakers—even when both parents work (Mize et al., 2021). It is worthwhile to consider how the pandemic might reshape parental roles for all parents. The United States tends to emphasize intensive parenting (e.g., great emotional investment and supervision) and romanticizes the "supermom" (Whiley et al., 2020). Research suggests that some working mothers found an increased caregiver role at odds with their identity, having previously constructed a motherhood role with clear family-work boundaries (Hertz et al., 2021). Interestingly, endorsement of intensive parenting declined significantly over the first month of school closures and stay-at-home orders (Forbes et al., 2022). Given the large number of mothers exiting the workforce, how will motherhood identity be reconciled as families move toward a postpandemic homeostasis (Whiley et al.,

2020)? COVID-19 is presenting heterosexual families with a unique opportunity to weaken the gender norms that typically divide unpaid labor (Alon et al., 2020), with fathers increasing their homemaker role, as many have during the pandemic (Ruppanner et al., 2021). Moreover, how same-sex parents are negotiating roles is largely unknown, offering another important avenue of research.

Effects on Young Children

Early in the pandemic, working mothers reported increased stress due to financial worries, uncertainty about the future, social isolation, relationship dissatisfaction, health, child care and education, and working from home while caring for children (Brown et al., 2020). Parenting stress experienced during the pandemic has been uniquely linked with quality of life, including the parents' health, safety, and social relationships (Limbers et al., 2020), which has the potential for spill over in the parent-child subsystem. Indeed, at least one study indicates an association between cumulative stressors faced by parents and children's psychological well-being (Gassman-Pines et al., 2020). However, as of this writing, much of the published research on the impact of the pandemic on children's outcomes has focused on documenting children's psychological states and experiences. For example, some studies suggested that children experienced higher rates of depression, anxiety, and externalizing behaviors, particularly in the early months of the pandemic (Patrick et al., 2020; Sama et al., 2021). Other studies have focused on how children's daily activities (physical activity, time spent on schooling, reading with adults) changed as a result of stay-at-home orders (Barnett et al., 2020; Dunton et al., 2020). Undoubtedly, many other child outcomes were impacted by the pandemic, as their entire worlds changed literally overnight: Schools closed, extracurricular activities stopped, socializing opportunities were reduced, and the grown-ups were anxious or distressed (see Chapter 2 for more on how the pandemic changed life and Chapter 3 for a summary of pandemic-related policies). For some children, the pandemic meant increased time with at least one parent or family member. For others, such as children of essential workers, the pandemic meant more time apart. While research is needed to identify the many ways in which children have been impacted by the pandemic, future research will also need to examine these issues from an FST lens, focusing on the changes within the parent-child subsystem and how these changes interact with societal structures (James et al., 2018).

LESSONS LEARNED AND MOVING RESEARCH FORWARD

For families with young children, FST offers a perspective of the COVID-19 pandemic in which family systems have been forced to adapt to an uncharted context, with mothers taking much of the burden. As evidenced in this chapter, research since the pandemic indicates that resources, mental health, parenting support, and intersecting oppressions all play a role in individual and system well-being. Centering maternal mental health as a salient variable within the family system will help conceptualize other system elements that interact with maternal depression, anxiety, and loneliness. For example, COVID-19 has provided families with a massive opportunity to overhaul work and family roles and boundaries within the system. Researchers can also focus on postpandemic relationship quality in the marital/romantic subsystem, including how pandemic-related stress has strained system functioning and potential effects on children. Additionally, to move FST research forward, it is critical for researchers to consider that family systems' interactions with the environment are situated in historical time and societal structures (James et al., 2018). Families of color have faced disproportionate effects of COVID-19 as well as heightened racial violence. When examining within-system processes, researchers must consider how racist structures influence the "structure and patterns" within systems (James et al., 2018, p. 424).

Similarly, the pandemic has caused major employment and earning setbacks for women—particularly women of color. In the United States, *any* discussion of unemployed mothers returning to the workforce must start with expanding access to affordable, quality child care (Dingel et al., 2020). COVID-19 has laid bare just how essential child care is to system homeostasis. It has also highlighted the importance of reconceptualizing "day care" as quality, affordable 0–5 education that pays living wages to well-trained teachers. Researchers have an unprecedented opportunity to advocate for subsidized child care as infrastructure that is vital to the economy—especially when all pandemic research thus far suggests that overloading mothers' unpaid care work is untenable for system functioning (Whiley et al., 2020). In fact, it would benefit all postpandemic recovery efforts to take a family systems approach. For example, there will likely be many initiatives to help children make up losses sustained during the pandemic; however, these efforts will be limited if parents' well-being and oppressions are not accounted for as well.

Other research topics suggested by an examination of the pandemic's impact on family systems include

1. Impacts on family roles for same-sex and more egalitarian parents
2. Women's reduced presence in the workforce as it relates to the motherhood role
3. Compounding effects of the stress associated with heightened racism and disparities on pandemic recovery
4. Shifts in less intensive parenting styles and associations with parenting stress
5. How children's reactions to the pandemic influenced family systems
6. How the pandemic and concurrent racial strife in the United States have compounded the stress felt by some families, and the results of this stress on family functioning
7. Family systems approaches to postpandemic recovery efforts

It is clear that using FST as a frame for viewing families in the context of the COVID-19 pandemic is beneficial and has the potential to move research on families forward. This brief review has elucidated the impact of the pandemic on mothers in particular. Within the United States, the deficiency of policies that effectively support parenting have been laid bare by the pandemic. Researchers can study these deficiencies and examine impacts on family systems, but until policies change, the family system remains vulnerable to massive disruptions such as those caused by COVID-19.

CONCLUSION

Moving forward, U.S. families will continue to face unprecedented challenges in this new pandemic recovery context. COVID-19 has made visible many inequities in family life, particularly the lack of structural support for mothers with young children. The tenets of FST explain how maternal mental health, parenting, relationships, and child development are linked within the family system and interact with pandemic life. Despite the setbacks mothers have faced recently, COVID-19 has also presented the United States with an opportunity to reevaluate the family, work, education, and child care arenas to derive programs and policies that better support mothers with young children.

REFERENCES

Alon, T., Doepke, M., Olmstead-Rumsey, J., & Tertilt, M. (2020). The impact of COVID-19 on gender equality. *Covid Economics: Vetted and Real-Time Papers, 4*, 62–85. https://www.nber.org/papers/w26947

Bick, A., & Blandin, A. (2020). Real-time labor market estimates during the 2020 coronavirus outbreak [Unpublished manuscript]. University of Arizona. http://dx.doi.org/10.2139/ssrn.3692425

Barnett, S., Jung, K., & Nores, M. (2020). *Young children's home learning and preschool participation experiences during the pandemic: NIEER 2020 preschool learning activities survey: Technical report and selected findings.* National Institute for Early Education Research. https://nieer.org/wp-content/uploads/2020/11/NIEER_Tech_Rpt_July2020_Young_Childrens_Home_Learning_and_Preschool_Participation_Experiences_During_the_Pandemic-AUG2020.pdf

Brown, S. M., Doom, J. R., Lechuga-Pena, S., Watamura, S. E., & Koppels, T. (2020). Stress and parenting during the global COVID-19 pandemic. *Child Abuse and Neglect, 110*(Pt. 2), Article 104699. https://doi.org/10.1016/j.chiabu.2020.104699

Centers for Disease Control and Prevention. (2021, May 26). Risk for COVID-19 infection, hospitalization, and death by race/ethnicity. https://stacks.cdc.gov/view/cdc/105453

Collins, C., Landivar, L. C., Ruppanner, L., & Scarborough, W. J. (2020). COVID-19 and the gender gap in work hours. *Gender, Work, and Organization, 28*(S1), 101–112. https://doi.org/10.1111/gwao.12506

Cox, M. J., & Paley, B. (1997). Families as systems. *Annual Review of Psychology, 48*(1), 243–267. https://doi.org/10.1146/annurev.psych.48.1.243

Dingel, J. I., Patterson, C., & Vavra, J. (2020). Childcare obligations will constrain many workers when reopening the U.S. economy (Working Paper No. 2020-46). Becker Friedman Institute for Economics at the University of Chicago. https://bfi.uchicago.edu/wp-content/uploads/BFI_WP_202046.pdf

Dunton, G. F., Do, B., & Wang, S. (2020). Early effects of the COVID-19 pandemic on physical activity and sedentary behavior in children living in the U.S. *BMC Public Health*, *20*(1), 1–13. https://doi.org/10.1186/s12889-020-09429-3

Feinberg, M. E., Solmeyer, A. R., & McHale, S. M. (2012). The third rail of family systems: Sibling relationships, mental and behavioral health, and preventive intervention in childhood and adolescence. *Clinical Child and Family Psychology Review*, *15*, 43–57. https://doi.org/10.1007/s10567-011-0104-5

Forbes, L. K., Lamar, M. R., Speciale, M., & Donovan, C. (2022). Mothers' and fathers' parenting attitudes during COVID-19. *Current Psychology*, *41*, 470–479. https://doi.org/10.1007/s12144-021-01605-x

Friedman, M., & Satterthwaite, E. (2021). Same storm, different boats: Some thoughts on gender, race, and class in the time of COVID-19. In F. J. Green & A. O'Reilly (Eds.), *Mothers, mothering, and COVID-19: Dispatches from the pandemic* (pp. 53–63). Demeter Press.

Gassman-Pines, A., Ananat, E. O., & Fitz-Henley J. (2020). COVID-19 and parent-child psychological well-being. *Pediatrics*, *146*, e2020007294. https://doi.org/10.1542/peds.2020-007294

Gould, E., Perez, D., & Wilson, V. (2020). Latinx workers—particularly women—face devastating job losses in the COVID-19 recession. Economic Policy Institute. https://www.epi.org/publication/latinx-workers-covid/

Gould, E., & Wilson, V. (2020). Black workers face two of the most lethal preexisting conditions for coronavirus—racism and economic inequality. Economic Policy Institute. https://www.epi.org/publication/black-workers-covid/

Heggeness, M. L., & Fields, J. M. (2020). Working moms bear brunt of home schooling while working during COVID-19. U.S. Census Bureau American counts: Stories behind the numbers. https://www.census.gov/library/stories/2020/08/parents-juggle-work-and-child-care-during-pandemic.html

Hertz, R., Mattes, J., & Shook, A. (2021). When paid work invades the family: Single mothers in the COVID-19 pandemic. *Journal of Family Issues*, *42*(9), 2019–2045. https://doi.org/10.1177/0192513X20961420

Hibel, L. C., Boyer, C. J., Buhler-Wassmann, A. C., & Shaw, B. J. (2021). The psychological and economic toll of the COVID-19 pandemic on Latina mothers in primarily low-income essential worker families. *Traumatology*, *27*(1), 40–47. http://dx.doi.org/10.1037/trm0000293

Holmes, E. K., Sasaki, T., & Hazen, N. L. (2013). Smooth versus rocky transitions to parenthood: Family systems in developmental context. *Family Relations*, *62*(5), 824–837. https://doi.org/10.1111/fare.12041

Kazak, A. E., & Noll, R. B. (2004). Child death from pediatric illness: Conceptualizing intervention from a family/systems and public health perspective. *Professional Psychology: Research and Practice*, *35*(3), 219–226. https://doi.org/10.1037/0735-7028.35.3.219

Kluwer, E. S. (2010). From partnership to parenthood: A review of marital change across the transition to parenthood. *Journal of Family Theory & Review*, *2*(2), 105–125. https://doi.org/10.1111/j.1756-2589.2010.00045.x

James, A. G., Coard, S. I., Fine, M. A., & Rudy, D. (2018). The central roles of race and racism in reframing family systems theory: A consideration of choice and time. *Journal of Family Theory & Review, 10*(2), 419–433. https://doi.org/10.1111/jftr.12262

Johnson, V. K. (2001). Marital interaction, family organization, and differences in parenting behavior: Explaining variations across family interaction contexts. *Family Process, 40*(3), 333–342. https://doi.org/10.1111/j.1545-5300.2001.4030100333.x

Limbers, C. A., McCollum, C., & Greenwood, E. (2020). Physical activity moderates the association between parenting stress and quality of life in working mothers during the COVID-19 pandemic. *Mental Health and Physical Activity, 19*, Article 100358. https://doi.org/10.1016/j.mhpa.2020.100358

Lopez, L., Hart, L. H., & Katz, M. H. (2021). Racial and ethnic disparities related to COVID-19. *JAMA, 325*(8), 719–720. https://jamanetwork.com/journals/jama/article-abstract/2775687

Luetke, M., Hensel, D., Herbenick, D., & Rosenberg, M. (2020). Romantic relationship conflict due to the COVID-19 pandemic and changes in intimate and sexual behaviors in a nationally representative sample of American adults. *Sex & Marital Therapy, 46*(8), 747–762. https://doi.org/10.1080/0092623X.2020.1810185

Lyttelton, T., Zang, E., & Musick, K. (2020). Gender differences in telecommuting and implications for inequality at home and work. SSRN. http://dx.doi.org/10.2139/ssrn.3645561

McHale, J. P., & Lindahl, K. M. (2011). *Coparenting: A conceptual and clinical examination of family systems.* American Psychological Association.

Mehta, A., Cohen, S. R., & Chan, L. S. (2009). Palliative care: A need for a family systems approach. *Palliative & Supportive Care, 7*(2), 235–243. https://doi.org/10.1017/S1478951509000303

Mize, T., Kaufman, G., & Petts, R. J. (2021). Visualizing shifts in gendered parenting attitudes during COVID-19. *Socius, 7*, 1–3. https://doi.org/10.1177%2F23780231211013128

Mongey, S., Pilossoph, L., & Weinberg, A. (2020). Which workers bear the burden of social distancing policies? (NBER Working Paper 27085). National Bureau of Economic Research. https://www.nber.org/papers/w27085

Mousavi, S. F. (2020). Psychological well-being, marital satisfaction, and parental burnout in Iranian parents: The effect of home quarantine during COVID-19 outbreaks. *Frontiers in Psychology, 11*, 1–11. https://doi.org/10.3389/fpsyg.2020.553880

Novacek, D. M., Hampton-Anderson, J. N., Ebor, M. T., Loeb, T. B., & Wyatt, G. E. (2020). Mental health ramifications of the COVID-19 pandemic for Black Americans: Clinical and research recommendations. *Psychological Trauma: Theory, Research, Practice, and Policy, 12*(5), 449–451. https://psycnet.apa.org/doi/10.1037/tra0000796

Olson, D. H. (2000). Circumplex model of marital and family systems. *Journal of Family Therapy, 22*(2), 144–167. https://doi.org/10.1111/1467-6427.00144

Patrick, S. W., Henkhaus, L. E., Zickafoose, J. S., Lovell, K., Halvorson, A., Loch, S., Letterie, M., & Davis, M. M. (2020). Well-being of parents and children during the COVID-19 pandemic: A national survey. *Pediatrics, 146*, e2020016824. https://doi.org/10.1542/peds.2020-016824

Pietromonaco, P. R., & Overall, N. C. (2021). Applying relationship science to evaluate how the COVID-19 pandemic may impact couples' relationships. *American Psychologist*, 76(3), 438–450. https://doi.org/10.1037/amp0000714

Piquero, A. R., Jennings, W. G., Jemison, E., Kaukinen, C., & Knaul, F. M. (2021). Domestic violence during the COVID-19 pandemic: Evidence from a systematic review and meta-analysis. *Journal of Criminal Justice*, 74, 101806. https://doi.org/10.1016/j.jcrimjus.2021.101806

Robin, A. L., & Foster, S. L. (2002). *Negotiating parent-adolescent conflict: A behavioral-family systems approach*. Guilford Press.

Ruppanner, L., Tan, X., Scarborough, W., Landivar, L. C., & Collins, C. (2021). Shifting inequalities? Parents' sleep, anxiety, and calm during the COVID-19 pandemic in Australia and the United States. *Men and Masculinities*, 24(1), 181–188. https://doi.org/10.1177%2F1097184X21990737

Sama, B. K., Kaur, P., Thind, P. S., Verma, M. K., Kaur, M., & Singh, D. D. (2021). Implications of COVID-19 induced nationwide lockdown on children's behavior in Punjab, India. *Child: Care, Health, and Development*, 47(1), 128–135. https://doi.org/10.1111/cch.12816

Shierholz, H. (2021). U.S. labor shortage? Unlikely. Here's why. Economic Policy Institute. https://www.epi.org/blog/u-s-labor-shortage-unlikely-heres-why/

Shim, R. S., & Starks, S. M. (2021). COVID-19, Structural racism, and mental health inequities: Policy implications for an emerging syndemic. *Psychiatric Services*. Advance online publication. https://doi.org/10.1176/appi.ps.202000725

Trask, B. S. (2017). Alleviating the stress on working families: Promoting family-friendly workplace policies (Policy Brief, Vol. 2). National Council on Family Relations. https://www.ncfr.org/sites/default/files/2017-01/ncfr_policy_brief_january_2017.pdf

Turliuc, M. N., & Candel, O. S. (2021). Not all in the same boat. Socioeconomic differences in marital stress and satisfaction during the COVID-19 pandemic. *Frontiers in Psychology*, 12. Advance online publication. https://doi.org/10.3389/fpsyg.2021.635148

Von Bertalanffy, L. (1975). *Perspectives on general system theory: Scientific-philosophical studies*. George Braziller.

U.S. Census. (2020). Current population survey, 2020 annual social and economic supplement. https://www.census.gov/data/tables/2020/demo/families/cps-2020.html

Van Gasse, D., & Mortelmans, D. (2020). Reorganizing the single-parent family system: Exploring the process perspective on divorce. *Family Relations*, 69(5), 1100–1112. https://doi.org/10.1111/fare.12432

Whiley, L. A., Sayer, H., & Juanchich, M. (2020). Motherhood and guilt in a pandemic: Negotiating the "new" normal with a feminist identity. *Gender, Work & Organization*, 28(S2), 612–619. https://doi.org/10.1111/gwao.12613

Whitchurch, G. G., & Constantine, L. L. (2004). Systems theory. In P. G. Boss, W. J. Doherty, R. LaRossa, W. R. Schumm, & S. K. Steinmetz (Eds.), *Sourcebook of family theories and methods: A contextual approach* (pp. 325–352). Springer.

White, J. M., Martin, T. F., & Adamsons, K. (2019). *Family theories: An introduction* (5th ed.). Sage.

Yavorsky, J. E., Qian, Y., & Sargent, A. C. (2021). The gendered pandemic: The implications of COVID-19 for work and family. *Sociology Compass*, 15(6), e12881. https://doi.org/10.1111/soc4.12881

30

Dreams in the Times of the COVID-19 Pandemic

Theoretical Perspectives on the Way the Pandemic Affects Dream Contents

JARNO TUOMINEN, ANTTI REVONSUO, AND KATJA VALLI ■

INTRODUCTION

Simultaneously with the outbreak of the SARS-CoV2 (severe acute respiratory syndrome coronavirus 2) (i.e., the coronavirus that causes COVID-19), a different, more internal phenomenon began cropping up across the globe: People started to report vivid and weird dreams (Gorman, 2020). It seemed the changes to our everyday lives (see Chapter 2) also bore an effect on our nightly experiences. As such, the question about the relationship between dream contents and our waking environments and experiences that has been actively debated at least since Aristotle became acutely visible. As with several other research topics, the COVID-19 pandemic allowed for an unexpected naturalistic, large-scale study design to address questions previously beyond practical or ethical reach. In this chapter, we briefly summarize the various theoretical viewpoints on dreams, relate them to the COVID-19 pandemic, and propose a way forward for the dream sciences. As several research groups have undertaken dream report collection during the pandemic, we aim to simultaneously increase the rigor of dream science and bring the various strands of theories under a unified research program. Our aim, however, reaches beyond dreaming. We consider dreaming as a token example that combines a variety of problems in explaining psychological phenomena in a particularly distinct form.

Jarno Tuominen, Antti Revonsuo, and Katja Valli, *Dreams in the Times of the COVID-19 Pandemic* In: *The Social Science of the COVID-19 Pandemic*. Edited by: Monica K. Miller, Oxford University Press. © Oxford University Press 2024.
DOI: 10.1093/oso/9780197615133.003.0030

DREAM THEORIES

What *are* dreams and why *do* we have them? These questions have preoccupied great minds throughout millennia. Likely due to both their commonality and their ephemeral nature, several theories for dreaming have been developed. In fact, as recently as the year 2000, leading figures claimed that far from a covering[1] theory, there is not even a consensus on what counts as dreaming or how the concept should be defined (Hobson et al., 2000; Nielsen, 2000). From the outset, such a situation might seem discouraging. However, since the turn of the millennium, views on the definition of dreaming have shifted toward a new idea that is universally shared in dream research. The overall, universal *form* of dreaming described as a "dream world" or a "being-in a-world" experience is now widely accepted, although several different terms are used in the literature to capture this idea, for instance, world-analogue; virtual reality; world-simulation; or spatiotemporal hallucination that occurs during sleep. That provides the form and definition of dreams, yet the function seems more difficult to pin down.

Do Dreams Have Functions?

How should the term *function* be understood? One way is to distinguish between dreams serving either a biological or a psychological function. Biological function refers to a view that dreams have likely served an evolutionarily beneficial function in our species' history. The topic is too wide in scope to review here, but for example, the high level of brain activity required to generate complex conscious experiences such as dreams has an energy cost. Thus, unless dreaming has a function, it is difficult to explain why the brain wastes metabolic energy for generating dreams. Such a waste should have been under a negative selection pressure during evolution given the general drive for efficiency. This has led to the development of three major strands of evolutionarily proposed functions: those that emphasize dreams as enhancing survival through simulating threatening events (Revonsuo, 2000), those that propose social functions for dreams (for an overview, see, e.g., Revonsuo et al., 2016a), and those that propose a more general simulation function for dreams (e.g., Bulkeley, 2019; Hobson et al., 2014; Hoel, 2021). Conversely, several theories consider dreams as not functional in an evolutionary sense but to serve a psychological purpose, more akin to that of psychotherapy. Most notably, these include the ideas that dreams are a continuation of waking thought (for a review, see Schredl, 2019) or aid in the regulation of emotions (for a review, see Horton & Malinowski, 2019). The modern emotion regulation theories (ERTs) seem to have been partly inspired by Freud's theory, although they have moved far beyond it. The theories see the function of dreaming as the containment, assimilation, and transformation of powerful negative emotions to positive or neutral ones. When this function fails, nightmares and bad dreams surface.

Dreams as a Subject of Scientific Study

Extant dream theories can be seen to preside in a specific stage of science. This is visible in the way they progress and deal with anomalies. Until recently, the theories themselves have been built by analogues or by "Baconian" data collection, from which theories are then inferred. They have often dealt with anomalies by adding exceptions or additional explanatory layers. For example, Freud revised his theory several times when met with findings incompatible with the original proposals (e.g., adding the impact of negative wake events as exceptions to wish fulfillments). The continuity hypotheses have similarly been expanded and modified by various authors, leading to an ongoing fierce debate on what exactly should be continuous (Domhoff, 2017; Schredl, 2017). This of course is not necessarily problematic per se; theories should be revised when faced with unexpected or contradictory findings. Additional auxiliary hypotheses do, nevertheless, weaken the explanatory power of the theories. However, the problem in dream theories rests on the other side: They have proven very limited in producing precisely formulated, scientifically informative, and empirically testable hypotheses. Theories should be clear enough to produce falsifiable, that is, risky predictions that further our understanding beyond mere post hoc description and interpretation of the data. When theories are not specific enough to generate such hypotheses yet are so malleable as to be able to incorporate any and all findings, they have failed as progressive scientific theories as they have no genuine explanatory power. We have argued elsewhere (Revonsuo et al., 2016b) that the best way forward in dream science is to derive directly conflicting predictions and empirically testable hypotheses from competing theories already before data collection. Consequently, the data from the empirical tests will show which of the rival theories is supported by the evidence and which ones are not. Dream science will make progress when we revise, discard, and combine theoretical views, guided by the strict empirical testing of rival theories against each other.

COVID-19 PANDEMIC AND DREAMING

How should researchers approach the study of dreams during the COVID-19 pandemic? In this chapter, we summarize previous and existing research that could provide some instruction on how best to approach this topic. We then consider two of the functional theories more specifically as case examples of theory-driven hypothesis formation and propose a way forward.

The Impact of the Pandemic and the Mitigation Efforts

While there is no previous literature on how historical pandemics such as the influenza of 1918 (i.e., the Spanish flu), the Ebola outbreak, the SARS virus, or other diseases have affected people's dream contents, there is some indication on the effects from other large-scale events. Traumatic events have been categorized in three subcategories: natural disasters (e.g., floods, earthquakes), man-made disasters (e.g., wars, terrorism), and violence perpetrated by an attachment figure (e.g., intimate partner violence, child abuse) (Luyten & Fonagy, 2019). Arguably, most of dream research on the impact of traumatic events has concentrated on the second category. For example, Hartmann and Brezler (2008) carried out a dream study that by chance was perforated by the 9/11 World Trade Center attacks. This allowed them to assess how the media coverage impacted people's dreams. Similarly, Major Hopkins collected dream diaries at the Laufen prisoner of war camp during the World War II (Barrett et al., 2013), and a retrospective assessment on the impact of the concentration camps for dreams has been conducted concerning holocaust survivors (Bergman et al., 2020). Further, the effect of inter- or intrastate conflict was assessed in the dream contents of Kurdish and Palestinian children (Valli et al., 2005, 2006) and in dissidents in Germany during the Nazi regime (Beradt, 1966). There are also numerous studies on post-traumatic nightmares in war veterans (e.g., Schreuder et al., 2000; Wilmer, 1996). However, while these traumatic events group to the second category of trauma, the situation with regard to the COVID-19 or similar future pandemics is less clear. In general, a viral outbreak can be considered to reside in the first category as there is no intentional agent behind the virus itself. Considering the mechanism of infection, we soon move to the second category as the virus is spread via human-to-human interaction. The situation is further complicated by the mitigation efforts that aim to control the spread of the disease. Social distancing, closure of public spaces and services, and the subsequent increase in secondary traumatic events (e.g., the two- to-fourfold increase in domestic abuse, increased unemployment; see Chapters 26 and 29) could also include the third category of trauma.

Threat Simulation Theory as an Example for Theory-Driven Hypothesis Formation

From the viewpoint of the threat simulation theory (TST) of dreaming (Revonsuo, 2000) the SARS-CoV-2 virus itself presents a salient threat. However, when considering the environment of evolutionary adaptedness—meaning the natural environment that presented various selection pressures for the human populations for tens of thousands of years—pandemics of this scale are likely not to have been a common acquaintance given the overall very low population size and density with relatively sparse intertribal social exchange. Thus, while the difference between a pandemic and a more geographically constrained deadly disease would be a matter of semantics, the effects of deadly communicable viral diseases for small communities were potentially destructive. However, the type of threat that microbial diseases presented for humans in the ancestral environment is quite different from the threats presented by concrete enemies such as predators, tribal warfare, competition for scarce resources and mating opportunities, and destructive natural forces. As microbes are enemies invisible to human perceptual systems, arguably the first line of biological defense against them is anatomical and physiological (protective membranes, immune responses) rather than psychological or behavioral. Only some phobias and aversions, such as disgust against foul-smelling foods or avoidance of feces or otherwise contaminated objects, have evolved to enhance avoidance of the invisible microbial threats. Our threat perception mechanisms and threat avoidance strategies are mostly specialized to detect and avoid concrete, perceptible macroscopic enemies, which were abundant in the ancestral environments. Thus, our evolved threat simulation system during dreaming should also be expected to mostly simulate concrete, macroscopic threats and behavioral strategies that are efficient against such threats.

This would lead to possible tentative hypotheses with regard to TST. First, based on previous research (e.g., Lafrenière et al., 2018), we can expect the increased stress, anxiety, and fear generated by the pandemic most likely to lead to an activation of the threat simulation system and generate more threatening dreams in general. Perhaps more interestingly, TST would predict a longitudinal change in dream content when the situation persists, with more imagery related to the specific current context (e.g., mask use, mass gatherings, contamination) and with incorporation into the context of each individual person's own life (e.g., unemployment, illness of close others). However, dreams would be unlikely to simulate the illness of the dreamer or subsequent health consequences, as such simulation would be functionally pointless as there is no behavioural avoidance strategy that could be rehearsed in dreams at that point. In other words, the simulation of oneself being ill in the dream will not subsequently make falling ill less likely or recovery from a disease more likely in waking life. In contrast, the continuity hypothesis should predict that whatever has occurred in waking life will be incorporated into dream life. The ERTs predict that dreams should try to "heal" or alleviate the negative emotional impact of waking life. Thus, the three theories, threat simulation versus continuity versus emotion regulation, will each issue different predictions about how our dream life will respond to the pandemic.

Social Simulation Theory as an Example for Theory-Driven Hypothesis Formation

While TSTs, and for some aspects ERTs, are arguably the theoretical frameworks that have most to say about the direct impact of the pandemic, the view is broadened when we consider the effects of the mitigation efforts. In this case, the key environmental factor to consider is the alteration of social life. Whereas there are no dream report data from previous pandemics, and the data on the impact of SARS-CoV-2 are only beginning to be published, there is at least some indication on likely effects of the mitigation efforts. One interesting example that could further theoretical clarification is provided by the assessment of the impact of social distancing measures. Tuominen and colleagues (2022) evaluated how social isolation affects dream contents. In their study, participants spent days in social seclusion on a remote island in the Finnish archipelago while their dream contents were systematically collected. The research specifically assessed hypotheses proposed by the social simulation theory (SST) (Revonsuo et al., 2016a) and found support for the *strengthening hypothesis*, which predicts a drastic decrease in social interactions to invoke simulations aimed to regain social belonging to our most important groups. In other words, they found the proportion of close relationships in dreams to increase at the expense of interactions with unknown characters. This study gives an interesting vantage point into the likely outcomes of social isolation while the negative experiences and real-life threat to actual social groups were minimized. Thus, it only tracked what would happen to our dreams if we voluntarily saw fewer people. With regard to COVID-19, the situation is more complex, yet similar trends should be detectable. SST would thus predict an increase in the most important social bonds in our dreams in order to strengthen the support network of the individual given a potentially catastrophic situation. Similarly, even as the mitigation efforts of social distancing minimize or remove daily social interactions, they would likely be continued in our dreams. In the previously mentioned seclusion, when the amount of waking social situations dropped to zero, the amount of dream social simulation, however, remained relatively constant, suggesting mere waking replay not to constitute a likely explanation for social dream contents. In situations where belongingness is actually threatened and people feel lonely, as is the case for many during this current pandemic, SST's *compensation hypothesis* suggests the number of social simulations to actually increase in dreams compared to prepandemic levels (Tuominen, Revonsuo, & Valli, 2019). This would allow dreamers to practice relevant social skills, strengthen existing or probable social bonds, and thus allow for more adaptive social behavior in waking life. Furthermore, dreams should increasingly begin to simulate those relevant social behaviors that have changed, such as social distancing in order to recalibrate social schemas, scripts, or internal working models.

How to Design Data Collection to Allow for Comparisons and Contrasts

How, then, can we separate dream contents chosen specifically for a given function from mere replay or continuation of wake experiences? First, it depends on how we frame this continuity. If we consider dreams to reflect wake experiences, it follows that the same amount of given contents and behaviors would be present in both the waking life and the dream life. From previous research that has compared actual wake reports or situations with corresponding dream contents, however, we already know this not to be the case (McNamara et al., 2005; Tuominen et al., 2022; Tuominen, Stenberg, et al., 2019; Valli et al., 2008). Dreams seem to be biased toward certain kinds of contents, most notably those of a social and/or threatening nature. An alternative view would be to note that dreams do not exactly *mirror* waking life, but rather reflect our current concerns and mental processes, especially what we worry about and think about during wakefulness. In this case, the comparative data would not be reports of waking events, but reports of internal states, such as daydreaming and mind wandering (see e.g., Blagrove et al., 2019; Carr & Nielsen, 2015; Sikka et al., 2021). Indeed, here the comparison with dreams seems more likely. For instance, Mar and colleagues (2012) found approximately 73% of people always or frequently had social daydreams. During the COVID-19 pandemic, a combined approach would thus seem recommendable: Simultaneously collect reports during the same data collection period from both waking life (mind wandering, daydreaming, experience sampling) and dream life (systematically collected dream reports). This allows for fruitful comparisons between the continuity and discontinuity of waking concerns and contents on the one hand and to more specifically trace the events that affect corresponding change in dream contents on the other hand (and vice versa; see, e.g., Selterman et al., 2014, for how dreams affect subsequent waking behavior). When the data collected are commensurable, they can be contrasted and the differences in various conscious experiences highlighted more clearly.

LESSONS LEARNED: HOW TO PROCEED?

The COVID-19 pandemic has affected the contents of people's dreams, invoking a newfound interest in the interplay between external and internal worlds and thus brought to bear on the possible functions of dreaming. Consequently, research into COVID-19 dreams is an active topic yet still plagued by the lack of shared practices and/or criteria for data collection or for adversarial hypothesis testing. COVID-19 has provided a spontaneous naturalistic experiment that can shed light on topics previously beyond reach. Careful data collection and hypothesis formation during this pandemic can help evaluate long-held disputes within the dream science and help situate dreaming in relation to other phenomena, such as daydreaming or mind wandering. Currently, there are already some publications on the impact of the COVID-19 pandemic on dreams. From the viewpoint of TST, continuity hypotheses, and ERT it is interesting to note that the frequency of nightmares has increased, and dreams have incorporated pandemic-related imagery, especially in females (Jiang et al., 2020; Musse et al., 2020; Pesonen et al., 2020; Scarpelli et al. 2021). Iorio and colleagues (2020) found a fifth of the dreams (collected using the most recent dream method) contained explicit references to the pandemic and strong negative emotions. Those who had known people who had either fallen ill or died of COVID-19 reported higher emotional intensity. Kilius and colleagues (2021) further found female students reported more aggressive social interactions compared to normative data from mid-20th century. Specific changes in contents were reported by MacKay and DeCicco (2020), who found COVID dreams included more animal, food, head, changes in location, and virus-related imagery. A computational assessment of Brazilian dream reports found a higher proportion of words related to anger and sadness, as well as cleanliness and contamination, compared to controls (Mota et al., 2020) and associated with social isolation and its negative psychological consequences. Those who have been the most affected by the COVID-19 pandemic also reported more negative dreams and pandemic-related imagery (Schredl & Bulkeley, 2020).

In conclusion, data collection is active, and the mounting data present an unprecedented possibility to truly propel dream research forward. These studies have used various theoretical assumptions, and while support has been found for TST, SST, continuity hypotheses, and ERT, no sustained overarching approach has been shared. The use of preregistered competitive hypotheses, "adversarial" collaboration between researchers with varying theoretical assumptions, and precise, testable, and risky predictions derived from the competing theories help move the whole field into a more advanced level. Combined with commensurable data collection methodology between cultures on the one hand and between various experimental states on the other hand allows for fruitful comparisons and contrasts. In hindsight, such cataclysmic events have proven valuable in other multidisciplinary efforts as well. For example, the dream experiences collected by Beradt (1966) from dissenting Germans during the Nazi regime have allowed us to understand a whole other level of influence an oppressive regime effects on its population. By gaining an understanding of the way dreams reflect external circumstances, we might be able to also use them to catch those at an increased risk for developing a mental health issue and focus preventive efforts prior to them reaching a diagnostic cut point. While research on predicting the mental health outcomes from dream reports is yet to be carried out, dreams have been proposed to serve as markers for mental health in general (e.g., Sikka et al., 2018), and reductions in depressive symptoms are correlated with corresponding change in the affective content of dreams (Riemann et al., 1990; Schredl et al., 2009). Interestingly, graph analyses of dream reports can be used to identify bipolar illness with higher accuracy than psychometric scores or wake reports (Mota et al., 2014). Longitudinal dream report data collection during major emergencies allows for testing the predictive power of such methods.

CONCLUSION

The COVID-19 pandemic has uniquely affected practically every person on Earth. In the wake of this human disaster is carried an opportunity for a deeper understanding of the relation between our internal experiences and the external circumstances. Here, we have focused on the special case of dreaming as it exemplifies several of the problems ingrained in the study of human experience in general but showcases them in an especially marked form. Dreams are private, accessible only retroactively, and underscore the difference between the first-person lived experience of the dream and the third-person observation of this phenomenon. In this chapter, we have called for a more systematic approach to collecting and using dream reports from the COVID-19 pandemic. In dream research, this could help untangle some long-standing theoretical disputes and clarify very basic-level questions of the function of dreaming. Here, we have presented a few options on theory-driven hypotheses from theories that propose an evolutionary function for dreaming as examples that could then be contrasted with corresponding rival or baseline hypotheses. From the view of the pandemic, understanding the impact such events have on the private internal experiences of individuals allows for an added layer of analysis. There is some indication that such data could be used, for example, on earlier identification of persons likely to develop mental health problems and ideally allow for early prevention of more persistent or severe psychological distress. Given the global nature of the pandemic, systematizing and standardizing the approaches for data gathering would allow for very interesting cross-cultural comparisons. With regard to the evolutionarily informed theories, such as TST and SST, such comparisons would form a crucial test as they both predict the mechanisms for dream content selection to be universal in (at least) humans.

NOTE

1. The term *covering* here denotes a theory that provides inferences and thus aims at understanding in addition to mere explanation (see, e.g., Rohrlich, 1994).

REFERENCES

Barrett, D., Sogolow, Z., Angela, O. H., Panton, J., Grayson, M., & Justiniano, M. (2013). Content of dreams from WWII POWs. *Imagination, Cognition and Personality*, *33*(1), 193–204. https://doi.org/10.2190/IC.33.1-2.g

Beradt, C. (1966). *Das dritte reich des traums*. Suhrkamp Verlag.

Bergman, M., MacGregor, O., Olkoniemi, H., Owczarski, W., Revonsuo, A., & Valli, K. (2020). The Holocaust as a lifelong nightmare: Posttraumatic symptoms and dream content in Polish Auschwitz survivors 30 years after WWII. *American Journal of Psychology*, *133*(2), 143–166. https://doi.org/10.5406/amerjpsyc.133.2.0143

Blagrove, M., Edwards, C., van Rijn, E., Reid, A., Malinowski, J., Bennett, P., Carr, M., Eichenlaub, J.-B., McGee, S., Evans, K., & Ruby, P. (2019). Insight from the consideration of REM dreams, non-REM dreams, and daydreams. *Psychology of Consciousness: Theory, Research and Practice*, *6*(2), 138–162. http://dx.doi.org/10.1037/cns0000167

Bulkeley, K. (2019). Dreaming is imaginative play in sleep: A theory of the function of dreams. *Dreaming*, *29*(1), 1–21. https://doi.org/10.1037/drm0000099

Carr, M., & Nielsen, T. (2015). Daydreams and nap dreams: Content comparisons. *Consciousness and Cognition*, *36*, 196–205. https://doi.org/10.1016/j.concog.2015.06.012

Domhoff, G. W. (2017). The invasion of the concept snatchers: The origins, distortions, and future of the continuity hypothesis. *Dreaming*, *27*(1), 14–39. https://doi.org/10.1037/drm0000047

Gorman, A. (2020, September 1). Welcome to my nightmare: Researchers to investigate the strange world of Covid dreams. *The Guardian*. https://www.theguardian.com/lifeandstyle/2020/sep/01/welcome-to-my-nightmare-researchers-to-investigate-the-strange-world-of-covid-dreams

Hartmann, E., & Brezler, T. (2008). A systematic change in dreams after 9/11/01. *Sleep*, *31*(2), 213–218. https://doi.org/10.1093/sleep/31.2.213

Hobson, J. A., Hong, C. C. H., & Friston, K. J. (2014). Virtual reality and consciousness inference in dreaming. *Frontiers in Psychology, 5,* 1133. https://doi.org/10.3389/fpsyg.2014.01133

Hobson, J. A., Pace-Schott, E. F., & Stickgold, R. (2000). Dreaming and the brain: Toward a cognitive neuroscience of conscious states. *Behavioral and Brain Sciences*, *23*(6), 793–842. https://doi.org/10.1017/s0140525x00003976

Hoel, E. (2021). The overfitted brain: Dreams evolved to assist generalization. *Patterns*, *2*(5), 100244. https://doi.org/10.1016/j.patter.2021.100244

Horton, C. L., & Malinowski, J. E. (2019). Emotion regulation in dreaming. In K. Valli, R. J. Hoss, & R. P. Gongloff (Eds.), *Dreams: Understanding biology, psychology and culture* (Vol. 2, pp. 105–111). ABC-CLIO.

Iorio, I., Sommantico, M., & Parrello, S. (2020). Dreaming in the time of COVID-19: A quali-quantitative Italian study. *Dreaming*, *30*(3), 199–215. https://doi.org/10.1037/drm0000142

Jiang, W., Ren, Z., Yu, L., Tan, Y., & Shi, C. (2020). A network analysis of post-traumatic stress disorder symptoms and correlates during the COVID-19 pandemic. *Frontiers in Psychiatry*, *11*. https://doi.org/10.3389/fpsyt.2020.568037

Kilius, E., Abbas, N. H., McKinnon, L., & Samson, D. R. (2021). Pandemic nightmares: COVID-19 lockdown associated with increased aggression in female university students' dreams. *Frontiers in Psychology*, *12*, 562. https://doi.org/10.3389/fpsyg.2021.644636

Lafrenière, A., Lortie-Lussier, M., Dale, A., Robidoux, R., & De Koninck, J. (2018). Autobiographical memory sources of threats in dreams. *Consciousness and Cognition*, *58*, 124–135. https://doi.org/10.1016/j.concog.2017.10.017

Luyten, P., & Fonagy, P. (2019). Mentalizing and trauma. In *Handbook of mentalizing in mental health practice* (pp. 79–99). American Psychiatric Association Publishing.

MacKay, C., & DeCicco, T. L. (2020). Pandemic dreaming: The effect of COVID-19 on dream imagery, a pilot study. *Dreaming*, *30*(3), 222–234. https://doi.org/10.1037/drm0000148

Mar, R. A., Mason, M. F., & Litvack, A. (2012). How daydreaming relates to life satisfaction, loneliness, and social support: The importance of gender and daydream content. *Consciousness and Cognition*, *21*(1), 401–407. https://doi.org/10.1016/j.concog.2011.08.001

McNamara, P., McLaren, D., Smith, D., Brown, A., & Stickgold, R. (2005). A "Jekyll and Hyde" within. *Psychological Science*, *16*(2), 130–136. https://doi.org/10.1111/j.0956-7976.2005.00793.x

Musse, F. C. C., de Siqueira Castro, L., Sousa, K. M. M., Mestre, T. F., Teixeira, C. D. M., Pelloso, S. M., Poyares, D., & de Barros Carvalho, M. D. (2020). Mental violence: The COVID-19 nightmare. *Frontiers in Psychiatry*, *11*, 579289. https://doi.org/10.3389/fpsyt.2020.579289

Mota, N. B., Furtado, R., Maia, P. P., Copelli, M., & Ribeiro, S. (2014). Graph analysis of dream reports is especially informative about psychosis. *Scientific Reports*, *4*(1), 1–7. https://doi.org/10.1038/srep03691

Mota, N. B., Weissheimer, J., Ribeiro, M., de Paiva, M., Avilla-Souza, J., Simabucuru, G., Chaves, M. F., Cecchi, L., Cirne, J., Cecchi, G., Rodrigues, C., Copelli, M., & Ribeiro, S.

(2020). Dreaming during the Covid-19 pandemic: Computational assessment of dream reports reveals mental suffering related to fear of contagion. *PloS One, 15*(11), e0242903. https://doi.org/10.1371/journal.pone.0242903

Nielsen, T. A. (2000). A review of mentation in REM and NREM sleep: "Covert" REM sleep as a possible reconciliation of two opposing models. *Behavioral and Brain Sciences, 23*(6), 851–866.https://doi.org/10.1017/s0140525x0000399x

Pesonen, A. K., Lipsanen, J., Halonen, R., Elovainio, M., Sandman, N., Mäkelä, J. M., Antila, M., Béchard, D., Ollilla, H. M., & Kuula, L. (2020). Pandemic dreams: Network analysis of dream content during the COVID-19 lockdown. *Frontiers in Psychology, 11*, 2569. https://doi.org/10.3389/fpsyg.2020.573961

Revonsuo, A. (2000). The reinterpretation of dreams: An evolutionary hypothesis of the function of dreaming. *Behavioral and Brain Sciences, 2*(6), 877–901. https://doi.org/10.1017/S0140525X00004015

Revonsuo, A., Tuominen, J., & Valli, K. (2016a). Avatars in the machine: Dreaming as a simulation of social reality. In T. Metzinger & J. Windt (Ed.). *Open MIND: Philosophy of mind and the cognitive sciences in the 21st century* (Vol. 2, pp. 1295-1322). MIT Press.

Revonsuo, A, Tuominen, J., & Valli, K. (2016b). The simulation theories of dreaming: How to make theoretical progress in the dream sciences. In T. Metzinger & J. Windt (Eds.), *Open MIND: Philosophy of mind and the cognitive sciences in the 21st century.* (Vol. 2, pp. 1341-1348). MIT Press.

Riemann, D., Low, H., Schredl, M., Wiegand, M., Dippel, B., & Berger, M. (1990). Investigations of morning and laboratory dream recall and content in depressive patients during baseline conditions and under antidepressive treatment with trimipramine. *Psychiatry Journal of the University of Ottawa, 15*(2), 93–99.

Rohrlich, F. (1994). Scientific explanation: From covering law to covering theory. *PSA: Proceedings of the Biennial Meeting of the Philosophy of Science Association, 1*, 69–77. https://doi.org/10.1086/psaprocbienmeetp.1994.1.193012

Scarpelli, S., Alfonsi, V., Mangiaruga, A., Musetti, A., Quattropani, M. C., Lenzo, V., Freda, M. F., Lemmo, D., Vegni, E., Borghi, L., Saita, E., Cattivelli, R., Cestelnuovo, G., Plazzi, G., De Gennaro, L., & Franceschini, C. (2021). Pandemic nightmares: Effects on dream activity of the COVID-19 lockdown in Italy. *Journal of Sleep Research, 30*(5), e13300. https://doi.org/10.1111/jsr.13300

Schredl, M. (2017). Theorizing about the continuity between waking and dreaming: Comment on Domhoff (2017). *Dreaming, 27*(4), 351–359. https://doi.org/10.1037/drm0000062

Schredl, M. (2019). Continuity hypothesis of dreaming. In K. Valli, R. J. Hoss, & R. P. Gongloff (Eds.), *Dreams: Understanding biology, psychology and culture* (Vol. 2, pp. 88–94). ABC-CLIO.

Schredl, M., Berger, M., & Riemann, D. (2009). The effect of trimipramine on dream recall and dream emotions in depressive outpatients. *Psychiatry Research, 167*, 279–286. https://doi.org/10.1016/j.psychres.2008.03.002

Schredl, M., & Bulkeley, K. (2020). Dreaming and the COVID-19 pandemic: A survey in a U.S. sample. *Dreaming, 30*(3), 189–198. https://doi.org/10.1037/drm0000146

Schreuder, B. J., Kleijn, W. C., & Rooijmans, H. G. (2000). Nocturnal re-experiencing more than forty years after war trauma. *Journal of Traumatic Stress, 13*(3), 453–463. https://doi.org/10.1023/A:1007733324351

Selterman, D. F., Apetroaia, A. I., Riela, S., & Aron, A. (2014). Dreaming of you: Behavior and emotion in dreams of significant others predict subsequent relational behavior. *Social Psychological and Personality Science, 5*(1), 111–118. https://doi.org/10.1177/1948550613486678

Sikka, P., Pesonen, H., & Revonsuo, A. (2018). Peace of mind and anxiety in the waking state are related to the affective content of dreams. *Scientific Reports, 8,* 12762. https://doi.org/10.1038/s41598-018-30721-1

Sikka, P., Valli, K., Revonsuo, A., & Tuominen, J. (2021). The dynamics of affect across the wake-sleep cycle: From waking mind-wandering to night-time dreaming. PsyArxiv. https://doi.org/10.31234/osf.io/f9av6

Tuominen, J., Olkoniemi, H., Revonsuo, A., & Valli, K. (2022). "No man is an island": Effects of social seclusion on dream contents and REM sleep. *British Journal of Psychology, 113*(1), 84–104. https://doi.org/10.1111/bjop.12515

Tuominen, J., Revonsuo, A., & Valli, K. (2019). Social simulation theory. In K. Valli, R. J. Hoss, & R. P. Gongloff (Eds.), *Dreams: Understanding biology, psychology and culture* (Vol. 2, pp. 132–136). ABC-CLIO.

Tuominen, J., Stenberg, T., Revonsuo, A., & Valli, K. (2019). Social contents in dreams: An empirical test of the social simulation theory. *Consciousness and Cognition, 69,* 133–145. https://doi.org/10.1016/j.concog.2019.01.017

Valli, K., Revonsuo, A., Pälkäs, O., & Punamäki, R. L. (2006). The effect of trauma on dream content—A field study of Palestinian children. *Dreaming, 16*(2), 63–87. https://doi.org/10.1037/1053-0797.16.2.63

Valli, K., Revonsuo, A., Pälkäs, O., Ismail, K. H., Ali, K. J., & Punamäki, R. L. (2005). The threat simulation theory of the evolutionary function of dreaming: Evidence from dreams of traumatized children. *Consciousness and Cognition, 14*(1), 188–218. https://doi.org/10.1016/S1053-8100(03)00019-9

Valli, K., Strandholm, T., Sillanmäki, L., & Revonsuo, A. (2008). Dreams are more negative than real life—Implications for the function of dreaming. *Cognition and Emotion, 22*(5), 833–861. https://doi.org/10.1080/02699930701541591

Wilmer, H. A. (1996). The healing nightmare: War dreams of Vietnam veterans. In D. Barrett (Ed.), *Trauma and dreams* (pp. 85–99). Harvard University Press.

FURTHER READING

Revonsuo, A. (2006). *Inner presence: Consciousness as a biological phenomenon.* MIT Press

Valli, K., & Hoss, R. J. (Eds.) (2019). *Dreams: Understanding biology, psychology and culture* (Vol. 1). ABC-CLIO.

Windt, J. M. (2015). *Dreaming: A conceptual framework for philosophy of mind and empirical research.* MIT Press.

Zadra, A., & Stickgold, R. (2021). *When brains dream: Exploring the science and mystery of sleep.* W. W. Norton.

31

Past Victimization and Responses to the COVID-19 Pandemic

MICHAŁ BILEWICZ AND MARIA BABIŃSKA ■

The recent COVID-19 crisis had a hard impact on economies and societies all over the world. With more than 4 million deaths globally, it might be considered one of the deadliest pandemics in history. Even though the COVID-19 pandemic was a global phenomenon, it did not affect all human societies in the same way. In some countries (like Peru or Mexico), the case-fatality ratio reached 9%, whereas in others (like Iceland, United Arab Emirates, or Singapore) it was less than 0.5% (Dong et al., 2020). It is obvious that these differences could be attributed to wealth inequality and variability in health systems efficiency. Numerous health, economical, and societal consequences of the COVID-19 crisis disproportionately affected vulnerable populations and lower-income countries (Bundervoet et al., 2021). At the same time, however, effective responses to the pandemic were also determined by psychological factors such as trust, healthy relationships, proneness to misinformation and conspiracy theories, effective leadership, and effective persuasion (van Bavel et al., 2020). These factors also varied between countries and cultures, and their impact on preventive behavior and public health is fundamental.

Among many societal determinants of trust, adherence to norms, and belief in conspiracy theories, one seems highly obvious: historical victimization. Groups that were historically disadvantaged and marginalized, such as Black Americans, were also more at risk during the pandemic (Kim & Bostwick, 2020; see Chapters 24 and 25 for more on the disproportionate impact on marginalized groups). In this chapter, we examine how past victimization could impact people's responses to and experiences of the COVID-19 pandemic. Based on psychological theorizing, as well as research on minority groups and historically victimized nations, we define the ways through which historical victimization could affect the way people interpreted the epidemic situation and behaved in the face of the pathogenic threat. Ultimately, a person's group membership can shape their experiences during the pandemic.

Michał Bilewicz and Maria Babińska, *Past Victimization and Responses to the COVID-19 Pandemic* In: *The Social Science of the COVID-19 Pandemic*. Edited by: Monica K. Miller, Oxford University Press. © Oxford University Press 2024.
DOI: 10.1093/oso/9780197615133.003.0031

THE ROLE OF NATIONAL HISTORY IN PERCEIVING PRESENT-DAY EVENTS

History has since long been considered a key framework people use for understanding contemporary social and political events. Marcus Tullius Cicero named history "a life's teacher" (*Historia est Magistra Vitae*), and this metaphor accurately describes the fundamental role history plays in our common interpretations of facts and behaviors. Liu and Hilton (2005) analyzed the way people commemorate important events from national histories and developed a concept of "group charters." They suggested that the common representations of history define the way people would like to view their national group (the position of a given nation in international relations): its moral status and goals that the collective might see in its future.

The historical role of a victim is one of the essential roles in which nations view their past. In countries that have an imperial past (e.g., England, Spain), the history of being a global superpower (e.g., United States, Russia), or the history of being a perpetrator of inhumanities and war instigator (e.g., Germany, Japan), the dominant perception of history would not include elements of collective victimization. Members of such nations would most likely view their own nation as a perpetrator of crimes and colonizer of others—this leading to the problems of collective shame, guilt, or regret (Imhoff et al., 2012). In contrast, in countries that were historically conquered, colonized, or occupied, as well as among disadvantaged minority groups—a different representation of history prevails: the one of being a victim.

A history of being a collective victim of wars, occupations, atrocities, or discrimination has a fundamental impact on the way people interpret current events. Although this impact is contingent on one's construal of historical victimization, there are some shared consequences of victimhood that determine levels of trust, beliefs in conspiracies, and perception of national authorities (Bilewicz & Liu, 2020). However, the attitude toward other nations, minorities, rival groups, and past enemies depends largely on the way people view their victimhood—whether they perceive national victimization in exclusive versus inclusive terms and how they view the perpetrators and bystanders (Bilali & Vollhardt, 2019).

Past victimization is a collective experience, but there is also important variability in the extent to which people think about their nation being victimized. For some of them, the history of victimization is central to their identity, and they consider these events in national history essential. For others, past victimization is not as important, and they tend to focus more on present-day issues and orient toward the future rather than being constrained by past grievances. This individual variability in the subjective importance of historical victimization is often named "historical trauma salience": an extent to which traumatic narratives are salient for an individual (Skrodzka et al., 2021). Both socially shared victimization and an individual focus on victims' past can severely affect people's behavior in the situation of epidemic threat.

Past Victimization and the Tendency to Believe in Conspiracy Theories

A single traumatic event can cause severe psychological consequences, but often it leads to mobilization and mobilization of behavior, known as post-traumatic growth. At the same time, people who suffered from frequent acts of discrimination or were victims of massive crimes targeting their groups, such as genocides or ethnic cleansing, often adapt to these realities. They develop a specific mindset that interprets further experiences as subsequent acts of victimization (Bar-Tal et al., 2009). This is because such trauma is socially shared and endures for a long period of time. Therefore, people tend to adapt to the traumatic reality in which their nations function for a prolonged time (Bilewicz & Liu, 2020).

One of the serious consequences of past victimization is the tendency to interpret reality using conspiracy theories. For instance, a study performed in Greece (Pantazi et al., 2022) found that people focused on past victimization of the Greek nation were more likely to believe in financial conspiracies (a plot of bankers as being responsible for the economic crisis of 2009). This effect was particularly pronounced among Greeks highly identified with their nation. The more they identified with being Greek, the more their focus on past victimization fueled conspiracy accounts of current events. Similarly, in Poland, highly identifying people, when reminded about past victimization of their nation, also interpreted current events in a more conspiratorial way. A study of people's explanations of the Smoleńsk air disaster (Bilewicz et al., 2019), in which a Polish Air Force flight crashed with the country's president on board, found that the tendency to interpret this event in a conspiratorial way was determined by people's focus on national victimhood. People who perceived national history as constant victimization would interpret the aviation accident as an intended action against the nation. More importantly, conspiracy theories in such a society create a "traumatic rift"—a strong polarization between the believers and nonbelievers, ultimately leading to a long-lasting intractable conflict.

Conspiracy theories about COVID-19 have been widespread since the beginning of the pandemic, suggesting that COVID-19 was intentionally created by China as a means of economic rivalry with the United States or that the COVID-19 pandemic is a hoax developed by liberal intellectuals and ideologically motivated scientists in order to limit civil liberties (Douglas, 2021). Such theories are known to reduce social distancing—a pattern observed in both correlational (Biddlestone et al., 2020) and longitudinal studies (Bierwiaczonek et al., 2020)—as well as other protective behaviors crucial to public health in times of a pandemic, from handwashing (Oleksy et al., 2021) to vaccination (Earnshaw et al., 2020). Therefore, the popularity of conspiracy theories in victimized societies and disadvantaged social groups is not only a political issue, but also a large public health problem that makes such societies particularly vulnerable to infectious diseases.

Past Victimization and Mistrust

The paradox of conspiracy theories in victimized groups is that they tend to be adaptive for such societies. A shared deprivation of control and long-time disadvantage creates a more general mindset that gives meaningful interpretations of people's environment. Nations and minorities that were constantly targeted by enemies or majority groups quite correctly view the intentions of others as hostile. The correlation between the sense of victimhood (perception of one's nation as being a victim, rather than perpetrator, across history), and the tendency to believe in conspiracy theories is particularly visible in societies that have a factual history of collective trauma (Bilewicz & Liu, 2020). In such societies, victimhood beliefs also reduce trust in political institutions and government (see Chapter 18 for more on trust in COVID-19). People living in historically colonized or occupied countries tend to perceive the existing institutions as agents of external power. Such mistrust has been extremely dangerous in times of the COVID-19 pandemic as it made public health policies ineffective: People did not believe in the honest intentions of their health ministries and other state agencies.

This problem has been addressed for many decades by clinical psychologists working with ethnic minorities and disadvantaged groups. In one of the studies, they found that the cultural mistrust of African Americans often leads to their unequal access to counseling and psychotherapy (Whaley, 2001). As a result of long-lasting racial discrimination and unfair treatment, Black Americans developed a strong distrust that inhibited their intention to take part in counseling and psychotherapy and reduced their willingness to self-disclose (among those who decided to become clients of White-dominated counseling and therapeutic institutions).

During a pandemic, countries with high levels of social trust have a clear advantage over the ones with low trust. In times when compliance with public health appeals is necessary, social trust becomes inevitable. In the regions of Europe with the highest levels of social trust people followed health-related orders and procedures (e.g., reduced mobility; Bargain & Aminjonov, 2020). Interestingly, COVID-19-related threats made many people in Europe more authoritarian. However, different aspects of authoritarianism were boosted by the COVID-19 threat in countries with high and low levels of trust (Bilewicz et al., 2023). In high-trust nations, people afraid of the pandemic became highly obedient to authorities and followed their political leadership. In low-trust nations, people scared by COVID-19 became more hostile toward dissidents and deviants (authoritarian aggression), but this reaction was not matched with high obedience to authorities and norms. When people cannot rely on their authorities, the pandemic threat leads to maladaptive reactions. This is a common experience of victimized groups and societies around the world.

Past Victimization and Control Deprivation

The position of a collective victim can be also viewed as a fundamental threat to the sense of personal control. Being a member of a strong and powerful group is an important source of a person's sense of control and agency. Historically victimized groups often suffer from the feeling that their community cannot effectively help them in overcoming their everyday problems. When thinking about history, they can generate an impression that people cannot effectively control their life and environment. Such thinking often leads to a heightened belief in conspiracy theories and other irrational beliefs (Kay et al., 2009). For example, when people are reminded about uncontrollable aspects of their lives, they start believing that other ethnic groups are in control of politics, media, and the economy (Kofta et al., 2020). Conspiracy theories seem to compensate for the general feeling of uncontrollability: "If I cannot control the reality, then some other forces must have control over it!"

People from historically victimized groups construe the history of their group as constantly deprived of control: They view others as controlling the fate of their nation. When interpreting contemporary events, they use the same schema, regardless of the current situation of their group. This has been clearly visible in times of the COVID-19 epidemic. Nations with a long history of victimization viewed the pandemic as a subsequent control loss. People who viewed events in their nation's history as being a result of external forces rather than their own national agency tended to interpret COVID-19 as a result of a conspiracy. This in turn led to underestimation of health risks, mistrust, and less protective behavior (Babińska & Bilewicz, 2021). The COVID-19 pandemic is itself a severe threat to personal control: People cannot effectively predict what will happen in the future; many of them lose jobs and other sources of income due to restrictions. Among historically victimized groups, this control deprivation could have particularly strong adverse effects.

COVID-19 AND HISTORICAL TRAUMA

Historical victimization is a large-scale societal problem, but it also has clear consequences for individual people's mental health. It is estimated that 22% of people living in conflict zones suffer from mental health problems (Charlson et al., 2019). Even after these conflicts are over, populations living in such areas still suffer from depression, anxiety, and post-traumatic stress disorder (Daud et al., 2005). In many traumatized populations, post-traumatic stress disorder is transgenerationally transmitted—through both narratives and epigenetic transmission. This is why in many historically victimized groups (e.g., native people, minorities) higher levels of substance use, affective disorder, and conduct disorder have been observed more frequently than in other populations (Ehlers et al., 2013). This phenomenon has been often named *historical trauma*, as it is the group's history that directly affects its current mental health problems. Historical trauma is a combination of two psychological phenomena: salience of historical victimization and traumatic symptoms. The more historical crimes are cognitively salient, the more symptoms can be observed among members of such groups. For instance, among Iraqi Kurds, those who frequently emphasized the historical victimization of their communities, such as the loss of their ancestral lands, tended to experience more severe traumatic symptoms related to this historical victimization. These symptoms included feelings of helplessness and various negative emotions. Consequently, individuals with higher levels of these traumatic symptoms were more likely to have ongoing mental health challenges, including conditions like depression, stress, and anxiety (Skrodzka et al., 2021).

The situation of the pandemic might affect historically victimized groups' mental health in twofold ways. First, it makes historical trauma more salient, as many aspects of the epidemic situation could remind them of historical victimization. More so, as pathogen stress induces ethnocentrism and authoritarianism (Tybur et al., 2016), minority groups might observe more hostile reactions from majorities. The situation in which majority groups become more authoritarian and stress their coherence can be a reminder of historical contexts in which minorities were excluded, harmed, or killed. This, in turn, makes the historical trauma more salient and—indirectly—leads to further deterioration of mental health.

In 2020, WHO drew attention to the risk of social stigma related to COVID-19. Such stigma was described as "the negative association between a person or group of people who share certain characteristics and a specific disease" (WHO, 2020). Labeling the virus as "the China virus" or "the Wuhan virus" was common not only among laypeople, but also in the media and among politicians. Such descriptions pointed to historically discriminated minority groups as being associated with the new pathogen. The omnipresence of such language could lead to even higher levels of anxiety among historically victimized groups.

The second important aspect of the epidemic situation regarding minorities' mental health is general increased anxiety, stress, and depression in such groups. Regardless of majorities' attitudes and behavior, the situation of social isolation (due to distancing) and lockdowns could amplify the already existing mental health problems in minority populations. Social isolation could be particularly difficult for people with major depressive disorder. Another mental health effect of the epidemic among victimized groups is the increased sense of threat from the pathogen itself. Recently psychologists and psychiatrists defined COVID stress syndrome as a multifaceted phenomenon that includes fear of infection and fear of coming into contact with objects or surfaces contaminated with the coronavirus; fear of socioeconomic effects of the pandemic; fear of foreigners who might be possibly be infected; compulsive checking information about the pandemic and reassurance seeking; and typical traumatic stress symptoms related to pandemic (Taylor, 2021). Members of victimized groups have a natural tendency to react to such situations with higher anxiety; therefore, all aspects of the COVID stress syndrome would be particularly visible in such groups.

VICTIMHOOD-DRIVEN PREJUDICE

Although members of the historically victimized groups obviously suffer from the epidemic situation, such a situation could also lead to further victimization of other people by historically victimized groups. This vicious cycle of victimization has been well-documented in social psychology (Bar-Tal et al., 2009; Klar et al., 2013). The focus on past victimization is a psychological ground for intergroup hostility, although it can also foster reconciliation and intergroup harmony (Bilali & Vollhardt, 2019). Much of that depends on how people construe their victimhood. It can be perceived in exclusive terms ("they did it only to us") or in more inclusive ones ("people did it to other people"). For example, there are four distinctive lessons learned from the history of the Holocaust among contemporary Israelis (Klar et al., 2013): "never be a passive victim," "never forsake your brothers," "never be passive bystander," and "never be a perpetrator." Some of them are based on more exclusive understanding of ingroups' victimhood and lead to a more aggressive approach to other groups (e.g., never be a passive victim), whereas others are based on inclusive construals of victimhood, leading to peaceful coexistence with others and intergroup altruism (e.g., never be a passive bystander).

One of the key factors determining people's lessons from past victimhood is their sense of threat, particularly threat to their mere existence. When people are anxious about their individual survival (Jonas & Fritsche, 2013) or the survival of their group (Wohl et al., 2010), they might view others as enemies and mobilize all resources to confront them. The situation of an epidemic elicits death anxiety, which is a well-known antecedent of conformist and group-focused behaviors. Such a threat would motivate people to interpret their own victimhood also in a group-based, collectivistic manner rather than a more inclusive, universalistic one. In fact, during the COVID-19 epidemic acts of anti-immigrant or homophobic crimes and violence were observed in countries that have a long history of victimhood (e.g., anti-Arab riots in Israel, attacks against Asians and Ukrainians in Poland; see Chapter 23 for more about COVID-19-related violence against minority groups). The period following the COVID-19 outbreak in several historically marginalized societies in Eastern Europe, including Hungary, Romania, Poland, and Slovakia, witnessed a noticeable increase in state-level discrimination against both gay individuals and the Roma community.

FUTURE RESEARCH ON PANDEMIC IN HISTORICALLY VICTIMIZED SOCIETIES

Although the COVID-19 epidemic inspired an ample amount of cross-cultural research on human behavior in times of a pandemic, the attention has been focused predominantly on individual characteristics that are potential candidates for key determinants of human health behavior. This approach creates a risk of overlooking the societal-level and historical determinants of people's willingness to vaccinate, engage in protective behaviors (wearing masks, washing hands, etc.), and trust health providers and state institutions.

We strongly believe that future large-scale, cross-cultural research should take into account the historical context of people's behavior, addressing past grievances and experiences of victimization and discrimination. It is essential to examine the role of these objective determinants of current behavior, as well as their indirect effects through such psychological processes as specific victimhood beliefs, conspiracy theories, mistrust, and collective/individual sense of control. In such analyses, psychologists should be accompanied by historians, political scientists, and sociologists to provide essential expertise on societal-level processes that determine behavior beyond well-known cultural factors such as collectivism/individualism or self-construals. In order to explain the role of victimization in human reactions to pathogen threat, such collaboration would be inevitable.

CONCLUSION

The epidemic of COVID-19 has affected different populations in highly unequal ways. As in many other severe global crises, historically disadvantaged groups were mostly affected. In this chapter, we provided evidence that groups with an experience of collective violence, such as genocides, cleansing, wars, violent conflicts, and occupations, generated a specific mindset that guides their behavior, emotions, and cognitions. After long experience of living in such adverse environments, disadvantaged groups developed strategies that allow them to understand the situation and deal with everyday victimization. These strategies include a generalized lack of trust in institutions and conspiracy theories explaining political and social reality. In the situation of a global pandemic, such as the COVID-19 epidemic, these strategies became extremely maladaptive, as they lowered trust in authorities and institutions, disobedience to health restrictions, irrational behavior, stockpiling supplies, and belief in antivaccination conspiracy theories and pseudoscience. We believe that a greater focus on the victimhood-based mindset of historically disadvantaged groups is not only a moral responsibility for contemporary societies, but also a prerequisite to successful confrontation with potential future global challenges, such as pandemic diseases.

ACKNOWLEDGMENT

This work was developed within the project "Language as a Cure: Linguistic Vitality as a Tool for Psychological Well-Being, Health and Economic Sustainability," which is carried out within the team program of the Foundation for Polish Science co-financed by the European Union under the European Regional Development Fund. The work of the second author was supported by the Polish National Science Centre (NCN) grant 2018/31/N/HS6/02875.

REFERENCES

Babińska, M., & Bilewicz, M. (2021). Perceived group control in history and political collective action [Manuscript in preparation].

Bargain, O., & Aminjonov, U. (2020). Trust and compliance to public health policies in times of COVID-19. *Journal of Public Economics*, *192*, 104316. https://doi.org/10.1016/j.jpubeco.2020.104316

Bar-Tal, D., Chernyak-Hai, L., Schori, N., & Gundar, A. (2009). A sense of self-perceived collective victimhood in intractable conflicts. *International Review of the Red Cross*, *91*(874), 229–258. https://doi.org/10.1017/S1816383109990221

Bavel, J., Baicker, K., Boggio, P. S., Capraro, V., Cichocka, A., Cikara, M., Crockett, M. J., Crum, A. J., Douglas, K. M., Druckman, J. N., Drury, J., Dube, O., Ellemers, N., Finkel, E. J., Fowler, J. H., Gelfand, M., Han, S., Haslam, S. A., Jetten, J., . . . Willer, R. (2020). Using social and behavioural science to support COVID-19 pandemic response. *Nature Human Behaviour*, *4*(5), 460–471. https://doi.org/10.1038/s41562-020-0884-z

Biddlestone, M., Green, R., & Douglas, K. M. (2020). Cultural orientation, power, belief in conspiracy theories, and intentions to reduce the spread of COVID-19. *British Journal of Social Psychology*, *59*(3), 663–673. https://doi.org/10.1111/bjso.12397

Bierwiaczonek, K., Kunst, J. R., & Pich, O. (2020). Belief in COVID-19 conspiracy theories reduces social distancing over time. *Applied Psychology: Health and Well-Being*, *12*(4), 1270–1285. https://doi.org/10.1111/aphw.12223

Bilali, R., & Vollhardt, J. R. (2019). Victim and perpetrator groups' divergent perspectives on collective violence: Implications for intergroup relations. *Advances in Political Psychology*, *40*(Suppl. 1), 75–108. https://doi.org/10.1111/pops.12570

Bilewicz, M., Bulska, D., Winiewski, M., & Fritsche, I. (2023). Obedience to authorities is not unconditional: Differential effects of COVID-19 threat on three facets of RWA in Poland and Germany. *Social and Personality Psychology Compass*, *17*(9), e12800. https://doi.org/10.1111/spc3.12800

Bilewicz, M., & Liu, J. (2020). Collective victimhood as a form of adaptation: A world system perspective. In J. Ray Vollhardt (Ed.), *The social psychology of collective victimhood* (pp. 120–140). Oxford University Press. https://doi.org/10.1093/oso/9780190875190.003.0006

Bilewicz, M., Witkowska, M., Pantazi, M., Gkinopoulos, T., & Klein, O. (2019). Traumatic rift: How conspiracy beliefs undermine cohesion after societal trauma? *Europe's Journal of Psychology*, *15*(1), 82. https://doi.org/10.5964/ejop.v15i1.1699

Bundervoet, T., Dávalos, M. E., & Garcia, N. (2021). The short-term impacts of COVID-19 on households in developing countries (Policy Research Working Paper 9582). World Bank. https://doi.org/10.1596/1813-9450-9582

Charlson, F. J., Ommeren, M. V., Flaxman, A. D., Cornett, J. A., Whiteford, H., & Saxena, S. (2019). New who prevalence estimates of mental disorders in conflict settings: A systematic review and meta-analysis. *Lancet*, *394*(10194), 240–248. https://doi.org/10.1016/s0140-6736(19)30934-1

Daud, A., Skoglund, E., & Rydelius, P.-A. (2005). Children in families of torture victims: Transgenerational transmission of parents' traumatic experiences to their children. *International Journal of Social Welfare*, *14*(1), 23–32. https://doi.org/10.1111/j.1468-2397.2005.00336.x

Dong, E., Du, H., & Gardner, L. (2020). An interactive web-based dashboard to track COVID-19 in real time. *Lancet. Infectious Diseases*, *20*(5), 533–534. https://doi.org/10.1016/S1473-3099(20)30120-1

Douglas, K. M. (2021). COVID-19 conspiracy theories. *Group Processes & Intergroup Relations*, *24*(2), 270–275. https://doi.org/10.1177/1368430220982068

Earnshaw, V. A., Eaton, L. A., Kalichman, S. C., Brousseau, N. M., Hill, E. C., & Fox, A. B. (2020). COVID-19 conspiracy beliefs, health behaviors, and policy support. *Translational Behavioral Medicine*, *10*(4), 850–856. https://doi.org/10.1093/tbm/ibaa090

Ehlers, C. L., Gizer, I. R., Gilder, D. A., Ellingson, J. M., & Yehuda, R. (2013). Measuring historical trauma in an American Indian community sample: Contributions of substance dependence, affective disorder, conduct disorder and PTSD. *Drug and Alcohol Dependence*, *133*(1), 180–187. https://doi.org/10.1016/j.drugalcdep.2013.05.011

Imhoff, R., Bilewicz, M., & Erb, H.-P. (2012). Collective regret versus collective guilt: Different emotional reactions to historical atrocities. *European Journal of Social Psychology*, *42*(6), 729–742. https://doi.org/10.1002/ejsp.1886

Jonas, E., & Fritsche, I. (2013). Destined to die but not to wage war: How existential threat can contribute to escalation or de-escalation of violent intergroup conflict. *American Psychologist*, *68*(7), 543. https://doi.org/10.1037/a0033052

Kay, A. C., Whitson, J. A., Gaucher, D., & Galinsky, A. D. (2009). Compensatory control: Achieving order through the mind, our institutions, and the heavens. *Current Directions in Psychological Science*, *18*(5), 264–268. https://doi.org/10.1111/j.1467-8721.2009.01649.x

Kim, S. J., & Bostwick, W. (2020). Social vulnerability and racial inequality in COVID-19 deaths in Chicago. *Health Education & Behavior*, *47*(4), 509–513. https://doi.org/10.1177/1090198120929677

Klar, Y., Schori-Eyal, N., & Klar, Y. (2013). The "never again" state of Israel: The emergence of the Holocaust as a core feature of Israeli identity and its four incongruent voices. *Journal of Social Issues*, *69*(1), 125–143. https://doi.org/10.1111/josi.12007

Kofta, M., Soral, W., & Bilewicz, M. (2020). What breeds conspiracy antisemitism? The role of political uncontrollability and uncertainty in the belief in Jewish conspiracy. *Journal of Personality and Social Psychology*, *118*(5), 900–918. https://doi.org/10.1037/pspa0000183

Liu, J. H., & Hilton, D. J. (2005). How the past weighs on the present: Social representations of history and their role in identity politics. *British Journal of Social Psychology*, *44*(4), 537–556. https://doi.org/10.1348/014466605X27162

Oleksy, T., Wnuk, A., Maison, D., & Łyś, A. (2021). Content matters. Different predictors and social consequences of general and government-related conspiracy theories on COVID-19. *Personality and Individual Differences*, *168*, 110289. https://doi.org/10.1016/j.paid.2020.110289

Pantazi, M., Gkinopoulos, T., Witkowska, M., Klein, O., & Bilewicz, M. (2022). "Historia est magistra vitae"? The impact of historical victimhood on current conspiracy beliefs. *Group Processes & Intergroup Relations*, *25*(2), 581–601. https://doi.org/10.1177/1368430220968898

Skrodzka, M., Sosnowski, P., Bilewicz, M., & Stefaniak, A. (2021). Group identification attenuates the effect of historical trauma on mental health: A study of Iraqi Kurds. *American Journal of Orthopsychiatry*, *91*(6), 693–702. https://doi.org/10.1037/ort0000571

Whaley, A. L. (2001). Cultural mistrust: An important psychological construct for diagnosis and treatment of African Americans. *Professional Psychology: Research and Practice*, *32*(6), 555–562. https://doi.org/10.1037/0735-7028.32.6.555

Wohl, M. J., Branscombe, N. R., & Reysen, S. (2010). Perceiving your group's future to be in jeopardy: Extinction threat induces collective angst and the desire to strengthen the ingroup. *Personality and Social Psychology Bulletin, 36*(7), 898–910. https://doi.org/10.1177/0146167210372505

World Health Organisation (2020, February) *A guide to preventing and addressing social stigma associated with COVID-19.* https://www.who.int/publications/m/item/a-guide-to-preventing-and-addressing-social-stigma-associated-with-covid-19

Taylor, S. (2021). COVID stress syndrome: Clinical and nosological considerations. *Current Psychiatry Reports, 23*, 19. https://doi.org/10.1007/s11920-021-01226-y

Tybur, J. M., Inbar, Y., Aarøe, L., Barclay, P., Barlow, F. K., Barra, M. d., Becker, D. V., Borovoi, L., Choi, I., Choi, J. Y., Consedine, N. S., Conway, A., Conway, J., Conway, P., Adoric, V. C., Demirci, D. E., Fernández, A. I., Marques, R. C., . . . Žeželj, I. (2016). Parasite stress and pathogen avoidance relate to distinct dimensions of political ideology across 30 nations. *Proceedings of the National Academy of Sciences of the United States of America, 113*(44), 12408–12413.

FURTHER READING

Bilali, R., & Vollhardt, J. R. (2019). Victim and perpetrator groups' divergent perspectives on collective violence: Implications for intergroup relations. *Advances in Political Psychology, 40*(Suppl. 1), 75–108. https://doi.org/10.1111/pops.12570

Bilewicz, M., & Liu, J. (2020). Collective victimhood as a form of adaptation: A world system perspective. In J. Ray Vollhardt (Ed.), *The social psychology of collective victimhood* (pp. 120–140). Oxford University Press. https://doi.org/10.1093/oso/9780190875190.003.0006

Pantazi, M., Gkinopoulos, T., Witkowska, M., Klein, O., & Bilewicz, M. (2022). "Historia est magistra vitae"? The impact of historical victimhood on current conspiracy beliefs. *Group Processes & Intergroup Relations, 25*(2), 581–601. https://doi.org/10.1177/1368430220968898

Outcomes After the Pandemic

32

Leadership and the COVID-19 Pandemic

YVONNE STEDHAM AND STEVEN MUELLER ■

The devastation of COVID-19 took the world and its leaders by surprise. The virus spread faster than scientists and government officials could learn about it. It became clear quickly that many people were going to die, while details on how the virus spread remained unknown. All of these unknowns led to uncertainty and hysteria. Many societies around the world cried out for bold leadership to save them.

Crises are an important opportunity to reveal key factors of effective leadership that can affect outcomes, such as how quickly the pandemic ends and how many people perish. In this chapter, we demonstrate that the most successful leaders during the COVID-19 pandemic were able to influence others to forgo their self-interests for communal benefits. This notion of leadership has been labeled in the academic community as transformational leadership.

TRANSFORMATIONAL LEADERSHIP

Leadership research spans various fields, such as management, psychology, political science, and sociology. The existing leadership models are categorized into two groups: transactional and transformational. Transactional leadership models are focused on the leader and grounded on the assumption that the leader's impact depends on an exchange relationship between the leader and a person. These early models identified leader qualities and behaviors to predict leader effectiveness (Judge & Piccolo, 2004). Recognizing that leadership effectiveness could also depend on the situational context, research evolved and produced complex contingency models that were of great theoretical but little practical value.

Yvonne Stedham and Steven Mueller, *Leadership and the COVID-19 Pandemic* In: *The Social Science of the COVID-19 Pandemic*. Edited by: Monica K. Miller, Oxford University Press. © Oxford University Press 2024.
DOI: 10.1093/oso/9780197615133.003.0032

Eventually, leadership scholars completely shifted their focus away from the leader and toward a focus on the followers. It became clear leading is about influencing, and influence involves trust and authentic relationships that go beyond merely "exchange" and "transaction." This shift from transactions to trust and authenticity led to models of leadership referred to collectively as transformational leadership (Bass & Riggio, 2006; Dirks & Ferrin, 2002). These transformational leadership models are at the core of this chapter's conversation about leadership.

What Is Transformational Leadership?

A transformational leader is attentive to the needs and motives of the followers and helps them reach their fullest potential (Judge & Piccolo, 2004). Most importantly, such leaders not only transcend their own self-interest but also inspire others to transcend their self-interest for the benefit of the community.

What Does a Transformational Leader Do?

Four sets of transformational leadership behaviors have been discerned (Avolio et al., 1999; Bass & Riggio, 2006). The first set of behaviors represents *individualized consideration*. Effective leaders truly know and care about each of their followers. Followers know that they play a role in reaching shared goals, that they are important to the "mission." The leader communicates such care by sincerely wanting to know their followers' needs and values. Once identified, transformational leaders respond in a way that honors these needs and values (Bass & Riggio, 2006). As such, interactions with the followers are personalized. Therefore, leaders portraying individualized consideration are empathetic and practice good listening, provide learning opportunities, and delegate tasks to develop follower skills.

The second set of transformational leadership behaviors relates to the leader's ability to be a role model for followers and is referred to as *idealized influence.* The leader is seen as principled—following high ethical standards—and as charismatic (Bass & Riggio, 2006). The leader "walks the talk" and exhibits behavioral consistency, resulting in follower trust and respect for the leader. At the same time, the leader is confident and assertive and takes risks. Based on the desire to emulate the leader who they admire, these characteristics and behaviors shape followers' own values and morality! When a leader reflects individualized consideration and idealized influence, followers know they are valuable and are motivated to act morally.

However, these two behavioral sets are insufficient on their own to motivate followers to act. So, how do transformational leaders motivate followers to act? *Inspirational motivation* behaviors, such as creating team spirit and optimism, enable the leader to communicate meaning or value in the task to the follower.

The inspirationally motivating leader must create a sense of community and a common goal (Bass & Riggio, 2006). In addition to inspirational motivation, an effective transformational leader will *intellectually stimulate* their followers and allow for an environment in which followers can be creative and perform at the top of their ability. Intellectually stimulating behaviors include encouraging followers to question and challenge assumptions, reframe problems, and refrain from criticizing novel ideas (Bass & Riggio, 2006).

LEADERSHIP DURING COVID-19

Right at the start of the COVID-19 pandemic, attempting to reduce uncertainty, worried people began searching for answers to their questions about the disease using any available information sources. The power of today's technology and its impact on information accessibility differentiates the COVID-19 pandemic from any prior crises.

In order to build trust and alleviate uncertainty, timely and transparent communication became a leader's primary task. This task proved to be extremely difficult as much misinformation about COVID-19 was distributed online and created mass confusion (see Chapter 36 for more about COVID-19 and misinformation). Misinformation, information that is false or out of context but presented as fact, was widespread. Intentional misinformation, referred to as disinformation, caused serious harm. Due to a vacuum of factual information regarding the disease, people swarmed to nontraditional sources of information with the hope of learning new information to protect themselves. Disinformation campaigns were intended to divide, place blame, and create chaos and confusion. This led to decreased safety guideline adherence and an environment that perpetuated selfish and destructive behaviors. Misinformation and disinformation became so problematic that the World Health Organization declared that we were fighting an infodemic alongside the COVID-19 pandemic.

This infodemic further intensified the need for leaders who could remain calm and focused, maintain integrity, admit when mistakes were made, and consistently provide relevant and credible information. In the following sections, we first summarize research on leadership during the COVID-19 pandemic and then provide specific examples of leaders to demonstrate the implementation of transformational leadership behaviors and how they potentially affected the outcomes of the COVID-19 pandemic.

COVID-19 Leadership Research: Relevant Findings

The nature of COVID-19, a deadly airborne disease, and its global scope required a level of collaboration and coordination among individual people, organizations, and countries and their governments not seen in over a century. Managing and finding a solution to the pandemic meant prioritization of common interest over self-interest, requiring a shift from self-enhancement to self-transcendence. Therefore, during COVID-19, it became a leader's most important responsibility to get people to understand that the pandemic could only be managed and solved if all people focus on the common interest. This requires an inspirational shift from self-interest toward collaborating and working together (see Chapter 13 for more about self-interest and COVID-19).

The leaders who effectively managed the pandemic did exactly that. To determine how they did this, we reviewed several 2020 peer-reviewed leadership articles regarding the COVID-19 pandemic. The majority of these articles were in medical, public health, healthcare, and management journals. Two primary themes emerged: (1) the need for transparent, frequent, and timely communication and (2) consistent leader behaviors that instilled trust in their followers, fostered collaboration, and built a sense of community. These two themes align with the core transformational leadership behaviors and the unique infodemic-induced requirements.

Nearly all of the articles specifically addressed the value of communication during this crisis. Beilstein et al. (2021) described "good" communication as empathetic, honest, transparent, and understandable; able to build trust; and able to foster resilience. Effective communication should clearly differentiate between assumptions and facts. Information updates and timely redirection are also considered critical. These comments were echoed by Lagowska et al. (2020), who added that leaders should publicly defend their staff and show bounded optimism. The idea of tampered optimism was also mentioned by Crayne and Medeiros (2020), who differentiated between charismatic, ideological, and pragmatic leadership in response to COVID-19, using Angela Merkel (German chancellor) as an example for a pragmatic leader. They quoted Merkel as saying: "It is true that the latest numbers . . . as high as they are, very cautiously give a bit of hope. However, it is definitely too soon to recognize a definite trend." (p. 466). Nicola et al. (2020) emphasized the importance of communication for planning and coordination purposes. They specifically reminded leaders to be mindful of the importance to continually inform, update, and promote its population on the existence of known, proven, and recommended guidelines and interventions to protect the general public and speed recovery. Furthermore, they stressed: "They must refrain from communicating any false or non-evidence-based scientific information that may lead to panic and negative health outcomes."

Collectively, these authors described communication that reflects transformational leadership behaviors. For example, Beilstein et al.'s (2021) description of "good" communication aligns well with *individualized consideration* and *idealized influence*. Similarly, recommended tempered optimism, admission of mistakes, defending staff in public, and repeated emphasis on transparency are examples for *idealized influence*. *Intellectual stimulation* is represented by Nicola et al.'s (2020) assertion that communication needs to be science based and accurate. These types of communications reduce uncertainty and increase trust in the leader, resulting in an increased willingness to follow the leader's recommendations.

Consideration of Longstaff and Yang's (2008) warning is appropriate here. They asserted that all attempts to distribute information were in vain if people do not trust the message or the sender of the message. They suggested that building trust requires repeated and consistent engagement over time. Therefore, leaders who had a "trust deficit" at the start of the pandemic were at a disadvantage regarding communication effectiveness.

The second theme emerging from research on leadership during COVID-19 relates to leader behaviors that instill trust and foster collaboration and a sense of community in followers. Ajzenman et al. (2023) found strong support for the importance of the leader's modeling the expected social distancing behaviors. This "walking-the-talk" behavior had a strong effect on followers' social distancing preferences and is a perfect example of an *idealized influence behavior*. Providing another example for idealized influence, Bleich et al. (2020) found that, as the pandemic started, leaders were clearly held to higher standards and were expected to shift their attention from simply implementing public policy to formulating policy. Several of the articles explicitly addressed *inspirational motivation*, emphasizing the leader's responsibility to get people to collaborate and transcend their self-interest by showing empathy and engaging in self-sacrificing behavior (Haslam et al., 2021; Lagowska et al., 2020; Shingler-Nace, 2020).

Articles on gender differences in COVID-19 leadership showed that women and men differed in their approach. Coscieme et al. (2020) found that countries led by women fared generally better than countries led by men. The reasons mentioned for women's leadership success during the pandemic are that they listened to health experts, they acted quickly if necessary, and they were generally more engaged in social equality and well-being issues. Similarly, Sergent and Stajkovic (2020) concluded that women did a better job, including the female U.S. governors, because they had more empathy and emphasized communal needs. Haslam et al. (2021) integrated those results into their identity leadership framework by focusing on shared identity and considering followers to be partners and thinking of power as power through others rather than power over others. In contrast, however, Windsor et al. (2020) argued that the effectiveness of female leadership was not about gender, but about culture, including cultural attitudes about women in power. Specifically, they found that having a woman leader in power did not make a country fare better during the pandemic unless the country also had the cultural values that supported female leadership. Hence, it was those countries that respected feminine traits such as caring for and nurturing others that fared better.

COVID-19 Leadership Examples

In addition to presenting empirical evidence in support of the effectiveness of transformational leadership during COVID-19, much anecdotal evidence exists. For example, Adam Silver,[1] the commissioner of the National Basketball Association, took the bold and challenging decision to suspend the professional basketball league season on March 11, 2020, the same day the World Health Organization declared COVID-19 a pandemic. This action was early and decisive and sent a message to Americans how serious the situation was, and that safety considerations outweighed the profits of entertainment. By this action, he was *modeling* the importance of transcending self-interest, making money, for the benefit of securing safety. Rachael Bedard,[2] a physician who worked as the senior director of geriatrics and complex-care services at the Rikers Island jail complex in New York City, used Twitter to garner attention to the prison systems' vulnerability to the deadliness of this disease (see Chapter 43 for more on the effects of the pandemic on prisons). Her actions heightened awareness of the dangers COVID-19 brought to the prison system and likely helped bring the concept of depopulating the prison to the forefront of conversations across states as a possible response to reducing spread of the virus among the prison populations. This action exemplifies *individualized consideration* and demonstrates that a transformational leader is concerned with all followers and their needs.

Despite numerous examples of transformational leadership during this time of crisis, we decided to focus on a few leaders that enacted such notable change that lives were impacted for the better because of their transformative prowess. One such leader was Katie Porter, a first-term Democrat House Representative from the state of California. Her actions during COVID-19 led to various headlines, such as "How Rep. Katie Porter, at a Coronavirus Hearing, May Have Saved Your Life" in the *Arizona Republic*[3] to "Katie Porter Grilling the CDC Chief Is the Leadership We Desperately Need" in *GQ*.[4] Katie Porter is a true exemplar of transformational leadership. On March 12, 2021, Katie Porter was provided a 5-minute opportunity to question the director of the Centers for Disease Control and Prevention (CDC), Dr. Robert Redfield, during a House Oversight and Reform Committee hearing. In short, her tenacity, empathy, and preparedness led to free COVID-19 testing for all Americans, regardless of whether citizens had insurance or not.

During this hearing, as well as many other hearings, using her whiteboard and marker, Katie Porter reflects *intellectual stimulation*. She broke down complex issues, questioned assumptions, and clarified otherwise unclear concepts to challenge whoever she was facing during these hearings. Rep. Porter also reflects *individualized consideration*; she was well versed in the role, authority, and responsibilities of the person she was speaking to in order to inspire consequential actions. During her questioning of Dr. Redfield, she came prepared: She had found an obscure federal statute that provided the CDC director the authority to immediately waive the cost of COVID-19 testing for everyone.

Rep. Porter also enacted inspirational motivation and idealized influence. Inspirational motivation was demonstrated through her appeals to both reason and empathy. Through reason, Rep. Porter explained to Dr. Redfield his ability and power to save lives through the statute (42 CFR 71.30). Through empathy, Rep. Porter highlighted the fear many Americans harbored regarding prohibitive costs of testing and obtaining treatment, such as with her statement to Dr. Redfield: "Fear of these costs are going to keep people from being tested, from getting the care they need and from keeping their communities safe." Last, Rep.

Porter demonstrated idealized influence through her tenacity to fight for what was right. When Dr. Redfield's answer was evasive, suggesting his team was looking into the issue, she would reclaim her time and insisted on a response. Dr. Redfield eventually responded: "I think you're an excellent questioner, so my answer is yes." Rep. Porter followed this answer with the following response, speaking to Dr. Redfield and the American people: "Excellent! Everybody in America hear that—you are eligible to go get tested for coronavirus and have that covered, regardless of insurance."

Mike DeWine, the Republican governor of Ohio, also exemplified transformational leadership. Many leaders in the Republican Party rallied against science, safety, and health protocols during this pandemic. Governor DeWine had to face extraordinary challenges to balance support of his party and the lives and well-being of his constituents. In fact, DeWine issued a statement, "Open Letter to Ohioans," urging citizens to put aside their political divisions and rise to higher ground to fight COVID-19. Mike DeWine was the first governor in the country to close schools, based on the advice of scientific leaders, and to declare a state of emergency, which enabled resources for the state to react and respond to the virus more quickly.

Mike DeWine engaged in intellectual stimulation through his actions as one of the first state leaders to start live daily coronavirus updates to keep citizens informed. During these updates, DeWine reflected a sense of calmness and control, announcing new policies while explaining the decisions he and his team made. Governor DeWine would even occasionally use humor as an outreach of human connection and relatability during an incredibly difficult and serious time for all. In a time of misinformation, DeWine even tweeted daily about false rumors regarding COVID-19 to clarify the truths and evidence.

Mike DeWine exhibited individualized consideration by acknowledging that a "one-size-fits-all" model would not work in the state of Ohio. He delegated and requested local leaders, including county commissioners, mayors, local hospital leaders, health commissioners, business and religious leaders, to come together, calling them "COVID defense teams," to develop strategies appropriate for their communities to reduce community spread. In addition to the "Open Letter to Ohioans" initiative, Governor DeWine demonstrated inspirational motivation by regularly reaching out to leaders in areas of high spread, such as in Cuyahoga County, offering to help in any way that was needed. He stated[5]: "We'll bring people together. And we'll just kind of talk and we'll exchange ideas. I'll be there. My team will be there to listen to your concerns, listen to where you need us to help you."

Last, Governor DeWine exhibited idealized influence by serving as a role model and adhering to ethical principles and standards. He regularly wore his mask during press briefings except when he was speaking. When many conservative states were ending their stay-at-home orders, DeWine provided the science-based argument about why these orders were necessary and had to continue. He closely listened to the recommendations of Dr. Amy Acton, who served as the director of the Ohio Department of Health throughout the early months of the pandemic.

Due to conservative opposition to public health safety guidelines, Dr. Acton became the target of the growing animosity of these restrictions. Some of these people began protesting outside of Dr. Acton's home and threatening her and her family's lives. DeWine did not tolerate these attacks, stating: "I'm the elected official who ran for office. I'm the one who makes policy decisions. Members of my Cabinet work hard, but I set the policy." Regarding the threats, he stated: "To bother the family of Dr. Acton, that's not fair game. It's not right. It's not necessary. The buck stops here. I'm the responsible person."

In addition to these examples of exceptional leadership in the United States, there are many leaders who exhibited transformational leadership across the world. The prime minister of New Zealand (Jacinda Ardern) and chancellor of Germany (Angela Merkel) both earned much respect from their citizens due to their competence and transparency. In the middle of March 2020, Ardern provided an 8-minute televised speech, implementing a four-level COVID-19 alert system. This four-level system was familiar to citizens as it was modeled on the fire risk system in New Zealand. This allowed quick clarity regarding the guidelines of how the government would respond and what was expected of citizens. At the time of her speech, there were 52 confirmed cases, and the country was placed at the second alert level. When the confirmed infection rate nearly quadrupled in 4 days, the alert level was raised to the highest level of 4, and the country went into lockdown. Infection rates dropped quickly, even the *Washington Post*[6] headlined an article: "New Zealand Isn't Just Flattening the Curve. It's Squashing It."

In March 2020, Merkel gave a live and unscheduled address. In her speech, she expressed that she trusted Germans to listen to the science and clarified that everyone had a responsibility to follow the recommendations, reflecting intellectual stimulation. By referencing World War II, Merkel reminded the German people that Germany was able to recover from the devastating consequences of the war by working together and persevering. She provided further inspirational motivation when she stated: "I firmly believe that we will pass this test if all citizens genuinely see this as their task." Sentiments like these allowed the country to enter lockdown as a community in solidarity. Last, Merkel demonstrated idealized influence through transparency, sharing what she and the scientific community did and did not know about the virus throughout the pandemic. This level-headed, honest approach provided the German people with a sense of calmness and togetherness during a frightening time.

LESSONS LEARNED: PREVENTING LEADERSHIP FAILURES

One "lesson learned" is that leaders who effectively addressed the pandemic did so by engaging in transformational leadership behaviors. This implies that it may be time to reflect on the potential or current leaders in our organizations, communities, and societies. Would they be the people who could bring their followers together during a crisis? Are they transformational leaders?

A second lesson learned focuses on understanding that leadership during a crisis is about reducing fear and uncertainty through gaining followers' trust. Trust is to believe despite uncertainty (Misztal, 2001) and is defined as the willingness to be vulnerable (Mayer et al., 1995). Therefore, everything a leader says or does has to be evaluated in terms of its potential impact on people's trust in the leader. The specifics learned here are that the four sets of transformational leadership behaviors (individualized consideration, idealized influence, inspirational motivation, and intellectual stimulation) facilitate trust and must be practiced and cultivated.

A third lesson learned involves one of the idealized influence behaviors: modeling the desired behavior. Based on the COVID-19 leadership research and the examples provided in this chapter, it is very clear that it was extremely powerful and important that leaders consistently engaged in the mitigation behaviors they condoned. The lesson learned is to not underestimate the importance of behavioral integrity. Leaders who make promises or statements that are not followed by actions, or leaders who do not "walk the talk," cause permanent damage to trust.

A fourth lesson learned is that the leader's primary task is to reduce uncertainty through providing accurate, frequent, and reliable information. Preempting mis- and disinformation, the leader must stay ahead as the primary source for transparent, relevant, up-to-date information (see Chapter 36 for more on "prebunking" misinformation).

A final lesson learned is that the leader must remember that societal problems can only be solved through collective action. This is quite a challenge for leaders because as they work to inspire their followers to a shared goal, they must address their followers' motivations to act egotistically and based on self-interest out of fear and uncertainty during times of crises. The leader must be the first to demonstrate self-sacrificing behavior in favor of the community and inspire others to also transcend their self-interests for the good of all.

FUTURE RESEARCH: LEADERSHIP PREPAREDNESS

Many strengths and weaknesses in leadership were uncovered through the challenges associated with the pandemic. We encourage scholars to conduct research that supports the development of leaders who are prepared to lead effectively during a crisis such as a pandemic. In the following, we present some general research topics that may shape future research.

How to Recognize People With Transformational Leadership Potential

Although the research on transformational leadership is extensive (Judge & Piccolo, 2004), much of it focuses on the impact of such leadership rather than its antecedents. Charisma, extraversion, and emotional intelligence have been

among the few characteristics studied and shown to be related to transformational leadership or transformational leadership emergence (Barling et al., 2000;
Judge et al., 2002).

Transformational leaders are identified by their behaviors. Bass and Avolio
(2000) developed a leadership assessment tool that includes 36 behavioral
statements, the Multifactor Leadership Questionnaire. This is the standard instrument used in transformational leadership research. The challenge is that currently
there is no proven way to early on identify individuals who may have the potential
to become a transformational leader. This is an obstacle to ensuring that the "right
person is in the right place at the right time." Any research that could provide
insights into transformational leadership predictors would be extremely helpful.

What Are Best Practices for the Development of Transformational Leadership Behavior?

Transformational leaders are effective because they engage in behaviors that gain
followers' trust. These behaviors can be developed. But how are behaviors related
to, for example, idealized influence cultivated? Some interesting research on novel
ways for leadership development has gained momentum, including programs
based on mindfulness and identity (Ibarra, et al., 2010; Kuechler & Stedham,
2018; Stedham & Skaar, 2019).

What Is Unique About Transformational Leadership Communication?

Leadership and communication are intimately intertwined, yet interdisciplinary
research across these two areas is scarce. We encourage collaboration between
scholars to explore how transformational leaders can ensure efficient and effective utilization of the communication technology available today. For example,
Miftari (2018) explained that transformational leadership communication has
undergone rapid changes with social media but failed to elaborate what the specific implications of these changes are.

CONCLUSION

The leadership challenges of the COVID-19 pandemic offered an important opportunity to reveal key factors of effective leadership that have potential to affect
the outcome of the pandemic (e.g., number of deaths). The uncertainty-induced
fear people experienced resulted in unbridled self-interest and called for leaders
who would be able to inspire people to come together and focus on the well-
being of all by engaging in the recommended mitigation processes. Such transformational leaders were able to gain followers' trust by acting with integrity

and transparency, engaging in self-sacrificing behavior, walking the talk, and communicating accurately and frequently. Future research should focus on how the world can be better prepared for the next crisis by having such transformational leaders in place and ready to act.

NOTES

1. https://hbr.org/2020/04/what-good-leadership-looks-like-during-this-pandemic
2. https://fortune.com/worlds-greatest-leaders/2020/rachael-bedard/
3. https://www.azcentral.com/story/opinion/op-ed/ej-montini/2020/03/12/how-rep-katie-porter-covid-19-hearing-may-have-saved-your-life/5039363002/
4. https://www.gq.com/story/katie-porter-grilling-cdc-chief
5. https://www.cleveland.com/open/2020/10/gov-mike-dewines-new-plan-to-encourage-local-leaders-to-make-community-plans-to-cut-coronavirus-spread.html
6. https://www.washingtonpost.com/world/asia_pacific/new-zealand-isnt-just-flattening-the-curve-its-squashing-it/2020/04/07/6cab3a4a-7822-11ea-a311-adb1344719a9_story.html

REFERENCES

Ajzenman, N., Cavalcanti, T., & Da Mata, D. (2023). More than words: Leaders' speech and risky behavior during a pandemic (SSRN 3482908). *American Economic Journal: Economic Policy, 15*(3), 351–371. https://doi.org/10.1257/pol.20210284

Avolio, B. J., Bass, B. M., & Jung, D. I. (1999). Re-examining the components of transformational and transactional leadership using the multifactor leadership. *Journal of Occupational and Organizational Psychology, 72*(4), 441–462. https://doi.org/10.1348/096317999166789

Barling, J., Slater, F., & Kelloway, E. K. (2000). Transformational leadership and emotional intelligence: An exploratory study. *Leadership & Organization Development Journal, 21*(3), 157–161. https://doi-org.unr.idm.oclc.org/10.1108/01437730010325040

Bass, B. M., & Avolio, B. J. (2000). *MLQ: Multifactor Leadership Questionnaire* (2nd ed.). Mind Garden. https://doi.org/10.1037/t03624-000

Bass, B. M., & Riggio, R. E. (2006). *Transformational leadership.* Psychology Press. https://doi.org/10.4324/9781410617095

Beilstein, C. M., Lehmann, L. E., Braun, M., Urman, R. D., Luedi, M. M., & Stüber, F. (2021). Leadership in a time of crisis: Lessons learned from a pandemic. *Best Practice & Research Clinical Anaesthesiology, 35*(3), 405–414. https://doi.org/10.1016/j.bpa.2020.11.011

Bleich, M. R., Smith, S., & McDougle, R. (2020). Public policy in a pandemic: A call for leadership action. *The Journal of Continuing Education in Nursing, 51*(6), 250–252. https://doi.org/10.3928/00220124-20200514-03

Coscieme, L., Fioramonti, L., Mortensen, L. F., Pickett, K. E., Kubiszewski, I., Lovins, H., McGlade, J., Ragnarsdóttir, K. V., Roberts, D., Costanza, R., De Vogli, R., &

Wilkinson, R. (2020). Women in power: Female leadership and public health outcomes during the COVID-19 pandemic. *MedRxiv*, 2020-07. https://doi.org/10.1101/2020.07.13.20152397

Crayne, M. P., & Medeiros, K. E. (2021). Making sense of crisis: Charismatic, ideological, and pragmatic leadership in response to COVID-19. *American Psychologist*, 76(3), 462–474. https://doi.org/10.1037/amp0000715

Dirks, K. T., & Ferrin, D. L. (2002). Trust in leadership: Meta-analytic findings and implications for research and practice. *Journal of Applied Psychology*, 87(4), 611–628. https://doi.org/10.1037/0021-9010.87.4.611

Haslam, S. A., Steffens, N. K., Reicher, S. D., & Bentley, S. V. (2021). Identity leadership in a crisis: A 5R framework for learning from responses to COVID-19. *Social Issues and Policy Review*, 15(1), 35–83. https://doi.org/10.31234/osf.io/bhj49

Ibarra, H., Snook, S., & Guillen Ramo, L. (2010). Identity-based leader development. *Handbook of Leadership Theory and Practice*, 657, 678. https://doi.org/10.5860/choice.48-0370

Judge, T. A., Bono, J. E., Ilies, R., & Gerhardt, M. W. (2002). Personality and leadership: A qualitative and quantitative review. *Journal of Applied Psychology*, 87(4), 765. https://doi.org/10.1037/0021-9010.87.4.765

Judge, T. A., & Piccolo, R. F. (2004). Transformational and transactional leadership: A meta-analytic test of their relative validity. *Journal of Applied Psychology*, 89(5), 755. https://doi.org/10.1037/0021-9010.89.5.755

Kuechler, W., & Stedham, Y. (2018). Management education and transformational learning: The integration of mindfulness in an MBA course. *Journal of Management Education*, 42(1), 8–33. https://doi.org/10.1177/1052562917727797

Lagowska, U., Sobral, F., & Furtado, L. M. G. P. (2020). Leadership under crises: A research agenda for the post-Covid-19 era. *BAR-Brazilian Administration Review*, 17(2), 1–5. https://doi.org/10.1590/1807-7692bar2020200062

Longstaff, P. H., & Yang, S. U. (2008). Communication management and trust: Their role in building resilience to "surprises" such as natural disasters, pandemic flu, and terrorism. *Ecology and Society*, 13(1), Article 3. https://doi.org/10.5751/es-02232-130103

Mayer, R. C., Davis, J. H., & Schoorman, F. D. (1995). An integrative model of organizational trust. *Academy of Management Review*, 20(3), 709–734. https://doi.org/10.5465/amr.1995.9508080335

Miftari, V. (2018). Transformational leadership communication in developing countries' business environment. *Journal of History Culture and Art Research*, 7(2), 259–264.

Misztal, B. A. (2001). Trust and cooperation: the democratic public sphere. *Journal of Sociology*, 37(4), 371–386. https://doi.org/10.1177/144078301128756409

Nicola, M., Sohrabi, C., Mathew, G., Kerwan, A., Al-Jabir, A., Griffin, M., Agha, M., & Agha, R. (2020). Health policy and leadership models during the COVID-19 pandemic—A review. *International Journal of Surgery*, 81, 122–129. https://doi.org/10.1016/j.ijsu.2020.07.026

Sergent, K., & Stajkovic, A. D. (2020). Women's leadership is associated with fewer deaths during the COVID-19 crisis: Quantitative and qualitative analyses of United States governors. *Journal of Applied Psychology*, 105(8), 771–783. https://doi.org/10.1037/apl0000577

Shingler-Nace, A. (2020). COVID-19: When leadership calls. *Nurse Leader*, 18(3), 202–203. https://doi.org/10.1016/j.mnl.2020.03.017

Stedham, Y., & Skaar, T. B. (2019). Mindfulness, trust, and leader effectiveness: A conceptual framework. *Frontiers in Psychology*, *10*, 1588. https://doi.org/10.3389/fpsyg.2019.01588

Windsor, L. C., Yannitell Reinhardt, G., Windsor, A. J., Ostergard, R., Allen, S., Burns, C., Giger, J., & Wood, R. (2020). Gender in the time of COVID-19: Evaluating national leadership and COVID-19 fatalities. *PLoS One*, *15*(12), e0244531. https://doi.org/10.1371/journal.pone.0244531

FURTHER READING

Nohria, N., & Khurana, R. (Eds.). (2010). *Handbook of leadership theory and practice.* Harvard Business Press. https://doi.org/10.5860/choice.48-0370

Northouse, P. G. (2021). *Leadership: Theory and practice.* SAGE Publications.

Schyns, B., & Schilling, J. (2013). How bad are the effects of bad leaders? A meta-analysis of destructive leadership and its outcomes. *The Leadership Quarterly*, *24*(1), 138–158. https://doi.org/10.1016/j.leaqua.2012.09.001

33

Terror Management During and After the COVID-19 Pandemic

DYLAN E. HORNER, ALEX SIELAFF, TOM PYSZCZYNSKI, AND JEFF GREENBERG ▪

In his book *The Plague*, Albert Camus (1947/1975) provides a telling illustration of people's unique way of dealing with their awareness of disease and vulnerability: "Everybody knows that pestilences have a way of recurring in the world; yet somehow we find it hard to believe in ones that crash down on our heads from a blue sky. There have been as many plagues as wars in history; yet always plagues and wars take people equally by surprise" (p. 37). Throughout the COVID-19 pandemic, people around the world were inundated with constant reminders of death. Whether at the forefront of people's focal attention or as a lingering backdrop of death-related concerns, this awareness likely affected most people's attitudes and behaviors during the pandemic. Terror management theory (TMT; Greenberg et al., 1986; Routledge & Vess, 2019) suggests that awareness of the inevitability of death is a unique psychological problem that people manage by employing two distinct systems of defense. During the pandemic, such methods of managing death awareness were put to the test, as myriad personal, social, and political issues disrupted the day-to-day lives of almost everyone and strained systems that people use to keep anxiety at bay. This chapter discusses TMT and its relation to how people responded to the COVID-19 pandemic and the implications of this analysis for understanding postpandemic outcomes and directions for future research.

TERROR MANAGEMENT THEORY

Terror management theory provides a theoretical and empirical framework for understanding how people manage the awareness of death, and this perspective

Dylan E. Horner, Alex Sielaff, Tom Pyszczynski, and Jeff Greenberg, *Terror Management During and After the COVID-19 Pandemic* In: *The Social Science of the COVID-19 Pandemic*. Edited by: Monica K. Miller, Oxford University Press.

could shed light on the diverse attitudes and behaviors people exhibited during the pandemic. Before delving into this issue, this section provides an overview of the theory, highlights key empirical findings, and briefly covers implications of TMT for understanding how virus-related threats affect people's behavior by motivating terror management defenses.

Theoretical Background

Based largely on the work of cultural anthropologist Ernest Becker (1973), TMT posits that humankind's sophisticated cognitive abilities lead to awareness of the inevitability of death, which engenders a potential for debilitating anxiety, referred to as existential terror. As highlighted by Becker, this awareness of mortality can be a potent source of potential existential concern: "What does it mean to be a self-conscious animal? The idea is ludicrous . . . to have emerged from nothing, to have a name, consciousness of self, deep inner feelings, an excruciating inner yearning for life and self-expression—and with all this yet to die" (p. 87). As such, to manage this potential for anxiety, early humans developed cultural worldviews, systems of meaning that imbue life with significance and provide hope of immortality. Cultural worldviews provide conceptions of reality that answer basic questions about life and death, standards for valued behavior, and the promise of literal or symbolic immortality to those who believe in their worldview and live up to its standards. When people live up to these standards, they gain a sense of personal value and enduring significance. In other words, they garner self-esteem, affording them the sense that they are on the path to obtaining their worldview-prescribed immortality—transcending death either literally (e.g., through reincarnation or an afterlife) and/or symbolically (e.g., by living on through one's legacy, family, accomplishments). Close relationships help validate these worldviews and support self-esteem, as well as bolster a sense of legacy through offspring or an extended social group. Thus, in short, maintaining faith in one's cultural worldview, striving toward self-esteem, and maintaining close relationships help defend against the potentially terrifying awareness of mortality.

Three Core Hypotheses

Terror management theory offers three core hypotheses that have guided research to assess its validity (for a review, see Schimel et al., 2019). First, the *mortality salience (MS) hypothesis* states that if certain psychological structures—such as self-esteem, worldviews, and close relationships—serve to shield people from death-related anxieties, then reminders of death (making mortality more salient) should motivate people to cling more strongly to these structures and defend them against threats. Indeed, a large body of research has shown that MS motivates people to uphold and defend their bases of value and meaning. For example, MS increases hostility and aggression toward those with different beliefs; boosts self-esteem striving in worldview-relevant domains; and increases desire for off-spring and efforts to maintain close relationships (for a review, see Routledge & Vess, 2019).

Second, the *anxiety-buffer hypothesis* posits that if certain psychological structures serve to shield people against death awareness, then bolstering or affirming them should reduce death-related anxiety and mitigate defensive responses to MS. For example, high dispositional or experimentally bolstered self-esteem reduces both self-reported and physiological indicators of anxiety in response to threats and prevents MS-induced defensiveness and harm to well-being (e.g., Routledge et al., 2010).

Finally, the *death-thought accessibility (DTA) hypothesis* states that if psycho-logical structures function to buffer against death awareness, then undermining or threatening these structures should increase the accessibility of death-related cognition and bolstering them should reduce such thoughts. Indeed, research has found that threats to self-esteem, worldviews, and close relationships increase DTA, that bolstering these entities reduces DTA, and that the conditions that in-crease DTA are the same conditions that lead to increased worldview defense, self-esteem striving, and commitment to close relationships (for review, see Hayes et al., 2010).

Dual-Process Model of Defense

Terror management theory posits a dual-process model of defense, such that people defend against awareness of death in different ways depending on whether or not death thought is in focal attention. Specifically, the dual-process model suggests that when people are consciously focused on death-related informa-tion, they first engage in pseudorational or problem-solving strategies aimed at minimizing the perceived or actual threat of death. This might entail increasing health-oriented behavior, denying one's vulnerability, or suppressing death-oriented thoughts. These tactics—referred to as *proximal defenses*—enable people to become distracted or psychologically distanced from explicit thoughts of death; that is, they push the problem of death out of current conscious awareness. However, after being removed from focal attention, death thoughts remain cogni-tively accessible, as reflected in a resurgence of DTA following proximal defense. This heightened DTA sets the stage for *distal defenses*, which include efforts to de-fend and affirm one's cultural worldview and self-esteem (for a review, see Kosloff et al., 2019).

TMT Research on Illness-Related Threats

Some previous TMT research has shed light on how virus-related mortality threats impact terror management processes. For instance, Arrowood et al. (2017) found that reminders of Ebola increased DTA, which in turn motivated increased worldview defense. Similarly, Arndt et al. (2007) found that reminders of cancer increased DTA, and Bélanger et al. (2013) found that reminders of the swine flu virus (i.e., H1N1) increased worldview defense. These findings suggest that real-world health threats of mortality can increase DTA and subsequently lead to defensive terror management processes.

TERROR MANAGEMENT DURING THE PANDEMIC

As described above, people manage the potential for anxiety associated with awareness of death through two distinct systems. When death-related thoughts are conscious and in focal attention, people use proximal strategies aimed at minimizing their perceived vulnerability and pushing death into the distant future; when such thoughts are out of focal attention but still cognitively accessible, people instead engage in distal defenses geared toward upholding their worldviews and self-esteem. This section discusses how these two forms of defense were employed during the pandemic.

Proximal Defenses: Managing Conscious Death Thought

When thoughts of death are in focal attention, people attempt to push them out of conscious awareness. Doing so sometimes entails suppressing such thoughts; however, the barrage of virus-related information in the media during the pandemic, as well as changes to people's daily lives due to mandates and safety regulations, made suppressing death thoughts difficult, if not impossible. However, by adhering to prescriptions provided by the medical community, people were able, at least to some extent, to assuage conscious concerns about contracting the virus and potential death. For instance, surveys suggested that over 80% of Americans followed health guidelines to some extent (e.g., practicing social distancing, sheltering in place),[1] and a high prevalence of mask wearing was evident in many regions worldwide.[2] People also altered their daily routines to include additional cleaning and disinfecting procedures, as well as socially distanced or remote activities. These forms of proximal defense afforded the sense that the risk of infection and death can be directly minimized through improved health-oriented behaviors.

Another form of proximal defense observed during the pandemic was the subjective minimization of *perceived* threat; in other words, rather that minimizing the risk of infection, some people trivialized the level of risk posed by COVID-19 itself. For example, some argued that the virus was much less contagious than health experts suggested[3] or that it was only dangerous for elderly individuals or those with other health conditions.[4] Another common strategy was to question the veracity of statistics and other information provided by medical authorities (e.g., arguing that hospitals inflated infection reports for financial reasons or that the media exaggerated the dangers of the disease for political reasons). Indeed, although many Americans changed holiday plans due to COVID-19, a third of adults made little to no adjustments.[5]

Distal Defenses: Managing Nonconscious Death Thought

The proximal defenses noted above helped to alleviate, even if only momentarily, conscious concerns about death and COVID-19. Additionally, although death-related thoughts concerning the virus were pervasive, it is likely that such concerns were not *always* in focal attention but were still highly accessible. Thus, DTA was likely high during the pandemic, and many of the attitudes and behaviors seen during the pandemic were forms of distal defense aimed at managing this nonconscious but accessible death thought. Specifically, people strived to uphold and affirm their worldviews as well as maintain a sense of value and meaning.

One example of such distal defense was the seemingly increased polarization between conservatives and liberals in the United States. For instance, liberals tended to hold more confidence in the scientific community[6] and viewed COVID-19 as much more dangerous than conservatives.[7] Such divergence in attitudes likely represented an attempt to manage the backdrop of DTA due to the pandemic. Moreover, previous research has found that death awareness motivates both liberals and conservatives to respond in politically oriented ways, defending values and positions consistent with their respective ideological orientations (e.g., Kosloff et al., 2010). In this vein, partisan defenses during the pandemic extended beyond dealings with the virus and likely intensified concerns with other social issues and increased the motivation for things such as protests in support of the Black Lives Matter movement among many liberals[8] and claims of fraud in results of the 2020 presidential election among many conservatives.[9]

Aside from politically oriented defenses, people strived to maintain a sense of meaning and value in their lives in other ways as well. Given that the pandemic hampered many people's bases of self-worth and meaning—such as financial goals, career pursuits, and social connections—finding new ways to derive value and meaning from life was important. People accomplished this by engaging in new hobbies, redesigning social events to sustain meaningful relationships (e.g., online get-togethers), striving toward important goals through new modalities (e.g., online schooling, socially distanced exercising), and working together to prevent the spread of the virus. For example, celebrities exemplified and promoted safety measures such as staying at home and wearing masks,[10] and people banded together on social media to promote handwashing and social distancing. Through such behaviors, a "new norm" of safety measures emerged that was embraced by some and actively rejected and protested by others; as noted above, political orientation was a powerful predictor of which side of this issue people embraced.

Though the distinction between proximal and distal defenses is an important one, people's responses to the pandemic showed that the attitudes and values that make up people's worldviews, and are thus usually associated with distal defenses, can affect proximal defenses. The prominent role that political ideology played in people's willingness to take precautions to reduce the spread of the virus showed that distal defenses sometimes affect the specific forms that proximal defenses take. It could be that this was especially likely to occur during the COVID-19 pandemic because politicians and pundits politicized the virus and promoted different ideas about how people should respond. In addition, the ubiquitous nature of the pandemic and its consequences, and the fact that so many aspects of life were affected by it, could have made it a frequent topic of people's thoughts and conversations and thus a likely domain for distal defenses to play out.

TERROR MANAGEMENT AFTER THE PANDEMIC: LESSONS LEARNED AND MOVING FORWARD

Death-related concerns were dramatically brought to people's attention during the pandemic, and myriad personal, social, and political issues emerged that likely threatened people's worldviews and self-esteem during a time when the protection these entities usually provided was needed more than ever. In addition to the many terror management defenses seen during the pandemic, postpandemic functioning will likely continue to be shaped by such forces. This section explores how various postpandemic outcomes can be understood through a terror management perspective.

Proximal Defenses: Avoiding Threats and Maintaining Health

As noted above, the pandemic highlighted distinct differences in how people proximally defended against the threat of COVID-19. One possibility following the pandemic is that the high death toll will underpin the importance of emphasizing the seriousness of specific future threats, and people's responses to such threats might be more proactive rather than dismissive. Some research has found that—regardless of being primed with MS, COVID-19, or a control topic—those who viewed COVID-19 as a serious issue reported relatively high intentions to engage in healthy behaviors (e.g., handwashing, mask wearing, social distancing). However, for those who viewed COVID-19 as a less serious threat, whose intentions for health-promoting behavior were low, brief contemplation of their thoughts about COVID-19 and how it would affect them increased their health behavior intentions and to a level not different from those who viewed the virus as more serious (Horner et al., 2023). These findings suggest that encouraging people to contemplate how a disease could affect them could help motivate people who are prone to minimize such threats to endorse intentions for healthier behavior more strongly.

Distal Defenses: Maintaining Purpose and Defending Meaning

During the pandemic, people's day-to-day lives were disrupted, and their worldviews and sources of self-esteem were strained. After the pandemic, people will likely be motivated to reinstate a sense of structure to their lives, as well as reaffirm a sense of personal value and meaning. These distal defenses will help people keep death-related anxiety at bay after the COVID-19 pandemic, and it will be important that such defenses can encompass benevolent and prosocial values.

PERCEIVED ORDER AND STRUCTURE

The pandemic introduced uncertainty to people's lives, and issues that once seemed clearly defined were put into disarray and uncertainty. In addition, proximal defenses were often at odds with distal defenses. For example, lockdowns to curtail the spread of the virus (proximal defense) disrupted people's careers and abilities to provide for themselves and their families (distal defense). Another example was that, although health experts adamantly emphasized the importance of staying at home and engaging in measures to prevent the spread of COVID-19, there was also a simultaneous effort to encourage advocacy for police reform and racial justice through protesting in large gatherings.[11] As a result of these conflicting forces, clear and structured conceptions of what people deemed "good" or "right" were strained.

From a terror management perspective, clear conceptions of the world help to quell death-related anxieties because they help to minimize ambiguity and offer a sense of consistency needed to maintain faith in people's terror-assuaging worldviews. Given that the pandemic threatened many people's conceptions of the world, some people might be motivated to reinstate a sense of order, especially those high in personal need for structure (PNS). Previous research has found that MS motivates worldview defense and greater preference for just-world interpretations among those high in PNS; in contrast, MS leads those low in PNS toward creativity and openness to nontraditional ideas (e.g., Landau et al., 2004; Routledge & Juhl, 2012). Thus, varying proclivities for structure will likely impact how people navigate the milieu of social and personal unrest after the pandemic, and this postpandemic functioning might be improved by promoting a sense of structure that simultaneously encompasses prosocial values, benevolence, and openness to constructive change.

INGROUP DEFENSE

Another issue during the pandemic was avoidance of perceived outgroups. For instance, research found that MS led U.S. participants during the pandemic to rate American takeout food as safer to eat relative to other cuisine, including Chinese food (McCabe & Erdem, 2021). Even worse, the linking of the pandemic to China, with terms like "Chinese virus," led to a dramatic increase in hate crimes against Asians and Asian Americans.[12] These actions mirror prior TMT research finding that death awareness leads to not only more favorable evaluations of domestic rather than foreign products but also increased racism and stereotyping (e.g., Jonas et al., 2005; Schimel et al., 1999).

Thus, one issue following the pandemic might be continued avoidance or derogation of perceived outgroups. People will be rebuilding disrupted lives following the death of friends and family, changes in or loss of employment, and isolation from valued close others. The resulting backdrop of death thought due to these undermined psychological buffers could heighten the need for distal terror management defenses to uphold one's ingroup. Thus, it might be important to emphasize a sense of widely shared collective experience following the pandemic, such that people expand their ingroup to include a wider array of people and can consequently buffer against this heightened DTA in more prosocial ways.

Research has found that emphasizing shared experiences and goals can reduce hostile reactions to reminders of death. A series of studies by Motyl et al. (2011) found that MS decreased prejudice and increased tolerance when participants were prompted to recall memories or view activities that they shared with people from other cultures. In a related vein, Pyszczynski et al. (2012) found that, when one's ingroup was expanded to encompass humanity (e.g., by considering global climate change rather than a more localized issue), MS increased support for peacemaking and decreased support for defensive militaristic action in ongoing conflicts. Accordingly, postpandemic strides toward more encompassing worldviews and greater interconnectedness with others could help facilitate intergroup cooperation.

WORK AND CAREER DOMAINS

As people adjust to postpandemic life, many will continue to be unemployed or will be navigating changes in their jobs and careers. For example, many people will return to in-person duties and work longer shifts; others will remain at home or work remotely; and others will have modified workloads and routines. In any case, people striving for a sense of value in their work and career might face many barriers. It will therefore be important for them to have supports in place to either help them find jobs after the pandemic or feel competent and cared for in their current employment (e.g., peer support from colleagues, administrative efforts toward employee well-being). Indeed, during the pandemic, death anxiety was tied to higher psychological distress among nonworking people (Shakil et al., 2022). Research has also found that MS increases people's desire to work, and that imagining employment for a cherished job prevents MS-induced DTA and defensiveness (Yaakobi, 2015).

DISRUPTED SOURCES OF MEANING

Anxiety buffer disruption theory (ABDT; Pyszczynski & Kesebir, 2011), a clinically oriented extension of TMT that deals specifically with trauma, could provide insight for the more extreme end of the spectrum for postpandemic outcomes. This perspective suggests that post-traumatic stress disorder (PTSD) could be a result of a person experiencing something so traumatic that it shatters their worldview, resulting in a disrupted anxiety buffer system and the adoption (implicitly or explicitly) of the perspective that nothing can protect them. ABDT research (for a review, see Pyszczynski & Kesebir, 2011) has shown that people who went through a traumatizing experience who either had a PTSD diagnosis or had vulnerability factors for PTSD did not display typical terror management responses to reminders of death, and this effect was found in diverse countries, including Iran, the Ivory Coast, Poland, and the United States. More recent work (Vail et al., 2018) found that affirming participants' worldviews prevented typical MS-induced DTA, but only for those low in post-traumatic stress symptoms. That is, those high in post-traumatic stress symptoms did not experience any palliative effects of self-affirmation, suggesting that their anxiety buffer was not functioning effectively.

These findings suggest that, for some people, pandemics might sufficiently challenge assumptions of their worldviews regarding the safety and benevolence of the world to the point that their anxiety buffers are rendered ineffective, leaving them vulnerable to increased death-related cognition and psychological distress. Thus, after the pandemic, it will be especially important for therapeutic treatments to focus on restoring effective anxiety buffer functioning for those severely affected by COVID-19 experiences.

POTENTIAL DIRECTIONS FOR FUTURE RESEARCH

People's day-to-day lives were changed due to COVID-19 and will continue to be different in many ways after the pandemic. Moving forward, researchers should consider the significant impact that the pandemic has had on people's lives and conduct research to help understand long-term outcomes that could follow. This section offers some potential directions for future research to increase understanding of these issues.

Individual and Personal Outcomes

One striking shift in people's lives during the pandemic was the inability or difficulty to gather with others. Initially, public gatherings were prohibited and then later strictly regulated, resulting in an abrupt disruption of social interactions that are important bases for people's sense of personal worth and meaning. Some adapted to these changes and managed to maintain social interactions, albeit through online communications and virtual gatherings and parties. Future research might explore the extent to which these online relationships afford a sense of meaning, whether they do this as well as in-person interactions, and whether different online platforms are more useful in this regard.

Another shift that occurred for many people during the pandemic was the development of new sources of meaning and self-worth. For example, people developed new hobbies (e.g., bread making, reading, art, poetry, yoga) and shared these interests with others, either through socially distanced activities or through social media and online platforms. Such activities might have provided people with a renewed sense of value and meaning in life, and some people might continue to pursue these interests long after the pandemic. Research could explore whether certain pressures or individual differences were predictive of people's search for meaning through new pursuits; identify what types of activities people maintain after the pandemic and how this impacts well-being; and investigate the extent to which people have integrated these changes with other duties, jobs, and relationships. Such research might help reveal what types of changes are likely to occur (and for whom) during stressful periods like a pandemic, and this would be useful in helping people prepare for and manage death-related concerns in the future.

Political and Social Outcomes

As the pandemic was unfolding, an intense focus on social and economic injustice was triggered by the death of George Floyd[13] and other related tragedies. Although some of the responses to these incidents involved looting and vandalism, there was also a large effort through peaceful protests and organized demonstrations to advocate for police reform and accountability. One avenue for future research will be to investigate whether these ideals and related values (e.g., diversity, inclusion, equity) become integrated broadly into people's worldviews and whether people uphold these issues in the years to come. Previous research has found that when prosocial values—such as pacifism, benevolence, and tolerance—are viewed as culturally important, MS leads people to uphold these values in their attitudes and behaviors (e.g., Jonas et al., 2008). As topics like diversity, equity, and accountability move to the forefront of social movements and political campaigns, people across the globe could find ways to meaningfully contribute to such causes and gain a sense of purpose and value. Future research might explore the conditions and individual differences that predict support for these values.

CONCLUSION

The COVID-19 pandemic heightened people's awareness of mortality and led to various proximal and distal defenses aimed at managing death-related anxieties and concerns. TMT offers a framework for understanding how postpandemic functioning could entail further defenses to support health and sustain perceptions of personal value and meaning. Future research should explore how such defenses are maintained, how proximal and distal defenses can work together rather than be in opposition to each other, and whether certain attitudes and behaviors provide more psychological equanimity than others for managing death thought after the pandemic.

NOTES

1. https://www.axios.com/coronavirus-social-distancing-lockdown-polling-7c27d86f-bb4b-4cbf-aedf-cfdd26799fd1.html
2. https://socialdatascience.umd.edu/global-trends-of-mask-usage-in-19-million-adults/
3. https://news.harvard.edu/gazette/story/2020/10/what-caused-the-u-s-anti-science-trend/
4. https://theprint.in/health/covid-19-mainly-kills-old-people-so-do-most-other-diseases/416931/
5. https://www.pewresearch.org/fact-tank/2020/12/22/as-cdc-warned-against-holiday-travel-57-of-americans-say-they-changed-thanksgiving-plans-due-to-covid-19/
6. https://www.pewresearch.org/science/2020/05/21/trust-in-medical-scientists-has-grown-in-u-s-but-mainly-among-democrats/
7. https://news.gallup.com/poll/311408/republicans-skeptical-covid-lethality.aspx?utm_source=alert&utm_medium=email&utm_content=morelink&utm_campaign=syndication
8. https://www.pewsocialtrends.org/2020/06/12/amid-protests-majorities-across-racial-and-ethnic-groups-express-support-for-the-black-lives-matter-movement/
9. https://time.com/5926883/trump-supporters-storm-capitol/
10. https://www.usmagazine.com/celebrity-news/pictures/celebrities-take-precautions-during-coronavirus-outbreak-pics/
11. https://www.politico.com/news/magazine/2020/06/04/public-health-protests-301534
12. https://www.usatoday.com/story/news/nation/2021/02/27/asian-hate-crimes-attacks-fueled-covid-19-racism-threaten-asians/4566376001/
13. https://www.nytimes.com/2020/05/31/us/george-floyd-investigation.html

REFERENCES

Arndt, J., Cook, A., Goldenberg, J. L., & Cox, C. R. (2007). Cancer and the threat of death: The cognitive dynamics of death-thought suppression and its impact on behavioral health intentions. *Journal of Personality and Social Psychology*, *92*(1), 12–29.http://dx.doi.org/10.1037/0022-3514.92.1.12

Arrowood, R. B., Cox, C. R., Kersten, M., Routledge, C., Shelton, J. T., & Hood, R. W., Jr. (2017). Ebola salience, death-thought accessibility, and worldview defense: A terror management theory perspective. *Death Studies*, *41*(9), 585–591.https://doi.org/10.1080/07481187.2017.1322644

Becker, E. (1973). *The denial of death*. Free Press.

Bélanger, J. J., Faber, T., & Gelfand, M. J. (2013). Supersize my identity: When thoughts of contracting swine flu boost one's patriotic identity. *Journal of Applied Social Psychology*, *43*, 153–155. https://doi.org/10.1111/jasp.12032

Camus, A. (1947/1975). *The plague* (S. Gilbert, Trans.). Vintage Books.

Greenberg, J., Pyszczynski, T., & Solomon, S. (1986). The causes and consequences of a need for self-esteem: A terror management theory. In R. F. Baumeister (Ed.), *Public self and private self* (pp. 189–212). Springer.

Hayes, J., Schimel, J., Arndt, J., & Faucher, E. H. (2010). A theoretical and empirical review of the death-thought accessibility concept in terror management research. *Psychological Bulletin*, *136*(5), 699–739. http://dx.doi.org/10.1037/a0020524

Horner, D. E., Sielaff, A., Pyszczynski, T., & Greenberg, J. (2023). The role of perceived level of threat, reactance proneness, political orientation, and coronavirus salience on health behavior intentions. *Psychology & Health*, *38*(5), 647–666. https://doi.org/10.1080/08870446.2021.1982940.

Jonas, E., Fritsche, I., & Greenberg, J. (2005). Currencies as cultural symbols—An existential psychological perspective on reactions of Germans toward the euro. *Journal of Economic Psychology*, *26*(1), 129–146. https://doi.org/10.1016/j.joep.2004.02.003

Jonas, E., Martens, A., Kayser, D. N., Fritsche, I., Sullivan, D., & Greenberg, J. (2008). Focus theory of normative conduct and terror-management theory: The interactive impact of mortality salience and norm salience on social judgment. *Journal of Personality and Social Psychology*, *95*(6), 1239–1251. https://doi.org/10.1037/a0013593

Kosloff, S., Anderson, G., Nottbohm, A., & Hoshiko, B. (2019). Proximal and distal terror management defenses: A systematic review and analysis. In C. Routledge & M. Vess (Eds.), *Handbook of terror management* (pp. 31–63). Elsevier Academic Press.

Kosloff, S., Greenberg, J., Weise, D., & Solomon, S. (2010). The effects of mortality salience on political preferences: The roles of charisma and political orientation. *Journal of Experimental Social Psychology*, *46*(1), 139–145.https://doi.org/10.1016/j.jesp.2009.09.002

Landau, M. J., Johns, M., Greenberg, J., Pyszczynski, T., Martens, A., Goldenberg, J. L., & Solomon, S. (2004). A function of form: Terror management and structuring the social world. *Journal of Personality and Social Psychology*, *87*(2), 190–210.http://dx.doi.org/10.1037/0022-3514.87.2.190

McCabe, S., & Erdem, S. (2021). The influence of mortality reminders on cultural in-group versus out-group takeaway food safety perceptions during the COVID-19 pandemic. *Journal of Applied Social Psychology*, *51*(4), 363–369. https://doi.org/10.1111/jasp.12740

Motyl, M., Hart, J., Pyszczynski, T., Weise, D., Maxfield, M., & Siedel, A. (2011). Subtle priming of shared human experiences eliminates threat-induced negativity toward Arabs, immigrants, and peace-making. *Journal of Experimental Social Psychology*, *47*, 1179–1184. https://doi.org/10.1016/j.jesp.2011.04.010

Pyszczynski, T., & Kesebir, P. (2011). Anxiety buffer disruption theory: A terror management account of posttraumatic stress disorder. *Anxiety, Stress, & Coping*, *24*(1), 3–26.https://doi.org/10.1080/10615806.2010.517524

Pyszczynski, T., Motyl, M., Vail, K. E., Hirschberger, G., Arndt, J., & Kesebir, P. (2012). Drawing attention to global climate change decreases support for war. *Peace and Conflict: Journal of Peace Psychology*, *18*(4), 354–368.http://dx.doi.org/10.1037/a0030328

Routledge, C., & Juhl, J. (2012). The creative spark of death: The effects of mortality salience and personal need for structure on creativity. *Motivation and Emotion*, *36*, 478–482.https://doi.org/10.1007/s11031-011-9274-1

Routledge, C., Ostafin, B., Juhl, J., Sedikides, C., Cathey, C., & Liao, J. (2010). Adjusting to death: The effects of mortality salience and self-esteem on psychological well-being, growth motivation, and maladaptive behavior. *Journal of Personality and Social Psychology*, *99*(6), 897–916. http://dx.doi.org/10.1037/a0021431

Routledge, C., & Vess, M. (2019). *Handbook of terror management.* Elsevier Academic Press.

Schimel, J., Hayes, J., & Sharp, M. (2019). A consideration of three critical hypotheses. In C. Routledge & M. Vess (Eds.), *Handbook of terror management* (pp. 1–30). Elsevier Academic Press.

Schimel, J., Simon, L., Greenberg, J., Pyszczynski, T., Solomon, S., Waxmonsky, J., & Arndt, J. (1999). Stereotypes and terror management: Evidence that mortality salience enhances stereotypic thinking and preferences. *Journal of Personality and Social Psychology, 77*(5), 905–926. http://dx.doi.org/10.1037/0022-3514.77.5.905

Shakil, M., Ashraf, F., Muazzam, A., Amjad, M., & Javed, S. (2022). Work status, death anxiety and psychological distress during COVID-19 pandemic: Implications of the terror management theory. *Death Studies, 46*(5), 1100–1105. https://doi.org/10.1080/07481187.2020.1865479

Vail, K. E., Morgan, A., & Kahle, L. (2018). Self-affirmation attenuates death-thought accessibility after mortality salience, but not among a high post-traumatic stress sample. *Psychological Trauma: Theory, Research, Practice, and Policy, 10*(1), 112–120.http://dx.doi.org/10.1037/tra0000304

Yaakobi, E. (2015). Desire to work as a death anxiety buffer mechanism. *Experimental Psychology, 62*(2), 110–122. https://doi.org/10.1027/1618-3169/a000278

FURTHER READING

Greenberg, J., Vail, K., & Pyszczynski, T. (2014). Terror management theory and research: How the desire for death transcendence drives our strivings for meaning and significance. In A. J. Elliot (ed.), *Advances in motivation science* (Vol. 1, pp. 85–134). Elsevier Academic Press.

Pyszczynski, T., Lockett, M., Greenberg, J., & Solomon, S. (2021). Terror management theory and the COVID-19 pandemic. Journal of Humanistic Psychology, *61*(2), 173–189.https://doi.org/10.1177/0022167820959488

Solomon, S., Greenberg, J., & Pyszczynski, T. (2015). The worm at the core: On the role of death in life. Random House.

Vail, K. E., Juhl, J., Arndt, J., Vess, M., Routledge, C., & Rutjens, B. T. (2012). When death is good for life: Considering the positive trajectories of terror management. *Personality and Social Psychology Review, 16*(4), 303–329. https://doi.org/10.1177/1088868312440046

34

Harnessing Moral Cognition to Save Lives

JUSTIN F. LANDY AND ALEXANDER D. PERRY ■

Research has clearly shown the importance of public health behaviors (PHBs) like mask wearing and social distancing for limiting the spread of COVID-19 and thus limiting negative outcomes (e.g., minimizing the number of lives lost to the disease; IHME COVID-19 Forecasting Team, 2021). Although a Harris poll from October 2020 found that 90% of Americans wore a mask at least "sometimes" when they were outside their home, only 61% reported "always" doing so, and these numbers were notably higher than in previous polls.[1] Moreover, a Gallup poll from the same time showed that people have engaged in *less* social distancing behavior as the pandemic has progressed.[2] Thus, despite the importance of PHBs in minimizing the death toll of the pandemic, many people had not fully embraced these behaviors. In other words, lives have been needlessly lost, and will continue to be, due to people not engaging in PHBs. Our focus here is to offer theory-related suggestions on how to minimize negative pandemic outcomes.

We think that part of why people have not fully embraced PHBs is because of the messaging surrounding them. In particular, we think that the messaging surrounding PHBs has not been informed by what is known about how people think about moral issues and therefore has not motivated people to engage in PHBs as effectively as it could have (see Chapters 10 and 14 for treatments of nonmoral aspects of messaging in the pandemic). We draw on research on moral cognition and identify three ways in which messaging promoting PHBs could be improved. We argue that people will be more persuaded by messages encouraging them to engage in PHBs that (a) highlight risks to people of all ages; (b) draw attention to specific, identifiable, victims; and (c) use tailored moral messaging. Granted, implementing these suggestions is not likely to be effective in persuading people who doubt the existence of COVID-19, so these suggestions are aimed less toward persuading those people and more toward persuading people who acknowledge

Justin F. Landy and Alexander D. Perry, *Harnessing Moral Cognition to Save Lives* In: *The Social Science of the COVID-19 Pandemic*. Edited by: Monica K. Miller, Oxford University Press. © Oxford University Press 2024.
DOI: 10.1093/oso/9780197615133.003.0034

the pandemic, but need to be prompted to engage in PHBs. This chapter raises new questions for basic and applied research in moral psychology, provides actionable strategies for promoting PHBs in this pandemic and future public health crises, and highlights the importance of understanding how people think about morality for minimizing negative outcomes during the pandemic.

MISTAKES MADE IN MORAL MESSAGING

Moral psychology is an interdisciplinary field that empirically studies how people think about ethical issues. Although the COVID-19 pandemic is a public health crisis, we argue that it also has clear moral aspects to it. The pandemic has required people to sacrifice their own desires and freedoms in order to promote the greater good to an extent unparalleled in recent memory. In fact, because engaging in PHBs (in particular mask wearing) is primarily aimed at protecting *others* from the virus, deciding whether to do so is arguably as much a moral decision as it is a health decision. Therefore, we suggest that one way to effectively encourage people to engage in PHBs is to appeal to their morals. Indeed, messaging promoting PHBs has frequently emphasized moral reasons for engaging in them, usually that mask wearing and social distancing can save other people's lives.[3,4] This emphasis on moral concerns is reasonable, as merely conceiving of an attitude as rooted in one's moral values can align a person's behavior with that attitude (Luttrell et al., 2016). This suggests that the more a person sees their attitude toward PHBs as being related to their moral values, the more likely they are to act in accordance with that attitude. Unfortunately, messaging surrounding PHBs has not been sufficiently informed by insights from moral psychology and might not be motivating people as effectively as it could. In this portion of our chapter, we identify three well-known principles from the study of moral cognition that could be harnessed to motivate engagement in PHBs and identify examples of how, so far, they have *not* been harnessed effectively.

People Value Younger Lives More Than Older Lives

The risk of dying from COVID-19 is much greater for the elderly than for other age groups (Centers for Disease Control and Prevention [CDC], 2023).[5] Of course, the risk of dying for younger people is nonzero and increases if they have preexisting chronic health conditions.[6] We are just beginning to understand the deleterious long-term effects of the virus on younger patients who do not die,[7] but it is clear that the virus is most lethal for older people. This is probably why much of the messaging surrounding the consequences of the COVID-19 pandemic has focused on the risks it poses to older people.[8,9,10]

However, a great deal of research indicates that people do not value all human lives equally. In particular, less moral value is placed on the lives of elderly people than the lives of younger people (see, e.g., Cropper et al., 1994; Dolan et al., 2005;

Goodwin & Landy, 2014; Johannesson & Johansson, 1997; Lewis & Charny, 1989; Li et al., 2010; Ratcliffe, 2000; Rodríguez & Pinto, 2000; Tsuchiya et al., 2003). Indeed, this is even true among older people themselves, indicating that this pattern of valuing lives is quite general and widespread, at least in Western societies (Busschbach et al., 1993; Li et al., 2010). Thus, the people with the highest risk of death from the pandemic are precisely the people whose continued survival is least valued by society. This could decrease willingness to engage in PHBs. For instance, people strongly prefer to act to save the life of a 10-year-old child rather than a 70-year-old adult (Goodwin & Landy, 2014). Therefore, by highlighting that PHBs mainly protect older people, messaging might not engage with people's moral concerns, which are primarily directed toward the young.

People Are Moved by Identifiable Victims, Not Statistics

Much of the messaging about the COVID-19 pandemic has highlighted grim statistics about the number of confirmed cases and the number of deaths due to the virus.[11,12,13] The reason for this emphasis on numbers seems obvious: The numbers are staggering. As of early 2021, the U.S. CDC (2021) reported over 28 million total cases and over 500,000 total deaths in the United States, and the World Health Organization (2021) reported over 115 million confirmed cases and 2.5 million deaths worldwide. Intuitively, the presentation of numbers like this should encourage people to engage in PHBs to protect themselves and others.

The problem with this intuitive view is that a great deal of research has shown that people are moved more by specific, salient victims than they are by statistics. This "identifiable victim effect" has been extensively studied in the domain of charitable giving, and the findings are extremely consistent: People give more money to help a single, identified victim than they do to help victims who are not identified (Lee & Feeley, 2016). There seem to be many reasons for this (Jenni & Loewenstein, 1997; Kogut & Ritov, 2011), but one important one is that identifiable victims elicit stronger emotional responses (i.e., empathy) than unidentified, "statistical victims" (Small & Loewenstein, 2003; Small et al., 2007).

Relatedly, people do not seem to fully recognize differences between large numbers of statistical victims, especially when there is a rapid increase in the numbers, a phenomenon known as *scope neglect* (Baron & Greene, 1996; Fetherstonhaugh et al., 1997). In a particularly famous study, three groups of participants were asked how much of a tax increase they would be willing to accept in order to save endangered birds (Desvousges et al., 1993). One group was told the tax would save 2,000 birds, another, 20,000 birds, and a third, 200,000 birds. The mean responses were $80, $78, and $88, respectively. Thus, multiplying the number of birds to be saved by 10 had little to no effect on participants' willingness to pay to save them. Thus, people are primarily moved by specific, identifiable victims and do not respond very differently to very different numbers of statistical victims.

People Differ in Which Moral Values Motivate Them

As noted above, much of the moral messaging around PHBs has emphasized that they can save other people's lives. For many of us, minimizing the horrific outcomes of the pandemic is *the* central moral concern in this crisis. However, this "one-size-fits-all" approach to moral messaging may not be equally effective at motivating everyone. According to a theoretical framework known as Moral Foundations Theory, political liberals and conservatives possess different constellations of values (see Chapter 37 in this volume for more on this theory). Liberals primarily concern themselves with care (i.e., preventing harm to all other people) and fairness, and conservatives show greater concern for loyalty to ingroups like one's family and nation, respect for legitimate authority, and bodily and sexual purity. This claim has received considerable empirical support (see, e.g., Graham et al., 2009; Haidt & Graham, 2007; Landy, 2016).

Moreover, research on another theoretical approach, the Model of Moral Motives, has shown that liberals are more prescriptive in their moral motives (i.e., they focus on promoting desirable behaviors in the interest of social justice), and conservatives are more proscriptive in their moral motives (i.e., they focus on restraining undesirable behaviors in the interest of social order). Again, this claim has received considerable support (see Janoff-Bulman et al., 2008, 2009).

Moral messaging promoting PHBs has generally emphasized the potential to save the lives of anonymous strangers by engaging in desirable PHBs. Whereas liberals are likely to be moved by appeals of this sort, given the importance they place on preventing harm to everyone and on promoting desirable behaviors, conservatives could find these appeals to be less persuasive. Indeed, both public opinion polls[14,15] and academic research (Makridis & Rothwell, 2020; Nowlan & Zane, 2022) have found that liberals are more likely than conservatives to engage in PHBs like mask wearing and social distancing. There are probably many reasons for this, but one contributing factor could be that messaging encouraging these behaviors is aligned more closely with liberals' morality than conservatives' morality. Given these differences in moral values and motivations across the political spectrum, messaging on PHBs could have different persuasive effects depending on how the message is framed. Tailoring moral messages to fit different groups' unique moralities is known as "moral reframing"; we return to how this strategy could be effective in the context of the COVID-19 pandemic below.

LESSONS LEARNED: HOW TO IMPROVE PANDEMIC-RELATED MORAL MESSAGING

Thus far, we have seen that, although much messaging promoting PHBs has tried to appeal to people's morals, it has often done so in ways that are misguided and disconnected from insights from moral psychology. Specifically, messaging has

(a) focused on risks to older people, whose lives are less valued than younger people; (b) emphasized statistics rather than identifiable victims; and (c) primarily appealed to the morality of political liberals by making prescriptive appeals about preventing harm to anonymous strangers. We now propose potential remedies to each of these mistakes, rooted in prior research. The remedies we propose have not been directly tested in the context of pandemics before (with the exception of one preliminary result relating to identifiable victims; see Draw Attention to Specific, Identifiable Victims), meaning that they also generate testable hypotheses for future research. Specifically, we argue that messaging about PHBs should (a) highlight risks to people of all ages; (b) draw attention to specific, identifiable victims; and (c) use tailored moral messaging. These suggestions are rooted in prior research on how people value lives, the identifiable victim effect, and scope neglect, and moral foundations theory, the model of moral motives, and moral reframing, respectively.

Highlight Risks to People of All Ages

As reviewed above, people place greater value on the continued survival of younger, rather than older, people. Therefore, in addition to informing the public about risks to older people, pandemic-related messaging should also emphasize that the virus poses serious risks of death or long-term complications to young people as well. Drawing attention to these risks could increase people's motivation to act to save lives (i.e., their willingness to engage in PHBs).

The prediction that emphasizing risks to younger people will increase willingness to engage in PHBs like mask wearing and social distancing in a pandemic has not been directly tested, but it is consistent with prior research. For instance, Vietri et al. (2012) found that participants were more willing to be vaccinated against influenza when doing so protected more people from contracting the disease, even if they were not at risk themselves (i.e., if they could spread the virus as carriers but were themselves immune to its symptoms). That is, when faced with situations where they could *do more good*, people were more willing to vaccinate themselves to help others. Of course, this study did not directly test the prediction above for several reasons. First, it dealt with influenza, which is a less contagious and less deadly disease than COVID-19; COVID-19 killed more people in 2020 than influenza has since 2016.[16] Second, the study examined intentions to vaccinate, which is a one-and-done (or two-and-done, in some cases) behavior, rather than willingness to engage in PHBs like mask wearing and social distancing, which must be adhered to consistently whenever one is in public. Third and most importantly, this study did not examine the effect of the ages of the people to be helped. But, the research reviewed above shows that people place greater value on younger people's continued survival. Thus, we expect that when people are thinking about how their behavior can benefit younger people, not just the elderly, they will think about this in the same way that they think about protecting more people in Vietri et al.'s (2012) study: as *doing more good*. Therefore, they will be more willing to engage in behaviors including not only vaccination, but also everyday PHBs. Directly testing this prediction is of the utmost importance for future research on messages encouraging PHBs.

Draw Attention to Specific, Identifiable Victims

As reviewed, people are more moved by identifiable victims than they are by statistical victims. This suggests that, in the context of the COVID-19 pandemic, people will react more strongly to a single, identifiable person who is at risk from the disease than they will to statistical information. Simply put, people probably do not see 500,000 deaths due to COVID-19 as all that much worse than 50,000 deaths or even 5,000 deaths. So, continuously presenting people with statistics of this sort is unlikely to increase willingness to engage in PHBs. Instead, we suggest that harnessing the power of the identifiable victim effect could be a viable way to increase compliance with PHBs. If people are presented with a particular, sympathetic victim of the pandemic, the empathy they feel for this person could motivate them to wear masks and social distance.

This prediction seems reasonable in light of the research on charitable giving reviewed in this chapter so far. Insofar as altering one's usual routine by wearing a mask or social distancing is perceived as a "cost" to be paid to help someone else, in the same way that a charitable donation is, then willingness to pay this cost would likely be increased when attention is drawn to an identifiable victim rather than bland statistics. Indeed, one recent study found that drawing attention to identifiable, vulnerable people at risk from the pandemic increased behavioral intentions to engage in social distancing, compared to a control message that just reminded people to engage in social distancing, though no condition with statistical victims was included (Lunn et al., 2020). Another recent project showed that framing messages in terms of identifiable (as compared to statistical) victims increased donations to help those affected by the pandemic (van Esch et al., 2021). Most directly, a very recent study found a small effect of drawing attention to identifiable (vs. statistical) victims on reported intentions to engage in PHBs, though this effect was overwhelmed by an effect of participants' preexisting philosophical beliefs (Byrd & Białek, 2021). However, considering that it is easier to adjust messaging than it is to change deep-rooted ethical principles, we still consider emphasizing identifiable victims to be important when designing messages aimed at promoting PHBs.

Use Tailored Moral Messaging

We have pointed out already that political liberals and conservatives differ in their moral values and motives and in the rates at which they engage in PHBs. Specifically, it is known that conservatives value loyalty, respect for authority, and purity more than liberals, whereas liberals primarily value care and fairness (Graham et al., 2009), and that conservatives are more proscriptive in their moral motives, while liberals are more prescriptive in their moral motives (Janoff-Bulman et al., 2008). Because the moral foundation of care and prescriptive morality involve behaviors that help others by alleviating their suffering or advancing their well-being, it is not surprising that people who emphasize this value and motive would be more likely to engage in PHBs. Thus, current messaging aligns more with the morality of liberals, which might partially explain why they engage in PHBs more than conservatives.

So, what are we to do about this political divide? We think that developing tailored moral messaging that promotes PHBs using the language of conservative morality could increase willingness to engage in these behaviors among conservatives. In particular, we think that appealing to conservative moral concerns with loyalty is likely to be more effective than just focusing on care. Instead of highlighting that PHBs can save the lives of anonymous strangers, messages could emphasize that they can save the lives of one's family, and that people need to "do their part" for the good of their nation. Messages emphasizing that engaging in PHBs is part of being a member of important ingroups (e.g., one's family and one's nation) might be more persuasive to conservatives than current messages are. Similarly, messages that are framed proscriptively as opposed to prescriptively will be more effective at persuading conservatives.

These predictions are rooted in previous research on "moral reframing." Simply put, when a position is framed as being consistent with one's moral values, one becomes more accepting of the position and the person advocating it. For instance, conservatives expressed greater support for universal healthcare (a typically liberal political position) after reading an argument for it framed in terms of purity (a conservative value) rather than fairness (a liberal value). Similarly, liberals expressed greater support for increased military spending (a typically conservative political position) when an argument for it was framed in terms of fairness rather than loyalty and authority (Feinberg & Willer, 2015). Moral reframing has similarly been shown to moderate support for political candidates (Voelkel & Feinberg, 2018) and has been applied speculatively to increasing support for environmental causes (Rottman et al., 2015).

To our knowledge, moral reframing has not been applied to increasing support for PHBs. But, given that it has successfully increased support for universal healthcare among conservatives, we think it is reasonable to predict that it could also increase support for PHBs. A patriotic image of Uncle Sam (appealing to loyalty and patriotism) wearing a face mask reminding people "don't leave home without it" (a proscriptive appeal) would likely be much more effective at motivating conservatives than current messaging, which tends to use prescriptive language and emphasize protecting anonymous strangers. Testing this prediction would extend prior research on moral reframing to the context of the pandemic and provide another method for encouraging PHBs.

CONCLUSION

There is no doubt that the COVID-19 pandemic is a moral crisis as much as a medical one, and that engaging in PHBs is as much (or more) about unselfishly helping others as it is about protecting oneself. Unfortunately, much of the messaging surrounding the pandemic has not been sufficiently informed by insights from moral psychology and has therefore been less effective at promoting PHBs like mask wearing and social distancing than it could have been. We have offered three suggestions for improving this messaging: highlight risks to people of all ages; draw attention to specific, identifiable, victims; and use tailored moral messaging. The first suggestion draws on research showing that people place greater moral value on saving the lives of younger people rather than older people. The second is rooted in research showing that people are more moved by, and more willing to incur costs to help, identifiable victims than statistical victims. The final suggestion derives from research showing that liberals and conservatives differ in their moral values and motives, and that presenting arguments that are congruent with the target audience's morality can increase support for political positions. We have hypothesized that following these suggestions will lead to increased intentions to engage in PHBs and thus more actual compliance. Although these predictions have (for the most part) not yet been directly tested, they are rooted in considerable prior research. So, we think that implementing these suggestions should not be delayed until after these predictions have been empirically verified. Indeed, we think that the people who craft messages about the pandemic—the media, politicians, community leaders, and scientific authorities—would do well to take these suggestions to heart and design messages that are likely to engage and motivate as many people as possible. We speculate that the most effective messages might combine all three of these suggestions by drawing attention to a young, identifiable victim and tailoring the message's language to the moral values and motives of the target audience.

Notably, the suggestions we have presented here are unlikely to be effective in persuading people who believe that COVID-19 is a hoax, or similar conspiracy theories, to engage in PHBs. Conspiratorial thinking is an active and fascinating area of research (see, e.g., Alper et al., 2021; Swami et al., 2014), but falls outside the scope of this chapter. Our suggestions are likely to be most effective at promoting PHBs among people who accept that the pandemic is real but need to be motivated to do their part to fight it.

In summary, the present chapter presents actionable, empirically grounded recommendations for people crafting messages about the pandemic, generates new research hypotheses for basic and applied psychology research, and highlights the importance of informing public messaging with insights from the study of moral cognition. By drawing on these insights and properly designing messages to harness them, we might just be able to save more lives, both in this pandemic, and future crises.

NOTES

1. https://consumer.healthday.com/infectious-disease-information-21/coronavirus-1008/mask-use-by-americans-now-tops-90-37-poll-finds-762360.html
2. https://news.gallup.com/poll/322064/americans-social-distancing-habits-tapered-july.aspx
3. https://www.cnn.com/2020/06/01/health/review-masks-social-distancing-covid-19-wellness/index.html
4. https://www.cnn.com/2020/06/12/health/coronavirus-mask-wellness-trnd/index.html
5. https://www.statnews.com/2020/03/30/what-explains-coronavirus-lethality-for-elderly/
6. https://www.nytimes.com/2020/12/16/opinion/covid-deaths-young-adults.html
7. https://www.nbcnews.com/health/health-news/young-people-are-risk-severe-covid-19-illness-n1240761
8. https://wwmt.com/news/coronavirus/covid-19-data-shows-elderly-minorities-most-at-risk-in-michigan
9. https://www.tampabay.com/news/health/2020/07/21/covid-cases-among-floridas-elderly-continue-to-soar/
10. https://www.medicalnewstoday.com/articles/the-impact-of-the-covid-19-pandemic-on-older-adults
11. https://www.heart.org/en/news/2020/12/16/covid-19-is-the-big-story-in-mortality-statistics-but-not-the-only-one
12. https://www.cnn.com/2020/11/12/health/coronavirus-fall-surge-statistics/index.html
13. https://www.bbc.com/news/world-51235105
14. https://news.gallup.com/poll/315590/americans-face-mask-usage-varies-greatly-demographics.aspx
15. https://consumer.healthday.com/infectious-disease-information-21/coronavirus-1008/mask-use-by-americans-now-tops-90-37-poll-finds-762360.html
16. https://www.cnn.com/2020/10/06/health/flu-covid-19-deaths-comparison-trnd/index.html

REFERENCES

Alper, S., Bayrak, F., & Yilmaz, O. (2021). Psychological correlates of COVID-19 conspiracy beliefs and preventive measures: Evidence from Turkey. *Current Psychology, 40*, 5708–5017. http://dx.doi.org/10.1007/s12144-020-00903-0

Baron, J., & Greene, J. (1996). Determinants of insensitivity to quantity in valuation of public goods: Contribution, warm glow, budget constraints, availability, and prominence. *Journal of Experimental Psychology: Applied, 2*(2), 107–125. http://dx.doi.org/10.1037/1076-898X.2.2.107

Busschbach, J. J. V., Hessing, D. J., & De Charro, F. T. (1993). The utility of health at different stages in life: A quantitative approach. *Social Science & Medicine, 37*(2), 153–158. http://dx.doi.org/10.1016/0277-9536(93)90451-9

Byrd, N., & Białek, M. (2021). Your health vs. my liberty: Philosophical beliefs dominated reflection and identifiable victim effects when predicting public health recommendation compliance during the COVID-19 pandemic. *Cognition, 212,* 104649. https://doi.org/10.1016/j.cognition.2021.104649

Centers for Disease Control and Prevention (CDC). (2023). COVID-19 risks and information for older adults. https://www.cdc.gov/aging/covid19/index.html

Centers for Disease Control and Prevention (CDC). (2021). COVID data tracker. https://covid.cdc.gov/covid-data-tracker/#cases_casesinlast7days

Cropper, M. L., Aydede, S. K., & Portney, P. R. (1994). Preferences for life saving programs: How the public discounts time and age. *Journal of Risk and Uncertainty, 8,* 243–265. http://dx.doi.org/10.1007/BF01064044

Desvousges, W. H., Johnson, F. R., Dunford, R. W., Boyle, K. J., Hudson, S. P., & Wilson, K. N. (1993). Measuring natural resource damages with contingent valuation: Tests of validity and reliability. In J. A. Hausman (Ed.), *Contingent valuation: A critical assessment* (pp. 91–159). Elsevier. http://dx.doi.org/10.1016/B978-0-444-81469-2.50009-2

Dolan, P., Shaw, R., Tsuchiya, A., & Williams, A. (2005). QALY maximisation and people's preferences: A methodological review of the literature. *Health Economics, 14*(2), 197–208. http://dx.doi.org/10.1002/hec.924

Feinberg, M., & Willer, R. (2015). From gulf to bridge: When do moral arguments facilitate political influence? *Personality and Social Psychology Bulletin, 41*(12), 1665–1681. http://dx.doi.org/10.1177/0146167215607842

Fetherstonhaugh, D., Slovic, P., Johnson, S. M., & Friedrich, J. (1997). Insensitivity to the value of human life: A study of psychophysical numbing. *Journal of Risk and Uncertainty, 14,* 283–300. https://doi.org/10.1023/A:1007744326393

Goodwin, G. P., & Landy, J. F. (2014). Valuing different human lives. *Journal of Experimental Psychology: General, 143*(2), 778–803. http://dx.doi.org/10.1037/a0032796

Graham, J., Haidt, J., & Nosek, B. A. (2009). Liberals and conservatives rely on different sets of moral foundations. *Journal of Personality and Social Psychology, 96*(5), 1029–1046. http://dx.doi.org/10.1037/a0015141

Haidt, J., & Graham, J. (2007). When morality opposes justice: Conservatives have moral intuitions that liberals may not recognize. *Social Justice Research, 20*(1), 98–116. http://dx.doi.org/10.1007/s11211-007-0034-z

IHME COVID-19 Forecasting Team. (2021). Modeling COVID-19 scenarios for the United States. *Nature Medicine, 27*(1), 94–105. http://dx.doi.org/10.1038/s41591-020-1132-9

Janoff-Bulman, R., Sheikh, S., & Baldacci, K. G. (2008). Mapping moral motives: Approach, avoidance, and political orientation. *Journal of Experimental Social Psychology, 44*(4), 1091–1099. https://doi.org/10.1016/j.jesp.2007.11.003

Janoff-Bulman, R., Sheikh, S., & Hepp, S. (2009). Proscriptive versus prescriptive morality: Two faces of moral regulation. *Journal of Personality and Social Psychology, 96*(3), 521–537. https://doi.org/10.1037/a0013779

Jenni, K., & Loewenstein, G. (1997). Explaining the identifiable victim effect. *Journal of Risk and Uncertainty, 14,* 235–257. https://doi.org/10.1023/A:1007740225484

Johannesson, M., & Johansson, P.-O. (1997). Is the valuation of a QALY gained independent of age? Some empirical evidence. *Journal of Health Economics, 16*(5), 589–599. http://dx.doi.org/10.1016/S0167-6296(96)00516-4

Kogut, T., & Ritov, I. (2011). The identifiable victim effect: Causes and boundary conditions. In D. M. Oppenheimer & C. Y. Olivola (Eds.), *The science of giving: Experimental approaches to the study of charity* (pp. 133–145). Psychology Press.

Landy, J. F. (2016). Representations of moral violations: Category members and associated features. *Judgment and Decision Making, 11*(5), 496–508.

Lee, S., & Feeley, T. H. (2016). The identifiable victim effect: A meta-analytic review. *Social Influence, 11*(3), 199–215. http://dx.doi.org/10.1080/15534510.2016.1216891

Lewis, P. A., & Charny, M. (1989). Which of two individuals do you treat when only their ages are different and you can't treat both? *Journal of Medical Ethics, 15*(1), 28–34. http://dx.doi.org/10.1136/jme.15.1.28

Li, M., Vietri, J., Galvani, A. P., & Chapman, G. B. (2010). How do people value life? *Psychological Science, 21*(2), 163–167. http://dx.doi.org/10.1177/0956797609357707

Luttrell, A., Petty, R. E., Briñol, P., & Wagner, B. C. (2016). Making it moral: Merely labeling an attitude as moral increases its strength. *Journal of Experimental Social Psychology, 65*, 82–93. http://dx.doi.org/10.1016/j.jesp.2016.04.003

Lunn, P. D., Timmons, S., Belton, C. A., Barjaková, M., Julienne, H., & Lavin, C. (2020). Motivating social distancing during the COVID-19 pandemic: An online experiment. *Social Science and Medicine, 265*, 113478. https://doi.org/10.1016/j.socscimed.2020.113478

Makridis, C., & Rothwell, J. T. The real cost of political polarization: Evidence from the COVID-19 pandemic (2020, June 29). SSRN. https://ssrn.com/abstract=3638373; http://dx.doi.org/10.2139/ssrn.3638373

Nowlan, L., & Zane, D. M. (2022). Getting conservatives and liberals to agree on the COVID-19 threat. *Journal of the Association for Consumer Research, 7*(1), 72–80. http://dx.doi.org/10.1086/711838

Ratcliffe, J. (2000). Public preferences for the allocation of donor liver grafts for transplantation. *Health Economics, 9*(2), 137–148. http://dx.doi.org/10.1002/(SICI)1099-1050(200003)9:2%3C137::AID-HEC489%3E3.0.CO;2-1

Rodríguez, E., & Pinto, J. L. (2000). The social value of health programmes: Is age a relevant factor? *Health Economics, 9*(7), 611–621. https://doi.org/10.1002/1099-1050(200010)9:7<611::AID-HEC540>3.0.CO;2-R

Rottman, J., Keleman, D., & Young, L., (2015). Hindering harm and preserving purity: How can moral psychology save the planet? *Philosophy Compass, 10*(2), 134–144. http://dx.doi.org/10.1111/phc3.12195

Small, D. A., & Loewenstein, G. (2003). Helping *a* victim or helping *the* victim: Altruism and identifiability. *Journal of Risk and Uncertainty, 26*, 5–16. https://doi.org/10.1023/A:1022299422219

Small, D. A., Loewenstein, G., & Slovic, P. (2007). Sympathy and callousness: The impact of deliberative thought on donations to identifiable and statistical victims. *Organizational Behavior and Human Decision Processes, 102*(2), 143–153. https://doi.org/10.1016/j.obhdp.2006.01.005

Swami, V., Voracek, M., Stieger, S., Tran, U. S., & Furnham, A. (2014). Analytic thinking reduces belief in conspiracy theories. *Cognition, 133*(3), 572–585. http://dx.doi.org/10.1016/j.cognition.2014.08.006

Tsuchiya, A., Dolan, P., & Shaw, R. (2003). Measuring people's preferences regarding ageism in health: Some methodological issues and some fresh evidence. *Social Science & Medicine, 57*(4), 687–696. http://dx.doi.org/10.1016/S0277-9536(02)00418-5

van Esch, P., Cui, Y., & Jain, S. P. (2021). The effect of political ideology and message frame on donation intent during the COVID-19 pandemic. *Journal of Business Research*, *125*, 201–213. https://doi.org/10.1016/j.jbusres.2020.12.040

Vietri, J. T., Li, M., Galvani, A. P., & Chapman, G. B. (2012). Vaccinating to help ourselves and others. *Medical Decision Making*, *32*(3), 447–458. http://dx.doi.org/10.1177/0272989X11427762

Voelkel, J. G., & Feinberg, M. (2018). Morally reframed arguments can affect support for political candidates. *Social Psychological and Personality Science*, *9*(8), 917–924. http://dx.doi.org/10.1177/1948550617729408

World Health Organization. (2021). WHO coronavirus disease (COVID-19) dashboard. https://covid19.who.int/

FURTHER READING

Day, M. V., Fiske, S. T., Downing, E. L., & Trail, T. E. (2014). Shifting liberal and conservative attitudes using moral foundations theory. *Personality and Social Psychology Bulletin*, *40*(12), 1559–1573. http://dx.doi.org/10.1177/0146167214551152

Feinberg, M., & Willer, R. (2019). Moral reframing: A technique for effective and persuasive communication across political divides. *Social and Personality Psychology Compass*, *13*(12), e12501. http://dx.doi.org/10.1111/spc3.12501

Janoff-Bulman, R., & Carnes, N. C. (2013). Surveying the moral landscape: Moral motives and group-based moralities. *Personality and Social Psychology Review*, *17*(3), 219–236. http://dx.doi.org/10.1177/1088868313480274

Small, D. A. (2015). On the psychology of the identifiable victim effect. In I. G. Cohen, N. Daniels, & N. Eyal (Eds.), *Identified versus statistical lives: An interdisciplinary perspective* (pp. 13–23). Oxford University Press. http://dx.doi.org/10.1093/acprof:oso/9780190217471.003.0002

35

A Failure of Fear

Liabilities of Looseness During COVID-19

MICHELE J. GELFAND, XINYUE PAN, AND ALEX LANDRY ■

In early 2020, as COVID-19 spread across the globe, it became clear that, although countries were universally affected by the pandemic, their ability to manage it was highly variable. Countries like the United States, Italy, and Brazil had far more cases and deaths per million as compared to China, Singapore, and South Korea, which were better able to contain the virus. Such variation is surely determined by multiple factors, including differences in government responses, demographics, and economic vulnerabilities. Here, we focus on *cultural liabilities* that affected countries responses during COVID-19, with a specific focus on the strength of social norms, or cultural tightness-looseness (for discussions of other cultural factors that affected COVID-19 outcomes, see Chapter 16 this volume, and Ashraf, 2021; Bazzi et al. 2021; Fernandez-Perez et al., 2021; Frey et al., 2020; Huynh, 2020; Lu et al., 2021; Ozkan et al., 2021; Salvador et al., 2020; Wang, 2021). The central thesis that we expound on in this chapter is that tightening social norms during a collective threat is an adaptive evolutionary response. Yet some cultures, particularly loose ones, were slower to tighten, creating what we call a *cultural evolutionary mismatch*. We discuss how the threat signal that typically facilitates tightening during threat was misperceived and/or manipulated in loose cultures, which resulted in worse health outcomes (i.e., COVID-19 cases and deaths) as of late fall 2020 (see Chapter 25 of this volume for more on health disparities). We conclude with a discussion of how to prevent these global health disparities in future pandemics.

THE EARLY WARNINGS

In March 2020, we began to worry about cultural liabilities during COVID-19. In an op-ed we wrote in the *Boston Globe*, we warned: "To survive the coronavirus,

Michele J. Gelfand, Xinyue Pan, and Alex Landry, *A Failure of Fear* In: *The Social Science of the COVID-19 Pandemic*. Edited by: Monica K. Miller, Oxford University Press. © Oxford University Press 2024. DOI: 10.1093/oso/9780197615133.003.0035 we need to tighten up. It is not just about medicine. It is about culture" (Gelfand, 2020a). Indeed, as the virus began to spread across the globe and in our home country of the United States, we already witnessed highly divergent reactions. In the United States, we saw conflicting, unstandardized, and uncoordinated responses and even hoarding and egocentric behavior. Universities and public schools were reluctant to cancel classes, and testing efforts remained slow, cumbersome, and haphazard (Gelfand, 2020a). Meanwhile, in China and South Korea, people were more organized and swiftly began to abide by new physical distancing measures and mask wearing to contain the virus. While there are many differences between these countries, we reasoned that they could be due, in part, to differences in cultural norms that pre-dated the pandemic.

The gist is this: All cultures have social norms or unwritten rules for social behavior.

We abide by dress codes, discipline our kids, and do not cut in line not because these are legislative codes but because they help our society function. Social norms, in fact, are one of humans' greatest inventions: They help us predict our behavior and coordinate in unprecedented ways as compared to our animal cousins. But researchers have shown that some cultures abide by social norms quite strictly; they are *tight*. Others are *loose*—with a more relaxed attitude toward rule breakers. While this distinction was discussed many decades ago by anthropologists (Pelto, 1968), it was recently found to explain variation in modern societies. Specifically, in our study of 33 nations, we found that countries such as China, Singapore, South Korea, Norway, Germany, and Austria tended to veer tighter, while countries such as Brazil, Spain, the United States, Italy, and Greece tended to veer looser. Moreover, variation in tightness-looseness was tied to cultures' histories of social and ecological threat. As compared with loose cultures, tight cultures tended to have higher historical rates of natural disasters, disease prevalence, resource scarcity, and invasions. From an evolutionary perspective, following rules can help groups to survive chaos and crisis. On the flip side, looser groups that have faced fewer threats can thus afford to be more permissive. These patterns were later replicated in nonindustrial societies (Jackson, et al., 2020) and among different regions in the United States (Harrington & Gelfand, 2014) and China (Chua et al., 2019). To be sure, not all tight cultures have had a chronic threat and not all loose cultures have experienced chronic safety. Moreover, threat is not the only predictor of tightness. For example, Talhelm and English (2020) found that societies that rely on rice farming, which requires a high level of coordination, were tighter than those that relied on wheat farming, which enables more flexibility. Cultures low on mobility also tend to be tighter (Harrington & Gelfand, 2014; Thomson et al., 2018). On the other hand, cultures that have diversity and norms for debate evolve to be looser (Gelfand, 2018).

Notably, neither tight nor loose is inherently better or worse. As groups tighten to deal with coordination needs, they also experience a number of trade-offs associated with *order* versus *openness*. In particular, tight cultures tend to have more order—that is, more monitoring and less crime (Gelfand et al., 2011); more uniformity (Gelfand, 2018); higher self-regulation (e.g., less debt, alcoholism, and obesity; Gelfand, 2018); and a preference for strong, independent leaders (Aktas et al., 2016)—but lower levels of openness. By contrast, loose cultures tend to have less order but more openness, that is, less prejudice toward stigmatized groups (Jackson et al., 2019), higher creativity (Chua et al., 2015), higher openness to change (De et al., 2017), and a preference for visionary team leaders (Aktas et al., 2016; see Chapter 32 of this volume for more on leadership during the pandemic). In a sense, one's culture's strengths can be another's liability and vice-a-versa (see Figure 35.1).

This naturally raised the question: During a global pandemic, which requires large-scale cooperation and coordination, would tight cultures have an advantage given that they are used to sacrificing liberty for rules to deal with collective threat? Alternatively, a lot of our own research suggested that *all* cultures naturally tighten when there is a collective threat. In another op-ed published in *The Hill*, we raised this distinct optimistic possibility—namely, that we have tightened temporarily during threats in the past, like during 9/11 (Gelfand, 2020b). Indeed, our own research was supportive of that view. In a number of experimental studies, we "primed" collective threats, such as natural disasters, terrorism, or disease—and found that people were more likely to desire tight norms as compared to control conditions (see Chapter 39 for more on collective response to the pandemic). For example, in one study, participants were randomly assigned to read a school newspaper article about a terrorist threat warning system that was being implemented at either one's own university or another university in a different country. We found that participants who were primed with threats to their own territory had a stronger desire to punish social norm violators and showed more ethnocentric attitudes (Gelfand & Lun, 2013). Likewise, people who reported

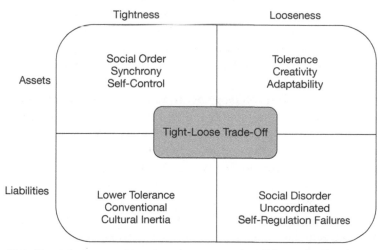

Figure 35.1 The tight-loose order versus openness trade-off. [From "Cultural Evolutionary Mismatches in Response to Collective Threat," by M. J. Gelfand, 2021, *Current Directions in Psychological Science, 30*(5), p. 402 (https://doi.org/10.1177/096372 14211025032). Copyright 2021 by the Author(s)].

feeling threatened—whether from natural disasters, terrorism, pathogens, debt, immigration, an attack from North Korea or Iran—also desired greater tightness, as found in other field studies (Jackson et al., 2019).

Our evolutionary game theory (EGT) models also found that, as threat increased, agents rapidly cooperated and coordinated and also punished agents who defected. For example, Roos et al. (2015) varied levels of threat in the environment and examined its impact on the evolution of tightness. Threat was implemented by subtracting a certain amount from everyone's payoff, which resembles the idea that threat reduces people's resources. They found that different degrees of norm strength were evolutionarily adaptive to different levels of threat. Specifically, in a society with higher threat, the population evolved to be tighter: There were more contributions to the group tasks and more responsible punishment toward the norm violators. These models have also shown that temporary increases in objective threat caused norm strength to increase until the threat subsided. These results were also replicated when the agents were put in a scenario in which they needed to *coordinate* to gain high payoffs, for example, two cars driving toward each other needed to coordinate which side of the road to take. In the coordination game, there are two options of behaviors—Action A and Action B. Either action is equally likely to become the norm at the beginning, but once one norm has emerged, agents who do the opposite of the majority will become norm violators. Again, in our models, a higher threat level led to the evolution of more coordination and norm enforcers. These results indicated that different levels of cultural tightness naturally adapted to different levels of ecological threat.

Despite the insights from these models and experiments, they are limited in two fundamental ways. First, the threat in these EGT models and experiments was *clear and objective*—in other words, the threat signal was easy to see. But COVID-19 was a more abstract threat, and it was invisible, which, unlike 9/11 or warfare, could be easier to ignore and reduce the associated tightening response. Second, and relatedly, our models did not examine whether some groups responded *faster* than others to collective threat. Was it possible that loose cultures take longer to tighten than tight ones?

Our computer science-psychology began to develop new simulations to test this in March 2020. We reasoned that given that looseness is an evolutionary adaptation to low-threat environments, if the level of threat in the environment increased fast within a short period, loose cultures may show an *evolutionary mismatch*. The concept of evolutionary mismatch, which originated in evolutionary biology, refers to the idea that traits that evolved in organisms in one environment can be highly disadvantageous in a different environment. Evolutionary mismatch theory has been applied to diverse human phenomena, including obesity, drug addiction, and gambling, among other topics, as reviewed in the excellent book, *Mismatch* by Ronald Giphart and Mark van Vugt (2018). Here we started to think about how this concept may relate to cultural vulnerabilities during a collective threat. Could the loose traits, which are great for innovation and tolerance, be a hindrance in coping with a collective threat like COVID-19?

To examine this, we first developed an agent-based model and compared the change of cooperative behavior in tight versus loose cultures when they encountered an increasing threat (Gelfand et al., 2021). In our model, agents were embedded in a social network and decided whether to conduct a behavior that was costly to perform but would lead to a higher payoff for others (i.e., a cooperative behavior). Such a game generally reflects scenarios in the COVID-19 pandemic, where people can perform a costly behavior to benefit others, such as wearing a mask or self-quarantining. We then created two kinds of populations: One represented a tight culture where the agents faced strong pressure to conform with the major behavior in the neighborhood. The other represented a loose culture where the agents faced little pressure to conform. We then increased the level of threat in the environment gradually as in Roos et al. (2015) and compared the agents' reactions to threat in tight versus loose cultures. As seen in Figure 35.2, we found that as threat escalated, agents in both tight and loose cultures became more cooperative. However, and tellingly, compared with tight cultures, loose cultures were much slower to react to the threat escalation and ultimately had lower cooperation and survival rates. In another model we created, we found compared with tight cultures, loose cultures again reacted to the threat slower and, as a result, ultimately had a higher level of threat. These results suggested that looseness may be a liability during times of collective threat (Pan et al., 2020).

Computational models, of course, are wonderful at examining cultural dynamics but they are limited in having overly simplifying assumptions and only examining artificial agents. So as COVID-19 continue to spread, we began to collect data to examine whether cultures were naturally tightening and whether tighter cultures were better able to limit COVID-19 cases and deaths. In one large-scale study, we capitalized on data that we had collected on tight-loose in 57 countries prior to the pandemic. We quickly organized the team to collect data again on tight-loose right after the pandemic hit in early March through June 2020 (Andrighetto et al., 2023). The data found that, while all nations increased their handwashing rates, there was very little change in reported tightness. If anything,

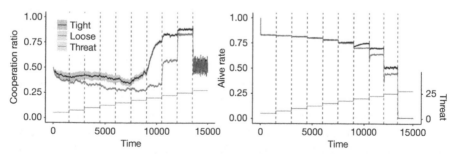

Figure 35.2 Cooperation and survival rates under threat in tight versus loose cultures. [From "The Relationship Between Cultural Tightness–Looseness and COVID-19 Cases and Deaths: A Global Analysis Supplementary Appendix," by M. Gelfand, J. Jackson, X. Pan, D. Nau, D. Pieper, E. Denison, M. Dagher, P. Van Lange, C. Chiu, and M. Wang, 2021, *The Lancet Planetary Health, 5*(3), p. 10. Copyright 2021 by the Author(s)].

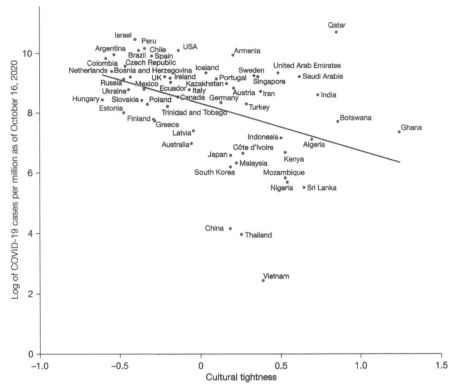

Figure 35.3 The association of cultural tightness and logged cases per million (October 16, 2020). [Adapted from "The Relationship Between Cultural Tightness–Looseness and COVID-19 Cases and Deaths: A Global Analysis" by M. Gelfand, J. Jackson, X. Pan, D. Nau, D. Pieper, E. Denison, M. Dagher, P. Van Lange, C. Chiu, and M. Wang, 2021, *The Lancet Planetary Health*, 5(3), p. e137. Copyright 2021 by the Author(s)].

there was a negligible *decrease* in tightness right after the pandemic hit, perhaps reflecting the early chaos and hoarding that we saw happening in some countries.

We then started to collect data on COVID-19 cases and deaths per capita (published by Our World in Data, 2020) and found some striking patterns: By the late fall 2020, countries that had looser norms prepandemic had five times the cases and almost nine times the deaths per capita as compared to tighter norms (see Figures 35.3 and 35.4). We also controlled for many other factors that could be linked to COVID-19 cases and deaths to see if tightness still explained variation. These factors included, for example, a country's level of testing per case, wealth, inequality, population density, age, climate, government stringency, and authoritarianism, among other factors. The effects of tightness-looseness were robust to these factors (see also Cao et al., 2020, who found similar results with a different tightness measure). Remarkably, our research showed that people in loose cultures had far less fear of the COVID-19 virus throughout 2020, even as cases skyrocketed. In tight nations, 70% of people were very scared of catching the virus. In loose cultures, only 49% were. During a devastating global pandemic—where

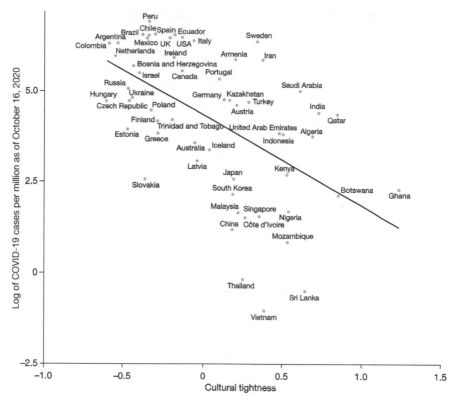

Figure 35.4 The association of cultural tightness and logged deaths per million (October 16, 2020). [Adapted from "The Relationship Between Cultural Tightness–Looseness and COVID-19 Cases and Deaths: A Global Analysis" by M. Gelfand, J. Jackson, X. Pan, D. Nau, D. Pieper, E. Denison, M. Dagher, P. Van Lange, C. Chiu, and M. Wang, 2021, *The Lancet Planetary Health*, 5(3), p. e140. Copyright 2021 by the Author(s)].

calibrating our levels of fear to the collective threat is critical—this is a clear cultural evolutionary mismatch. Like our computational models, this suggests that people in cultures that are adapted to low levels of danger did not respond as swiftly to the "threat signal" embodied by the pandemic when it came.

How COVID-19 Weaponized Culture

COVID-19 weaponized loose traits, most notably the questioning of rules. While rule breaking is useful for creativity in times of safety, it can be highly problematic during times of emergencies. We witnessed countless citizens continue holding parties, shopping maskless, and scoffing at the virus. When the fear reflex *was* triggered, it was directed at the very behaviors that could help contain the pandemic: Many people feared lockdowns and mask mandates more than the virus itself. Indeed, later research found that people in tight cultures were more responsive to descriptive norms to engage in behaviors that protected against COVID-19

(Fischer & Karl, 2022) and ultimately had less anxiety about COVID-19 (Burkova et al., 2021). Meanwhile, perceived looseness of norms was associated with non-compliance (Kleitman et al., 2021).

Loose traits surely enabled the cultural mismatches that we saw during COVID-19. But the threat signal also got hijacked by poor leadership who failed to adequately sound the alarm that the threat was dire. In the United States, U.S. President Donald Trump wishfully said: "Just stay calm. It will go away" on March 10, 2020 (Wolfe & Dale, 2020). After testing positive, he tweeted: "Feeling really good! Don't be afraid of Covid" (Reuters Staff, 2020). Trump's repeated downplaying helps explain why conservative states, who generally lean tight (Harrington & Gelfand, 2014) and respond to threats faster, have been at the forefront of COVID denialism. Tragically, they followed their leader over their instincts. Similarly, British Prime Minister Boris Johnson boasted about shaking hands with COVID-19 patients and otherwise made light of the crisis (Mason, 2020). Perhaps not surprisingly, in studies reported by King's College in London, only 1 in 10 citizens who were exposed to a confirmed COVID-19 carrier followed orders to quarantine for 2 weeks (Matthews & Chalmers, 2020).

It is important to note that not all tight cultures responded effectively. Some, like India, loosened prematurely, with devastating consequences. Moreover, there are downsides to tightening during COVID-19. For example, as people feared COVID and desired more tightening, they also had more negative attitudes toward immigrants (Mula et al., 2022). Likewise, research found that while groups who tightened in response to discussions of COVID-19 had less workplace deviance, increases in tightness also dampened creativity (Qin et al., 2021)—reflective of the aforementioned order versus openness trade-off. There is even some evidence that tight cultures, which were able to successfully deal with COVID-19, have had lower vaccination rates, perhaps due to higher levels of complacency (Ng & Tan, 2023). Finally, it is also worth noting that not all loose cultures got the threat signal wrong. New Zealand is an example of a country that veers loose, yet with great leadership and people willing to follow the rules, they were able to limit COVID-19 cases and deaths far more than other loose cultures. They had what we have called *tight-loose ambidexterity*—the ability to tighten under threat and loosen when it is safe.

CONCLUSION

As this volume attests, we have learned many valuable psychological, political, and economic lessons from COVID-19. Here we focus on how culture influenced health outcomes during COVID-19. The data suggest that as compared to tight cultures, loose cultures suffered worse outcomes in terms of COVID-19 cases and deaths and, also ironically, had less fear of the virus by later fall 2020.

These global disparities in health outcomes suggest that we need to build *cultural intelligence* to continue to fight COVID-19 and to deal with future collective threats. First, we need to develop more effective messaging. We tighten quickly in response to vivid, concrete threats, such as warfare. For example, on 9/11, Americans tightened quickly: We locked cockpit doors, tightened security protocols at airports, and passed the Patriot Act to strengthen our surveillance capabilities. The threat was very clear and impossible to ignore. By contrast, because germs are invisible and abstract, they do not trigger anxiety in the same way. Public health officials need to make COVID's dangers vivid and have clear and consistent communication about the levels of threat. To be sure, simply scaring people can backfire: When feeling helpless, people may adopt a defensive, passive posture. To empower people to action, we need to be candid about COVID symptoms while also emphasizing that with the right behaviors, we have the efficacy to reduce the threat, just as our computational models have shown. Likewise, given that people in loose cultures have generally enjoyed much more latitude, they might experience much more psychological reactance to being asked to follow more rules. Interventions are needed to help people in loose cultures maintain a sense of psychological autonomy during times of crisis.

Second, it is important to stress the time-limited nature of strict rules—namely, that tightening is temporary. Particularly for people uncomfortable with rules, we need to emphasize that the faster we tighten, the faster we will reduce the threat and the faster we will restore freedom. The computational models we have run illustrate this, and ample behavioral evidence during COVID-19 illustrates that groups can and did follow this general principle with great success. While we need to be tight on rules to stop the spread of germs, it is worth noting that we need to recruit the benefits of creativity (that come from looseness), particularly as it pertains to novel technical solutions to fight the virus. During COVID-19, we witnessed many creative ways to detect the virus, such as developing sensors in sewage, as well as novel ways to stay connected with loved ones, afforded by Zoom and other technology. The rapid development of a COVID-19 vaccine was built on decades of creativity of scientists all around the globe. Finding ways to be tight *and* loose during collective threats will be critical to successfully deal with future threats.

Finally, we need to cultivate a sense of trust in government and in each other and collective efficacy. The *Washington Post* profiled one small town that exemplified this approach (Jamison, 2020). Tangier Island is known for its religious, conservative population. For months, it was free of cases. But when the outbreak hit, it united in a powerful display of public health coordination. Resident Reta Pruitt captured the town's ethos: "They're taking it serious now. But that's the whole trouble: The first time, we weren't serious about it." An evolutionary mismatch was thwarted just in time by compassion and coordination.

COVID-19 was deadly enough without dividing us or using some of our cultural traits against us. By recognizing some of the cultural traps we have fallen into, we can leverage smarter strategies to successfully navigate future collective threats.

REFERENCES

Aktas, M., Gelfand, M. J., & Hanges, P. J. (2016). Cultural tightness–looseness and perceptions of effective leadership. *Journal of Cross-Cultural Psychology*, *47*(2), 294–309. https://doi.org/10.1177/0022022115606802

Andrighetto, G., Szekely, A., Guido, A., Gelfand, M. J., Abernathy, J. Arikan, G., Aycan, Z., Barrera, D., Basnight-Brown, D., Belaus, A., Berezina, E., Boski, P., Blumen, S., Borges Rodrigues, R., Thi Thu Bui, H., Camilo Cárdenas, J., Cekrlija, D., de Barra, M., Pde Zoys, P., . . . Eriksson, K. (2023). Norm change and disease across the globe [Manuscript under review].

Ashraf, B. N. (2021). Stock markets' reaction to COVID-19: Moderating role of national culture. *Finance Research Letters*, *41*, 101857. https://doi.org/10.1016/j.frl.2020.101857

Bazzi, S., Fiszbein, M., & Gebresilasse, M. (2021). "Rugged individualism" and collective (in)action during the COVID-19 pandemic. *Journal of Public Economics*, *195*, 104357. https://doi.org/10.1016/j.jpubeco.2020.104357

Burkova, V. N., Butovskaya, M. L., Randall, A. K., Fedenok, J. N., Ahmadi, K., Alghraibeh, A. M., Allami, F. B. M., Alpaslan, F. S., Al-Zu'bi, M. A. A., Bicer, D. F., Cetinkaya, H., David, O. A., Donato, S., Dural, S., Erickson, P., Ermakov, A. M., Ertuğrul, B., Fayankinnu, E. A., Fisher, M. L., . . . Zinurova, R. I. (2021). Predictors of anxiety in the COVID-19 pandemic from a global perspective: Data from 23 countries. *Sustainability*, *13*(7), 4017. https://doi.org/10.3390/su13074017

Cao, C., Li, N., & Liu, L. (2020). Do national cultures matter in the containment of COVID-19? *International Journal of Sociology and Social Policy*. *40*(9), 939–961. https://doi.org/10.1108/IJSSP-07-2020-0334

Chua, R. Y. J., Huang, K. G., & Jin, M. (2019). Mapping cultural tightness and its links to innovation, urbanization, and happiness across 31 provinces in China. *Proceedings of the National Academy of Sciences of the United States of America*, *116*(14), 6720–6725. https://doi.org/10.1073/pnas.1815723116

Chua, R. Y. J., Roth, Y., & Lemoine, J.-F. (2015). The impact of culture on creativity: How cultural tightness and cultural distance affect global innovation crowdsourcing work. *Administrative Science Quarterly*, *60*(2), 189–227. https://doi.org/10.1177/0001839214563595

De, S., Nau, D. S., & Gelfand, M. J. (2017, May). Understanding norm change: An evolutionary game-theoretic approach. *Proceedings of the 16th Conference on Autonomous Agents and MultiAgent Systems*, *60*(2), 1433–1441. http://dl.acm.org/citation.cfm?id=3091125.3091323

Fernandez-Perez, A., Gilbert, A., Indriawan, I., & Nguyen, N. H. (2021). COVID-19 pandemic and stock market response: A culture effect. *Journal of Behavioral and Experimental Finance*, *29*, 100454. https://doi.org/10.1016/j.jbef.2020.100454

Fischer, R., & Karl, J. A. (2022). Predicting behavioral intentions to prevent or mitigate COVID-19: A cross-cultural meta-analysis of attitudes, norms, and perceived behavioral control effects. *Social Psychological and Personality Science*, *13*(1), 264–276. https://doi.org/10.1177/19485506211019844

Foster, K. R. (2004). Diminishing returns in social evolution: The not-so-tragic commons. *Journal of Evolutionary Biology*, *17*(5), 1058–1072. https://doi.org/10.1111/j.1420-9101.2004.00747.x

Frey, C. B., Chen, C., & Presidente, G. (2020). Democracy, culture, and contagion: Political regimes and countries responsiveness to Covid-19. *Covid Economics, 18*, 1–20.

Gelfand, M. J. (2018). *Rule makers, rule breakers: How tight and loose cultures wire our world*. Scribner.

Gelfand, M. J. (2020a, March 13). To survive the coronavirus, the United States must tighten up. *Boston Globe*. https://www.bostonglobe.com/2020/03/13/opinion/surv ive-coronavirus-united-states-must-tighten-up/

Gelfand, M. J. (2020b, March 28). America's cultural weapon against COVID-19. *The Hill*. https://thehill.com/opinion/national-security/489973-americas-cultural-wea pon-against-covid-19

Gelfand, M. J., Jackson, J. C., Pan, X., Nau, D., Pieper, D., Denison, E., Dagher, M., Van Lange, P. A. M., Chiu, C.-Y., & Wang, M. (2021). The relationship between cultural tightness–looseness and COVID-19 cases and deaths: A global analysis. *The Lancet Planetary Health, 5*(3), e135–e144. https://doi.org/10.1016/S2542-5196(20)30301-6

Gelfand, M. J., & Lun, J. (2013). Ecological priming: Convergent evidence for the link between ecology and psychological processes. *Behavioral and Brain Sciences, 36*(5), 489–490.

Gelfand, M. J., Raver, J. L., Nishii, L., Leslie, L. M., Lun, J., Lim, B. C., Duan, L., Almaliach, A., Ang, S., Arnadottir, J., Aycan, Z., Boehnke, K., Boski, P., Cabecinhas, R., Chan, D., Chhokar, J., D'Amato, A., Ferrer, M., Fischlmayr, I. C., . . . Yamaguchi, S. (2011). Differences between tight and loose cultures: A 33-nation study. *Science, 332*(6033), 1100–1104. https://doi.org/10.1126/science.1197754

Giphart, R., & van Vugt, M. (2018). *Mismatch: How our Stone Age brain deceives us every day (and what we can do about it)*. Robinson.

Harrington, J. R., & Gelfand, M. J. (2014). Tightness–looseness across the 50 united states. *Proceedings of the National Academy of Sciences of the United States of America, 111*(22), 7990–7995. https://doi.org/10.1073/pnas.1317937111

Huynh, T. L. D. (2020). Does culture matter social distancing under the COVID-19 pandemic? *Safety Science, 130*, 104872. https://doi.org/10.1016/j.ssci.2020.104872

Jackson, J. C., Gelfand, M., & Ember, C. (2020). A global analysis of cultural tightness in non-industrial societies. *Proceedings of the Royal Society B: Biological Sciences, 287*, 20201036. https://doi.org/10.31234/osf.io/9s57z

Jackson, J. C., van Egmond, M., Choi, V. K., Ember, C. R., Halberstadt, J., Balanovic, J., Basker, I. N., Boehnke, K., Buki, N., Fischer, R., Fulop, M., Fulmer, A., Homan, A. C., van Kleef, G. A., Kreemers, L., Schei, V., Szabo, E., Ward, C., & Gelfand, M. J. (2019). Ecological and cultural factors underlying the global distribution of prejudice. *PLoS One, 14*(9), e0221953. https://doi.org/10.1371/journal.pone.0221953

Jamison, P. (2020, December 22). On a Trump-loving island in the Chesapeake, a virus outbreak unites instead of divides. *Washington Post*. https://www.washingtonpost.com/dc-md-va/2020/12/22/tangier-island-covid-outbreak-trump/

Kleitman, S., Fullerton, D. J., Zhang, L. M., Blanchard, M. D., Lee, J., Stankov, L., & Thompson, V. (2021). To comply or not comply? A latent profile analysis of behaviours and attitudes during the COVID-19 pandemic. *PLoS One, 16*(7), e0255268. https://doi.org/10.1371/journal.pone.0255268

Lu, J. G., Jin, P., & English, A. S. (2021). Collectivism predicts mask use during COVID-19. *Proceedings of the National Academy of Sciences of the United States of America, 118*(23), e2021793118. https://doi.org/10.1073/pnas.2021793118

Mason, R. (2020, May 5). Boris Johnson boasted of shaking hands on day Sage warned not to. *The Guardian.* https://www.theguardian.com/politics/2020/may/05/boris-johnson-boasted-of-shaking-hands-on-day-sage-warned-not-to

Matthews, S., & Chalmers, V. (2020, September 25). Only one in FIVE Britons with symptoms of Covid-19 are self-isolating. *Daily Mail Online.* https://www.dailymail.co.uk/news/article-8771807/Only-one-FIVE-Britons-tell-tale-symptoms-Covid-19-self-isolating-study-reveals.html

Mula, S., Di Santo, D., Resta, E., Bakhtiari, F., Baldner, C., Molinario, E., Pierro, A., Gelfand, M. J., Denison, E., Agostini, M., Bélanger, J. J., Gützkow, B., Kreienkamp, J., Abakoumkin, G., Khaiyom, J. H. A., Ahmedi, V., Akkas, H., Almenara, C. A., Atta, M., . . . & Leander, N. P. (2022). Concern with COVID-19 pandemic threat and attitudes towards immigrants: The mediating effect of the desire for tightness. *Current Research in Ecological and Social Psychology, 3*, 100028.

Ng, J. H., & Tan, E. K. (2023). COVID-19 vaccination and cultural tightness. *Psychological Medicine, 53*(3), 1124–1125. https://doi.org/10.1017/S0033291721001823

Our World in Data. (2020). Retrieved from https://ourworldindata.org/coronavirus-data

Ozkan, A., Ozkan, G., Yalaman, A., & Yildiz, Y. (2021). Climate risk, culture and the Covid-19 mortality: A cross-country analysis. *World Development, 141*, 105412. https://doi.org/10.1016/j.worlddev.2021.105412

Pan, X., Nau, D., & Gelfand, M. (2020). Cooperative norms and the growth of threat: Differences across tight and loose cultures. In 2020 7th International Conference on Behavioural and Social Computing (BESC) (pp. 1–6). Bournemouth, U.K. https://doi.org/10.1109/BESC51023.2020.9348297

Pelto, P. J. (1968). The differences between "tight" and "loose" societies. *Trans-Action, 5*(5), 37–40. https://doi.org/10.1007/BF03180447

Qin, X., Yam, K. C., Chen, C., Li, W., & Dong, X. (2021). Talking about COVID-19 is positively associated with team cultural tightness: Implications for team deviance and creativity. *Journal of Applied Psychology, 106*(4), 530–541. https://doi.org/10.1037/apl0000918

Reuters Staff. (2020, October 5). Trump says will leave hospital on Monday, "Don't be afraid of Covid." *Reuters.* https://www.reuters.com/article/healthcare-coronavirus-trump-leave-int-idUSKBN26Q2TI

Roos, P., Gelfand, M., Nau, D., & Lun, J. (2015). Societal threat and cultural variation in the strength of social norms: An evolutionary basis. *Organizational Behavior and Human Decision Processes, 129*, 14–23. https://doi.org/10.1016/j.obhdp.2015.01.003

Salvador, C. E., Berg, M. K., Yu, Q., San Martin, A., & Kitayama, S. (2020). Relational mobility predicts faster spread of COVID-19: A 39-country study. *Psychological Science, 31*(10), 1236–1244.

Talhelm, T., & English, A. S. (2020). Historically rice-farming societies have tighter social norms in China and worldwide. *Proceedings of the National Academy of Sciences of the United States of America, 117*(33), 19816–19824. https://doi.org/10.1073/pnas.1909909117

Thomson, R., Yuki, M., Talhelm, T., Schug, J., Kito, M., Ayanian, A. H., Becker, J. C., Becker, M., Chiu, C., Choi, H.-S., Ferreira, C. M., Fülöp, M., Gul, P., Houghton-Illera, A. M., Joasoo, M., Jong, J., Kavanagh, C. M., Khutkyy, D., Manzi, C., . . . Visserman, M. L. (2018). Relational mobility predicts social behaviors in 39 countries and is tied to historical farming and threat. *Proceedings of the National Academy of Sciences of*

the United States of America, 115(29), 7521–7526. https://doi.org/10.1073/pnas.171
3191115

Wang, Y. (2021). Government policies, national culture and social distancing during the
first wave of the COVID-19 pandemic: International evidence. *Safety Science*, *135*,
105138. https://doi.org/10.1016/j.ssci.2020.105138

Wolfe, D., & Dale, D. (2020, October 31). "It's going to disappear": A timeline of Trump's
claims that Covid-19 will vanish. *CNN*. https://www.cnn.com/interactive/2020/10/
politics/covid-disappearing-trump-comment-tracker/

FURTHER READING

Gelfand, M. J. (2021). Cultural evolutionary mismatches in response to collective threat.
Current Directions in Psychological Science, *30*(5), 401–409. https://doi.org/10.1177/
09637214211025032

Pan, X., Nau, D., & Gelfand, M. (2020, November). Cooperative norms and the growth
of threat: Differences across tight and loose cultures. In 2020 7th International
Conference on Behavioural and Social Computing (BESC) (pp. 1–6). Bournemouth,
U.K. https://doi.org/10.1109/BESC51023.2020.9348297

Van Bavel, J. J., Baicker, K., Boggio, P. S., Capraro, V., Cichocka, A., Cikara, M., Crockett,
M. J., Crum, A. J., Douglas, K. M., Druckman, J. N., Drury, J., Dube, O., Ellemers,
N., Finkel, E. J., Fowler, J. H., Gelfand, M., Han, S., Haslam, S. A., Jetten, J., . . . &
Willer, R. (2020). Using social and behavioural science to support COVID-19 pan-
demic response. *Nature Human Behaviour*, *4*(5), 460–471. https://doi.org/10.1038/
s41562-020-0884-z

36

Fake News and the COVID-19 Pandemic

SANDER VAN DER LINDEN AND JON ROOZENBEEK ■

The COVID-19 pandemic has been accompanied by a significant amount of misleading and outright false information. In some cases, this involves financial scams, such as a company selling "BioShield" USB sticks that they claimed offered protection against supposedly harmful 5G radiation,[1] which became a topic of concern after false rumors about a link between 5G and COVID-19 symptoms went viral.[2] In other cases, the harms of COVID-19 misinformation are physical, for example, when dozens of people died from methanol poisoning in Iran because of the false belief that drinking it could cure the disease (Delirrad & Mohammadi, 2020). Worryingly, belief in misinformation about the virus has also been linked to lower intentions to get vaccinated (Roozenbeek, Schneider, et al., 2020), even posing a potential threat to future herd immunity (Loomba et al., 2021). As such, the spread of misinformation has the potential to affect the outcome of the pandemic: How soon things go back to normal, for example, depends in part on whether herd immunity is achieved.

All of this provides a clear incentive to limit the spread of COVID-19 misinformation. In doing so, however, we run into several issues related to problem definition (what counts as misinformation?) and how to effectively tackle it. This chapter first briefly explores the conceptual issue of defining the problem of misinformation and why fact-checking and debunking on their own are not a sufficient solution. Next, we examine the social psychological theory of inoculation to preemptively debunk (or "prebunk") misinformation in order to prevent it from going viral and taking hold in the first place. Finally, we detail how our own program of research has been used by governments, the World Health Organization (WHO), and the United Nations to fight COVID-19 misinformation at scale.

Sander van der Linden and Jon Roozenbeek, *Fake News and the COVID-19 Pandemic* In: *The Social Science of the COVID-19 Pandemic*. Edited by: Monica K. Miller, Oxford University Press. © Oxford University Press 2024. DOI: 10.1093/oso/9780197615133.003.0036

DEFINING THE PROBLEM OF MISINFORMATION

A commonly used definition of "fake news" is "fabricated information that mimics news media content in form, but not in organizational process or intent" (Lazer et al., 2018). However, exclusively focusing on fabricated content is problematic, as some false news is entirely harmless (e.g., satirical news), while true information can be presented in a misleading and harmful way (van der Linden & Roozenbeek, 2020). For example, within the context of the COVID-19 pandemic, not only objectively false stories such as the aforementioned 5G BioShield scam make the rounds online, but also stories that are not exactly fake but so stripped of relevant context that they are highly misleading. For example, the Centers for Disease Control and Prevention (CDC) mentioned a "plausible causal relationship between the J&J/Janssen COVID-19 Vaccine and a rare and serious adverse event—blood clots with low platelets—which has caused deaths."[3] This sounds serious at the surface level, but the CDC also provided the statistics for the likelihood of such an event: "As of May 11, 2021, more than 9 million doses of the J&J/Janssen COVID-19 Vaccine have been given in the United States. Through continuous safety monitoring, CDC and FDA [Food and Drug Administration] identified 28 confirmed reports of people who got the J&J/Janssen COVID-19 Vaccine and later developed TTS [thrombocytopenia syndrome]." In other words, in mid-May 2021, there were 28 confirmed cases of vaccine-related thrombosis out of 9 million vaccinations (not all of those affected died as a result), a probability of 0.000003% or about 1 in 320,000. For comparison, the odds of dying in a motor vehicle accident in any given year are about 1 in 8,000.[4] However, this did not prevent the *Chicago Tribune* from publishing a story with the headline "A 'Healthy' Doctor Died Two Weeks After Getting a COVID-19 Vaccine; CDC Is Investigating Why."[5] Despite the cause of this doctor's death being unknown at the time of publication, and the *Tribune* later adding an update to the story saying that there was not enough evidence to "rule out or confirm the vaccine was a contributing factor," the story was shared millions of time across social media.[6] Such misleading content is all the more problematic because research shows that using moral-emotional language in social media content increases its potential to go viral (Berriche & Altay, 2020; Brady et al., 2017; Rathje et al., 2021). In other words, even defining what counts as COVID-19 misinformation is a tough nut to crack. For the purpose of this chapter, we define misinformation as information that is either intentionally or unintentionally manipulative.

FACT-CHECKING, CONTINUED INFLUENCE, AND ILLUSORY TRUTH

An intuitive way to combat misinformation is through fact-checking. Initiatives that debunk false and misleading stories proliferating online abound and can range from independent fact-checking organizations such as Snopes and Full Fact to Facebook's third-party fact-checking program.[7] Such debunking initiatives are generally useful and more or less effective at what they seek to accomplish, provided they take into account the scientific literature on how to make post hoc corrections as effective as they can be. Stephan Lewandowsky and colleagues recently published a useful step-by-step guide on how to do this: "Debunking Handbook" (Lewandowsky et al., 2020).

However, even when done perfectly, debunking suffers from several psychological limitations that hamper its efficacy as a way to fight misinformation online. First of all, research has shown that false rumors can spread further, faster, and deeper than true information on social media (Vosoughi et al., 2018), although this might not necessarily be the case for news about COVID-19 (Cinelli et al., 2020). In some contexts, misinformation could thus outpace fact checks in terms of their potential reach. Second, the continued influence effect, a well-known finding from psychology, suggests that people can continue to rely on misinformation even after it has been debunked (Ecker et al., 2020; Lewandowsky et al., 2012). In other words, even if someone is exposed to a correction after seeing the original misinformation, this might not fully undo the damage as people continue to rely on the misinformation when forming judgments. Third, repeated exposure to misinformation can increase people's belief in it, even if they know it is false, a phenomenon known as the "illusory truth effect" (Fazio et al., 2015). What this means is that if someone sees the same false story multiple times on their social media feed, its perceived reliability could be strengthened, thus reducing the potential effectiveness of a subsequent fact check. For all of these reasons, it stands to reason that "prevention is better than cure."

INOCULATION THEORY AND PREBUNKING

These problems with post hoc corrections therefore raise an interesting possibility: Is it possible to prevent exposure to misinformation from being effective in the first place? To investigate this question, misinformation researchers have turned to inoculation theory as a way to preemptively debunk (or "prebunk"). Developed in the 1960s by social psychologist William McGuire, inoculation theory is based on a medical analogy (McGuire & Papageorgis, 1961a, 1962; Papageorgis & McGuire, 1961). Medical vaccines (traditionally) are weakened versions of a pathogen that, after being introduced to the body, trigger the production of an immune response, thus building resistance against future infection. Psychological inoculations work much the same way: By preemptively presenting a person with a psychological "vaccine" (consisting of a warning of an impending attack on one's beliefs and a preemptive refutation, a "prebunk"), a thought process is triggered that is akin to "mental antibodies," which engenders psychological resistance against future exposure to misinformation (Compton, 2013; Papageorgis & McGuire, 1961). Over the years, a large body of evidence and (meta)studies has been amassed showing that inoculation theory is a robust framework for conferring resistance against unwanted persuasion (Banas & Rains, 2010; Lewandowsky & van der Linden, 2021).

Traditionally, inoculation research has focused mainly on so-called prophylactic inoculations, or inoculations against persuasive arguments that people had no prior exposure to. McGuire believed that psychological inoculations would be most effective when applied to so-called germ-free beliefs (truisms that people generally do not hear many arguments against, e.g., the idea that brushing your teeth is beneficial; see McGuire, 1964). A shortcoming of this paradigm is that it can only be tested in settings that are quite far removed from society, for example, by prescreening people into the experiment based on their prior attitudes. In the context of online misinformation, this "no prior exposure" clause is an unrealistic assumption, as people commonly have prior beliefs (e.g., about politics) that misinformation taps into. In addition, there is often no way of knowing if people have already been exposed to a particular piece of misinformation (Lewandowsky & van der Linden, 2021). To address these issues, researchers have begun to explore the feasibility of *therapeutic* inoculations: the idea that inoculation treatments can be effective even when people already have prior attitudes about the topic of the inoculation (Compton, 2019; Wood et al., 2012).

A second recent innovation within inoculation research that has proven to be useful in terms of the scalability of the theory is a move away from issue-based toward logic- or technique-based inoculations (Cook et al., 2017; Roozenbeek & van der Linden, 2018). Traditional inoculation research has mostly focused on individual persuasive attacks (e.g., the conspiracy theory that COVID-19 was bioengineered in a military lab in Wuhan, China). But in the context of online misinformation, this is impractical, as researchers cannot reasonably anticipate exactly what specific misinformation will go viral and design inoculation messages accordingly. Instead, researchers have explored whether it is possible to inoculate people against the manipulation techniques that are commonly used in online misinformation, such as constructing conspiracy theories (i.e., blaming a small, secretive, and nefarious group of people for large societal problems) or the use of excessively emotional language to evoke fear or outrage, fueling intergroup polarization, or artificially amplifying the reach of certain content by using bots or fake "likes" (van der Linden & Roozenbeek, 2020). If people can be inoculated against these techniques, they might recognize them in the social media content that they come across, and update their judgment of the veracity of this content accordingly. Such an approach circumvents the need to prebunk individual examples of misinformation, and since the approach tackles epistemologically dubious content (which makes use of logical fallacies, e.g.), it could be less likely to be perceived as biased or partisan.

PREBUNKING AGAINST COVID-19 MISINFORMATION

Here, we discuss how to leverage inoculation theory to prebunk misinformation about COVID-19, focusing on the use of online games as the metaphorical "syringe" of the inoculation treatment. We also discuss the results of one of our studies about *Go Viral!* (a "fake news" game against COVID-19 misinformation that we developed).

Games as "Active" Inoculation

Starting in 2018, we began to look for creative ways to apply technique-based inoculations against misinformation in the real world. To do so, we developed a series of free browser games in which players take on the role of fake news creators. There are multiple advantages to this approach: (1) Rather than simply being exposed to misinformation techniques (e.g., by reading them), players make choices throughout the game that either reward them with more points or punish them by taking points away, thus prompting them to think proactively about how misinformation techniques are used and generate their own counterarguments, an approach known as "active" inoculation (McGuire & Papageorgis, 1961b; Roozenbeek & van der Linden, 2018); (2) playing an inoculation game engages active experiential learning through perspective taking and might confer long-term benefits in terms of improving people's ability to spot misinformation (Maertens et al., 2021); (3) a game allows for players to be inoculated against multiple misinformation techniques at once (Roozenbeek & van der Linden, 2019); and last, (4) the games are not static interventions and can be dynamically adapted to changing circumstances (e.g., by including a scenario about COVID-19 misinformation).

In 2018, we launched *Bad News* (www.getbadnews.com), in collaboration with the Dutch antimisinformation platform DROG and design agency Gusmanson. Over the course of six scenarios (or "badges"), players grow from anonymous social media users to fake news tycoons, wreaking havoc on the media land-scape in the process. In so doing, they learn six common misinformation techniques: impersonating fake accounts, using emotional language, fueling intergroup polarization, spreading conspiracies, discrediting opponents through ad hominem attacks, and trolling people to evoke a response (Roozenbeek & van der Linden, 2019). Since its launch, *Bad News* has been translated to more than 20 languages and has been played more than 1.2 million times. In 2020, in collaboration with DROG, Gusmanson, and the Global Engagement Center in Washington, D.C., we launched *Harmony Square* (https://harmonysquare.game/en), a game about political disinformation and polarization. Over the course of a series of studies, we found that game players find misinformation significantly less reliable after playing (Roozenbeek & van der Linden, 2019), even if participants had never encountered the misinformation before (Roozenbeek et al., 2021); were significantly more confident in their ability to assess the reliability of mis-information on their feed (Basol et al., 2020); and were significantly less likely to report being willing to share misinformation with other people in their net-work (Roozenbeek & van der Linden, 2020). We also found that similar inocu-lation effects are conferred across cultures and languages (Roozenbeek, van der Linden, & Nygren, 2020). In terms of the longevity of the observed inoculation effects, we found that people remained significantly better at spotting manipula-tion techniques in social media content for at least 1 week after playing (Maertens et al., 2021). This "immunity" lasted up to 3 months when participants were assessed at regular intervals each week. We see these prompts as motivational "booster shots," topping up people's immunity to misinformation by staying engaged. Overall, these findings provide support for the idea of using inoculation games as a way to reduce susceptibility to misinformation.

Prebunking Against COVID-19 Misinformation: *Go Viral!*

After it became clear that misinformation about COVID-19 had the potential to cause significant societal harm, we began working with the Cabinet Office of the United Kingdom to develop a game similar to *Bad News* and *Harmony Square* but specifically about COVID-19 misinformation. This new game, *Go Viral!* (www.goviralgame.com) was launched in October 2020 and takes about 5 minutes to play and inoculates people against three common techniques used to spread misinformation about COVID-19: fearmongering, fake experts, and conspiracy theories. Players start out as anonymous social media users, and over the course of three scenarios are slowly lured into an online echo chamber where misinformation and outrage-evoking content about COVID-19 proliferate widely. In the first scenario, "The Fearmongerer," players learn how to increase engagement with the content they produce by using emotionally evocative language (Berriche & Altay, 2020; Brady et al., 2017; Rathje et al., 2021). After doing so, they are invited to join *Not Co-Fraid*, a group of online "truth-tellers." In the next scenario, "My Imaginary Expert," players build their credibility as Not Co-Fraid's newest member by backing up their claims by quoting fake experts such as Dr. Hyde T. Paine from the "University of Life." By misleading people into believing that their content is endorsed by (nonexisting) experts (Cook et al., 2017; Roozenbeek & van der Linden, 2019), players gain popularity within the group. At the end of the scenario, they become a moderator for Not Co-Fraid. In the final scenario, "Master of Puppets," players create a conspiracy theory about COVID-19 (Roozenbeek, Schneider, et al., 2020). After picking a target (e.g., a nongovernmental organization, the government, or one Bob from New York), they begin to accuse it of nefarious activities and "hiding the truth," which results in large-scale protests and a full-blown escalation of their conspiracy. In short, during the game players are forewarned about the dangers of fake news by getting a glimpse of some of harmful consequences firsthand. Players are also exposed to weakened or "microdoses" of the techniques used to spread misinformation in a simulated social media environment, strong enough to trigger the production of cognitive "antibodies" but not so strong as to actually persuade or dupe people. An example is provided in Figure 36.1.

To test the efficacy of *Go Viral!* as a way to reduce susceptibility to COVID-19 misinformation, we ran two large-scale studies, recently published in the journal *Big Data & Society* (Basol et al., 2021). For Study 1, we implemented a voluntary survey within the *Go Viral!* game environment. At the start and at the end of the game, game players who agreed to participate in the survey rated on a scale from 1 to 7, 1 being "not at all manipulative" and 7 being "very manipulative" the manipulativeness of a series of six Twitter posts about COVID-19 Figure 36.2 shows what the survey looks like in the game environment.

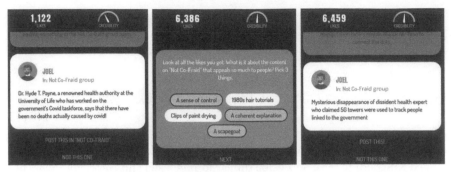

Figure 36.1 Screenshots from the *Go Viral!* game showing example of the player (in this case "Joel") gaining "likes" by making use of the "fake expert" (left panel) and "conspiracy" techniques (middle and right panels).

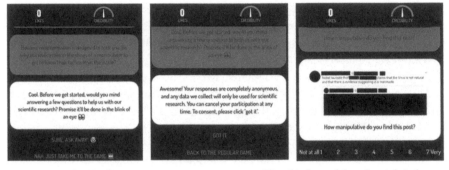

Figure 36.2 *Go Viral!* in-game survey environment. The third panel (on the right) shows an example of a survey item containing misinformation. (Reprinted with permission from Basol, et al., 2021.)

Three of the Twitter posts were real tweets from reputable news organizations (e.g., the BBC and Associated Press) and did not contain any misinformation. The other three were examples of misinformation taken from fact-checking websites that made use of one of the three techniques learned in the game (emotional language, using fake experts, or conspiracy theories). We hypothesized that game players would find the misinformation tweets significantly more manipulative post-gameplay, while rating the tweets containing real news as equally manipulative, resulting in improved ability to discern manipulative from nonmanipulative social media content. Figure 36.3 shows the results.

Figure 36.3 shows that the data supported our hypothesis: We found a significant pre-post increase in the perceived manipulativeness of COVID-19 misinformation, but no change for real news, thus significantly improving truth discernment or people's ability to discern fact from fiction. In Study 2, we addressed a number of important open questions that we could not answer in Study 1. First, we tested *Go Viral!* against a control group (in which participants played *Tetris*). Second, aside from looking at the perceived manipulativeness

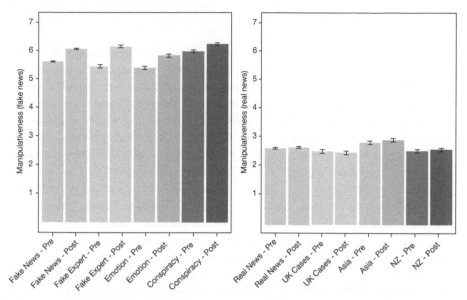

Figure 36.3 Results from study 1 from Basol, et al., (2021). The left graph shows the perceived manipulativeness of COVID-19 misinformation before (Pre) and after (Post) playing *Go Viral!* The right graph shows the perceived manipulativeness of real news about COVID-19, also before and after playing. (Reprinted with permission from Basol, et al., 2021.)

of COVID-19 misinformation, we also looked at whether the game improved people's confidence at spotting misinformation and whether playing it reduced participants' willingness to share misinformation with people in their network. Third, we tested whether the game was equally effective in different languages (English, French, and German). Fourth, we followed up with our participants 1 week after they took part in the study and again assessed their ability to spot COVID-19 misinformation to check whether playing the game conferred long-term benefits. Fifth, and most importantly, we tested the *Go Viral!* game against a series of prebunking infographics about COVID-19 misinformation, developed by UNESCO (United Nations Educational, Scientific, and Cultural Organization),[8] to see if both "active" and "passive" prebunking interventions could be effective at mitigating susceptibility to COVID-19 misinformation. We again found highly robust results: Playing the game significantly increased the perceived manipulativeness of COVID-19 misinformation, increased their confidence in their ability to spot manipulative content, and reduced their willingness to share misinformation with others, compared to the control group (with the first two effects still significant 1 week after playing). The first two effects were also observed for the passive UNESCO infographics and were similar across different languages. Overall, these findings showed robust support for the use of gamified prebunking as a way to reduce people's susceptibility to COVID-19 misinformation at scale.

LESSONS LEARNED

Scholars have urged psychological scientists to test their theories specifically in the context of COVID-19 (Van Bavel et al., 2020). Although psychological inoculation started out as a scientific theory, validated initially through laboratory studies, it eventually culminated in a real-world intervention to combat misinformation about COVID-19 "in the wild." The game was developed in collaboration with game designers and the U.K. Cabinet Office, which provided valuable input about how to translate a scientific theory into practice. Since then, the game has been played more than 350,000 times and was translated by the government into 10 languages via strategic collaborations with universities and governments around the world. The game has become part of the WHO's *Stop the Spread* campaign[9] to fight the ongoing infodemic as well as the United Nation's *Verified* campaign, garnering over 200 million impressions on social media.[10] What we have learned is that in order to fight misinformation in the real world, we need to translate theories from the laboratory into fun, educational, and scalable interventions. But like the COVID-19 virus, misinformation continues to evolve into new and more virulent strains. In response, we need dynamic and "living" interventions that can be updated and deployed in real time. In the words of Defense Against the Dark Arts teacher Professor Severus Snape: "Our defenses must therefore be as flexible and inventive as the arts we seek to undo."

CONCLUSION

In this chapter, we have explored some of the difficulties with defining and tackling COVID-19 misinformation. We discussed how inoculation theory and preemptive debunking (prebunking) have emerged as novel mechanisms for reducing misinformation susceptibility at scale. Finally, we have illustrated how our program of research used gamification in collaboration with governments and international organizations to build psychological resistance against COVID-19 misinformation. Of course, important open questions remain. For example, in order to follow inoculation theory to its logical conclusion, we need to move from cognitive immunity at the individual level to societal herd immunity. Future research will need to provide crucial insights into what level of psychological immunity is required, at what scale, and for how long in order to confer long-term societal resistance against misinformation.

ACKNOWLEDGMENT

Both authors contributed equally to this work. Authorship order was determined via coin toss.

NOTES

1. https://www.bbc.co.uk/news/technology-52810220
2. https://www.bbc.co.uk/news/technology-52370616
3. https://www.cdc.gov/coronavirus/2019-ncov/vaccines/safety/adverse-events.html
4. https://www.iii.org/fact-statistic/facts-statistics-mortality-risk
5. https://www.chicagotribune.com/coronavirus/fl-ne-miami-doctor-vaccine-death-20210107-afzysvqqjbgwnetcy5v6ec62py-story.html
6. https://www.npr.org/2021/03/25/980035707/lying-through-truth-misleading-facts-fuel-vaccine-misinformation?t=1621596471521
7. https://www.cjr.org/analysis/five-days-of-facebook-fact-checking.php
8. https://en.unesco.org/themes/gced/thinkbeforesharing
9. https://www.who.int/news-room/feature-stories/detail/fighting-misinformation-in-the-time-of-covid-19-one-click-at-a-time
10. https://twitter.com/un/status/1314370997525643264?lang=en

REFERENCES

Banas, J. A., & Rains, S. A. (2010). A meta-analysis of research on inoculation theory. *Communication Monographs, 77*(3), 281–311. https://doi.org/10.1080/03637751003758193

Basol, M., Roozenbeek, J., Berriche, M., Uenal, F., McClanahan, W., & van der Linden, S. (2021). Towards psychological herd immunity: Cross-cultural evidence for two prebunking interventions against COVID-19 misinformation. *Big Data and Society, 8*(1). https://doi.org/10.1177/20539517211013868

Basol, M., Roozenbeek, J., & van der Linden, S. (2020). Good news about *Bad News*: Gamified inoculation boosts confidence and cognitive immunity against fake news. *Journal of Cognition, 3*(1), Article 2. https://doi.org/https://doi.org/10.5334/joc.91

Berriche, M., & Altay, S. (2020). Internet users engage more with phatic posts than with health misinformation on Facebook. *Palgrave Communications, 6*(1), 1–9.

Brady, W. J., Wills, J. A., Jost, J. T., Tucker, J. A., & Van Bavel, J. J. (2017). Emotion shapes the diffusion of moralized content in social networks. *Proceedings of the National Academy of Sciences of the United States of America, 114*(28), 7313–7318. https://doi.org/10.1073/pnas.1618923114

Cinelli, M., Quattrociocchi, W., Galeazzi, A., Valensise, C. M., Brugnoli, E., Schmidt, A. L., Zola, P., Zollo, F., & Scala, A. (2020). The COVID-19 social media infodemic. *Scientific Reports, 10*(1), 16598. https://doi.org/10.1038/s41598-020-73510-5

Compton, J. (2013). Inoculation theory. In J. P. Dillard & L. Shen (Eds.), *The SAGE handbook of persuasion: Developments in theory and practice* (2nd ed., pp. 220–236). Sage Publications. https://doi.org/10.4135/9781452218410

Compton, J. (2019). Prophylactic versus therapeutic inoculation treatments for resistance to influence. *Communication Theory, 30*(3), 330–343. https://doi.org/10.1093/ct/qtz004

Cook, J., Lewandowsky, S., & Ecker, U. K. H. (2017). Neutralizing misinformation through inoculation: Exposing misleading argumentation techniques reduces their influence. *PLoS One, 12*(5), 1–21. https://doi.org/10.1371/journal.pone.0175799

Delirrad, M., & Mohammadi, A. B. (2020). New methanol poisoning outbreaks in Iran following COVID-19 pandemic. *Alcohol and Alcoholism, 55*(4), 347–348. https://doi.org/10.1093/alcalc/agaa036

Ecker, U. K. H., Lewandowsky, S., & Chadwick, M. (2020). Can corrections spread misinformation to new audiences? Testing for the elusive familiarity backfire effect. *Cognitive Research: Principles and Implications, 5*(1), 41. https://doi.org/10.1186/s41235-020-00241-6

Fazio, L., Brashier, N. M., Payne, B. K., & Marsh, E. J. (2015). Knowledge does not protect against illusory truth. *Journal of Experimental Psychology: General, 144*(5), 993–1002. https://doi.org/10.1037/xge0000098

Lazer, D. M. J., Baum, M. A., Benkler, Y., Berinsky, A. J., Greenhill, K. M., Menczer, F., Metzger, M. J., Nyhan, B., Pennycook, G., Rothschild, D., Schudson, M., Sloman, S. A., Sunstein, C. R., Thorson, E. A., Watts, D. J., & Zittrain, J. L. (2018). The science of fake news. *Science, 359*(6380), 1094–1096. https://doi.org/10.1126/science.aao2998

Lewandowsky, S., Cook, J., Ecker, U. K. H., Albarracín, D., Amazeen, M. A., Kendeou, P., Lombardi, D., Newman, E. J., Pennycook, G., Porter, E., Rand, D. G., Rapp, D. N., Reifler, J., Roozenbeek, J., Schmid, P., Seifert, C. M., Sinatra, G. M., Swire-Thompson, B., van der Linden, S., . . . Zaragoza, M. S. (2020). The debunking handbook 2020. Databrary. https://doi.org/10.17910/b7.1182

Lewandowsky, S., Ecker, U. K. H., Seifert, C. M., Schwarz, N., & Cook, J. (2012). Misinformation and its correction: Continued influence and successful debiasing. *Psychological Science in the Public Interest, 13*(3), 106–131. https://doi.org/10.1177/1529100612451018

Lewandowsky, S., & van der Linden, S. (2021). Countering misinformation and fake news through inoculation and prebunking. *European Review of Social Psychology, 32*(2), 348–384. https://doi.org/10.1080/10463283.2021.1876983

Loomba, S., de Figueiredo, A., Piatek, S. J., de Graaf, K., & Larson, H. J. (2021). Measuring the impact of COVID-19 vaccine misinformation on vaccination intent in the U.K. and USA. *Nature Human Behaviour, 5*, 337–348. https://doi.org/10.1038/s41562-021-01056-1

Maertens, R., Roozenbeek, J., Basol, M., & van der Linden, S. (2021). Long-term effectiveness of inoculation against misinformation: Three longitudinal experiments. *Journal of Experimental Psychology: Applied, 27*(1), 1–16. https://doi.org/10.1037/xap0000315

McGuire, W. J. (1964). Inducing resistance against persuasion: Some contemporary approaches. *Advances in Experimental Social Psychology, 1*, 191–229. https://doi.org/http://dx.doi.org/10.1016/S0065-2601(08)60052-0

McGuire, W. J., & Papageorgis, D. (1961a). The relative efficacy of various types of prior belief-defense in producing immunity against persuasion. *Journal of Abnormal and Social Psychology, 62*(2), 327–337.

McGuire, W. J., & Papageorgis, D. (1961b). Resistance to persuasion conferred by active and passive prior refutation of the same and alternative counterarguments. *Journal of Abnormal and Social Psychology, 63* (2), 326–332.

McGuire, W. J., & Papageorgis, D. (1962). Effectiveness of forewarning in developing resistance to persuasion. *Public Opinion Quarterly, 26*(1), 24–34. https://doi.org/10.1086/267068

Papageorgis, D., & McGuire, W. J. (1961). The generality of immunity to persuasion produced by pre-exposure to weakened counterarguments. *Journal of Abnormal and Social Psychology, 62*, 475–481.

Rathje, S., Van Bavel, J. J., & van der Linden, S. (2021). Out-group animosity drives engagement on social media. *Proceedings of the National Academy of Sciences of the United States of America, 118*(26), e2024292118. https://pubmed.ncbi.nlm.nih.gov/34162706/

Roozenbeek, J., Maertens, R., McClanahan, W., & van der Linden, S. (2021). Disentangling item and testing effects in inoculation research on online misinformation. *Educational and Psychological Measurement, 81*(2), 340–362. https://doi.org/10.1177/0013164420940378

Roozenbeek, J., Schneider, C. R., Dryhurst, S., Kerr, J., Freeman, A. L. J., Recchia, G., van der Bles, A. M., & van der Linden, S. (2020). Susceptibility to misinformation about COVID-19 around the world. *Royal Society Open Science, 7*(201199). https://doi.org/10.1098/rsos.201199

Roozenbeek, J., & van der Linden, S. (2018). The fake news game: Actively inoculating against the risk of misinformation. *Journal of Risk Research, 22*(5), 570–580. https://doi.org/10.1080/13669877.2018.1443491

Roozenbeek, J., & van der Linden, S. (2019). Fake news game confers psychological resistance against online misinformation. *Humanities and Social Sciences Communications, 5*(65), 1–10. https://doi.org/10.1057/s41599-019-0279-9

Roozenbeek, J., & van der Linden, S. (2020). Breaking *Harmony Square*: A game that "inoculates" against political misinformation. *The Harvard Kennedy School (HKS) Misinformation Review, 1*(8). https://doi.org/10.37016/mr-2020-47

Roozenbeek, J., van der Linden, S., & Nygren, T. (2020). Prebunking interventions based on "inoculation" theory can reduce susceptibility to misinformation across cultures. *The Harvard Kennedy School (HKS) Misinformation Review, 1*(2). https://doi.org/10.37016//mr-2020-008

Van Bavel, J. J., Baicker, K., Boggio, P. S., Capraro, V., Cichocka, A., Cikara, M., Crockett, M. J., Crum, A. J., Douglas, K. M., Druckman, J. N., Drury, J., Dube, O., Ellemers, N., Finkel, E. J., Fowler, J. H., Gelfand, M., Han, S., Haslam, S. A., Jetten, J., . . . Willer, R. (2020). Using social and behavioural science to support COVID-19 pandemic response. *Nature Human Behaviour, 4*(5), 460–471. https://doi.org/10.1038/s41562-020-0884-z

van der Linden, S., & Roozenbeek, J. (2020). Psychological inoculation against fake news. In R. Greifenader, M. Jaffé, E. Newman, & N. Schwarz (Eds.), *The psychology of fake news: Accepting, sharing, and correcting misinformation* (pp. 147–169). Psychology Press. https://doi.org/10.4324/9780429295379-11

Vosoughi, S., Roy, D., & Aral, S. (2018). The spread of true and false news online. *Science, 359*(6380), 1146–1151. https://doi.org/10.1126/science.aap9559

Wood, M. J., Douglas, K. M., & Sutton, R. M. (2012). Dead and alive: Beliefs in contradictory conspiracy theories. *Social Psychological and Personality Science, 3*(6), 767–773. https://doi.org/10.1177/1948550611434786

FURTHER READING

Compton, J., van der Linden, S., Cook, J., & Basol, M. (2021). Inoculation theory in the post-truth era: Extant findings and new frontiers for contested science, misinformation, and conspiracy theories. Social and Personality Psychology Compass, *15*(6), e12602.

McGuire, W. J. (1970). A vaccine for brainwash. *Psychology Today*, *3*(9), 37–64.

Roozenbeek, J., & van der Linden, S. (2021). A psychological vaccine against fake news: From the lab to worldwide implementation In N. Mazar & D. Soman (Eds.), *Behavioral Science in the Wild* (pp. 188–206). University of Toronto Press.

37

Will the COVID-19 Pandemic Influence People's Moral Beliefs and Behavior?

Insights From Parasite-Stress Theory and Moral Foundations Theory

MATTHEW P. WEST AND LOGAN A. YELDERMAN ■

If a friend offered you a sip of their drink *prior* to the COVID-19 pandemic, you might have accepted the offer and taken a sip from the same glass. If a friend offered you a sip of their drink *amidst* the pandemic, you might have felt a sense of disgust in your "gut" at the thought and declined the offer. The way you think and behave tends to be different when you face a high risk of catching an infectious disease compared to when you do not. This is the simple proposition made by parasite-stress theory (Thornhill & Fincher, 2014b; also Schaller, 2011). This chapter focuses on how parasite-stress theory, as well as moral foundations theory, might explain or predict some attitudinal and behavioral outcomes of the COVID-19 pandemic.

During the pandemic, some people formed "pandemic pods" (or "bubbles"), typically a group of individuals who would exclusively interact with each other without facial coverings.[1] Forming tight-knit groups with shared norms (or "rules") for behavior and avoiding outgroups are adaptive responses to the risk of infection according to parasite-stress theory, as well as others. The people in the pod reduce their risk of infection, but they also benefit from support of their pod members if an infection does occur ("insurance"). For example, members might help with child care while one member is bedridden. These pods, of course, rely on a level of trust and familiarity, maximizing the potential benefit of strengthening

Matthew P. West and Logan A. Yelderman, *Will the COVID-19 Pandemic Influence People's Moral Beliefs and Behavior?* In: *The Social Science of the COVID-19 Pandemic.* Edited by: Monica K. Miller, Oxford University Press.
© Oxford University Press 2024. DOI: 10.1093/oso/9780197615133.003.0037

the importance of the ingroup and providing a set of expectations that enhance ingroup cohesion (Benson et al., 2016; Kenworthy & Jones, 2009).

The thing about adaptive responses is that they often have "byproducts." Perhaps the most tragic and extreme cases are when responses are "triggered" by nonadaptive stimuli (cf. Haidt & Joseph, 2004, 2007). The blaring sounds of fire alarms in a building might lead most people to panic and rapidly exit a building, and the panic and rapid exit might have harmful consequences (e.g., trampling), regardless of the extent to which there is an actual threat of fire in the building. Analogously, ways of thinking and behaving that help people survive a specific threat, like pathogens, and pass on their genes can be triggered with consequences disproportionate to the actual risk. As many have noted, there is a reason why a common antecedent of genocides is rhetoric drawing an equivalence between a certain group of people and parasites, viruses, vermin, cockroaches, and so on (Smith, 2011). Other chapters in this book discuss how people and groups respond to threats (e.g., Chapter 9 and Chapter 47), and genocide is, of course, an extreme outcome. There are other, more insidious ways in which psychological and behavioral change in response to the risk of infectious disease might have consequences for people and groups.

This chapter is about the mundane, but nevertheless consequential, ways that the COVID-19 pandemic might have shifted people's psychology and behavior in the social world. We speculate that there might be a "conservative shift" in people's morality and, in turn, shifts in prejudice-related attitudes and behavior and punishment-related attitudes and behavior. First, we dive into the theoretical perspectives that this proposition is based in. After that, we apply these theories to explain how people's morality might be shaped by the COVID-19 pandemic and, in turn, outline some possible consequences of a conservative shift in morality. We then propose a number of testable hypotheses for future research.

PARASITE-STRESS THEORY AND MORAL FOUNDATIONS THEORY

Parasite-stress theory starts with the idea that humans have a "behavioral immune system," a term coined by Schaller (2011). In his conception, the behavioral immune system is responsible for processing information about the risk of infection and responding to that information by activating emotions, cognitions, and behavioral impulses (Schaller, 2011). The hypothetical example at the start of this chapter is an illustration of this sequence: The risk of infection might be considered high, you might experience the emotion of disgust, and you might decline to sip from the same glass as your friend. Parasite-stress theory takes a broader conception of the behavioral immune system, proposing numerous psychological and behavioral "defense" mechanisms (Thornhill & Fincher, 2014a). These mechanisms are evolutionary adaptations that serve the functional goals of both avoiding infection and minimizing the adverse effects of infection, and these mechanisms range from personality traits to residential habits (Thornhill &

Fincher, 2014a). What people think is right and wrong is one characteristic rooted in the behavioral immune system.

From an evolutionary perspective, the "name of the game" is ultimately passing on one's genes, and thus a morality that revolves around collective well-being is adaptive in the sense that it increases the chances of a group's long-term survival in the face of contagion. A notable byproduct we previously touched on is that the mechanisms that help people avoid and minimize the risk and deleterious effects of infectious diseases can also be applied to the social world (Kelly, 2011). People can associate ideas, physical characteristics, and behaviors with disease and respond accordingly (Tybur et al., 2013). One of the contributing reasons for this is that infectious diseases like COVID-19 are not directly observable, so people have to rely on things like cues, heuristics, and intuition; doing so means that people's inferences of risk might be inaccurate in many cases, and their behavior, while driven by the goal of avoiding and ameliorating the risk of infectious disease, might not necessarily achieve that goal.

Moral foundations theory, like parasite stress theory, is seated in an evolutionary perspective. The theory proposes that people have innate moral "foundations" (or intuitions) that developed in response to adaptive challenges (Haidt & Joseph, 2004, 2007). These moral foundations shape people's moral judgments. For instance, the protection and care of offspring is an adaptive challenge, so cognitions and behaviors associated with successful raising and protection of offspring began to shape and define the moral landscape, or moralize particular behaviors. A firefighter who rushes into a burning building to save a child would generally be judged a hero: Saving a child is moral because it serves to meet an adaptive challenge. Conversely, a person who murders a child would generally be judged a despicable monster: The immorality of harming children is even embedded in a variety of laws.[2]

Behaviors associated with meeting the adaptive challenge of surviving or avoiding disease are also moralized. One moral foundation posited by moral foundations theory, called "purity/sanctity," is rooted in the adaptive challenge of avoiding pathogens. Therefore, behaviors that help people avoid and mitigate the impacts of infections would be moral and behaviors that increase infection and transmission would be immoral (Tybur et al., 2013). The purity/sanctity foundation is one of three foundations—purity/sanctity, respect/authority, and ingroup/loyalty—referred to as the "binding foundations" because these foundations "bind" people together and emphasize collective well-being (Haidt et al., 2009). Two other foundations, harm/care and fairness/reciprocity, are referred to as the "individualizing foundations" because they emphasize individual well-being (Haidt et al., 2009). In line with parasite-stress theory, the greater the risk of infectious disease, the more people adhere to a "binding" morality (van Leeuwen et al., 2012). A morality that revolves around cleanliness, maintaining a hierarchical social order, and strong ingroup ties and outgroup avoidance is adaptive because it helps a group of people pass on their genes in the presence of infectious disease.

Together, parasite-stress theory and moral foundations theory provide a framework for understanding how people's psychology and behavior might have changed as a result of the COVID-19 pandemic. As this book attests, there are likely numerous ways that people's emotions, cognitions, and behaviors have changed as a result of the pandemic and associated events (e.g., Chapter 2), and much of this might be understood through the lens of theories like moral foundations theory (e.g., Chapter 37). This chapter takes a narrow focus on how people's morality might have shifted as a result of the pandemic and how that shift might have spurred change in how people think and act in relation to dissimilar "others" and people who violate norms.

THE "CONSERVATIVE SHIFT"

The term *conservative* means many things to many different people, including social scientists. Broadly speaking, we use the term to refer to a set of beliefs emphasizing resistance to change, adherence to traditional norms and authorities, and an acceptance of hierarchical intergroup relations (cf. Jost et al., 2003). This conceptualization of conservatism is thus distinct from political party affiliation and political identity, and it encompasses interrelated concepts like right-wing authoritarianism (Altemeyer, 1988), social dominance orientation (Pratto et al., 1994), and religious fundamentalism (Altemeyer & Hunsberger, 2004), all of which help magnify and fortify group boundaries. In theory, conservatism is an adaptive response to the risk of infectious disease because the beliefs promote durable ingroups and outgroup avoidance, which in turn help reduce the risk of infection and ameliorate the consequences of infection (Terrizzi et al., 2013; Thornhill & Fincher, 2014a).

Remember our point that when there is no directly observable "answer," people tend to rely on the available information. On a basic level, the world, and perhaps existence itself, can be terrifying. Threats and uncertainty abound. To some degree or another, everyone is motivated to think about the world in ways that make sense of those threats and uncertainties. Conservatism generally provides a stable set of answers to questions about a threatening and ambiguous world. While a bit hyperbolic, conservatism could be seen as a "survivor's guide" developed over generations and generations of humans experiencing and responding to uncertainty and threat. Some studies even suggested that a quarter to half of the variance in conservativism between people is explained by genetics (Hatemi & McDermott, 2012).

It is important to make the distinction between conservatism as a *trait* and conservatism as a *state*. In the literature drawing on parasite-stress theory and moral foundations theory, much attention has been paid to the former. These studies on individual and group differences in conservatism indicate that people who live in regions with higher risks of infection are more conservative and more strongly endorse the binding moral foundations (e.g., Thornhill & Fincher, 2014b; van Leeuwen et al., 2012), and that the binding foundations and conservatism are positively correlated (e.g., Kugler et al., 2014; Vaughan et al., 2019). The notion of a conservative shift, however, assumes that conservatism and its associated binding morality might change from one context to another. If conservatism and a binding morality are rooted in humans' behavioral immune system and help people survive and manage the threat of infectious diseases, we would expect people to be more conservative during the COVID-19 pandemic than prior to it. This would include both people who do and do not embrace traditional conservative beliefs and a binding morality. Albeit rhetoric, consider that the so-called Boston Bomber was sentenced to death in a state with the highest proportions of residents who identify as politically liberal in the United States (and that abolished the death penalty almost a half-century ago; the case was under federal jurisdiction).[3] The main point is that a conservative shift could occur temporarily *within* people and groups. The example also points to the potential paths from conservatism to other factors, namely punitiveness and prejudice. If the COVID-19 pandemic resulted in a conservative shift, there might also be shifts in punishment- and prejudice-related attitudes and behaviors (see Chapter 15 for more on political polarization during the pandemic).

The term *punitiveness*, like the term *conservatism*, can be a loaded and ambiguous term (e.g., Matthews, 2005). Here we use it to refer to people's punishment attitudes and decisions, with punishment meaning the infliction of suffering in response to wrongdoing (e.g., formal or informal norm violations). Conservatism and the binding foundations are associated with punitiveness (e.g., Vaughan et al., 2019). One reason this might be is that conservative beliefs and morality emphasize an "us" versus "them" mentality, which might fortify the distinction between "law-abiding citizens" and "criminals": Punishment, in some ways, can be a way of distancing oneself from them. Conservative beliefs and morality also emphasize reverence for and deference to authority and norms stemming therefrom ("law and order"), and crimes by definition violate formal authority and norms (i.e., law). Furthermore, crime and criminals are often associated with pathology; punishment metaphorically is a "treatment" to protect the group. Similar to our previous genocide example, it is not uncommon for people to describe those who commit especially egregious crimes as "monsters," "garbage," and "animals" (Butler, 2012; see Chapter 9 for more on moral disengagement). While speculative, it is possible that the pandemic played a role in greater support for charging police for crimes involving use of force. According to some polling, 65% of adults in the United States thought that police violence was treated too *leniently* by the justice system in 2020, an increase of over 20% compared to 2015.[4] While not definitive evidence, it is a notable shift that could be tied to some degree to the pandemic.

Prejudice is a more straightforward term meaning a negative judgment of a person because of that person's perceived or actual membership in a group (Crandall & Eshleman, 2003). Conservatism and the binding moral foundations are associated with prejudice (e.g., Park & Isherwood, 2011). Notably, prejudice and punitiveness are often linked. For example, judges and juries might think that one defendant is deserving of harsher punishment than another similarly situated defendant because of a negative evaluation of the former defendant's perceived group. Moreover, just as punishment might serve the evolutionary goal of perpetuating one's group, so might prejudice. We noted that punishment could be theoretically conceived as a way of distancing oneself from them; somewhat similarly, prejudice reifies group boundaries and can contribute to distancing in a very literal way (e.g., segregation or social distance; see Weitz, 1972). Generally speaking, prejudice encourages outgroup avoidance, which is an adaptive behavior in that it reduces the risk of contact with pathogens. Of course, prejudice-related behaviors have other consequences.

Prejudice-related behaviors have seemingly been a major topic in public discourse and media during the pandemic—prejudice in police behavior, prejudice in interpersonal violence and harassment, for instance. There were a number of protests and counterprotests, movements and countermovements. While it is hard to say to what extent the behavioral immune system's response to the COVID-19 pandemic played a role in hate crimes, for instance, an increase in hate crimes would align with a conservative, prejudiced, and punitive shift (see Chapter 23 for more on COVID-19-related prejudice and hate crime). Similarly, perhaps anti-immigrant sentiment has become more pronounced.

To briefly summarize, conservative beliefs and morality revolve on group well-being. As such, they are adaptive ways of thinking and encourage adaptive behaviors that help a group of people survive and manage the threat of infection. The pandemic might have resulted in a conservative shift, and in turn an increase in prejudice- and punishment-related attitudes and behavior, all of which would be temporary. To our knowledge, there are currently no published empirical studies applying parasite-stress theory to the COVID-19 pandemic, but we are not the first to suggest it.[5] Moreover, a number of recent studies have drawn on the concept of the behavioral immune system to understand attitudes and behavior during the COVID-19 pandemic (e.g., Schook et al., 2020). Nonetheless, the current literature is limited in a number of ways (e.g., cross-sectional designs), and no one has yet empirically tested the many provocative hypotheses associated with the "conservative shift" proposition. One obvious reason for this is that pandemics like the COVID-19 pandemic are quite rare. The title of this book includes the words "a call to action" because the COVID-19 pandemic is a rare opportunity to learn about human psychology and behavior in response to the risk of contagion. In the next section, we outline some hypotheses seated in a theoretical framework based on parasite-stress theory and moral foundations theory that future research could test.

Measuring the Conservative Shift and Its Possible Outcomes

We have proposed three interrelated "shifts" in psychology and behavior as a result of the increased risk of infection during the COVID-19 pandemic: a shift in conservative beliefs and morality, a shift in punishment-related attitudes and behavior, and a shift in prejudice-related attitudes and behavior. There are a number of ways these concepts could be operationalized and empirically investigated. We discuss some, but not all, possible hypotheses.

One basic hypothesis associated with the conservative shift is that people will more strongly hold conservative beliefs and more strongly endorse a binding morality during the pandemic than before it. This hypothesis could be tested with a "before/after" design, for instance, in which people's responses to survey items measuring conservatism and moral foundations are compared at some point prior to the COVID-19 pandemic and at some point during the pandemic. To strengthen validity, perhaps a difference-in-difference approach could be used. Naturally, the risk of infection tends to be concentrated in times (e.g., spikes in national infections) and places (e.g., rural vs. urban areas). In an ideal scenario, one might compare variation in conservatism across time in a location that experienced dynamic change in infections to a location with similar characteristics that experienced minimal or no change. Demonstrating causation is difficult, but this type of approach can help rule out potential confounding variables.

We mentioned that a conservative shift would be temporary, so other hypotheses could be posed about trends in conservatism (and characteristics thereof) across time. For example, one hypothesis might be that the trend line looks like a hill or mountain—increasing to a point and then decreasing—and one could compare the fit of different models. This would require a data set with conservatism repeatedly measured before, during, and after the pandemic (assuming there is an "after"). Such data might be nonexistent or rare, but longitudinal studies could provide insight into the behavioral immune system. How quickly do people's psychology and behavior change in response to the risk of infectious disease? How long does that change last? Are there residual changes? These are exciting questions that do not currently have very good answers.

Examining self-report measures of people's conservative beliefs and morality and how they correlate with different stages of the pandemic or the rate of COVID infections is one possible route, but there might be other creative and innovative routes readers can envision. Social media posts or search terms, for instance, could be coded and analyzed as measures of conservative beliefs and morality. Albeit a crude example, there is medium, positive correlation between search interest in the terms "God" and "infection" on Google since early 2020 in the United States.[6] As shown in Figure 37.1, the search interest trended parallel each other—notably, both peaked around the time that stay-at-home mandates were promulgated in the United States. Again, this is crude, but the point is that there might be a variety of unconventional ways to measure the conservative shift.

The approaches that could be used to examine a conservative shift could also be used to examine a shift in punishment-related attitudes. For instance, to test the hypothesis that people hold more punitive attitudes as a result of the COVID-19 pandemic, one might compare people's self-reported support for punitive criminal justice sanctions before, during, and after the pandemic. It might also be possible to examine a potential shift in punitive behaviors with measures like sentences, new legislation or policy, and voting behavior. In 2020, legislators in Nevada proposed a bill to abolish the death penalty, which, for the first time in Nevada's history, survived a policy committee and made it to a floor vote.[7] Amid

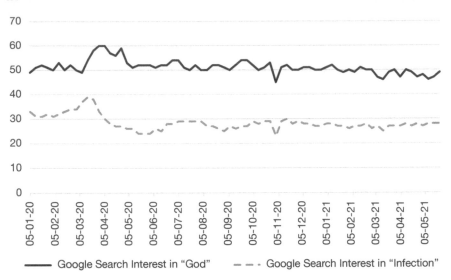

Note. Search interest ranges from 0 to 100 and reflects how popular a term is relative to its peak popularity in a time period and region. All data were obtained from Google Trends.

Figure 37.1 Trends in search interest in "God" and "infection" on Google in the United States.

the pandemic, the effort was rather unceremoniously snuffed out.[8] Like other select observations we have made, this could be entirely unrelated to the pandemic or related to the pandemic but not as a result of theoretical mechanisms tied to the behavioral immune system. Nonetheless, political behavior surrounding punishment-related legislation and policy might be one object of study for future research. One reason to mention it also is that there is a rich history of more qualitative approaches to understanding policy processes and decisions such as case studies. We have largely mentioned quantitative approaches, but qualitative designs would contribute to a deeper understanding of how people, organizations, and communities respond to the threat of infectious disease.

Dependent variables like the length of defendants' sentences are tied to what could be called "formal" punitiveness, governmental responses to lawbreaking. There is also what could be called "informal" or "extralegal" punitiveness, non-governmental responses to lawbreaking and unwritten rule breaking. Somewhat ironically, the binding foundations are associated with support for punitive legal sanctions for violent criminals, but at least one study suggested they are also associated with engaging in group violence (primarily driven by the ingroup/loyalty foundation; Silver & Silver, 2021). In some instances, group violence might be conceived as a form of punishment for violations of a codified or unwritten rule. Whether one calls it an insurrection or an instance of very aggressive tourism, the events of January 6, 2021, at the U.S. capitol seemingly involved a group of people attempting to dole out punishment in response to perceived lawbreaking. One hypothesis associated with the punishment shift is that the pandemic increased certain forms of group violence.

A shift in prejudice-related attitudes and behavior would also seem to contribute to or manifest itself in intergroup violence. The approaches we have discussed that could be applied to investigating a shift in conservatism and punishment-related attitudes and behavior could also be applied to investigating a shift in prejudice-related attitudes and behavior. People's responses to scales measuring prejudicial attitudes and people's reported comfort with and frequency of social interaction with dissimilar others, for instance, might have changed over time. We speculate, though, that the shifts in prejudice and punitiveness would be synergistic in a sense, or put another way, that the overall shift in prejudice and punitiveness would have greater consequences than the sum of the consequences of its constituent shifts (see Chapter 23). We previously noted that both prejudice and punishment fortify group boundaries and are ways of distancing us from them, and we just mentioned the study suggesting a positive link between a binding morality and group violence. A hate crime, for instance, can be conceived as the intersection of prejudice and (informal) punishment. Thus, one hypothesis based on the idea of shifts in punitiveness and prejudice is that there will be more incidents of hate crimes during the pandemic than prior to it (and/or some point after it). Similar hypotheses could be made with related dependent variables like "hate incidents" in general or forms of discrimination or harassment. At the time of this writing, July 2021, the rise in anti-Asian hate crimes and harassment during the pandemic is a subject of public discourse, and new hate crime legislation was recently passed.[9] This is a notable example because the origin of the pandemic might have provided a route for some people to rationalize their preexisting prejudicial feelings and express them by inflicting suffering for a perceived wrongdoing. Another example is the increased self-reporting of online harassment over a person's religious beliefs in 2020 when compared to 2017.[10]

Finally, hypotheses about indirect effects of the COVID-19 pandemic could be made. We basically proposed that the increased risk of infection would result in a conservative shift, which in turn would result in shifts in prejudice and punishment. Testing hypotheses about this proposed causal chain of events is exciting to think about, but perhaps the least feasible. As discussed below, future researchers will face difficulties in establishing causation. Nonetheless, we think it is worthwhile to empirically investigate potential links between shifts in moral psychology and behavior as a result of the pandemic. We were rather quick to dismiss testable hypotheses, but there might be data available to test hypotheses posing indirect effects, and qualitative studies could investigate a causal narrative.

Limitations

Perhaps the main difficulty of future research into the conservative shift is ruling out confounding factors, or "third variables." The risk of infection changed with the pandemic, but there were also a variety of other changes. For example, there was a presidential election in the United States around the start of the pandemic, and election periods tend to catalyze a focus on group identities and intergroup tensions. If a researcher compared a group of people's self-reported level of conservatism before and during the pandemic and observed a difference, the difference could be due to the pandemic, a third variable, or simply low measurement reliability. Including one or more comparison groups is probably the best route to exerting some degree of control, and collaborative research among social scientists across the globe would be especially advantageous. Admittedly, our examples throughout the chapter have been specific to the United States, but the pandemic is global.

Another difficultly, especially for hypotheses about relationships between shifts, is establishing time order. It is somewhat straightforward to establish variation in the risk of infection prior to other variations, but it will be difficult to establish that a conservative shift occurred prior to shifts in prejudice and punitiveness even if there are real-world shifts within people. A main reason for this, beyond presumably limited available data, is that we do not have well-refined expectations about timing: Say a group of people becomes more conservative from Day 1 to Day 30 in a linear fashion; if hate incidents peak on Day 7 and return to average on Day 15, is that shift an outcome of the conservative shift?

CONCLUSION

This chapter applied parasite-stress theory and moral foundations theory to understanding potential changes to people's moral psychology and behavior as a result of the COVID-19 pandemic. According to these theories, conservative beliefs and a binding morality are adaptive ways of thinking that promote behavior that serves the functional goals of avoiding and managing the risk of infectious disease. On a broad level, what helps a group *survive* might not help a society *thrive*. Conservative beliefs and a binding morality are associated with prejudice and punitiveness, and a shift in conservatism might come with shifts in behaviors like group-motivated violence. A theoretical framework–based parasite-stress theory and moral foundations theory present a provocative set of theoretical mechanisms that might explain a change in people's moral psychology and behavior as a result of the pandemic, but testing hypotheses based on it will be difficult in many cases, and when possible, internal validity might be weak. Despite barriers and limitations, future research has the potential to provide many insights into how people and groups react to the threat of disease, and that might help with preparing and responding more effectively to a future pandemic.

NOTES

1. https://www.theatlantic.com/health/archive/2020/11/pandemic-pod-bubble-concept-creep/617207/
2. For example, https://deathpenaltyinfo.org/stories/use-of-the-death-penalty-for-killing-a-child-victim.

3.   https://www.pewforum.org/religious-landscape-study/compare/political-ideol
     ogy/by/state/
4.   https://apnews.com/article/us-news-ap-top-news-racial-injustice-politics-police-
     728b414b8742129329081f7092179d1f
5.   https://blogs.lse.ac.uk/psychologylse/2020/06/19/the-power-of-the-crowd-a-post-
     pandemic-world/
6.   https://trends.google.com/trends/explore?geo=US&q=god,infection
7.   https://thenevadaindependent.com/article/nevada-assembly-votes-to-abolish-
     death-penalty-in-historic-move-bills-future-uncertain-in-senate
8.   https://thenevadaindependent.com/article/sisolak-democrats-spike-efforts-to-rep
     eal-the-death-penalty-in-nevada
9.   https://www.voanews.com/usa/anti-asian-hate-us-predates-pandemic
10. https://www.pewresearch.org/fact-tank/2021/02/01/about-one-in-five-americans-
     who-have-been-harassed-online-say-it-was-because-of-their-religion/

REFERENCES

Altemeyer, B. (1988). *Enemies of freedom: Understanding right-wing authoritarianism.* Jossey-Bass.

Altemeyer, B., & Hunsberger, B. (2004). A revised religious fundamentalism scale: The short and sweet of it. *The International Journal for the Psychology of Religion, 14*(1), 47–54. http://doi.org/10.1207/s15327582ijpr1401_4

Denson, A. J., Eys, M. A., & Irving, P. G. (2016). Great expectations: How role expectations and role experiences relate to perceptions of group cohesion. *Journal of Sport and Exercise Psychology, 38*(2), 160–172. http://doi.org/10.1123/jsep.2015-0228

Butler, B. M. (2012). Capital pretrial publicity as a symbolic public execution: A case report. *Journal of Forensic Psychology Practice, 12*(3), 259–269. http://doi.org/10.1080/15228932.2011.588522

Crandall, C. S., & Eshleman, A. (2003). A justification-suppression model of the expression and experience of prejudice. *Psychological Bulletin, 129*(3), 414–446. http://doi.org/10.1037/0033-2909.129.3.414

Haidt, J., Graham, J., & Joseph, C. (2009). Above and below left-right: Ideological narratives and moral foundations. *Psychological Inquiry, 20*(2–3), 110–119. http://doi.org/10.1080/10478400903028573

Haidt, J., & Joseph, C. (2004). How innately prepared intuitions generate culturally variable virtues. *Daedalus, 133*(4), 55–66. http://doi.org/10.1162/0011526042365555

Haidt, J., & Joseph, C. (2007). The moral mind: How five sets of innate intuitions guide the development of many culture-specific virtues, and perhaps even modules. In P. Carruthers, S. Laurence, & S. Stich (Eds.), *The innate mind* (Vol. 3, pp. 367–392). Oxford University Press.

Hatemi, P. K., & McDermott, R. (2012). The genetics of politics: Discovery, challenges, and progress. *Trends in Genetics, 28*(10), 525–533. http://doi.org/10.1016/j.tig.2012.07.004

Jost, J. T., Glaser, J., Kruglanski, A. W., & Sulloway, F. J. (2003). Political conservatism as motivated social cognition. *Psychological Bulletin, 129*(3), 339–375. https://doi.org/10.1037/0033-2909.129.3.339

Kelly, D. (2011). *Yuck! The nature and moral significance of disgust.* MIT Press.

Kenworthy, J. B., & Jones, J. (2009). The roles of group importance and anxiety in predicting depersonalized ingroup trust. *Group Processes & Intergroup Relations*, *12*(2), 227–239. http://doi.org/10.1177/1368430208101058

Kugler, M. B., Jost, J. T., & Noorbaloochi, T. (2014). Another look at moral foundations theory: Do authoritarianism and social dominance orientation explain liberal-conservative differences in "moral" intuitions? *Social Justice Research*, *27*(4), 413–431.

Matthews, R. (2005). The myth of punitiveness. *Theoretical Criminology*, *9*(2), 1362–4806. http://doi.org/10.1177/1362480605051639

Park, J. H., & Isherwood, E. (2011). Effects of concerns about pathogens on conservatism and anti-fat prejudice: Are they mediated by moral intuitions? *The Journal of Social Psychology*, *151*(4), 391–394. http://doi.org/10.1080/00224545.2010.481692

Pratto, F., Sidanius, J., Stallworth, L. M., & Malle, B. F. (1994). Social dominance orientation: A personality variable predicting social and political attitudes. *Journal of Personality and Social Psychology*, *67*(4), 741–763. http://doi.org/10.1037/0022-3514.67.4.741

Schaller, M. (2011). The behavioural immune system and the psychology of human sociality. *Philosophical Transactions of the Royal Society*, *366*(1583), 3418–3426. http://doi.org/10.1098/rstb.2011.0029

Schook, N. J., Sevi, B., Lee, J., Oosterhoff, B., & Fitzgerald, H. N. (2020). Disease avoidance in the time of COVID-19: The behavioral immune system is associated with concern and preventative health behaviors. *PLoS One*, *15*(8), e0238015. http://doi.org/10.1371/journal.pone.0238015

Silver, J. R., & Silver, E. (2021). The nature and role of morality in offending: A moral foundations approach. *Journal of Research in Crime and Delinquency*, *58*(3), 343–380. https://doi.org/10.1177/0022427820960201

Smith, D. L. (2011). *Less than human: Why we demean, enslave, and exterminate others*. Saint Martin's Press.

Terrizzi, J. A., Jr., Shook, N. J., & McDaniel, M. A. (2013). The behavioral immune system and social conservatism: A meta-analysis. *Evolution and Human Behavior*, *34*(2), 99–108. http://doi.org/10.1016/j.evolhumbehav.2012.10.003

Thornhill, R., & Fincher, C. L. (2014a). The parasite-stress theory of sociality, the behavioral immune system, and human social and cognitive uniqueness. *Evolutionary Behavioral Sciences*, *8*(4), 257–264. http://doi.org/10.1037/ebs0000020

Thornhill, R., & Fincher, C. L. (2014b). *The parasite-stress theory of values and sociality: Infectious disease, history and human values worldwide*. Springer.

Tybur, J. M., Lieberman, D., Kurzban, R., & DeScioli, P. (2013). Disgust: Evolved function and structure. *Psychological Review*, *120*(1), 65–84. http://doi.org/10.1037/a0030778

van Leeuwen, F., Park, J. H., Koenig, B. L., & Graham, J. (2012). Regional variation in pathogen prevalence predicts endorsement of group-focused moral concerns. *Evolution and Human Behavior*, *33*(5), 429–437. http://doi.org/10.1016/j.evolhumbehav.2011.12.005

Vaughan, T. J., Holleran, L. B., & Silver, J. R. (2019). Applying moral foundations theory to the explanation of capital jurors' sentencing decisions. *Justice Quarterly*, *36*(7), 1176–1205. http://doi.org/10.1080/07418825.2018.1537400

Weitz, S. (1972). Attitude, voice, and behavior: A repressed affect model of interracial interaction. *Journal of Personality and Social Psychology*, *24*(1), 14–21. https://doi.org/10.1037/h0033383

FURTHER READING

Choe, E., Srisarajivakul, E., Davis, D. E., DeBlaere, C., Van Tongeren, D. R., & Hook, J. N. (2019). Predicting attitudes towards lesbians and gay men: The effects of social conservatism, religious orientation, and cultural humility. *Journal of Psychology and Theology*, *47*(3), 175–186. http://doi.org/10.1177/0091647119837017

Fincher, C. L., & Thornhill, R. (2012). Parasite-stress promotes in-group assortative sociality: The cases of strong family ties and heightened religiosity. *Behavioral and Brain Sciences*, *35*(2), 61–119. http://doi.org/10.1017/S0140525X11000021

Hogg, M. A. (2007). Uncertainty–identity theory. *Advances in Experimental Social Psychology*, *39*, 69–126. http://doi.org/10.1016/S0065-2601(06)39002-8

McCann, S. J. (2008). Societal threat, authoritarianism, conservatism, and U.S. state death penalty sentencing (1977–2004). *Journal of Personality and Social Psychology*, *94*(5), 913. http://doi.org/10.1037/0022-3514.94.5.913

38

Looking Back on the COVID-19 Pandemic

Hindsight and Outcome Bias

HARTMUT BLANK* ∎

Long before the COVID-19 crisis is over, many people will have formed opinions about how well we—societies or countries, or even individual decision makers—have handled it. The main question I examine in this chapter is how such perceptions can be distorted by two biases—hindsight bias and outcome bias. Hindsight bias occurs when event outcomes seem more foreseeable and inevitable in hindsight than they appeared in foresight (Blank et al., 2007; Hawkins & Hastie, 1990). For instance, observers might find a second or third wave of the pandemic in a country inevitable and foreseeable in hindsight even though they did not necessarily see it coming before the event. Outcome bias, like hindsight bias, is a retrospective distortion of judgment, but it specifically pertains to judgments of the quality of event-related decision-making and to attributions of responsibility for bad event outcomes (rather than to the mere foreseeability of those outcomes; Baron & Hershey, 1988). In complex environments, even good decisions (in terms of taking all the relevant available information into account) can result in bad outcomes—but those decisions might then be perceived as flawed after the fact. Outcome bias is partly driven by hindsight bias in that

---

* I wrote this chapter in the summer of 2021, when the COVID-19 pandemic was still very much ongoing. Now, as this book goes to print in the summer of 2023, this pandemic is essentially, and thankfully, over. The delay, however, means that some of the factual statements appear premature or outdated. Still, I believe that it is better to leave the chapter as it is, as a snapshot in time, rather than re-writing it in hindsight with knowledge of the further developments. Moreover, all of the principal points I make in this chapter are not dependent on final outcomes and still hold.

Hartmut Blank, *Looking Back on the COVID-19 Pandemic* In: *The Social Science of the COVID-19 Pandemic*. Edited by: Monica K. Miller, Oxford University Press. © Oxford University Press 2024. DOI: 10.1093/oso/9780197615133.003.0038

decisions with "foreseeable" negative outcomes will be considered poor decisions, but the two biases are not the same (i.e., there are contributions of outcome valence to decision evaluation in excess of hindsight bias; see Blank et al., 2015, for a conceptual and empirical analysis). Because of their similarities, however, I treat them as broadly synonymous for the purposes of this chapter, focusing mostly on hindsight bias (as it is also involved in outcome bias) and drawing on outcome bias in its own right as required.

After a slightly more in-depth introduction of hindsight and outcome bias (including pointing out their implications for evaluations of individual and governmental COVID-19-related decisions), I highlight how hindsight perspectives can differ as a function of one's personal and political involvement and point out how hindsight bias has entered the political discourse itself. I then reflect on any lessons learned for future pandemics or similar crises and also discuss how the COVID-19 pandemic case can inform future research on hindsight and outcome bias. For example, all research on these biases to date used outcomes of single events with clearly defined outcomes. By contrast, there is no single "outcome" of the COVID-19 pandemic; multiple outcomes (e.g., physical health including deaths, mental health, social, economic) unfold over months and years as the situation develops.

HINDSIGHT BIAS

Hindsight bias was brought to the attention of psychologists through Baruch Fischhoff's groundbreaking work (e.g., Fischhoff, 1975; Fischhoff & Beyth, 1975) and swiftly developed into a "classical" bias of judgment and decision-making (see Blank et al., 2007; Hawkins & Hastie, 1990; Hoffrage & Pohl, 2003; for overviews). Three conceptually and empirically separable manifestations or "components" of hindsight bias can be distinguished (Blank et al., 2008): First are impressions of foreseeability, by which people think that outcomes were foreseeable in advance (or at least outcomes appear *more* foreseeable in hindsight than in foresight). In the case of negative outcomes, such perceptions often have unfavorable implications for decision makers. For example, in judicial contexts, foreseeability of potential negative outcomes suggests negligence, which can then lead to liability verdicts (Hastie et al., 1999; Oeberst & Goeckenjan, 2016). Similarly, the perceived foreseeability of negative COVID-19 outcomes would suggest that a government was negligent and acted recklessly in their handling of the situation (or, at the individual level, that a person acted recklessly when visiting friends and relatives—who shortly thereafter contracted COVID-19—while not being sure about having the virus themselves).

Second are impressions of inevitability; in hindsight, event outcomes appear more fixed and determined (and alternative outcomes less likely) than they really were. While this might sound similar to foreseeability at first glance, the crucial difference between the two is that inevitability refers to (perceived) objective reality (i.e., the real-world factors and reality constraints shaping possible event outcomes), whereas foreseeability is about what oneself or others knew, or could know, about this (i.e., the atmospheric forces driving the weather are principally well understood, but still the weather is often hard to predict). Accordingly, inevitability impressions also serve separate psychological functions, such as coping with loss and disappointment (Tykocinski, 2001): It makes a negative outcome more palatable if one can tell oneself in hindsight that there never was a real chance of a better outcome. In the context of the pandemic, strong impressions of inevitability might have helped coping with the loss of elderly relatives to COVID-19, particularly at the beginning of the pandemic when hardly anything was known about transmission, risk factors, and treatment, making the outcome seem inevitable indeed (not only, but particularly) in hindsight. For governmental decision makers, however, inevitability impressions would serve a quite different function, namely, the deflection of responsibility: If there was nothing that could have been done to avoid the first wave, for instance, then the government is not to blame. Conversely, if such inevitability impressions are contested, decision makers come under pressure to justify their performance; I return to this issue further in the chapter.

Third are hindsight memory distortions. The third "component" of hindsight bias reflects distorted remembering of earlier predictions (see Chapter 6 for on distorted memories related to COVID-19). For example, in the first demonstration of this memory bias (Fischhoff & Beyth, 1975), study participants provided estimates of the likelihoods of various conceivable outcomes of U.S. President Nixon's visit to China and the former Soviet Union. When recalling these estimates after the visit, they were systematically distorted toward the actual outcomes; that is, they were exaggerated on average for outcomes that did materialize and deflated for outcomes that did not materialize. Similarly, estimates of COVID-19 outcomes (e.g., deaths in a given country) made early in the pandemic might later be misremembered as being more in line with the actual outcomes (so far). In terms of pragmatic consequences in the context of the pandemic, hindsight memory distortions would seem similar to foreseeability impressions ("remembering" in hindsight that certain outcomes had been predicted implies that they were foreseeable), but generally their "moral" implications (e.g., for the conduct of decision makers) seem weaker and more indirect. For these reasons, they will not feature any further in this chapter.

In summary, hindsight bias comes in three varieties with different features and functions. Importantly, in the pandemic context (exaggerated, in hindsight), foreseeability impressions, when applied to decision makers, imply possible responsibility and blameworthiness. By contrast (exaggerated, in hindsight), inevitability impressions can help people cope with tragic COVID-19-related outcomes—but can also be used by decision makers to exculpate themselves from responsibility for negative outcomes. As discussed further in the chapter, these hindsight perceptions are just as much drivers of their moral consequences as they are themselves driven by the motivational and moral contexts in which individuals and decision makers find themselves during the pandemic.

OUTCOME BIAS

As previewed, outcome bias is similar to hindsight bias in that both are distortions of judgment that are driven by outcomes. The difference is that in outcome bias what is distorted is judgments about someone's (even one's own; Jones et al., 1997) performance or conduct (see reviews by Baron & Hershey, 1988; Rachlinski, 1988; Robbennolt, 2000). Hindsight bias can be indirectly involved in outcome bias, however. In an astute analysis, Baron and Hershey (1988) distinguished between outcome bias effects that were mediated through exaggerated perceptions of outcome probabilities (i.e., through hindsight bias) and effects that were triggered by the outcome in other ways. As an illustration of the first pathway, people can in hindsight exaggerate the foreseeability of a pandemic wave and as a result blame the government for not having prevented it. Alternatively, as an example for a direct outcome effect, people might be motivated (e.g., out of a desire for restorative justice, the need for a just world, or plain scapegoating) to punish a decision maker for a 50:50 (even in hindsight) decision that went wrong or conversely let them off if it went well.

In the context of the pandemic, such direct (not necessarily mediated through hindsight bias) outcome effects could feed into the desire of relatives of COVID-19 victims to see relevant decision makers investigated and punished. In the United Kingdom, for instance, a group of "COVID-19 Bereaved Families for Justice" demanded a public inquiry into the U.K. government's handling of the crisis,[1] particularly in the early stages (this could well find the government objectively at fault; the point here is about the mechanism underlying the subjective evaluation of the decision makers' performance). Importantly, and to emphasize the difference to hindsight-related, indirect outcome effects again, these direct effects are driven by outcome *valence* rather than outcome knowledge per se (see Blank et al., 2015; Tostain & Lebreuilly, 2008; for discussions).

The Flexible Role of Hindsight and Outcome Bias in the Context of the COVID-19 Pandemic

On the basis of the examples discussed above, it is difficult to imagine that there could be straightforward, uniform, and consistent hindsight and outcome bias effects in the context of the COVID-19 pandemic. Rather, the effects should vary depending on the particular nature of people's involvement in the situation—which also includes the possibility that in some or even many cases people's views will be more or less unbiased (as far as this can be established in the first place[2]). In fact, this heterogeneity of hindsight COVID-19 perceptions is far more interesting and relevant than any main, overarching hindsight or outcome bias.

Heterogeneous effects have been observed before in the hindsight literature; for example, people usually find positive but not negative decision outcomes or life events foreseeable in hindsight (Louie, 1999; Mark et al., 2003; Pezzo & Beckstead, 2008). This is easily understood via the wider implications of claims to foreseeability: If negative outcomes were foreseeable, why did the person make the decision regardless or fail to prepare for the event (e.g., a possible layoff; Mark & Mellor, 1991)? Moreover, people show more retroactive pessimism (i.e., inevitability perceptions of negative outcomes) in scenarios that imply little control over outcomes (Tykocinski & Steinberg, 2005), suggesting that there was nothing one could do and therefore the outcome was inevitable. Importantly, and adding to this heterogeneity, these perceptions depend on one's motivational involvement in the outcome from an actor perspective; observers and alternative stakeholders typically have different hindsight perceptions of the same situations (Mark et al., 2003).

In the current COVID-19 pandemic, heterogeneous hindsight perceptions are typically split along partisan lines. As an informal "case study" of partisan hindsight perceptions in the United Kingdom, I followed and collected general public comments on *BBC News* items related to the government handling of the COVID-19 crisis; I digest these comments here as an example of how hindsight perceptions can become polarized along political divides (I don't think this is particular to the United Kingdom; similar divides will be found in many countries; see Chapters 3 and 33 for more on the politics of COVID-19). There is no space here to analyze these comments in detail, but I outline the gist of the respective positions and illustrate them with some quotations.

The Hindsight Perspective of Government Critics

According to government critics, the COVID-19 threat, including a large number of COVID-19 deaths, was foreseeable and avoidable (i.e., not inevitable) in both the initial phase and certainly later stages. Specifically, at the beginning: "We could've seen what was happening in China, Italy [where the pandemic first started in Europe; H. B.], etc." Some also pointed to a pandemic simulation ("Exercise Cygnus") conducted by a previous government in 2016, which was available to the government when the COVID-19 pandemic started. Crucially: "Cygnus was done for a reason. It should never have been ignored in the way it was."[3] Implied in these claims to foreseeability is also that the worst outcomes could have been avoided, for instance, if Prime Minister Boris Johnson had not failed to attend five COBRA (the U.K. government's emergency committee) meetings in early 2020, had not let the Cheltenham horse racing festival go ahead in March (which was later identified as a superspreading event), had closed the airports, and had been quicker to impose a national lockdown (which eventually came on March 23, 2020).[4] Later comments echo these themes and suggest further developments that were foreseeable and should have been acted on: "Back in March we had plenty of warning—locked down late. Cases were still too high in June—came out of lockdown too early. Schools & Universities sent back—cases shot up. Tier system unfit for purpose—circuit breaker [a short national lockdown; H. B.] too late. Come out of circuit breaker too early to ensure crowded xmas shopping. People allowed to mix at xmas. Stupid."[5]

In summary, in the "critical hindsight view," the severity of the COVID-19 threat and the negative outcomes were foreseeable, and, consequently, these outcomes were not inevitable but avoidable.[6] Note that this is a remarkable combination of apparently contradictory hindsight perceptions (i.e., foreseeable but not inevitable) and certainly reinforces the idea that there is no one uniform hindsight effect (Blank et al., 2008). More interestingly, this combination might be characteristic for events within the realm of human action: The associated event outcomes are principally avoidable *because* they can be foreseen (and measures taken to prevent them).

The Hindsight Perspective of Government Defenders

Unsurprisingly, the hindsight view of government defenders (including most of the government itself) was very much the exact opposite of the critics' view. First, in this perspective the crisis and the negative outcomes were not foreseeable. For instance: "Did any country in the world have 'exact measures in place' to deal with an unknown pathogen?"[7] In addition to denying foreseeability (see the following material for a particularly interesting way of doing this), other comments suggested that the tragic outcomes were, to a large degree at least, inevitable. This comes in two varieties: First, government defenders point to other countries that supposedly did just as badly (also ignoring others that did clearly better, such as New Zealand or Taiwan), implying that this phenomenon was beyond the control of most agents (e.g., "What about France, Spain, Italy, Belgium? Germany are the exception to the rule. Most other European countries have fared about the same as the U.K., some slightly worse, some slightly better"[8]). Second, impressions of unavoidability (for the government) of negative outcomes were also strengthened through emphasizing other influences or agents at play, for example the public: "The main problem with this lockdown—after the first—is that so many will flout/ignore any & all compliance. . . . They will do anything & everything to avoid keeping themselves (& more importantly others) safe."[9] In summary, the hindsight picture painted by government defenders is very much along the lines of forces of nature (including the "irrational masses") against which one is powerless and which are largely unforeseeable (or, alternatively, foreseeability is irrelevant as one can't do anything about it anyway).

Hindsight Bias as a Defensive Political Weapon

In what must count as a stunning example of societal awareness of cognitive biases (at least when it suits one's purposes), the very concept of biased hindsight has been implicated in the debate on the government's handling of the COVID-19 crisis. Perhaps because the U.K. government's handling of the crisis is difficult to defend on objective grounds (the United Kingdom has one of the worst records in the first year of the pandemic, certainly among the G7 and European countries, in terms of both human cost and damage to the economy[10]), government defenders have taken to instead discrediting the critics' perspective as biased in hindsight (e.g., "Ain't hindsight great? It makes us all 'experts' "[11]). It appears that this move was spontaneously started by Prime Minister Boris Johnson himself. In a reply to critical questioning at Prime Minister's Questions in Parliament on July 8, 2020, he called opposition leader Sir Keir Starmer "Captain Hindsight," and he has continued to use the phrase ever since (e.g., very prominently at the Conservative Party conference in October 2020[12]), turning it into a political meme that has been widely shared by government defenders (e.g., "Keir Starmer The king of hindsight. If Boris tried to predict the lottery numbers, Keir would come out after the draw and say he should have predicted this"[13]). Government critics, of course, rejected the idea of biased hindsight (e.g., "It is simply wrong to say that Starmer has retrospectively suggested measures that the Govt. should have taken. He has done so in real time. He argued (at the time) that the first lock down was lifted too early. He argued (at that time) that the tiering and second lockdown should have been introduced earlier. He argued (at the time) that the Christmas relaxation was too much"[14]), and also tried to counter the Captain Hindsight meme (e.g., "I wonder what Johnson's nickname would be—'General Chaos' or 'Major Incompetence'?"[15]).

Hindsight Bias, Outcome Bias, and the COVID-19 Pandemic: Any Lessons to Be Learned?

Clearly, the political debate is already very much infused with the idea of biased hindsight (if not necessarily for the right reasons). Beyond this popularized version, can psychological science offer any further and perhaps more productive insights? I think three points are worth emphasizing: First, the Captain Hindsight jibe needs to be put into an enlightened scientific perspective. While hindsight bias is expected to be operative in many situations, exaggerating the foreseeability of outcomes in hindsight, it does not logically follow from this that these outcomes were completely unforeseeable to begin with. Assume, for the sake of argument, that it was possible to exactly quantify the foreseeability of outcomes; then, a certain negative outcome (e.g., the first COVID-19 wave in the United Kingdom) might have been 70% "objectively" foreseeable in foresight but 80% subjectively foreseeable in hindsight (i.e., hindsight bias accounting for the 10% increase in perceived foreseeability). Still, the actual foreseeability would be 70% in this case, not 0%. That is, hindsight bias does *not* automatically rule out "objective" foreseeability; it merely exaggerates it. Therefore, invoking hindsight bias to excuse bad government performance (where such has been displayed; this would need to be established independently, e.g., through systematic comparisons with other countries in similar situations) is not justified from a scientific point of view.

Second, there might be a lesson to be learned for attempts to *reduce* hindsight bias (which is of course desirable in terms of political and judicial fairness). With hindsight perceptions of the COVID-19 crisis and the government's handling of it being biased in opposite directions along political divides and depending on one's own involvement (e.g., decision maker or family of a victim), a good starting point for debiasing attempts—assuming some principal motivation to critically examine one's own views—would be *perspective-taking*. There is some evidence that this can work: In an experiment involving 157 U.S. judges, Anderson et al. (1997) completely *eliminated* hindsight bias in a civil liability case by asking the judges to consider possible outcomes for *alternative stakeholders* (applied to the COVID-19 context, this could mean, for instance, outcomes for people who lost their jobs in lockdown). In short, trying to view matters "from the other side" can help reduce bias, although it is worth pointing out that this has been a unique approach and needs replicating. More commonly, debiasing attempts focus on alternative outcomes (i.e., mentally simulating how the same decisions could have led to different outcomes, thus reducing inevitability impressions; e.g., Arkes et al., 1988); this and other debiasing techniques have been shown to be effective to some degree (see Giroux et al., 2016, for a review) and could be used in combination with perspective taking.

Finally, there is a general, more sobering message regarding learning lessons in the current COVID-19 crisis. The major reason why hindsight bias is considered problematic has always been that it limits people's ability to learn from experience (e.g., Fischhoff, 1980; see also Biais & Weber, 2009; Cassar & Craig, 2009, for empirical studies in applied contexts). In complex situations, learning from experience involves adapting one's (personal or collective) mental model of the subject to incoming new information. Hindsight bias undermines such updating by making it appear that one knew things all along, implying that there is no need to change one's model and approach. With some due caveats, it seems possible that such hindsight-induced complacency led some countries (e.g., Czechia, Germany, Greece, or Poland) that performed well during the first wave of the pandemic in spring 2020 to lower their guard and then suffer a massive second wave in the autumn. Likely, some relevant parameters had been missing, or had changed, from the models that informed these countries' initial approach. Perhaps the power of new virus variants to change the transmission dynamics had been underestimated, or the population's willingness to follow pandemic restrictions a second time around overestimated? In any case, the old approaches did not work anymore, and hindsight bias may partly be blamed for holding on to them for too long. In this very general sense, a good lesson to learn for the remainder of the COVID-19 crisis would be to "expect the unexpected"[16] and always be prepared to adapt one's working model(s) of the situation to new information (or even mere possibilities) sooner rather than later.

IMPLICATIONS FOR FUTURE RESEARCH ON HINDSIGHT AND OUTCOME BIASES

Some gaps in our knowledge about hindsight bias in complex societal crises have become apparent from the discussion in this chapter. It would be good, for instance, to know if the debiasing power of perspective taking generalizes beyond the one study in which it was investigated so far. It would also be desirable to more systematically explore the relation between hindsight bias and learning. Some researchers hold that hindsight bias can be a byproduct of successful learning, rather than an obstacle to it (Hoffrage et al., 2000), but we know little about the conditions under which one or the other effect is to be expected. Finally, one characteristic that distinguishes the current COVID-19 crisis from essentially all events that have been used as target events in hindsight bias research so far is its temporal extension: By the time this book is published, the world will be nearing or in the third year of the COVID-19 pandemic, and we still will not have any *final* outcomes. Compare this to typical events studied in hindsight bias research: They are all finished with final outcomes, and these outcomes will have developed over periods of minutes, hours (e.g., football matches), weeks, or months at most (e.g., liability cases in court). That is, next to nothing is known about how hindsight bias changes as a function of developing outcomes (Are hindsight perceptions cumulative? Or do they "crystallize" at some point and then remain more or less fixed? and so on), and therefore some proper ongoing, longitudinal research alongside developing events could yield important insights.

CONCLUSION

In the context of the COVID-19 crisis (or, probably, any complex and extended event with tragic consequences on a massive scale), hindsight bias and outcome bias manifest themselves in multiple different ways. To a large degree, hindsight perceptions are instances of motivated cognition (see Chapter 6) that depend, among other things, on one's political leanings and one's personal involvement in the situation. Hindsight bias has even entered the political discourse itself. Avoiding hindsight bias is difficult; it requires distancing oneself from one's own perspective and trying out alternatives to one's "time-tested" models of the situation.

NOTES

1. https://www.theguardian.com/world/2020/may/11/bereaved-families-seek-just ice-for-uk-victims-of-coronavirus; https://www.thetimes.co.uk/article/families-of-covid-dead-to-take-legal-action-to-force-inquiry-jnfp7j9lb
2. Strictly speaking, it is difficult, if not impossible, to establish the presence of genuine *bias* in the sense of a deviation of judgment from a normative or objective standard. Nobody knows how objectively inevitable a given outcome (or combination of outcomes; say, a pandemic wave of 50,000 COVID-19 deaths combined with a 10% decline of the economy) was, not least because the network of causal factors underlying it is complex and might never be known in its entirety. Relatedly, it is difficult to establish how foreseeable specific outcomes were at any point (this is not

least reflected, i.e., in the typically wide ranges of outcomes, e.g., deaths, provided by scientific prediction models). For these reasons, it is better to simply speak of hindsight *perceptions* or hindsight *effects* and then discuss these as a function of social, personality, and context, and other factors (we may occasionally still use the bias terminology, but in a loose manner of speaking, understanding that actual bias is hard to establish).

3. Comments by slim and BWhit480 on https://www.bbc.co.uk/news/uk-politics-54617148.
4. Comment by eobero on the same news item as in Note 3.
5. Comment by theythoughtwewouldnotnotice on https://www.bbc.co.uk/news/uk-politics-55529640.
6. In a rare critical moment, this was essentially confirmed by a member of the government, Home Secretary Priti Patel (https://www.bbc.co.uk/news/uk-politics-55733357).
7. Comment by Assynt on https://www.bbc.co.uk/news/uk-politics-54617148.
8. Comment by MrBlueSky on https://www.bbc.co.uk/news/uk-politics-54617148.
9. Comment by Sean on https://www.bbc.co.uk/news/uk-54783076.
10. See, for example, https://www.bbc.co.uk/news/business-57421886, https://www.ons.gov.uk/economy/grossdomesticproductgdp/articles/internationalcomparisonsofgdpduringthecoronaviruscovid19pandemic/2021-02-01
11. Comment by Aunties Magnum Hysteria on https://www.bbc.co.uk/news/uk-politics-55529640.
12. See, for example, https://www.bbc.co.uk/news/uk-politics-54435175.
13. Comment by fillhy on https://www.bbc.co.uk/news/uk-politics-55529640.
14. Comment by Nicholas John Grundy on https://www.bbc.co.uk/news/uk-politics-55733357.
15. Comment by olidab on https://www.bbc.co.uk/news/uk-politics-54435175.
16. The phrase is usually attributed to Heraclitus and/or Oscar Wilde.

REFERENCES

Anderson, J. C., Jennings, M. M., Lowe, D. J., & Reckers, P. M. (1997). The mitigation of hindsight bias in judges' evaluation of auditor decisions. *Auditing, 16,* 20–39.

Arkes, H. R., Faust, D., Guilmette, T. J., & Hart, K. (1988). Eliminating the hindsight bias. *Journal of Applied Psychology, 73,* 305–307. http://dx.doi.org/10.1037/0021-9010.73.2.305

Baron, J., & Hershey, J. C. (1988). Outcome bias in decision evaluation. *Journal of Personality and Social Psychology, 54,* 569–579. http://dx.doi.org/10.1037/0022-3514.54.4.569

Biais, B., & Weber, M. (2009). Hindsight bias, risk perception, and investment performance. *Management Science, 55,* 1018–1029. http://dx.doi.org/10.1287/mnsc.1090.1000

Blank, H., Diedenhofen, B., & Musch, J. (2015). Looking back on the London Olympics: Independent outcome and hindsight effects in decision evaluation. *British Journal of Social Psychology, 54,* 798–807. http://dx.doi.org/10.1111/bjso.12116

Blank, H., Musch, J., & Pohl, R. F. (2007). Hindsight bias: On being wise after the event. *Social Cognition, 25*, 1–9. http://dx.doi.org/10.1521/soco.2007.25.1.1

Blank, H., & Nestler, S., von Collani, G., & Fischer, V. (2008). How many hindsight biases are there? *Cognition, 106*, 1408–1440. http://dx.doi.org/10.1016/j.cognit ion.2007.07.007

Cassar, G., & Craig, J. (2009). An investigation of hindsight bias in nascent venture activity. *Journal of Business Venturing, 24*, 149–164. http://dx.doi.org/10.1016/j.jbusv ent.2008.02.003

Fischhoff, B. (1975). Hindsight foresight: The effect of outcome knowledge on judgment under uncertainty. *Journal of Experimental Psychology: Human Perception and Performance, 1*, 288–299. http://dx.doi.org/10.1037/0096-1523.1.3.288

Fischhoff, B. (1980). For those condemned to study the past: Reflections on historical judgment. *New Directions for Methodology of Social and Behavioral Science, 4*, 79–93.

Fischhoff, B., & Beyth, R. (1975). "I knew it would happen": Remembered probabilities of once-future things. *Organizational Behavior and Human Performance, 13*, 1–16. https://doi.org/10.1016/0030-5073(75)90002-1

Giroux, M. E., Coburn, P. I., Harley, E. M., Connolly, D. A., & Bernstein, D. M. (2016). Hindsight bias and law. *Zeitschrift für Psychologie, 224*, 190–203. http://dx.doi.org/10.1027/2151-2604/a000253

Hastie, R., Schkade, D. A., & Payne, J. W. (1999). Juror judgments in civil cases: Hindsight effects on judgments of liability for punitive damages. *Law and Human Behavior, 23*, 597–614. http://dx.doi.org/10.1023/A:1022352330466

Hawkins, S. A., & Hastie, R. (1990). Hindsight: Biased judgments of past events after the outcomes are known. *Psychological Bulletin, 107*, 311–327. http://dx.doi.org/10.1037/0033-2909.107.3.311

Hoffrage, U., Hertwig, R., & Gigerenzer, G. (2000). Hindsight bias: A by-product of knowledge updating? *Journal of Experimental Psychology: Learning, Memory, and Cognition, 26*, 566–581. http://dx.doi.org/10.1037/0278-7393.26.3.566

Hoffrage, U., & Pohl, R. (2003). Research on hindsight bias: A rich past, a productive present, and a challenging future. *Memory, 11*, 329–335. http://dx.doi.org/10.1080/09658210344000080

Jones, S. K., Yurak, T. J., & Frisch, D. (1997). The effect of outcome information on the evaluation and recall of individuals' own decisions. *Organizational Behavior and Human Decision Processes, 71*, 95–120. http://dx.doi.org/10.1006/obhd.1997.2714

Louie, T. A. (1999). Decision makers' hindsight bias after receiving favorable and unfavorable feedback. *Journal of Applied Psychology, 84*, 29–41. http://dx.doi.org/10.1037/0021-9010.84.1.29

Mark, M. M., Boburka, R. R., Eyssell, K. M., Cohen, L. L., & Mellor, S. (2003). I couldn't have seen it coming: The impact of negative self-relevant outcomes on retrospections about foreseeability. *Memory, 11*, 443–454. http://dx.doi.org/10.1080/0965821024 4000522

Mark, M. M., & Mellor, S. (1991). Effect of self-relevance of an event on hindsight bias: The foreseeability of a layoff. *Journal of Applied Psychology, 76*, 569–577. http://dx.doi.org/10.1037/0021-9010.76.4.569

Oeberst, A., & Goeckenjan, I. (2016). When being wise after the event results in injustice: Evidence for hindsight bias in judges' negligence assessments. *Psychology, Public Policy, and Law, 22*, 271–279. http://dx.doi.org/10.1037/law0000091

Pezzo, M. V., & Beckstead, J. W. (2008). The effects of disappointment on hindsight bias for real-world outcomes. *Applied Cognitive Psychology, 22*, 491–506. http://dx.doi.org/10.1002/acp.1377

Rachlinski, J. J. (1998). A positive psychological theory of judging in hindsight. *The University of Chicago Law Review, 65*, 571–625. http://dx.doi.org/10.2307/1600229

Robbennolt, J. K. (2000). Outcome severity and judgments of "responsibility": A meta-analytic review. *Journal of Applied Social Psychology, 30*, 2575–2609. http://dx.doi.org/10.1111/j.1559-1816.2000.tb02451.x

Tostain, M., & Lebreuilly, J. (2008). Rational model and justification model in "outcome bias." *European Journal of Social Psychology, 38*, 272–279. http://dx.doi.org/10.1002/ejsp.404

Tykocinski, O. E. (2001). I never had a chance: Using hindsight tactics to mitigate disappointments. *Personality and Social Psychology Bulletin, 27*, 376–382. http://dx.doi.org/10.1177/0146167201273011

Tykocinski, O. E., & Steinberg, N. (2005). Coping with disappointing outcomes: Retroactive pessimism and motivated inhibition of counterfactuals. *Journal of Experimental Social Psychology, 41*, 551–558. http://dx.doi.org/10.1016/j.jesp.2004.12.001

FURTHER READING

Alicke, M. D. (2000). Culpable control and the psychology of blame. *Psychological Bulletin, 126*, 556–574. https://doi.org/10.1037/0033-2909.126,4,556

Pezzo, M. V. (2011). Hindsight bias: A primer for motivational researchers. *Social and Personality Psychology Compass, 5*, 665–678. http://dx.doi.org/10.1111/j.1751-9004.2011.00381.x

39

World-Systems Analysis and the COVID-19 Pandemic

How the Structural Dynamics of the Capitalist World-Economy Exacerbate Societal Vulnerability and Undermine Collective Responses to External Shocks

MICHAEL TYRALA ■

World-systems analysis is an approach of historical macrosociology that revolutionized the study of modern social change by way of an ambitious framework and a sweeping metanarrative that combined to formulate a daring account of the history and development of the modern world-system—the capitalist world-economy (Arrighi, 1999; Chase-Dunn & Inoue, 2011; Williams, 2020). According to world-systems analysis, the structural dynamics of the capitalist world-economy—particularly the exploitative relations in the key spheres of production, circulation, and taxation—entrench and reproduce dangerous asymmetries of power within and between countries, which then translate into gaping economic, social, and political inequalities that lead to the immiseration of entire populations of the underprivileged and the marginalized, ultimately exacerbating societal vulnerability all across the world (Wallerstein, 1979, 1983, 1984). This important insight should be taken seriously even under normal circumstances given the high degree of instability and suffering that these inequalities have come to be associated with, but it gains even more relevance and urgency under the circumstances of catastrophic external shocks, especially globe-spanning ones that can only be addressed through collective responses and even more so when the responses are only as effective as the weakest link.

The COVID-19 pandemic is exactly that kind of an external shock. It is the most devastating event of the 21st century in terms of total number of deaths and long-term health outcomes; it triggered the sharpest and deepest economic contraction in the history of capitalism[1]; yet, the global response to it has mostly stood

Michael Tyrala, *World-Systems Analysis and the COVID-19 Pandemic* In: *The Social Science of the COVID-19 Pandemic*. Edited by: Monica K. Miller, Oxford University Press. © Oxford University Press 2024. DOI: 10.1093/oso/9780197615133.003.0039 out for its myriad failures, gaps, and delays in preparedness, communication, and decisive action.[2] Nearly 2 years into the pandemic, the virus itself shows no signs of abating, and the most recent projections by the International Monetary Fund (IMF) and the World Bank showed that the worst is yet to come in the form of severe economic and social crises with highly unequal impacts and dire political repercussions. Moreover, the one area in which the global response could initially be deemed at least a partial success—the relatively speedy development of effective vaccines—has now also turned into a failure due to the highly unequal global distribution of the vaccines. This chapter utilizes world-systems analysis to explain these outcomes, arguing that unless the underlying structural dynamics are radically transformed, future external shocks will be increasingly more difficult to deal with.

WORLD-SYSTEMS ANALYSIS

The foundations of world-systems analysis were laid down almost five decades ago by Immanuel Wallerstein (1974a, 1974b), but its intellectual forerunners date back much further. Despite being the source of countless original insights, world-systems analysis is a synthesis of continental European historicism (particularly Max Weber, Joseph Schumpeter, Karl Polanyi, and Fernand Braudel), Marxism and neo-Marxism (particularly Karl Marx and Antonio Gramsci), and Third World radicalism (particularly Raúl Prebisch and Frantz Fanon). It has emerged as one of the two main strands of historical macrosociology, but its influence has been felt throughout the social sciences, especially in the critical strands of international relations and international political economy. Like all successful research paradigms, world-systems analysis has not remained static over the decades. It has undergone several transformations and continues to evolve to this day. Consequently, there is no single unified world-systems consensus, but rather several distinct and sometimes contradictory world-systems perspectives (Amin, 2003; Arrighi, 2010; Babones, 2015; Chase-Dunn, 1998; Frank, 1998), although the original world-systems perspective developed and refined by Wallerstein (1974a, 1974b, 1979, 1983, 1984, 1991, 2003, 2014) remains dominant, and they all share a more or less common epistemological, conceptual, and theoretical basis. This section delves deeper into this common basis, starting with the main epistemological axiom of world-systems analysis, followed by an outline of the three main sets of concepts and theories that constitute its framework and metanarrative.

The Capitalist World-Economy as the Most Important Unit of Analysis

The main epistemological axiom of world-systems analysis is the insistence that in order to understand social reality, it should be studied holistically by capturing as much of its temporal and spatial complexity as possible: in other words, by taking into account all of its relevant historical and systemic factors (Wallerstein, 1974a, 1974b). In terms of research, the most important implication of this approach has been the substitution of the standard unit of analysis in the social sciences—the nation state—with the world-system itself. To clarify, the argument is not that social scientists should stop analyzing or comparing national or subnational histories, economies, polities, societies, populations, or any other lower order units, but that they should always keep in mind that all of these units are part of the same historical system, obeying its logic and its rules. As such, it is important to understand this logic and these rules and consider how they influence the units under scrutiny; otherwise, a considerable amount of analytical accuracy is sacrificed.

For the past several hundred years, the world-system in question has been the capitalist world-economy, the overarching priority of which is the endless accumulation of capital. The capitalist world-economy is a highly unequal system in which the success of those at the top—be they people or countries—is based on the exploitation of the labor and natural endowments of those at the bottom. For much of the history of the capitalist world-economy, this exploitation was carried out more bluntly by way of brutal repression at home and imperialism and colonialism abroad (Rodney, 1972), but gradually, the exploitation has also taken on a more sophisticated and polished form, as presented in the following outline of the approach's three main sets of concepts and theories.

The Axial Division of Labor

The first set of concepts and theories pertains to the axial division of labor, which divides production in the capitalist world-economy into core and peripheral production processes, with the pair relationally bound by an invisible axis (Wallerstein, 1979). Core production processes are capital intensive, requiring high-skilled labor and cutting-edge technology (e.g., information and communication technologies). They are the most profitable ones because they are the least accessible and thus subject to minimal competition, mostly run by global monopolies and oligopolies. Peripheral production processes are labor intensive, requiring only low-skilled labor and rudimentary technology (e.g., textile manufacturing). They are the least profitable ones because they are the most accessible and thus subject to the highest degree of competition.

When products and services enter into circulation, in other words when trade occurs, core processes are in a far stronger position than peripheral ones. This results in unequal exchange, a worldwide mechanism whereby surplus value—the profit that has been amassed through the exploitation of workers during production—constantly flows from the bottom to the top throughout the capitalist world-economy.

Aside from production and circulation, a similarly exploitative mechanism also operates in taxation (Robertson & Tyrala, 2022). The international tax system that is still in use today was set up in the late 1920s by Western colonial powers, which rigged it by skewing the allocation of taxing rights in their favor and then enshrining it in the system of bilateral tax treaties (Picciotto, 1992). This arrangement has eventually also come to enable widespread offshore tax evasion and avoidance by the capitalist classes and their multinational enterprises, eagerly assisted by the offshore-industrial complex comprising secretive tax havens and professional intermediaries from the accounting, legal, finance, banking, and other related sectors, which was likewise originally set up and continues to be overseen by many of the same Western powers (Ogle, 2017). According to the most recent estimates, this alone costs the world U.S. $427 billion in direct tax revenues every year, disproportionately affecting the working classes and developing countries (Cobham et al., 2020).

It is primarily through the exploitative relations in the key spheres of production, circulation, and taxation that the axial division of labor has led to the creation of a stark systemic hierarchy that divides the capitalist world-economy into core (developed), semiperipheral (emerging), and peripheral (developing) countries, depending to a large extent on the particular mixes of core and peripheral processes taking place within their territories, essentially determining their overall levels of power and development. There exists a certain degree of bounded dynamism within this division in that it is common for some countries to ascend and others to descend the rungs of the ladder, but the systemic hierarchy itself is set and constantly maintained with every successive cycle of capital accumulation. Hence, until there is a capitalist world-economy, there always exists an exploitative core, an exploited periphery, and in between them a semiperiphery that both exploits and is exploited (Wallerstein, 1984).

The Interstate System

The second set of concepts and theories pertains to the interstate system, which explains much of the bounded dynamism that takes place within the aforementioned systemic hierarchy (Wallerstein, 1983). States are important arenas of class struggle and play an indispensable role in cycles of accumulation by distorting the world market to favor their respective capitalist classes. The key determinant in their ability to do so is state power, the starting point of which, aside from natural and demographic endowments, is the modern bureaucratic apparatus, which leads to increasingly effective tax collection. Tax revenues then form the basis for the development of the productive, commercial, financial, cultural, diplomatic, military, and other capacities of the state. The more powerful states use these capacities to distort the world market, militarily through imperialism and colonialism, diplomatically through alliances and agreements, and economically through various forms of foreign and domestic coercion, regulation, taxation, and rule setting that reinforces the aforementioned exploitative relations. When a state succeeds in this endeavor, it attains a more favorable mix of core and peripheral processes and thus a more favorable position in the systemic hierarchy. Periodically, the ongoing rivalry between the most powerful core states ends in one of them achieving hegemony, a rare preeminent status characterized by simultaneous supremacy in so many domains of power that, for a time, it enables the hegemon to impose its own rules within the capitalist world-economy. This was once the case with Great Britain, and more recently with the United States, which is currently in the midst of its ongoing hegemonic decline (Wallerstein, 2003). Accordingly, it is state interference rather than the free market that is the more defining characteristic of capitalism. The free market is merely a product of ideology, one of the many myths used to legitimize capitalism.

The Dominant Geoculture

The third set of concepts and theories pertains to the dominant geoculture, which refers to the assortment of widely accepted truths, ideas, values, and norms that make up the ideological paradigm on which the capitalist world-economy functions and that constrains social action within it (Wallerstein, 1991). For most of the history of the capitalist world-economy, the dominant geoculture has been that of centrist liberalism, the middle-of-the-road ideology positioned between right-wing conservatism and left-wing radicalism. The fundamental difference between the three ideologies is how far and how fast they propose that progress in terms of class, racial, gender, and other traditional social hierarchies should go. Given the historical baseline of these hierarchies, what centrist liberalism delivered in practice was merely a milder form of bourgeois, White, male, and other forms of dominance. However, it also promised continued progress; so, through the combination of its moderating influence, repression, and co-option, it kept the antisystemic forces of both the right and the left in check, maintaining relative stability. This lasted until 1968, when the global wave of social unrest and general strikes in response to falling profitability and rising unemployment shattered the dominance of centrist liberalism over the two other ideologies, freeing them to reassert themselves. In an effort to retain control and stabilize the capitalist world-economy, the centrist liberal establishment strategically aligned with the antisystemic movements of the radical left on the sociocultural front, resulting in unprecedented progress on issues of race, gender, and sexuality; and with the antisystemic movements of the conservative right on the economic and political fronts, resulting in the global spread of neoliberalism, which by weakening the remaining curbs on the aforementioned exploitative relations reversed much of the progress achieved by the working classes and peripheral countries in the preceding decades and thus exacerbated societal vulnerability all across the world (Wallerstein, 2014).

WORLD-SYSTEMS ANALYSIS AND THE COVID-19 PANDEMIC

Despite the practically limitless research scope of world-systems analysis, the approach had not been directly applied to epidemics, pandemics, or the responses to them until only recently (Blinder et al., 2021). However, even from the abridged description of its framework and metanarrative presented here, it is clear that its insights, concepts, and theories can be deployed to enhance the understanding of numerous outcomes of the COVID-19 pandemic. This section highlights two clusters of outcomes that are emblematic of just how dangerous the asymmetries of power described by world-systems analysis really are. The first pertains to more general health, economic, and social inequalities and the second specifically to inequalities in vaccine development and distribution.

Health, Economic, and Social Inequalities

During the initial stages of the pandemic, the most obvious inequalities on display were those between national healthcare sectors (see Chapters 24 and 25 for more on inequalities related to the COVID-19 pandemic). As expected, most core countries have relatively well-staffed and well-equipped healthcare sectors, which helped save lives and bought their governments more time to flatten the curve (whether that time was always spent wisely is another matter), most peripheral countries barely have anything resembling modern healthcare sectors at all, and most semiperipheral countries fall somewhere in between. Nonetheless, because the pandemic had largely traced the circuits of capital as it spread,[3] it was core and semiperipheral countries that were initially the most affected. Going strictly by the number of reported COVID-19 deaths, which went beyond 3.7 million in May 2021, core countries accounted for 45% of the total, semiperipheral countries for 41%, and peripheral countries for the remaining 14%.[4] However, when attempting to quantify the pandemic's true death toll, it is not the number of reported COVID-19 deaths, but rather the number of excess deaths that provides the more comprehensive, accurate, and reliable measure. Excess deaths are defined as the difference between the number of observed deaths in a given time period and the expected number of deaths in the same time period had the pandemic never happened, thus capturing both the direct and the indirect death toll. Going by the number of excess deaths, which were estimated to have reached somewhere between 7 and 13 million in May 2021, core countries accounted for 14% of the total, semiperipheral countries for 34%, and peripheral countries for 52%. This already highlights just how unequally death and suffering have been distributed around the world, but it is only the beginning.

As the pandemic progresses and begins spilling over into what the IMF[5] and the World Bank[6] predicted to be severe economic and social crises, the inequalities are set to widen even further. This is partly because the core has been able to outspend the semiperiphery and the periphery by orders of magnitude when it comes to key policy responses such as stimulus and relief packages, job retention schemes, tax deferrals, rent freezes, eviction moratoriums, low-interest loans, loan payment pauses, and other measures,[7] and even though in some cases a disproportionate share of the benefits has been captured by the wealthy,[8] the spending has contributed significantly to cushioning the crushing blow of the unfolding crises. By 2025, the cumulative loss in output relative to the prepandemic projected path is expected to amount to U.S. $28 trillion,[9] but whereas these income losses over the 2020–2022 period are equivalent to 11% of 2019 per capita gross domestic product in core countries, they are expected to reach as much as 20% in most semiperipheral and peripheral countries. Moreover, these losses are disproportionately affecting the most vulnerable populations.[10] Earnings and employment impacts are being felt the most by younger and lower skilled workers, the informally employed, people of color, and women. At the same time, higher commodity prices have increased food, housing, and energy insecurity. Approximately 175 million people have fallen back into extreme poverty or are more undernourished than before. While public and private debt has risen across all country groups, peripheral countries and vulnerable populations are again hit the hardest because they have to borrow at higher interest rates, and debt servicing diverts funds from more pressing priorities. Meanwhile, the media have been filled with stories of the wealthy not only waiting out the pandemic from the relative safety of their second homes, yachts, and even private islands,[11] but also actually making record profits on which they often paid little to no tax.[12] Since the outbreak of the pandemic, the number of millionaires has increased by 5.2 million to 56.1 million globally, and billionaires saw their fortunes rise by 27%.[13]

The resulting tears in the social fabric have already begun to manifest in the form of dire political repercussions, leading to a further erosion of trust within and between societies and contributing to a festering of conspiratorial narratives targeting international institutions, governments, and the medical scientific community (see Chapters 18 and 36 for more on trust related to the COVID-19 pandemic). These conspiracies have not only helped foment political unrest, but also frustrated the effective implementation of even the most basic public health measures, let alone the mass vaccination programs, which experts agree are vital for ending the pandemic and that they stress needs to happen as urgently as possible because the longer the virus is allowed to spread, the higher the risk of new outbreaks featuring more transmissible and more severe variants that could evade existing vaccines. Given the emergence and persistence of the Delta variant, and the fact that April 2021 was the worst month on record yet in terms of global confirmed cases,[14] the prospect of this nightmare scenario materializing has become so real that the IMF and the World Bank now consider it to be the greatest threat to global recovery. This brings up another problem to contend with, one that is even more alarming than conspiracy-fueled vaccine hesitancy.

Inequalities in Vaccine Development and Distribution

Although vaccine development is a core process, due to its importance and urgency, there are currently over 300 COVID-19 vaccines being developed by dozens of core, semiperipheral, and even a few peripheral countries.[15] Nonetheless, the clear winners of the vaccine race—the ones whose vaccines have been administered the most and have reached Phase 4 trials—have predictably been the United States (Moderna, Janssen Pharmaceutical); the United States/Germany (Pfizer/BioNTech); the United Kingdom/Sweden (AstraZeneca/

Oxford); and China (Sinovac, Sinopharm, CanSino Biological), with most of the semiperiphery and the periphery at best only serving as either environments for clinical trials or as cheap manufacturing bases. Moreover, even though a significant portion of the funding used to develop these vaccines was public,[16] the vast majority of them are being sold for profit, and the profits have almost exclusively gone to the private sector, enriching a few individuals. Notable exceptions include the AstraZeneca/Oxford vaccine, which is being sold at cost, and companies like Sinopharm, which are majority state owned. However, it is the for-profit private sector model exemplified by Moderna that is more representative of the overall global trend. The Moderna vaccine, which is one of the most sophisticated and effective vaccines on the market, was almost completely publically funded,[17] and yet five of the nine new vaccine billionaires are associated with the company.[18]

Inequalities in vaccine development have naturally also begun to spill over into inequalities in the global distribution of the vaccines. The main reason behind this is that core and semiperipheral countries have much greater access to the vaccines, either because they developed them or because they possess the means to outbid peripheral countries when purchasing them. Of the 3.2 billion vaccine doses that had been administered as of June 2021, over 80% had gone to people in the core and parts of the semiperiphery and only 1% to people in the periphery. Even accounting for the donation pledges made by a few core and semiperipheral countries, a sufficient amount of vaccine doses is expected to reach peripheral countries only in 2023.[19] This not only increases the risk of further political unrest should new outbreaks call for a return of lockdowns or other restrictions, but also of the aforementioned nightmare scenario materializing. Despite these serious risks, core countries have been taking active steps to maintain their privileged access to the vaccines.

The most prominent example of this is their continued opposition to the temporary patent waiver on vaccines that India and South Africa officially applied for in October 2020 at the World Trade Organization (WTO).[20] The proposal finds widespread support with experts from the World Health Organization (WHO) and the global medical establishment,[21] global unions and civil society actors,[22] as well as most semiperipheral and peripheral countries,[23] but core countries and their pharmaceutical giants claim that such a patent waiver would not be helpful anyway because semiperipheral and peripheral countries lack the capacities and the expertise to significantly scale up global manufacturing while meeting the necessary quality standards. This convenient argumentation is unconvincing for at least three reasons.[24] First, there are over 140 companies in semiperipheral and peripheral countries with ample experience in vaccine manufacturing. In fact, many of them have managed to secure manufacturing contracts for the existing COVID-19 vaccines as soon as they were approved. A patent waiver would enable more of them to be drafted and begin manufacturing at least for their local populations. Second, the vaccines vary considerably in their efficacy. A patent waiver would likely increase the supply of the more efficacious vaccines and aid in the development of new vaccines. Third, the involvement of more developers and manufacturers would likely drive the prices of vaccines down. With the numerous upsides of the patent waiver so undeniable, and the only downside being a temporary hit to the profit margins of a few pharmaceutical giants, even the United States and France have eventually come around to supporting it. However, because decisions at the WTO generally require unanimity, and lobbying by the pharmaceutical giants has not let up, its passing remains highly unlikely. This was also confirmed at the June 2021 G7 summit, where the United Kingdom and Germany once again dismissed the patent waiver, pledging instead to increase their donations of vaccine doses.[25]

Meanwhile, vaccine hoarding by core countries has been reaching new proportions, especially as they have begun to administer booster shots. The United States, the United Kingdom, Canada, Australia, and members of the European Union have reportedly secured so many vaccine doses that they could vaccinate their populations four times over before many peripheral countries receive any at all.[26] As for the core's donation pledges, only a small fraction has actually been delivered as of September 2021, while 241 million of the stockpiled vaccine doses are at imminent risk of expiring.[27]

With demand so high and supply so low, the pharmaceutical giants have also become more brazen in their price gouging. Pfizer/BioNTech was accused of employing high-level bullying against at least two Latin American countries, which eventually turned to Russia and China for their vaccine needs,[28] and both Pfizer/BioNTech and Moderna have raised prices in their latest supply contracts.[29]

What these episodes reveal is not only the staggering global transfer of public funds to the private pockets of a few individuals, but also that most pharmaceutical giants and core countries would rather risk prolonging the pandemic than risk their profits and reduce the dependency of peripheral countries.

LESSONS LEARNED

The overarching lesson learned is that in order to reduce societal vulnerability and thus ensure that future external shocks will be dealt with more smoothly, it is crucial to radically transform the structural causes of inequality arising from the key spheres of production, circulation, and taxation. Minor fixes and tweaks addressing the proximate causes or impacts of these inequalities may contribute to a faster recovery and a return to the prepandemic normal, but it was that exact prepandemic normal that has made the pandemic so much worse than it had to be. The prepandemic normal was itself a period of an unfinished recovery from the Great Recession, a period beset by historically high levels of public and private debt[30]; high unemployment, underemployment, and precarious employment[31]; widespread extreme poverty[32]; and rampant inequality.[33] In short, the contemporary Holy Grail of the prepandemic normal is a Potemkin village global economy that has long been struggling, and a return to it is at best a pyrrhic victory.

The structural causes of inequality will need to be tackled from both the bottom, by eliminating extreme poverty, and the top, by redistributing excess wealth, which is even more important because it is only with the latter that the former can effectively be achieved. Moreover, what the COVID-19 pandemic has clearly shown is that redistribution needs to take place not only within countries, but between them as well. To attain these globally redistributive goals, there already exist several policy solutions that are too complex to discuss here in detail but are supported by hundreds and in some cases thousands of the most prominent experts and academics in the world. Key examples include democratizing and decommodifying work[34] (by empowering work councils to serve alongside boards as legitimate stakeholders with similar rights and by providing a universal jobs guarantee); introducing a global minimum wage[35] or a global universal basic income[36] that would set a floor for poverty (not uniform across countries, but based on a common formula to achieve a dignified living standard for everyone); and introducing a global maximum wealth cap[37] that would set an upper limit for how much wealth any individual is allowed to amass (again based on a common formula). The funding for this radical transformation of global society would come from the proceeds of a global wealth tax, a global financial transaction tax, and a global carbon tax.

None of these policy solutions are new. All of them are technically and financially feasible. And yet, at present, any single one of them (let alone the package as a whole) appears utopian, if not downright naïve. However, whether individually or as a package, they are no more utopian or naïve than the belief that the costs of the status quo will in the long term be any lower or that only minor incremental changes to it will be sufficient to adequately address future comparable external shocks, be they other pandemics, climate change, or something else entirely. On a positive note, one concrete step in this transformative direction was taken as recently as October 2021, when 136 countries representing 90% of the global economy struck a historic tax deal that includes a global minimum corporate tax rate of 15% to be paid by the world's largest and most profitable multinational enterprises,[38] many of which have been paying far below that for decades. This proves that transformative global action that seemed impossible only a few years ago is indeed possible, even though there is much further to go.

In terms of health, economic, and social inequalities, the lesson learned is that policy responses such as stimulus and relief packages work, but their effectiveness is directly proportional to how much is spent and whom it is spent on. Excess deaths, which are likely to cease in core countries after the pandemic but are likely to continue rising in semiperipheral and peripheral countries, are a case in point. Without the mitigating effects of these policy responses, the latter economies will likely take much longer to recover, further deepening existing power asymmetries.

In terms of inequalities in vaccine development and distribution, the lesson learned is that an automatic temporary patent waiver on vaccines for highly infectious diseases should be made into a global minimum standard. In fact, there is no good reason why such a patent waiver should not be permanent or why it should not apply to other life-saving vaccines as well, as was often discussed and even enforced in the past.[39] The main supposed downside of this step is that it might dissuade pharmaceutical companies from engaging in vaccine research. However, evidence from the prepandemic era suggests that vaccine research has long been severely underfunded because it is not considered by private-sector actors as lucrative enough due to the risks involved.[40] Moreover, the existing COVID-19 vaccines were already developed with significant public funding, and in some cases, such as Moderna and AstraZeneca/Oxford,[41] they were almost completely publically funded, which should make the latter's at-cost model of manufacturing and distribution the logical consequence rather than an example of corporate generosity. If even a temporary patent waiver cannot find consensus at the WTO, then every country that has not already done so should seriously consider nationalizing vaccine research,[42] or better still internationalizing it, perhaps under the auspices of the WHO. That way, the vaccines could become public goods, and even if they were sold for modest profits, the profits could immediately be channeled into more research or other public goods. Should private funding be considered indispensable due to the conditions in certain countries, then at the very least the ratio of public to private funding should be taken into account when distributing profits. In short, there are several models that are clearly superior to the typical for-profit private sector one exemplified by Moderna, in which the public spends billions to develop a vaccine and then has to spend billions more to purchase the vaccine at an inflated market rate without any commensurate financial return for its indispensable contribution. As before, retaining the status quo will only serve to deepen the existing power asymmetries further.

FUTURE RESEARCH

World-systems analysis posits that the regular functioning of the capitalist world-economy entrenches and reproduces dangerous power asymmetries within and between countries. The COVID-19 pandemic supercharged many of these patterns, making them more visible, while generating new data sources. As such, it represents an unprecedented opportunity to test many of the claims made by world-systems analysis, demonstrate structural inequalities and their real-world impacts, and thus strengthen calls for progressive policy change. What follows are just a few examples from within the two clusters of outcomes discussed above, although the expansive scope of world-systems analysis offers a much wider range of research avenues to pursue.

In terms of health, economic, and social inequalities, more research should be undertaken regarding the vast differences in the capacities of core, semiperipheral, and peripheral healthcare sectors, specifically as they relate to the pandemic. It will also be crucial to trace the patterns of excess deaths over time and see how closely they align with the expectations of world-systems analysis. More research should also be undertaken regarding the policy responses of different countries. What forms did these policy responses take? How effective were they in meeting their goals? How much was spent? Which social groups benefited the most and which the least? Will these experiences influence future policy, such as by normalizing regular transfer payments, various forms of rent control, or flexible work arrangements?

In terms of inequalities in vaccine development and distribution, more research should be undertaken regarding the amount of public funds that went into the development of the COVID-19 vaccines, including the funding of earlier scientific advances these vaccines are based on. More research should also be undertaken regarding the exact patterns of vaccine sales and donations. Which countries were able to secure which vaccines, how many, under what circumstances, when, and why? Have these patterns followed any existing relationships, such as former colonial powers selling or donating more vaccines to their former colonies or major powers using vaccine sales or donations as bargaining chips to further their interests? If the vaccine patents were waived, which countries would have the capacities and access to resources to commence manufacturing? What estimated effects would a patent waiver have on the global supply of vaccines, on their prices, and the potential to speed up research of other vaccines that are currently in different phases of development? Has vaccine distribution been subject to existing class, racial, gender, and other hierarchies? Are any of these results consistent across the capitalist world-economy or only for certain regions or countries?

CONCLUSION

World-systems analysis can explain how the structural dynamics of the capitalist world-economy have led to many of the highly unequal outcomes of the COVID-19 pandemic, from health, economic, and social inequalities to inequalities in vaccine development and distribution. The overarching lesson is stark but crucial. If the structural fundamentals are left unaddressed, the impacts of future comparable external shocks are bound to be even worse. Future research should scrutinize the structural causes of the current outcomes, expose their true societal cost, and use these data to strengthen existing calls for progressive policy change. This would contribute to making societies not only more resilient in times of crises, but also more stable and prosperous during normal periods.

NOTES

1. https://www.theguardian.com/business/2020/mar/25/coronavirus-pandemic-has-delivered-the-fastest-deepest-economic-shock-in-history
2. https://www.bbc.com/news/world-57085505
3. https://spectrejournal.com/how-just-in-time-capitalism-spread-covid-19/
4. https://www.brookings.edu/blog/future-development/2021/05/27/covid-19-is-a-developing-country-pandemic/
5. https://www.imf.org/en/Publications/WEO/Issues/2021/03/23/world-economic-outlook-april-2021
6. https://www.worldbank.org/en/publication/global-economic-prospects
7. https://www.imf.org/en/Topics/imf-and-covid19/Policy-Responses-to-COVID-19
8. https://time.com/5845116/coronavirus-bailout-rich-richer/

9. https://blogs.imf.org/2020/10/13/a-long-uneven-and-uncertain-ascent/
10. https://www.imperial.ac.uk/mrc-global-infectious-disease-analysis/covid-19/report-22-equity/
11. https://www.cnbc.com/2020/03/27/coronavirus-how-the-rich-are-self-isolating.html
12. https://www.propublica.org/article/the-secret-irs-files-trove-of-never-before-seen-records-reveal-how-the-wealthiest-avoid-income-tax
13. https://www.bbc.com/news/business-57575077
14. https://covid19.who.int/
15. https://www.who.int/publications/m/item/draft-landscape-of-covid-19-candidate-vaccines
16. https://www.forbes.com/sites/johnlamattina/2021/03/31/taxpayer-funded-research-and-the-covid-19-vaccine/
17. https://www.forbes.com/sites/judystone/2020/12/03/the-peoples-vaccine-modernas-coronavirus-vaccine-was-largely-funded-by-taxpayer-dollars/
18. https://www.oxfam.org/en/press-releases/covid-vaccines-create-9-new-billionaires-combined-wealth-greater-cost-vaccinating
19. https://www.nature.com/articles/d41586-021-01762-w
20. https://docs.wto.org/dol2fe/Pages/SS/directdoc.aspx?filename=q:/IP/C/W669.pdf&Open=True
21. https://www.theguardian.com/commentisfree/2021/mar/05/vaccination-covid-vaccines-rich-nations
22. https://www.globaljustice.org.uk/news/8668/
23. https://www.msf.org/countries-obstructing-covid-19-patent-waiver-must-allow-negotiations
24. https://www.politico.eu/article/waiving-patents-coronavirus-vaccine/
25. https://news.sky.com/story/g7-summit-boris-johnson-rejects-claims-of-moral-failure-on-vaccines-and-says-brexit-row-didnt-leave-sour-taste-in-cornwall-12331704
26. https://qz.com/2017272/rich-countries-are-buying-up-all-the-covid-19-vaccines/
27. https://www.bbc.com/news/world-us-canada-58640297
28. https://www.aljazeera.com/news/2021/3/11/investigation-pfizer-bullied-latin-american-nations
29. https://www.ft.com/content/d415a01e-d065-44a9-bad4-f9235aa04c1a
30. https://www.reuters.com/article/us-global-markets-debt-idUSKBN1XP1FB
31. https://www.ilo.org/global/about-the-ilo/newsroom/news/WCMS_670171/lang--en/index.htm
32. https://www.theguardian.com/commentisfree/2019/jan/29/bill-gates-davos-global-poverty-infographic-neoliberal
33. https://www.theguardian.com/global-development-professionals-network/2016/apr/08/global-inequality-may-be-much-worse-than-we-think
34. https://global.ilmanifesto.it/democratizing-work/
35. https://fpif.org/the-time-has-come-for-a-global-minimum-wage/
36. https://www.g20-insights.org/policy_briefs/building-global-citizenship-through-global-basic-income-and-progressive-global-taxation/
37. https://www.theguardian.com/commentisfree/2019/sep/19/life-earth-wealth-megarich-spending-power-environmental-damage

38. https://www.oecd.org/tax/oecd-secretary-general-tax-report-g20-finance-minist
     ers-october-2021.pdf
39. https://theconversation.com/the-us-drug-industry-used-to-oppose-patents-what-
     changed-161319
40. https://www.nbcnews.com/health/health-care/scientists-were-close-coronavirus-
     vaccine-years-ago-then-money-dried-n1150091
41. https://www.theguardian.com/science/2021/apr/15/oxfordastrazeneca-covid-vacc
     ine-research-was-97-publicly-funded
42. https://www.technologyreview.com/2002/05/01/275581/should-the-government-
     make-vaccines/

REFERENCES

Amin, S. (2003). *Obsolescent capitalism: Contemporary politics and global disorder.* Zed Books.

Arrighi, G. (1999). Globalization and historical macrosociology. In J. Abu-Lughod (Ed.), *Sociology for the twenty-first century: Continuities and cutting edges* (pp. 117–133). The University of Chicago Press.

Arrighi, G. (2010). *The long twentieth century: Money, power, and the origins of our times* (2nd ed.). Verso.

Babones, S. J. (2015). What *is* world-systems analysis? Distinguishing theory from perspective. *Thesis Eleven, 127*(1), 3–20.

Blinder, D., Zubeldía, L., & Surtayeva, S. (2021). Covid-19 and semi-periphery: Argentina and the global vaccines research and development. *Journal of World-Systems Research, 27*(2), 494–521.

Chase-Dunn, C. K. (1998). *Global formation: Structures of the world-economy* (2nd ed.). Rowman & Littlefield.

Chase-Dunn, C. K., & Inoue, H. (2011). Immanuel Wallerstein. In G. Ritzer & J. Stepnisky (Eds.), *The Wiley-Blackwell companion to major social theorists: Volume II—Contemporary social theorists* (pp. 395–411). Wiley-Blackwell.

Cobham, A., Garcia-Bernardo, J., Palanský, M., & Mansour, M. B. (2020, November 20). *The state of tax justice 2020: Tax justice in the time of COVID-19.* Tax Justice Network, the Global Alliance for Tax Justice, and Public Services International. https://www.taxjustice.net/reports/the-state-of-tax-justice-2020/

Frank, A. G. (1998). *ReORIENT: Global economy in the Asian age.* University of California Press.

Ogle, V. (2017). Archipelago capitalism: Tax havens, offshore money, and the state, 1950s–1970s. *The American Historical Review, 122*(5), 1431–1458.

Picciotto, S. (1992). *International business taxation: A study in the internationalization of business regulation.* Cambridge University Press.

Robertson, J., & Tyrala, M. (2022). *The uneven offshore world: Mauritius, India, and Africa in the global economy.* Routledge.

Rodney, W. (1972). *How Europe underdeveloped Africa.* Bogle-L'Ouverture Publications.

Wallerstein, I. M. (1974a). *The modern world-system: Capitalist agriculture and the origins of the European world-economy in the sixteenth century.* Academic Press.

Wallerstein, I. M. (1974b). The rise and future demise of the world capitalist system: Concepts for comparative analysis. *Comparative Studies in Society and History*, *16*(4), 387–415.

Wallerstein, I. M. (1979). *The capitalist world-economy*. Cambridge University Press.

Wallerstein, I. M. (1983). *Historical capitalism*. Verso.

Wallerstein, I. M. (1984). *The politics of the world-economy: The states, the movements and the civilizations*. Cambridge University Press.

Wallerstein, I. M. (1991). *Geopolitics and geoculture: Essays on the changing world-system*. Cambridge University Press.

Wallerstein, I. M. (2003). *The decline of American power: The U.S. in a chaotic world*. The New Press.

Wallerstein, I. M. (2014). Antisystemic movements, yesterday and today. *Journal of World-Systems Research*, *20*(2), 158–172.

Williams, G. P. (2020). *Contesting the global order: The radical political economy of Perry Anderson and Immanuel Wallerstein*. State University of New York Press.

FURTHER READING

el-Ojeili, C. (2015). Reflections on Wallerstein: The modern world-system, four decades on. *Critical Sociology*, *41*(4–5), 679–700.

Goldfrank, W. L. (2000). Paradigm regained? The rules of Wallerstein's world-system method. *Journal of World-Systems Research*, *6*(2), 150–195.

Wallerstein, I. M. (2000). *The essential Wallerstein*. The New Press.

Wallerstein, I. M. (2004). *World-systems analysis: An introduction*. Duke University Press.

40

Can COVID-19 Help Save the World?

The Consequence of the Pandemic for Changes in Climate Change Mitigation at the Institutional and Individual Levels

ADRIAN D. WÓJCIK AND MARZENA CYPRYAŃSKA ■

What will the postpandemic world be like? How will the pandemic change societies and the future of the world? Such questions started appearing in the public discussion at the beginning of the pandemic. They represent how the fear of the virus mingled with hope about changes in the future and how people were trying to find meaning in a tragic situation.

One thing seems inevitable: The world after COVID-19 is unlikely to be the world that existed before COVID-19. The pandemic seems to have made the future arrive faster. Many trends that were already underway in the world, such as the digital economy and digital behavior in general, have been accelerated during the pandemic. Also, independently of whether some things can be rebuilt, people might not want to rebuild them. For example, the World Economic Forum-Ipsos global survey, which was conducted in September 2020 with more than 21,000 adults from 27 countries, found that 86% of respondents preferred that the world would become more sustainable and equitable rather than return to how the world was before the COVID-19 crisis started.[1] The same was found for people's personal lives. Most respondents (72%) indicated that they wanted their lives to change significantly rather than to return to what their lives were like before the COVID-19 crisis.[2]

In addition to being a dramatic crisis that forced many unwanted changes in daily lives, the pandemic served as a warning. Specifically, the pandemic led many people to reflect on the world's condition and to consider how a world plagued by a pandemic can be made fairer, more sustainable, and more beautiful after

Adrian D. Wójcik and Marzena Cypryańska, *Can COVID-19 Help Save the World?* In: *The Social Science of the COVID-19 Pandemic.* Edited by: Monica K. Miller, Oxford University Press. © Oxford University Press 2024. DOI: 10.1093/oso/9780197615133.003.0040 the pandemic ends. This is what we call the postpandemic call for action, and it represents what can be observed in times of crisis. As noted by Rahm Emmanuel, chief of staff for President Barack Obama, when referring to the global financial crisis of 2008–2009: "You never want a serious crisis to go to waste," and whenever there is crisis people should look for a way to make it "an opportunity to do things that you think you could not before."

This chapter focuses on the challenges and opportunities for climate change mitigation that arise from the pandemic. At first glance, the COVID-19 pandemic and changes in the global climate do not seem to have much in common. The pandemic is an acute problem (it was unheard of before December 2019), and the effects of COVID-19 are immediate, are relatively easily measured, and shape people's daily experiences. In contrast, global climate change has been developing for decades, and its effects are measured in ways the average person cannot understand, and people cannot easily or readily identify how climate change affects them.

Nevertheless, the challenges posed by these two global problems have much in common. First, the solutions to each require coordinated, globalized, collective action. A COVID-19 variant in one country is a cause for concern in all countries. Similarly, a loss of biodiversity or excessive greenhouse gas emissions affects everyone. The climate is a global entity, and the interconnected nature of contemporary human society makes a virulent infection such as COVID-19 a global entity. Although countries can close their borders in an attempt to fight COVID-19, such strategies are short term, and unless a worldwide solution is found, countries that self-isolate will eventually experience economic, social, and political distress. Similarly, countries can make great strides to mitigate climate change in their borders, but climate change does not stop at borders.

Also, perhaps inevitably, the global nature of these two problems has led to their politicization despite the fact that understanding climate change and COVID-19 are scientific challenges. Scientists have known for decades that human activity has been changing the climate. There is no doubt about this among scientists. Similarly, there is a wealth of scientific evidence about how to contain the spread of infection. Admittedly, the novelty of COVID-19 made it difficult to develop vaccines in a few months, but there was available a wealth of scientific research about how to treat (and how not to treat) infections such as COVID-19.

Unfortunately, many politicians have reframed climate change mitigation and responding to the COVID-19 pandemic in terms of political choices. For such politicians, whether the climate is changing is viewed as a political question. Similarly, getting vaccinated is not about the science of vaccines, it is about personal, often politically motivated, views about vaccines and science in general. Although this is particularly visible in Brazil, in nearly every country there are movements that use populist, antiscience arguments to oppose climate change mitigation and COVID vaccination.

Indeed, the pandemic has shown that mass problems might not be resolved without the involvement of behavioral sciences (Van Bavel et al., 2020). The pandemic might encourage people to reflect on society and its problems and opportunities and might reveal what is unclear and needs to be understood to respond to the current world's challenges. In the following sections we summarize and describe (1) how social crises transform everyday behaviors, needs, and beliefs about the future; (2) how everyday behaviors can be influenced by social context (e.g., social norms); (3) the ways such social changes can be used to promote a more sustainable future; and (4) the mechanisms that contribute to sustaining individual behavioral changes.

PANDEMIC AS A GLOBAL LIFE DISRUPTOR

The global pandemic influenced virtually every aspect of all societies, and perhaps the most affected have been public health and the economy (Diffenbaugh et al., 2020). The day the first draft of this chapter was submitted (June 9, 2021) more than 174,700,000 people worldwide had been infected with COVID-19, and the COVID-19 death toll was estimated to be approximately 3.7 million. The restrictions implemented on mobility (lockdown to reduce the virus transmission, social distancing, and self-isolation) helped save human lives, but they had unprecedented socioeconomic consequences (Saadat et al., 2020). It is estimated that around 80% of the global workforce has been affected to some extent by lockdown measures, with substantial job losses and furloughs.[3]

The consequences of the pandemic also included the environment. Global consumption has fallen with reductions in traveling, shopping for discretionary items, and engaging in experience-based activities. The economic slowdown led to improvements in environmental quality, such as a reduction in ambient air pollution, water pollution, and noise pollution. Initially, the pandemic was discussed as a chance for nature to restore itself, but as the situation unfolded, the environmental consequences of the pandemic became more complex. For example, the pandemic led to an increase in medical waste production and plastic pollution (Ankit et al., 2021).

Nevertheless, taking into account environmental damage and benefits suggests that the pandemic has had positive environmental effects, particularly in reducing greenhouse gas (GHG) emissions due to economic decline. Although it is impossible to detect GHG emissions in the short term accurately, it has been estimated that, globally, GHG emissions fall by 5.4% in 2020. This is one of the most significant yearly emission reduction since World War II (Laughner et al., 2021).

Unfortunately, although the present reduction of GHG emissions is beneficial, it is not enough to mitigate climate change. To avoid ecological collapse, the current emissions drop will need to be sustained year after year to reach net-zero emissions by 2050. Moreover, it is important to note that the present reduction was the result of changes that were not meant to address climate change and were not meant to be permanent. The reduction was not the result of conscious decisions and persistent changes in behaviors, which means that it is likely that emissions will rebound once economies recover (Hepburn et al., 2020).

Representatives of the economic and business sectors agree that the current crisis can provide an opportunity for a large-scale green transformation. Across the world, various types of economic activities need to be restarted, and this presents a phenomenal opportunity to introduce environmentally sensitive practices into various business and other activities. If a business needs to restart, why not restart green? Accordingly, economic experts and representatives of G20 countries have stated that the economic recovery after COVID-19 has to include ecological elements like clean research and development and investment in clean energy infrastructure because it makes so much sense to do this now.

Nevertheless, it is not clear if there is or will be global support for such actions. For example, the recent reports of the development charity Tearfund, the Overseas Development Institute, and the International Institute for Sustainable Development were recently summarized in *The Guardian* (Laville, 2021). These reports were not optimistic. Specifically, the analyses reveal that between January 2020 and March 31, 2021 seven of the world's richest nations (G7) spent more money to support fossil fuels than clean forms of energy ($189 billion vs. $147 billion). The analyses strengthened the appeal made in the new report of the International Energy Agency[4]: "This gap between rhetoric and action needs to close if we are to have a fighting chance of reaching net zero by 2050 and limiting the rise in global temperatures to 1.5°C." This gap has many reasons, including political and economic conditions, as well as lobbying by the fossil fuel industry. The gap between rhetoric and action can be decreased if there is social pressure to change, social pressure that is based on social expectations, social needs, and finally, individual and collective action.

Although the green transformation depends heavily on systemic change, such as the introduction of carbon-reduction policies, it does not make the actions of individual people unimportant. The reduction of personal greenhouse gas emissions, support for climate change mitigation policies, and collective action that puts pressure on the system play essential roles in climate change mitigation. How the present pandemic crisis influences individual lifestyles, attitudes, beliefs, and needs will play crucial roles in future green transformation. Accordingly, we believe that to take advantage of these opportunities, we need to understand the dynamics of group behavior and how the pandemic-induced disruption of the global economy has influenced the daily lives of individual people, including their habitual (and often unstainable) behaviors. In the following sections, we describe some of the challenges and opportunities that we think are crucial to a widespread green transformation. We also point out those parts of social theory that need to be developed in order to solve the current environmental crisis.

THE PANDEMIC AS A DISRUPTOR OF DAILY HABITS AND THE POTENTIAL FOR INCREASING CLIMATE CHANGE MITIGATION BEHAVIOR

For some time, climate change researchers have been paying attention to the fact that increasing environmental awareness does not translate into changes in behaviors that mitigate climate change. There are many reasons for this (Gifford, 2011; Markowitz & Shariff, 2012), but what seems to be crucial is that climate change mitigation requires long-lasting changes, that is, permanent changes in daily habits. Habits are considered one of the most substantial obstacles to the lifestyle changes that can block new behaviors (Verplanken & Whitmarsh, 2021), and information campaigns are likely to be ineffective when they are not strong enough to disrupt everyday habits. Therefore, when considering the impact of the pandemic, it is important to understand the potential the disruptions of daily habits and lifestyle have for mitigating climate change (Monbiot, 2017).

The prolonged lockdowns and restrictions in commercial and business activities resulted in changing everyday behaviors, including a reduction in habitual behaviors that decrease sustainability (Whitmarsh et al., 2021). Probably one of the most tangible effects of the pandemic disruption of daily routines is that reactions to the pandemic included more environmentally friendly behaviors. For example, the pandemic lowered people's ecological footprint due to reductions in shopping and traveling.

This brought the planet some momentary relief; however, will such changes be continued when the pandemic is over? Existing research on attitude and behavior change suggests cautious optimism. It is unlikely that changes in behaviors forced by external factors will automatically become permanent habits that persist in the absence of these external factors. Many behaviors (including habits) are triggered automatically by environmental cues, but when those cues disappear, the behaviors that they elicited are likely to end or to be reduced considerably in magnitude and frequency (Verplanken & Orbell, 2019).

A critical issue in understanding the durability of changes elicited by the pandemic is whether the changes forced by the pandemic will be attributed to external or internal factors, including the perception of benefits from these changes. To the extent changes are seen as externally caused, it is less likely that the changes that occurred during the pandemic will be sustained after the pandemic ends. In contrast, the extent changes are seen as internally motivated are more likely to be sustained after the pandemic ends. In other words, it is unlikely that people will continue environmentally friendly behaviors if these changes are not accompanied by changes in attitudes, beliefs, and finally, the willingness to change their behaviors.

We present a few suggestions to help make a social transformation more ecologically friendly and more durable. First, whatever behavioral changes that occurred did not occur in an ecological vacuum. Globally, public support for policy change and various actions on climate change mitigation has gradually (although slowly) increased over the years, and it reached a peak before the pandemic. In many countries, government and corporate action in support of climate change mitigation have also increased over the past few years. Although the pandemic has slowed this acceleration, at the same time, it did not stop it.

What is important here is that the experience of the pandemic has not only broken daily habits but also challenged people's sense of security, stability, and predictability. In part this was due to the belief that the pandemic (or something like it) was foreseeable. This, combined with the adverse and painful outcomes of the pandemic, started increasing people's awareness of other phenomena that could have consequences worse than the pandemic.

As a result, the pandemic raised in the public discourse fundamental questions about the world's condition and future threats, which strengthened the common prepandemic feeling of "there is something wrong with the world today."[5] It also raised the concern for both individual people's health and the planet's condition, which can lead to decisions that combat climate change. Additionally, the results of opinion polls have found that people could notice uncongested streets and the return of wildlife and birdsong. Such observations can lead to questioning the desirability of what is called "normal," which is what was seen to be common and normative before pandemic. Also, people started appreciating the value of nature and being in nature (Naomi, 2020). Consistently, data from the cross-national research led by Open Society Foundations[6] show that most Western citizens are more interested in sustainability now than they were before the pandemic.

Such changes can make the COVID-19 crisis a turning point in progress on global climate change; however, the crucial factor here might be what people realized, thanks to pandemic experience, and their changes intentions, not necessarily what they were forced to do (or not to do) during the pandemic. Following this, we do not expect that whatever changes that occur will simply be a continuation of the changes in behavior that were forced by the pandemic; rather, we expect that changes will be manifested in looking for new ways to have more sustainable lifestyles, and this might be based more on approach motives than avoidance motives. This is what happens when people accept they need to change their lives (not simply need to solve a problem or avoid the threat) (Green, 2016).

Note that, at least at the beginning of the pandemic, in the face of an acute threat, people's behavior could be easily motivated by such basic factors as fear, especially when these behaviors are clearly related to protection from the threat (Cypryańska & Nezlek, 2020). In contrast, as the pandemic endured, resistance to restrictions and tendencies to deny the threat seemed to increase. To motivate long-term changes, particularly changes in lifestyle, changes in factors such as values, social and personal norms, and personal needs are required to motivate adaptive behaviors in response to immediate threats.

Therefore, to support the development of behavioral intentions it will be important for communicators to emphasize the rewards people will/can obtain by acting in a more sustainable fashion rather than emphasizing the costs they will incur if they do not act in a more sustainable fashion. We believe that how changes in daily behaviors that would mitigate climate change have been framed is not the best context to elicit desirable changes. Frequently, desirable changes have been framed in terms of sacrifices and resignations (e.g., limiting meat consumption, reducing consumption, and reducing traveling). We believe that more positive frames would be more effective (Bain et al., 2015).

ECOLOGICAL IDENTITY

Although there is a hope that a broad social transformation can occur after the pandemic, such a transformation must be grounded in not only the pandemic forced changes but also the enhanced environmental values. Current research suggests that maintaining the positive habit changes such as those that have occurred during the pandemic and expanding these changes to include other domains require strengthening ecological identity (Whitmarsh & O'Neill, 2010). Pro-environmental identity brings consistency and stability across different types of pro-environmental behaviors. As individuals adopt a stronger pro-environmental identity, this changes the support for pro-environmental behaviors from external, situational influences to more internal and stable dispositional influences.

Social psychology suggests two parallel paths that could strengthen pro-environmental identities shaped by the pandemic. The first is based mainly on personal (individual) identity. For example, according to Bem's (1972) self-perception theory, people sometimes infer their attitudes from their own behaviors. During the pandemic, the pro-environmental identity should emerge due to the restriction of everyday consumption. However, the process is unlikely to occur during the pandemic, as it is extremely easy to attribute one's behaviors to external influence.

A second way of strengthening pro-environmental identities created during the pandemic seems more promising. This possibility relies on social (collective) identity. Social identities are based on feelings of connectedness with other ingroup members, for example a nation or the ecological movement. To the extent an individual identifies as being a member of a group that consists of people who are environmentally aware, such an identity should provide support for pro-environmental actions and attitudes (see Chapter 16 for more on collective identity).

Nevertheless, adopting a pro-environmental collective identity alone is not enough to meet the challenges of climate change. Climate change mitigation requires both individual and collective action. An individual can adopt an environmentally friendly identity and behave in ways that are consistent with this identity, recycling, reducing the use of cars, and so forth; however, it is not clear how closely related pro-environmental behaviors in the private sphere are to support pro-environmental policies. Are/will decreasing levels of antienvironmental behaviors be associated with increased support for collective action?

INDIVIDUAL AND COLLECTIVE ACTIONS TO SOLVE THE ENVIRONMENTAL CRISIS

The available research suggests that pro-environmental individual behaviors are either weakly correlated or can be negatively correlated with collective action. For example, a cross-cultural study of European citizens found that actions in the collective and private spheres were independent (Johansson et al., 2018). At the same time, a Japanese study found that when people are reminded about their individual contributions to energy savings/conservation, their support for systematic action decreases (Werfel, 2017). Clearly, more research about such relationships is needed.

The general public's acceptance of new environmentally friendly policies will be needed to support the emerging agreement among societal leaders that the pandemic is an opportunity to move in a new and more environmentally friendly direction. For example, in September 2020 Ursula von der Leyen, president of the European Commission, declared that the postpandemic recovery should involve a more environmentally friendly transition connected with social justice. Moreover, this belief was supported by economic experts of the G20 countries. Specifically, the results of a survey of business representatives and economic experts of the G20 countries found that they believed that the economic recovery after COVID-19 has to include ecological elements such as clean research and development and investment in clean energy infrastructure (Hepburn et al., 2020).

Since the beginning of the pandemic, the postpandemic recovery has been presented (at least in Western countries) as inseparable from the green and pro-environmental transformation. What is not clear, however, is the extent to which average citizens believe that new environmental policies are beneficial to them. This is another line of research that needs to be developed: What individual differences are related to acceptance of the postpandemic green recovery?

Social scientists also need to focus on the collective level and treat the pandemic as a natural laboratory that allows researchers to capture processes at this level. Many responses to the pandemic were collective in nature. Even though many preventive methods such as social distancing and handwashing were individually based, the effectiveness of these measures depended on other people's behaviors. Moreover, individual actions communicated and strengthened specific collective identities. For example, refusing to wear masks during the pandemic became a sign of conservative ideology. Similarly, it is possible that refusing to engage in environmental actions will be a similar sign of political identity in the days to come.

There is also a need to understand how processes at the collective level such as social norms and values both influence and are influenced by individual-level behaviors, beliefs, and attitudes. For example, Fairbrother (2016) found that people who live in countries in which citizens believe that the government will act effectively to mitigate climate change are more willing to make sacrifices and to support financially pro-environmental actions than people who live in countries in which citizens do not think the government will act effectively to mitigate climate change. People who have strong pro-environmental attitudes will act accordingly and support pro-environmental policies only when they believe that the government will work effectively.

It is also likely that support for pro-environmental policies will depend on the rate of the postpandemic economic recovery. The influence of the rate of the recovery on the environment remains unclear and should be carefully examined.

In the short term, economic recovery can lead to increased environmental impact, but in the long term, the influence of economic recovery might not be positive. First, economic growth is usually positively related to postmaterialist values (Inglehart, 1977), which include environmental protection. Second, optimism about future living standards leads to support for more ambitious environmental policies (Fairbrother et al., 2021). It remains to be seen what the combined effects of these different influences will be.

CONCLUSION

Although the pandemic is one of the most stressful events of the 21st century, it provides insights into how we can deal with other global problems (e.g., the change in Earth's climate). The pandemic made more visible the importance of the behavioral and social sciences. Dealing with COVID-19 required knowledge that was beyond the mechanics of medicine and biology. Managing the pandemic required behavioral change, and this was best accomplished with guidance from behavioral scientists.

Behavioral change is also required to deal with the environmental crisis. The science of climate change and the solutions to it are well understood. There is little doubt among scientists about what is happening and what needs to be done to change the present situation and trajectory. Nevertheless, the commitment that is needed to mobilize the global public to solve the problem of climate change does not exist. Part of this is that the roles the behavioral sciences can play to solve global problems are not recognized and are underdeveloped (Overland & Sovacool, 2020). Another contributing factor is that the social sciences do not offer one-size-fits-all solutions. For example, local contexts need to be taken into account when formulating policy guidelines (IJzerman et al., 2020). Along these lines, it is crucial to expand scientific research beyond the traditional focus on WEIRD[7] populations.

The success of the behavioral sciences in helping to deal with the pandemic can change this. This success can also encourage researchers to focus more on applications of their work and on how their work can benefit society. Although behavioral science helped society deal with the pandemic, it also made more visible shortcomings in the existing research, particularly in terms of connections between individual and collective pro-environmental behaviors and institutional efficacy.

ACKNOWLEDGMENT

The author(s) disclose receipt of the following financial support for the research, authorship, and/or publication of this chapter: This work was supported by the National Science Center (Grant No. 2018/29/B/HS6/02826 and 2020/37/B/HS4/00988).

NOTES

1. IPSOS. (2020). How much is the world yearning for change after the COVID-19 crisis? https://www.ipsos.com/sites/default/files/ct/news/documents/2020-09/glo bal-yearning-for-change-after-the-covid-19-crisis-2020-09-ipsos.pdf
2. Russo, A., & Markovitz, G. (2020). Nearly 9 in 10 people globally want a more sustainable and equitable world post COVID-19. The World Economic Forum. https://www.weforum.org/press/2020/09/nearly-9-in-10-people-globally-want-a-more-sustainable-and-equitable-world-post-covid-19
3. ILO. (2021). ILO Monitor: COVID-19 and the world of work (7th ed). https://www.ilo.org/wcmsp5/groups/public/@dgreports/@dcomm/documents/briefingnote/wcms_767028.pdf
4. IEA. (2021). Net *zero* by 2050. A *roadmap for the global energy sector*. International Energy Agency; p. 3. https://iea.blob.core.windows.net/assets/4482cac7-edd6-4c03-b6a2-8e79792d16d9/NetZeroby2050-ARoadmapfortheGlobalEnergySec tor.pdf
5. Aerosmith. (1993). *Livin' on the Edge*. Geffen.
6. Eichhorn, J., Molthof, L., & Nicke, S. (2020). *From climate change awareness to climate crisis action*. Open Society–European Policy Institute.
7. Western, educated, industrialized, rich, and democratic (WEIRD) nations.

REFERENCES

Ankit, Kumar, A., Jain, V., Deovanshi, A., Lepcha, A., Das, C., Bauddh, K., & Srivastava, S. (2021). Environmental impact of COVID-19 pandemic: More negatives than positives. *Environmental Sustainability*, *4*, 447–454. https://doi.org/10.1007/s42 398-021-00159-9

Bain, P. G., Milfont, T. L., Kashima, Y., Bilewicz, M., Doron, G., Garðarsdóttir, R. B., Gouveia, V. V., Guan, Y., Johansson, L.-O., Pasquali, C., Corral-Verdugo, V., Aragones, J. I., Utsugi, A., Demarque, C., Otto, S., Park, J., Soland, M., Steg, L., González, R., . . . Saviolidis, N. M. (2015). Co-benefits of addressing climate change can motivate action around the world. *Nature Climate Change*, *6*, 154–157. https://doi.org/10.1038/nclimate2814

Bem, D. J. (1972). Self-perception theory. In L. Berkowitz (Ed.), *Advances in experimental social psychology* (pp. 1–62). Academic Press.

Cypryańska, M., & Nezlek, J. B. (2020). Anxiety as a mediator of relationships between perceptions of the threat of COVID-19 and coping behaviors during the onset of the pandemic in Poland. *PLoS One*, *15*(10), e0241464. https://doi.org/10.1371/jour nal.pone.0241464

Diffenbaugh, N. S., Field, C. B., Appel, E. A., Azevedo, I. L., Baldocchi, D. D., Burke, M., Burney, J. A., Ciais, P., Davis, S. J., Fiore, A. M., Fletcher, S. M., Hertel, T. W., Horton, D. E., Hsiang, S. M., Jackson, R. B., Jin, X., Levi, M., Lobell, D. B., McKinley, G. A., . . . Wong-Parodi, G. (2020). The COVID-19 lockdowns: A window into the earth system. *Nature Reviews Earth & Environment*, *1*(9), 470–481. https://doi.org/10.1038/s43017-020-0079-1

Fairbrother, M. (2016). Trust and public support for environmental protection in diverse national contexts. *Sociological Science, 3,* 359–382. https://doi.org/10.15195/v3.a17

Fairbrother, M., Arrhenius, G., Bykvist, K., & Campbell, T. (2021). Governing for future generations: How political trust shapes attitudes towards climate and debt policies. *Frontiers in Political Science, 3,* 656053. https://doi.org/10.3389/fpos.2021.656053

Gifford, R. (2011). The dragons of inaction: Psychological barriers that limit climate change mitigation and adaptation. *American Psychologist, 66*(4), 290–302. https://doi.org/10.1037/a0023566

Green, D. (2016). *How change happens.* Oxford University Press.

Hepburn, C., O'Callaghan, B., Stern, N., Stiglitz, J., & Zenghelis, D. (2020). Will COVID-19 fiscal recovery packages accelerate or retard progress on climate change? *Oxford Review of Economic Policy, 36,* 359–381. https://doi.org/10.1093/oxrep/graa015

IJzerman, H., Lewis, N. A., Przybylski, A. K., Weinstein, N., DeBruine, L., Ritchie, S. J., Vazire, S., Forscher, P. S., Morey, R. D., Ivory, J. D., & Anvari, F. (2020). Use caution when applying behavioural science to policy. *Nature Human Behaviour, 4*(11), 1092–1094. https://doi.org/10.1038/s41562-020-00990-w

Inglehart, R. (1977). Values, objective needs, and subjective satisfaction among Western publics. *Comparative Political Studies, 9*(4), 429–458. https://doi.org/10.1177/001041407700900403

Johansson Sevä, I., & Kulin, J. (2018). A little more action, please: Increasing the understanding about citizens' lack of commitment to protecting the environment in different national contexts. *International Journal of Sociology, 48*(4), 314–339. https://doi.org/10.1080/00207659.2018.1515703

Laughner, J. L., Neu, J. L., Schimel, D., Wennberg, P. O., Barsanti, K., Bowman, K. W., Chatterjee, A., Croes, B. E., Fitzmaurice, H. L., Henze, D. K., Kim, J., Kort, E. A., Liu, Z., Miyazaki, K., Turner, A. J., Anenberg, S., Avise, J., Cao, H., Crisp, D., . . . the rest of the Keck Institute for Space Studies "COVID-19: Identifying Unique Opportunities for Earth System Science" study team. (2021). Societal shifts due to COVID-19 reveal large-scale complexities and feedbacks between atmospheric chemistry and climate change. *Proceedings of the National Academy of Sciences, 118*(46), e2109481118. https://doi.org/10.1073/pnas.2109481118

Laville, S. (2021, June 2). G7 nations committing billions more to fossil fuel than green energy. *The Guardian.* https://www.theguardian.com/world/2021/jun/02/g7-nations-committing-billions-more-to-fossil-fuel-than-green-energy

Markowitz, E. M., & Shariff, A. F. (2012). Climate change and moral judgement. *Nature Climate Change, 2*(4), 243–247. https://doi.org/10.1038/nclimate1378

Monbiot, G. (2017). *Out of the wreckage: A new politics for an age of crisis.* Verso.

Naomi, A. S. (2020). Access to nature has always been important; with COVID-19, it is essential. *HERD: Health Environments Research & Design Journal, 13*(4), 242–244. https://doi.org/10.1177/1937586720949792

Overland, I., & Sovacool, B. K. (2020). The misallocation of climate research funding. *Energy Research & Social Science, 62,* 101349. https://doi.org/10.1016/j.erss.2019.101349

Saadat, S., Rawtani, D., & Hussain, C. M. (2020). Environmental perspective of COVID-19. *Science of the Total Environment, 728,* 138870. https://doi.org/10.1016/j.scitotenv.2020.138870

Van Bavel, J. J. V., Baicker, K., Boggio, P. S., Capraro, V., Cichocka, A., Cikara, M., Crockett, M. J., Crum, A. J., Douglas, K. M., Druckman, J. N., Drury, J., Dube, O.,

Ellemers, N., Finkel, E. J., Fowler, J. H., Gelfand, M., Han, S., Haslam, S. A., Jetten, J., . . . Willer, R. (2020). Using social and behavioural science to support COVID-19 pandemic response. *Nature Human Behaviour*, *4*(5), 460–471. https://doi.org/10.1038/s41562-020-0884-z

Verplanken, B., & Orbell, S. (2019). Habit and behavior change. In K. Sassenberg & M. L. W. Vliek (Eds.), Social psychology in action (pp. 65–78). Springer International Publishing. https://doi.org/10.1007/978-3-030-13788-5_5

Verplanken, B., & Whitmarsh, L. (2021). Habit and climate change. *Current Opinion in Behavioral Sciences*, *42*, 42–46. https://doi.org/10.1016/j.cobeha.2021.02.020

Werfel, S. H. (2017). Household behaviour crowds out support for climate change policy when sufficient progress is perceived. *Nature Climate Change*, *7*(7), 512–515. https://doi.org/10.1038/nclimate3316

Whitmarsh, L., & O'Neill, S. (2010). Green identity, green living? The role of pro-environmental self-identity in determining consistency across diverse pro-environmental behaviours. *Journal of Environmental Psychology*, *30*(3), 305–314. https://doi.org/10.1016/j.jenvp.2010.01.003

Whitmarsh, L., Poortinga, W., & Capstick, S. (2021). Behaviour change to address climate change. *Current Opinion in Psychology*, *42*, 76–81. https://doi.org/10.1016/j.copsyc.2021.04.002

FURTHER READING

Fritsche, I., Barth, M., Jugert, P., Masson, T., & Reese, G. (2018). A social identity model of pro-environmental action (SIMPEA). *Psychological Review*, *125*(2), 245–269. https://doi.org/10.1037/rev0000090

Lewandowsky, S., & Oberauer, K. (2021). Worldview-motivated rejection of science and the norms of science. *Cognition*, *215*, 104820. https://doi.org/10.1016/j.cognition.2021.104820

Reicher, S., & Bauld, L. (2021). From the "fragile rationalist" to "collective resilience": What human psychology has taught us about the COVID-19 pandemic and what the COVID-19 pandemic has taught us about human psychology. *Journal of the Royal College of Physicians of Edinburgh*, *51*(S1), S12–S19. https://doi.org/10.4997/JRCPE.2021.236

Conducting COVID-19 Pandemic Research

41

Scattered Black and Whites

The Importance of the Positive and Negative in the Mosaic of Human Experience

ELAINE KINSELLA AND RACHEL SUMNER ■

During the COVID-19 pandemic, many researchers were tackling research questions while, in parallel, living through their own personal pandemic experiences. In some ways, researchers hold "insider" status on pandemic research, yet in other ways, they are outsiders to the lived experiences of others. One particular challenge for researchers is, perhaps, to be inspired by our own and others' experiences, while also remaining open to the complexity that might be inherent in those experiences and associated questions. Researchers are influenced by their own life experiences, personal biases and assumptions, and disciplinary traditions—all of which can play out in the research space in a number of ways. In this chapter, we consider how social scientists can learn from their own experiences without limiting themselves to a narrow viewpoint by seeking out interdisciplinary collaborators and adopting both complementary and contrasting perspectives as a means of drawing greater meaning about the impact of key life events and experiences.

In part, we draw from our own experiences of conducting COVID-19 pandemic research. To provide context, we are psychologists that have developed from different traditions. We both research health and well-being, but each comes to this point from either a positive approach (heroism, positive psychology: E. K.) or a negative approach (stress, psychobiology: R. S.). Since March 2020, we have explored both the "light" side (looking at heroism, post-traumatic growth, sense of meaning in life) and the "dark" side (looking at stress, anxiety, and post-traumatic stress disorder [PTSD]) of the global pandemic[1]—assessing and interrogating these distinct social science theories and methods in our cross-sectional and longitudinal survey studies as well as qualitative interviews. Through our work together, we have found that these approaches are not sufficient in themselves,

Elaine Kinsella and Rachel Sumner, *Scattered Black and Whites* In: *The Social Science of the COVID-19 Pandemic*. Edited by: Monica K. Miller, Oxford University Press. © Oxford University Press 2024. DOI: 10.1093/oso/9780197615133.003.0041 and by combining perspectives, we are better able to plumb the depths of human experience to create a more holistic picture of the very complex social and emotional consequences of working through a crisis. We see the "two sides of the same coin" approach to be valid and important in this sort of research and not mutually exclusive in a project. In this chapter, we explore the benefits and challenges of drawing from multiple theoretical frames, as well as offering advice to researchers who are embarking on a longitudinal, multimethod project in an interdisciplinary team, not least during a major health crisis. The key takeaway messages from this chapter will be of interest to other researchers embarking not only on pandemic research, but also in a range of contexts involving significant, complex life experiences.

A COMPLICATED MOSAIC OF TRAUMA AND BENEFIT

Previous work on pandemics has typically focused on healthcare workers and with focus on measures of distress (e.g., Maunder, 2004; Tam et al., 2004). While previous pandemics and epidemics have not reached the same scale as the COVID-19 pandemic, one could argue that these studies were limited in scope by not considering other roles and experiences, as well as the breadth of variables considered. The various traditions within health and social psychologies that examine disasters or crises have historically taken a very uniformly negative perspective. The immediate assumption here is that a crisis must by definition be negative, that it will induce significant and profound harm to all involved, and that it will damage our health and well-being via a variety of biopsychosocial mechanisms. This is all true, of course; however, humans are also resilient and seek to make sense of their worlds and our experiences to mitigate these harms wherever possible (Rutter, 1993). In short, human experiences are rarely uniform or unidimensional.

Previous work on troubling and complex life events not surprisingly tended to focus on measures of distress. Yet, in more recent years, there has been an upsurge in work on post-traumatic growth and benefit finding—which shows that even after events that would typically be assumed to be experienced in an exclusively negative way, humans can show signs of positive adaptation. Within the domain of health psychology, for example, we have searched for real-life "models" of chronic stress to understand how sustained periods of stress can have an influence on a variety of measures of health, from the cell, to the person, to the population. One such model is found in caregiving, where someone is providing informal (i.e., unpaid and nonprofessional) care for a sick, elderly, or disabled relative (Allen et al., 2017). From markers of immune response to mortality rates, giving care has been suggested to be both profoundly stressful and harmful to health (Gouin et al., 2008). However, in attempting to understand the dynamics of this trajectory of harm, it has been discovered that a variety of aspects (e.g., with regard to the relationship between the caregiver and care recipient, the behavior of the care recipient, and the nature of function of care) can moderate or mediate that harm (e.g.,

Brown et al., 2009; Carmichael & Ercolani, 2016; Gallagher & Whiteley, 2013; Goins et al., 2011; Harmell et al., 2011). Over time, this has led to the development of research to understand the *benefits* of giving care: how caregivers can derive profound feelings of benefit within the role, by "giving back," making a difference, or otherwise finding fulfillment through meeting the needs of someone they love (e.g., Blum & Sherman, 2010; Kim et al., 2007; Roth et al., 2015). Each of these benefits has also been associated with important markers of health and well-being (Quinn & Toms, 2019), showing that while there has been plenty of negatives to uncover, the positives were also waiting to be found.

Similarly, work in the area of outcomes following critical events has for a long time focused on post-traumatic stress as a key endpoint. The emergence of post-traumatic growth as a concept changed much of this rhetoric, being described as a consequent reaction to traumatic events to instill "changes that are viewed as important, and that go beyond what was the previous status quo" (Tedeschi & Calhoun, 2004, p. 4). Taking the trauma out of the situation for a moment, growth is perhaps a very necessary and almost inevitable consequence to stress. Stress is inherently subjective not only between people (with similar events being appraised differently by different people), but also within people through processes of learning and habituation (Grissom & Bhatnagar, 2009). Humans are unique animals that not only encounter stress all the time, but also bring about stress in their own lives. People make themselves stressed in all manner of ways: from pushing occupational boundaries to pursuing leisure activities that are enormously physiologically and psychologically stressful. These types of stressors are usually in the domain of "eustress" (positive stress) and are appraised more positively (Nelson & Simmons, 2011); however, humans still put themselves in situations of threat as well, as exemplified through acts of heroism. The appraisal of stress has been the subject of much research over the years to understand the various psychological and biological outcomes of such events and whether there are unique differences between or within people that either do or do not confer negative consequences from stressors (Cacioppo et al., 1997; Norris et al., 2010). However, there is an inevitable function of existence that makes this very difficult to attain: People learn. The ability to adapt and learn from life events means that every stressful event is not only a potential to learn and grow, but also necessarily a cause of learning and growth (Park, 1998). This is related to the concept of resilience; however, resilience in itself tends to be situated within the context of it being a particular quality that people either do or do not have or that exists on some sort of scale between people. Instead, even in times of extreme stress, once people have survived, and there has been an appropriate period of time to facilitate reflection, there can be an acknowledgment of accomplishment, achievement, or—at the very least—strength from survival (Taylor, 1983).

Growth from serious psychological trauma is also ultimately possible. People are hardwired to learn from our experiences, and while traumatic experiences provide us with potentially extreme and dramatic examples of stress, our ability to adapt and continue is not only possible, but also inevitable. Of course, some people do suffer extreme psychological distress from traumatic events—and when this happens, and the pathological pattern of PTSD sets in, there is no amount of "positive thinking" that can reframe it. Interestingly, however, it is often this pathological reaction in PTSD that necessitates post-traumatic growth—with an understanding that growth might be directly proportional to the extent of trauma endured (Helgeson et al., 2006; see also Chapter 20 for more on mental health during the pandemic). It appears that the more research is conducted in the area, the more convincing the case is for growth to be a byproduct of being able to work through and adjust after a traumatic situation, provided that PTSD can be therapeutically managed and dealt with (Linley & Joseph, 2004). So here, it is important to remember that lived experience of trauma can be as much a product of time as it is of situation, with the opportunity for many suffering distressing reactions to the event, but then eventually emerging stronger or otherwise better adjusted (Olff et al., 2005).

This could also be important when considering that there are different types of trauma—that some can be discrete episodes (e.g., a car crash or a terrorist attack), but many can be chronic or cumulative (e.g., domestic abuse). An example of this more chronic and cumulative type of trauma would very well be in the context of front-line working in the pandemic, where the sustained effort has no foreseeable end and where waves or surges of distressing experiences ebb and flow across the trajectory of its course. Here, the ability to grow from this trauma must assuredly be a product of when that trauma ends and the various other aspects both mitigating and enhancing harm along the way. For example, we know that controllability over the event(s) and perceptions of loss and harm are associated with differing post-traumatic outcomes both psychologically and biologically (Olff et al., 2005), and also that repeated traumatic events have an impact on people's ability to cope in the longer term (Krause et al., 2008).

Indeed, coping is another fascinating area that is both adaptive and relative between and within people. Any one person might adopt different coping styles depending on the nature of the thing they are attempting to cope with, and— of course—sometimes the very nature of stressors themselves erode the ability to cope as well (Folkman & Lazarus, 1984). As an example, unemployment is considered to be a chronic stressor (much like caregiving) and comprises both a psychosocial form of stress, through stigma, lack of purpose, life structure, or role and a depreciation of means to cope, via financial means or emotional and social support from colleagues or distant friends (Bartley, 1994). However, people also tend to draw on the positives around us to allow us to cope during dark times, not as a point of successful adaptation, but as an innate necessity to prevent us from crumbling under the weight of our troubles. Both individually and collectively, humans seek to find the silver linings in order to keep going during times of prolonged mutual struggle (Shiota, 2006), yet these silver linings are often left out of research that seeks to understand the impact of such struggle.

Capturing this duality of human experience is not methodologically easy to wield. Researchers can become encumbered with needing to collect data on many more concepts and variables, which can be burdensome and requires sensitive handling with regard to presentation within a corpus of questionnaires.

Arguably, there is a need to avoid labeling others' experiences, where possible, before allowing them to label their own experiences. Researchers need to consider the role that researcher-led labeling and questioning during the research process might play in reconceptualizing or reframing the participants' own memories of a particular event. This places a duty on researchers to consider the questions being posed and how those questions are landing on their intended recipients through careful piloting and through public and patient involvement in research. In qualitative frameworks, there are very deep and complex ethical and practical navigations to be made in terms of how questions are phrased, in what order they appear in the schedule, and how they guide a conversation that not only is replete with opportunities to express thoughts and feelings, but also adequately attends to the fragility of the emotions being elicited. In quantitative analysis, a clear plan for how questions will be asked of the data is vital, an issue we have found to take more time than we had previously experienced with this work. In qualitative analysis, the consideration of data saturation becomes more complex, and the identification of themes perhaps less direct and clear. In reporting, there are issues of how the stories of the data can be cogently told, whether these comprise one paper or whether more manuscripts are needed to adequately communicate the findings. Finally, in broader dissemination and communication, there are further needs for sensitivity and careful planning. Is it the right time to be talking about pandemic positives? Is this the right or appropriate message for this audience? These complex considerations are perhaps why many studies might have previously adopted one approach or the other to reduce "noise" at every step of the research process. However, it is not impossible to incorporate, and our own experiences have shown us that this approach has provided a sum greater than the total of its parts at every stage.

For the purposes of our own research, we have understood the front-line workers' experiences to be stressful not only from the perspective of being on the front line, but also with the consideration that they might be separated from their families (to avoid infection and as a result of longer working hours), therefore, minimizing their social support. In addition, they have often needed to work against a rising tide of infection and death that largely exists beyond their control. They have often battled with discrepancies between official government and public health guidance and their own experiences "at the coalface," a parallel still playing out currently in many places. There have been times of being without meaningful protection, losing colleagues, being unable to achieve their goals of keeping others safe, and being confronted with apparent public dissent. However, there have also been times of enormous pride in their roles and their colleagues, gratitude to others around them, endurance through compassion, and many instances of joy, relief, and agape. Moreover, these experiences have occurred in disparate ways, being scattered through the trajectory of their front-line experience at different times, in different places, and in different ways. It is our hope that by the end of our project (whenever that end might be), we will be able to provide a record not only of the damage that has been done, but also a rubric by which mistakes in the future can be avoided to minimize harm. The latter is simply not possible without also examining those aspects of positive experience within. For something so complex, it is not simply enough to assert that negative aspects located in the dark should be removed, but we would also wish to see the potential for intervention, support, improvement—all of which can be derived from understanding what has come from the light.

Taken together, the very complex fallout of traumatic situations clearly requires both time and a deeper understanding of the dynamics of the individual (i.e., their personal coping resources) as well as the nature of the traumatic stressor itself (i.e., its duration, repetition, controllability, and incursion on varying aspects of the person's life). That is not to say, however, that they might not be able to cope or find growth throughout their experiences in their work. To this end, we have found not only that our participants have spoken of benefits such as being able to make a difference during such a phenomenal time, but also that they have experienced a newfound appreciation from the public and others in their community due to their essential roles (Kinsella et al., 2022). For some, this has reinvigorated their sense of purpose and meaning, a factor that is very much associated with positive outcomes in this same group (Sumner & Kinsella, 2021). The understanding of occupational stress has itself been far broadened by the divergence from viewing stress as the challenge-threat continuum, and that there is an "optimum" level of challenge in which workers can find sufficient challenge not to be bored, but also not to be exhausted. The Yerkes-Dodson law typifies an ideal level of stress encountered at work whereby people could thrive (Teigen, 1994). While not all essential workers envisaged being on the front line of an infectious disease pandemic, they work in roles that perform essential and helpful functions to people and societies, and they might conceivably thrive in some senses given the heightened onus (and in many cases, sincere appreciation) of their roles and their ability to act in some way. What we have found from our research thus far has been a complicated mosaic of trauma and benefit. Our participants speak of seemingly boundless personal tragedy, but also of heartwarming moments of fulfillment and hope (Kinsella et al., 2022). How they will fare through and beyond the pandemic is uncertain, but we are keen to find out.

LESSONS LEARNED: CAPTURING THE POSITIVE AND NEGATIVE IN THE MOSAIC OF HUMAN EXPERIENCE

It is as a result of the pandemic—and the way the pandemic has been experienced by *every* person, globally, that perhaps offers us an opportunity to reflect on the strengths of both adopting a human-centered approach to research and reflecting on the darker human aspects of our research that might need some further pondering. Researchers, like all people, are dynamic entities who are interacting with the world and whose experiences are evolving over time. They are situated in a particular social and cultural context and have their own expertise in a chosen field. From their discipline, they learn how to approach research, accumulate a body of specialist knowledge, learn particular theories and concepts, develop terminology and specialist language, and learn research methods that are appropriate to that particular discipline. The richness of their own experiences, as both human beings and researchers, lead to developing particular worldviews and research frames and the potential to explore fascinating avenues of scientific discovery. These often strong and passion-fueled beliefs can drive researchers to explore topics in more detail. Yet, the danger is that these experiences have the potential to lead researchers to adopt a narrow frame, to generate somewhat leading questions, and to have a tendency to focus on particular paradigms or "pet" theories that fit with familiar experiences.

Assumptions, biases, and disciplinary norms are part of the human side of research. Reflexivity is the formal term given to the process of examining our own beliefs, judgments, and practices during the research process (Finlay, 1998). While the practice of reflexivity is typically left in the domain of qualitative research, we (as predominantly quantitative researchers) can see the vital and valuable role that reflexivity can play in any research project, particularly where the subject matter relates to our own experiences and values. To do this effectively, researchers might need to consider how reflexive processes are built into the research process and our research team communications, along with plans for how to use these reflections to create high-quality research.

Our own experiences through the pandemic have reiterated to us the value and importance of considering multiple and sometimes contrasting theories relevant to the topic in question to help avoid the traps of narrow framing and to moderate some of our own biases and assumptions. Through open dialogue, researchers can widen their conception of the problem space, which leads to greater consideration of a wider range of potential solutions. As well as building self-awareness, researchers can actively seek opportunities to work with people who offer contrasting and complementary skills and perspectives. To really embrace this challenge of working in a diverse team, researchers simultaneously need to strive for an open communication culture within the project team where all viewpoints are respected and discussed and more senior or powerful colleagues invite the opinions and feedback of all others and explicitly discuss the power dynamics that exist within the team. From design, to data collection, to analysis and interpretation, there is a need to bring greater openness and discussion to the sources of influence on the work.

Finally, conducting research while living through a pandemic can be overwhelming and draining, as well as a source of meaning and purpose (see Chapter 45 of this book on the topic of emotional labor). The subject matter of our research can also be a source of frustration and pain in our personal life. For us, living through a global pandemic while tracking the well-being of front-line workers during the pandemic has, at times, produced uncertainty, self-doubt, and second-guessing. We have witnessed the pandemic through many pairs of eyes: as members of the public, as a mother, as a concerned family member of loved ones hit hard by the virus and repeated lockdowns, as children of vulnerable parents, as health researchers with insight into infectious disease and behavioral science, and finally, through the eyes of our participants: the front-line workers. Removing our own perspectives as people, and those impacted by the stories of our participants, from our most scientific selves has been anything between hard and impossible at times. We have tried to mitigate some of the more challenging aspects of this work through peer support and encouraging team members to take time out when things get too much. The benefit of working within a supportive, open team is being able to acknowledge how each member of the team is doing, both emotionally and psychologically, at any given point during the research process and to seek opportunities to delegate or scale back when required. Striving for balance—pulling back from being overwhelmed—is a work in progress.

CONCLUSION

We conclude with a message of hope: There are two sides of every coin that spins across the arc of human experience. While psychology has often leaned toward the dark, which is interesting and useful, it does not provide the full picture. Through our research during the COVID-19 pandemic, we have attempted to acknowledge the devastation and the tragedy, while also allowing a more holistic experience of the humanity in the experiences that our front-line workers have lived through to remain on record. Allowing for aspects of positive human coping and adaption to shine through does not detract from the very real suffering and trauma that people have faced. Humans have enormous capacity for resilience and growth, even throughout something as globally devastating as the COVID-19 pandemic. Indeed, our own research experiences to date have served as reminders that people often gravitate toward the light, even when life presents inconceivable challenges.

Throughout our continuing work we are exploring aspects of tragedy (i.e., PTSD, anxiety, burnout) alongside triumph (i.e., solidarity, post-traumatic growth, purpose, and meaning) to draw out the undulating patterns as they converge and diverge across the trajectory of this complex and unique period of our existence. Had we only forged ahead with documenting the trauma and negativity, we would have missed some of the beneficial recording of factors that support and help, along with some of the truly astonishing and humbling accounts of hope in dark times. Critically, as has been evidenced in related literature, we would have missed the contribution of *necessary* positive factors in the human response to prolonged stress and hardship. Whether these factors abound as a function of trauma or in spite of it we are not yet sure, but it is a valuable and important lesson to learn when attempting to take into account our front-line workers' experience of playing a vital role in a situation of this magnitude.

NOTE

1.   The CV19 Heroes project has tracked the well-being of front-line workers in the United Kingdom and Ireland since March 2020 (https://cv19heroes.com).

REFERENCES

Allen, A. P., Curran, E. A., Duggan, Á., Cryan, J. F., Chorcoráin, A. N., Dinan, T. G., Molloy, D. W., Kearney, P. M., & Clarke, G. (2017). A systematic review of the psychobiological burden of informal caregiving for patients with dementia: Focus on cognitive and biological markers of chronic stress. *Neuroscience & Biobehavioral Reviews, 73*, 123–164. https://doi.org/http://dx.doi.org/10.1016/j.neubiorev.2016.12.006

Bartley, M. (1994). Unemployment and ill health: Understanding the relationship. *Journal of Epidemiology and Community Health, 48*(4), 333–337. https://doi.org/10.1136/jech.48.4.333

Blum, K., & Sherman, D. W. (2010). Understanding the experience of caregivers: A focus on transitions. *Seminars in Oncology Nursing, 26*(4), 243–258. https://doi.org/http://dx.doi.org/10.1016/j.soncn.2010.08.005

Brown, S. L., Smith, D. M., Schulz, R., Kabeto, M. U., Ubel, P. A., Poulin, M., Yi, J., Kim, C., & Langa, K. M. (2009). Caregiving behavior is associated with decreased mortality risk. *Psychological Science, 20*(4), 488–494. https://doi.org/10.1111/j.1467-9280.2009.02323.x

Cacioppo, J. T., Gardner, W. L., & Berntson, G. G. (1997). Beyond bipolar conceptualizations and measures: The case of attitudes and evaluative space. *Personality and Social Psychology Review, 1*(1), 3. https://journals.sagepub.com/doi/10.1207/s15327957pspr0101_2?url_ver=Z39.88-2003&rfr_id=ori:rid:crossref.org&rfr_dat=cr_pub%3dpubmed

Carmichael, F., & Ercolani, M. G. (2016). Unpaid caregiving and paid work over life-courses: Different pathways, diverging outcomes. *Social Science & Medicine, 156*, 1–11. https://doi.org/http://dx.doi.org/10.1016/j.socscimed.2016.03.020

Finlay, L. (1998). Reflexivity: An essential component for all research? *British Journal of Occupational Therapy, 61*(10), 453–456.

Folkman, S., & Lazarus, R. S. (1984). *Stress, appraisal, and coping*. Springer Publishing Company.

Gallagher, S., & Whiteley, J. (2013). The association between stress and physical health in parents caring for children with intellectual disabilities is moderated by children's challenging behaviours. *Journal of Health Psychology, 18*(9), 1220–1231. https://doi.org/10.1177/1359105312464672

Goins, R. T., Spencer, S. M., McGuire, L. C., Goldberg, J., Wen, Y., & Henderson, J. A. (2011). Adult caregiving among American Indians: The role of cultural factors. *The Gerontologist, 51*(3), 310–320. https://doi.org/10.1093/geront/gnq101

Gouin, J. P., Hantsoo, L., & Kiecolt-Glaser, J. K. (2008). Immune dysregulation and chronic stress among older adults: A review. *Neuroimmunomodulation, 15*(4–6), 251–259. http://www.ncbi.nlm.nih.gov/pmc/articles/PMC2676338/pdf/nihms-109812.pdf

Grissom, N., & Bhatnagar, S. (2009). Habituation to repeated stress: Get used to it. *Neurobiology of Learning and Memory, 92*(2), 215–224. https://doi.org/https://doi.org/10.1016/j.nlm.2008.07.001

Harmell, A. L., Chattillion, E. A., Roepke, S. K., & Mausbach, B. T. (2011). A review of the psychobiology of dementia caregiving: A focus on resilience factors. *Current Psychiatry Reports, 13*(3), 219–224. https://doi.org/10.1007/s11920-011-0187-1

Helgeson, V. S., Reynolds, K. A., & Tomich, P. L. (2006). A meta-analytic review of benefit finding and growth. *Journal of Consulting and Clinical Psychology, 74*(5), 797–816. https://doi.org/10.1037/0022-006X.74.5.797

Kim, Y., Schulz, R., & Carver, C. S. (2007). Benefit finding in the cancer caregiving experience. *Psychosomatic Medicine, 69*(3), 283–291. https://doi.org/10.1097/PSY.0b013e3180417cf4

Kinsella, E. L., Hughes, S., Lemon, S., Stonebridge, N., & Sumner, R. C. (2022). "We shouldn't waste a good crisis": Constructions of the psychological impact of working through the first surge (and beyond) of COVID-19 by frontline workers in the UK and Ireland. *Psychology & Health, 22*(2), 151–177. https://doi.org/10.1080/08870446.2021.1928668

Krause, E. D., Kaltman, S., Goodman, L. A., & Dutton, M. A. (2008). Avoidant coping and PTSD symptoms related to domestic violence exposure: A longitudinal study. *Journal of Traumatic Stress, 21*(1), 83–90. https://doi.org/https://doi.org/10.1002/jts.20288

Linley, P. A., & Joseph, S. (2004). Positive change following trauma and adversity: A review. *Journal of Traumatic Stress, 17*(1), 11–21. https://onlinelibrary.wiley.com/doi/abs/10.1023/B%3AJOTS.0000014671.27856.7e

Maunder, R. (2004). The experience of the 2003 SARS outbreak as a traumatic stress among frontline healthcare workers in Toronto: Lessons learned. *Philosophical Transactions: Biological Sciences, 359*(1447), 1117. https://www.ncbi.nlm.nih.gov/pmc/articles/PMC1693388/pdf/15306398.pdf

Nelson, D. L., & Simmons, B. (2011). Savoring eustress while coping with distress: The holistic model of stress. In J. C. Quick & L. E. Tetrick (Eds.), *Handbook of occupational health psychology* (pp. 55–74). American Psychological Association.

Norris, C. J., Gollan, J., Berntson, G. G., & Cacioppo, J. T. (2010). The current status of research on the structure of evaluative space. *Biological Psychology, 84*(3), 422–436. https://doi.org/https://doi.org/10.1016/j.biopsycho.2010.03.011

Olff, M., Langeland, W., & Gersons, B. P. R. (2005). The psychobiology of PTSD: Coping with trauma. *Psychoneuroendocrinology, 30*(10), 974–982. https://doi.org/https://doi.org/10.1016/j.psyneuen.2005.04.009

Park, C. L. (1998). Stress-related growth and thriving through coping: The roles of personality and cognitive processes. *Journal of Social Issues, 54*(2), 267–277.

Quinn, C., & Toms, G. (2019). Influence of positive aspects of dementia caregiving on caregivers' well-being: A systematic review. *The Gerontologist, 59*(5), e584–e596.

Roth, D. L., Fredman, L., & Haley, W. E. (2015). Informal caregiving and its impact on health: A reappraisal from population-based studies. *The Gerontologist, 53*(2), 309–319. https://doi.org/10.1093/geront/gnu177

Rutter, M. (1993). Resilience: Some conceptual considerations. *Journal of Adolescent Health, 14*(8), 626–631.

Shiota, M. N. (2006). Silver linings and candles in the dark: Differences among positive coping strategies in predicting subjective well-being. *Emotion, 6*(2), 335.

Sumner, R. C., & Kinsella, E. L. (2021). Grace under pressure: Resilience, burnout, and wellbeing in frontline workers in the UK and Republic of Ireland during the SARS-Cov-2 pandemic. *Frontiers in Psychology, 11*, 576229. doi:10.3389/fpsyg.2020.576229.

Tam, C. W. C., Pang, E. P. F., Lam, L. C. W., & Chiu, H. F. K. (2004). Severe acute respiratory syndrome (SARS) in Hong Kong in 2003: Stress and psychological impact among frontline healthcare workers. *Psychological Medicine, 34*(7), 1197–1204. https://doi.org/10.1017/s0033291704002247

Taylor, S. E. (1983). Adjustment to threatening events: A theory of cognitive adaptation. *American Psychologist*, *38*(11), 1161.

Tedeschi, R. G., & Calhoun, L. G. (2004). Posttraumatic growth: Conceptual foundations and empirical evidence. *Psychological inquiry*, *15*(1), 1–18.

Teigen, K. H. (1994). Yerkes-Dodson: A law for all seasons. *Theory & Psychology*, *4*(4), 525–547.

FURTHER READING

Bregman, R. (2020). *Humankind: A hopeful history*. Bloomsbury Publishing.

Goldmann, E., & Galea, S. (2014). Mental health consequences of disasters. *Annual Review of Public Health*, *35*, 169–183.

Jetten, J. (2020). *Together apart: The psychology of COVID-19*. Sage.

Prati, G., & Pietrantoni, L. (2009). Optimism, social support, and coping strategies as factors contributing to posttraumatic growth: A meta-analysis. *Journal of Loss and Trauma*, *14*(5), 364–388.

On the Ethics of Social Science Research During a Pandemic

PHILIPP SCHOENEGGER AND THERON PUMMER ■

The emergence of SARS-CoV-2 (severe acute respiratory syndrome corona-virus 2) and the subsequent COVID-19 pandemic has led to numerous novel challenges for most aspects of modern life, from furloughs to lockdowns and social distancing (see Chapter 4 for more on pandemic-related ethics in daily life). Between January 1 and June 30, 2020, an estimated 23,634 academic papers on the topic of COVID-19 aimed at addressing and understanding various facets of this pandemic were published in peer-reviewed journals (Da Silva et al., 2021). The sheer volume of research in response to this pandemic, spanning the biomedical and social sciences, points to the urgent need for careful reflection on the moral challenges of this situation. In this chapter, we do just that, that is, specifically focus on the ethical challenges that this pandemic posed and continues to pose to research in the social sciences, such as trade-offs between participant welfare and scientific utility, the effects of quick ethics approval, and the role that social sciences ought to play in addressing this emergency.

Changes in research ethics have often been directly influenced by outside events that spurred reflection on the ethical guidelines of our research conduct in academic settings. Most notably perhaps was the Tuskegee syphilis study of 1972, in which several hundred poor and ill Black men from Alabama had been intentionally left untreated for 40 years. In response to the justified outcry, the U.S. Congress formed the National Commission for the Protection of Human Subjects of Biomedical and Behavioral Research, which then went on to compose the Belmont Report in 1978. This report ended up being a founding document for modern research ethics, aiming for the "identification of basic ethical principles" that ought to underlie research of human subjects, fundamentally altering the research ethics landscape. Even though the current pandemic might not lead to such a stark change in research ethics in the social sciences, we argue

Philipp Schoenegger and Theron Pummer, *On the Ethics of Social Science Research During a Pandemic* In: *The Social Science of the COVID-19 Pandemic*. Edited by: Monica K. Miller, Oxford University Press. © Oxford University Press 2024.
DOI: 10.1093/oso/9780197615133.003.0042

that this pandemic poses some unique ethical challenges to those basic principles that should not be overlooked and that could spur lasting change. Further, social scientists properly rising to the challenge during this emergency will benefit them in the future, as emergencies that are yet to come might pose similar dangers, and lessons learned in this context might be similarly applicable. Specifically, we investigate the following issues: (1) How does the notion of voluntary informed consent change in an emergency setting this like? (2) How should we think about the trade-off between scientific utility and subject welfare when conducting research? (3) What is the proper role of institutional review boards, and how should they think about speed and quality in reviewing submissions? (4) Is there a moral obligation of social scientists to be epistemically humble and openly communicate their findings with an adequate degree of uncertainty? This chapter discusses all four of these points and provides some guidance on how to conduct research in the future.

VOLUNTARY INFORMED CONSENT

One of the most tangible changes that this pandemic has necessitated for social science researchers is the move from laboratory and field experiments to the online domain. In addition to the methodological challenges raised by this move, some of which were discussed extensively prior to the pandemic (e.g., Chmielewski & Kucker, 2020; Kees et al., 2017), there are also a number of ethical challenges involved. In particular, the participants' informed and voluntary consent, aimed at ensuring that participants can make an informed decision and voluntarily consent to partaking in research, is markedly different in a pandemic compared to before. In this section, we outline these challenges to the notion of voluntary informed consent.

In a standard understanding of voluntariness, for an act to count as voluntary, one must be free from controlling influences when engaging in the action. Pointing to one way in which the current pandemic might make this concept morally problematic, Nelson and colleagues (2011) argued, albeit in a different context, that while a reduction in or even full lack of options does, by itself, not suffice for an action to be nonvoluntary per se, these situations might nevertheless lead to "deprivations of voluntariness that are morally problematic" (Nelson et al., 2011, p. 9). They went on to point out that if "subjects' economic disadvantage or lack of available alternatives or resources . . . is increased" (Nelson et al., 2011, p. 9), the moral challenge to voluntary consent is further heightened in a proportionate matter. The current pandemic not only removed a substantial number of options for participants by restricting the range of activities available in lockdown life, but also increased the economic disadvantage of not taking part in research for many people.

During 2020, lockdowns restricted opportunities of all sorts in a large number of countries and provinces, directly restricting the range of activities available to people and potential participants. Coupled with the harsh economic downturn that much of the world experienced, participants considering taking part in social science research now face a considerably altered choice environment. Not only are there fewer alternatives of employment and entertainment available to them, but also the participant payments and associated earned experimental endowments represent a more substantial potential income stream, especially to those who have lost their employment in this crisis. This, as Nelson et al. (2011) pointed out, is by itself not sufficient to classify participation as nonvoluntary, though it does raise relevant ethical challenges for our conception of voluntary consent that should not be disregarded.

It is worth pointing out, however, that the challenge here is less severe than it is within biomedical research, in which participants are expecting direct health benefits from participation in research all the while simultaneously hoping not to be in the no intervention arms of randomized controlled trials. This change in expectation and motivation highly distorts standard conceptions of consent and voluntariness, especially in situations like the current pandemic. Importantly, participants who are not chosen because of their fit for the research project at hand but simply because of the ease of access might be especially vulnerable for challenges of this nature in all areas of research.

While we have no reason to conclude that participants in general are not able to consent to social science research conducted in this pandemic, we must make clear the point that their participation could be compromised in an ethically relevant way: As researchers, we have to take extra care to design and advertise our research such that participants, irrespective of their background, can voluntarily and safely participate without making participation something one cannot pass up on or something that does not pay a fair participation wage. If we fail this balancing act, we risk imposing moral harm on our participants by compromising the notion of voluntary consent and by using them in a disrespectful way by exploiting their situations in order to further our research. However, if we contend with these challenges, we might acquire a richer and more robust conception of voluntary consent, which can help us prepare for future emergencies.

TRADE-OFFS BETWEEN SCIENTIFIC UTILITY AND SUBJECT WELFARE

One standard principle in research ethics is that research should not be justified only by its potential social utility. Rather, research has to be justified (at least) by recourse to three basic ethical principles: respect for persons, beneficence, and justice. A corollary of this is that research should not harm participants and that researchers ought to maximize possible benefits while minimizing possible harms to participants. The focus of this section is the trade-off that arises here, being one between scientific utility and subject welfare.

In this pandemic, the fundamental relationship between scientific utility and subject welfare has been put into focus in a unique way. This is because both the scientific utility of research conducted during this pandemic and subject welfare concerns have been fundamentally altered. On the former, research conducted during the pandemic promises to be relevant to directly addressing the current crisis, specifically linking scientific utility to the welfare. After all, finding successful behavioral interventions that promote, for example, mask wearing and social distancing might increase public welfare. Furthermore, much of this research is time sensitive in the sense that in order to gather informative data for this time period and to apply it in a timely manner to this emergency, one cannot retrospectively collect data once the risk profile has returned to normal, above and beyond concerns about external validity that such an approach would bring with it. Some argue that in emergencies like this, one ought to prioritize specific research over others at all cost. For example, Mormina et al. (2020) argued: "Research during emergencies should only be conducted if it has high social value" (p. 1) by providing support to the emergency responses, be it direct or indirect, thus arguing to focus on scientific utility.

On the concern for participant welfare, the risk profile for subject participation has changed significantly in this pandemic as well. Whereas the risk for participating in standard laboratory experiments was comparatively low before, inviting 20 people into a small computer room is nigh indefensible during this pandemic. As discussed before, one way to avoid this is to move to online research, which comes with its own challenges; but, for social science research that can only be conducted in person, the ethical challenge of weighing scientific utility with participant (and researcher) welfare are brought to the fore. For those agreeing with Mormina et al. (2020) that research should primarily be conducted if it directly helps address the current climate, most of social science research would be barred from being conducted. A second challenge to protecting subject welfare is that participants might understand participation as directly contributing to the public good, thereby further escalating the tension between these two concepts.

However, we argue that one should not need to be so crestfallen. Not all research conducted during a pandemic needs to directly address the pandemic and have high scientific value: Much powerful social science research is interesting and useful retrospectively (i.e., as a way to explain human behavior during this emergency post hoc, not necessarily as a guide through it with direct actionable recommendations). For example, some retrospective research without much direct relation to high social value might turn out to have high utility when it comes to dealing with future, similar emergencies. That is, some research projects might not have a high ex ante scientific value to address the pandemic, but could turn out conversely at a later point, and it is exceptionally hard to foresee these cases and consequences. For example, mask-related research (e.g., Eikenberry et al., 2020) might have been thought of as not addressing the pandemic directly in early March, when many institutional actors had not yet recognized the importance of mask wearing and were in fact opposing it. However, at a later point when this issue had been understood to be of exceptional importance, previous research and engagement proved invaluable, and research conducted during this emergency may inform future pandemic responses. This is why research, even in a pandemic, cannot simply be restricted to what we understand to be directly useful for resolving the emergency at any given point—because we simply cannot predict well enough which ideas will have that utility. As such, the main ethical challenge in this trade-off are the participant welfare issues, not necessarily the simple and direct scientific utility of the research conducted—protecting participants' welfare and safeguarding against failures to promote their interests maximally ought to be the main principle of research ethics, not a conception of useful research.

THE ROLE OF INSTITUTIONAL REVIEW BOARDS IN AN EMERGENCY

One unique challenge that has surfaced in this pandemic is that of the institutional review board's role in shaping the scientific response to the pandemic. From the very beginning of the pandemic, academics of all disciplines rushed to conduct research on some aspect of this emergency (cf. Da Silva et al., 2021). Faced with this sudden influx of applications, institutional review boards were overwhelmed and faced the following core trade-off in their decisions: Should they focus on a speedy process aimed at greenlighting as many acceptable research proposals as possible, or should they err on the side of caution and reject numerous submissions aimed at addressing this pandemic? This question interlinks with previously disused questions of the trade-off between scientific utility and participant welfare as well as that of consent (cf. Calia et al., 2020). In this section, we discuss the challenge that is posed to and by institutional review boards.

On the one hand, a lenient institutional review board could approve research projects that might fail to uphold ethical research standards in the light of the novel situations and the constraints faced. For example, if institutional review boards do not adapt their procedures to the new situations, challenges that arise precisely only in this situation could be overlooked. This threatens large-scale violations of ethical norms of research like the ones discussed above just because a large number of academic research proposals, some eventually fruitful, others futile, all aim to be conducted in a timely manner. A recent analysis suggested that between January and May 2020, papers broadly concerning COVID-19 were published eight times as quickly as comparable papers (Barakat et al., 2020). As an example of further ramifications, consider the finding by Besacon et al. (2020) that 8% of COVID-19 articles were submitted, reviewed, and accepted on the very same day. This raises serious questions as to the quality of review, further exacerbated by their additional finding that up to 43% of papers were flagged as having potential conflicts of interest, such as authors being editors at the journal that accepted the papers (Besacon et al., 2020). This suggests that, while a lenient institutional review board could lead to a high number of potentially useful research being accepted, there is the additional risk that a nonnegligible number of proposals risk violating ethical and scientific norms.

On the other hand, a restrictive institutional review board that slows approval processes in order to minimize the chance of allowing potentially harmful research might fail to prioritize research that would aim to alleviate the negative outcomes of the current pandemic and contribute to reducing its harmful effects. On this route, one is confronted with the challenge of how to weigh the upsides of a cautious process, namely, the reduction of risks to participants, against the possibility of blocking potentially valuable research and losing out on directly helpful research. As with so many situations of uncertainty, it is hard to foresee which research proposals will end up providing the insights needed to address this crisis, and reducing the amount of research conducted, for whatever reason, could further reduce the chance of valuable research being conducted (cf. Pundi et al., 2020). Such a restrictive institutional review board would prioritize participant welfare. However, recall that the most applicable social science research, almost by definition, is that with the highest external validity, which, in the current situation, comes with the highest risks for participants during this pandemic. This is because testing behavioral interventions in the field risks exposing participants to harms that online variants of these experiments would not. Exclusively optimizing for participant welfare thus risks defanging the ability of science to contribute to a substantial societal challenge, as emergencies bring with them myriad additional reasons why research could ultimately be harmful to subjects. It could be the case, as discussed previously, that most current research is unable to obtain as full a voluntary consent as was possible previously. Holding on to the highest standards thus could lead to a reduction in helpful scientific impact and further harm the public overall despite its intention to safeguard participant (and public) welfare.

We argue that this is a serious challenge, and that, overall, institutional review boards ought to try to balance the two extremes, with a focus on making sure they do not fall prey to an overly restrictive notion that we hold to be more dangerous. As Meagher et al. (2020) pointed out, cautious knowledge production can only be achieved by taking the long view. Doing that necessitates not only a careful consideration of participant welfare in novel contexts, but also continued focusing on the scientific utility of research that might often not be known ex ante, especially when the evidential basis of scientific findings relating to the topic being studied is simply unavailable at that moment (cf. Meagher et al., 2020).

THE ETHICS OF SOCIAL SCIENCE COMMUNICATION

The focus of this section is a challenge that presents itself in the context of communicating social science research to the public during this pandemic and more generally. In relation to the norms of communication, IJzerman et al. (2020) argued that social scientists ought to practice "extreme care [in] translating . . . findings to applications" (IJzerman et al., 2020, p. 1). They point to a number of methodological flaws in current social science research like a failure to test for stimulus generalizability, absence of validated scales, unreplicable studies, and too narrow a focus that does not take into account the historical, cultural, and structural factors that might impact the findings obtained. Taken together, they argue that we ought to be more cautious in applying social science findings to scenarios like the current situation primarily because we lack the certainty needed to do so (cf., e.g., Calia et al., 2020; Kowal et al., 2020; Bavel et al., 2020). This is especially important because some social science findings reported could have significant impact, such as a(n) (un-)successful messaging around vaccination campaigns. To put the above worry in slogan form, just because some research provides the best evidence available does not justify usage of this research as the gold standard or best practice and as such as the basis for policy recommendation. In fact, doing so could do significant harm despite the upside risk of this research in the current emergency.

In the remainder of this section, we wish to add a further, moral dimension to this general worry: Communicating findings with subpar evidential standards may threaten the public's trust in social science as the trust in politicians has already been shattered (Bramble, 2020, pp. 60–63; see Chapter 18 for more on trust related to the pandemic). If social scientists too confidently propose adoption of behavioral measures that end up failing or even backfiring, the public could soon distrust further messaging from social scientists, eroding not only trust but also the ability of future findings to impact behavior. As Hawley (2014) pointed out in her investigation of the more general issue of trust, distrust is not merely the absence of trust. Rather, distrust has an underlying normative dimension (Hawley, 2014, p. 3) that goes above and beyond that: It is not just the case that social science expertise could be thought of as unreliable, but rather as explicitly untrustworthy and could thus be viewed in a wholly different, negative light. That would present a substantive threat to scientists' ability to contribute to society in both the present and the future, a threat that ought to be taken seriously notwithstanding the methodological worries mentioned above.

As such, communicating findings that overstate their evidential basis has both practical and moral consequences. While untrusted social science findings might directly lead to lower adoption rates of recommendations in future applications and a general distrust of expertise in areas in which it might be warranted, Hawley argued that there is also an "intrinsic wrongness" (Hawley, 2014, p. 13) to violating trust by, in our example, communicating findings overzealously. It is the duty of social scientists to produce the best science possible and then to responsibly portray their findings with an adequate level of acknowledged uncertainty to their peers and the wider public in an attempt not to violate the trust the public has placed in us. We acknowledge that this raises an incentivization problem in which scientists who properly communicate their uncertainty first might be disadvantaged compared to their peers who continue to oversell. However, we believe that the individual costs of this move are substantially lower than the potential upside, and a great number of exemplary scholars already embody this ideal, although arguably this number is not high enough yet.

With this additional ethical challenge to communicating social science findings in this pandemic in mind, how should we communicate our findings to ensure we do not risk losing the public's trust and are seen as untrustworthy? How should one act in the light of a lack of scientific consensus on many topics? We claim that there are two values that social scientists ought to strive toward that would at least partially address this challenge: humility and openness.

First, social scientists ought to take the methodological worries of IJzerman et al. (2020) and all those pointing to them seriously and acknowledge the uncertainty inherent in their statements, in both standard peer-to-peer communication and especially in communication to the public and policymakers. Based on this acknowledgment of uncertainty, we argue that social scientists have a moral obligation to be epistemically humble about their findings and their applicability. Specifically, this includes the recommendation to always clearly articulate and communicate the uncertainty that underlies their statistical claims in clear and unmistakable terms. An epistemically humble communication of social science findings can still provide actionable evidence, but appreciates that its applications might be limited in scope and might not generalize as well to new contexts as an unqualified statement of its results might suggest. Communicating this directly would be a significant step toward (re-)establishing the trustworthiness of social scientists and their role in this pandemic.

Second, in order to retain or regain trust, social scientists ought to further embrace "open science" practices. Allowing open and free access to publications, data, and procedures are more important than ever in an emergency, as it allows for independent reproduction of findings as well as replication and reproduction attempts that do not rely on the main authors' willingness to share materials. This push for transparency, however advanced it may be at this moment, ought to be expanded. Yet, making flawed data sets publicly accessible may in itself pose a serious challenge (cf. Mormina et al., 2020), as does uploading documents before peer review (i.e., preprints) to archives that might be treated as established findings by journalists or the general public, which then recasts the above challenge. As such, while openness can undoubtedly help in addressing this challenge (cf. Hendriks et al., 2016), it ought to be done in a careful manner that ensures that no more harm is done in an attempt to establish the trustworthiness of social scientists in the context of this pandemic.

Overall, we conclude that if social scientists endorse the epistemic humility needed to properly communicate the numerous uncertainties involved in their findings, and if the values of openness are upheld and further expanded on, we can emerge from this crisis with a better understanding of the limitations of our research and our obligations to the public to further deserve their trust.

CONCLUSION

In this chapter, we have laid out four main ethical challenges for social science research in this pandemic. Specifically, we have discussed the altered landscape of informed voluntary consent, the novel trade-offs between scientific utility and subject welfare, the role of institutional review boards in the scientific response to the pandemic, and the moral obligation of social scientists to communicate their findings with a specific focus on the uncertainties involved and to make available their data and materials openly. We have argued that those challenges are both substantial and surmountable, and that an honest examination of them will leave the social sciences in a strong position to adequately respond to future emergencies of this kind.

REFERENCES

Barakat, A. F., Shokr, M., Ibrahim, J., Mandrola, J., & Elgendy, I. Y. (2020). Timeline from receipt to online publication for COVID-19 original research articles. medRxiv.https://www.medrxiv.org/content/10.1101/2020.06.22.20137653v1

Bavel, J. J. V., Baicker, K., Boggio, P. S., Capraro, V., Cichocka, A., Cikara, M., . . . & Willer, R. (2020). Using social and behavioural science to support COVID-19 pandemic response. *Nature Human Behaviour, 4*(5), 460–471.

Besacon, L., Peiffer-Smadja, N., Seagalas, C., Jiang, H., Masuzzo, P., Smout, Cd. A., Deforet, M., & Leyrat, C. (2020). Open science saves lives: Lessons from the COVID-19 pandemic. BioRxiv. https://www.biorxiv.org/content/10.1101/2020.08.13.249847v2.abstract

Bramble, B. (2020). *Pandemic ethics: 8 big questions of COVID-19.* Bartleby Books.

Calia, C., Reid, C., Guerra, C., Oshodi, A. G., Marley, C., Amos, A., Barrera, Pl., & Grant, L. (2020). Ethical challenges in the COVID-19 research context: A toolkit for supporting analysis and resolution. *Ethics & Behavior, 31*(1), 60–75. https://doi.org/10.1080/10508422.2020.1800469

Chmielewski, M., & Kucker, S. C. (2020). An MTurk crisis? Shifts in data quality and the impact on study results. *Social Psychological and Personality Science, 11*(4), 464–473. https://doi.org/10.1177/1948550619875149

Da Silva, J. A. T., Tsigaris, P., & Erfanmanesh, M. (2021). Publishing volumes in major databases related to Covid-19. *Scientometrics, 126*(1), 831–842. https://doi.org/10.1007/s11192-020-03675-3

Eikenberry, S. E., Mancuso, M., Iboi, E., Phan, T., Eikenberry, K., Kuang, Y., Kostelich, E., & Gumel, A. B. (2020). To mask or not to mask: Modeling the potential for face mask use by the general public to curtail the COVID-19 pandemic. *Infectious Disease Modelling, 5*, 293–308. https://doi.org/10.1016/j.idm.2020.04.001

Hawley, K. (2014). Trust, distrust and commitment. *Noûs, 48*(1), 1–20. https://doi.org/10.1111/nous.12000

Hendriks, F., Kienhues, D., & Bromme, R. (2016). Trust in science and the science of trust. In B. Blöbaum (Ed.), *Trust and communication in a digitized world* (pp. 143–159). Springer. https://doi.org/10.1007/978-3-319-28059-2_8

IJzerman, H., Lewis, N. A., Przybylski, A. K., Weinstein, N., DeBruine, L., Ritchie, S. J., Vazire, S., Forscher, P. S., Morey, R. D., Ivory, J. D., & Anvari, F. (2020). Use caution when applying behavioural science to policy. *Nature Human Behaviour, 4*(11), 1092–1094. https://doi.org/10.1038/s41562-020-00990-w

Kees, J., Berry, C., Burton, S., & Sheehan, K. (2017). An analysis of data quality: Professional panels, student subject pools, and Amazon's Mechanical Turk. *Journal of Advertising, 46*(1), 141–155. https://doi.org/10.1080/00913367.2016.1269304

Kowal, M., Bialek, M., & Groyecka-Bernard, A. (2020, December 11). Behavioural science is not good enough for building rockets, but still useful in crisis. https://socials

ciences.nature.com/posts/behavioural-science-is-not-good-enough-for-building-rockets-but-still-useful-in-crisis?badge_id=569-nature-human-behaviour

Meagher, K. M., Cummins, N. W., Bharucha, A. E., Badley, A. D., Chlan, L. L., & Wright, R. S. (2020, April). COVID-19 ethics and research. *Mayo Clinic Proceedings, 95*(6), 1119–1123. https://doi.org/10.1016/j.mayocp.2020.04.019

Mormina, M., Horn, R., Hallowell, N., Musesengwa, R., Lingou, S., & Nguqen, J. (2020). Guidance for research in response to humanitarian emergencies. Wellcome Centre for Ethics and Humanities. https://researchsupport.admin.ox.ac.uk/files/guidancef orresearchinresponsetopublichealthorhumanitarianemergenciespdf

Nelson, R. M., Beauchamp, T., Miller, V. A., Reynolds, W., Ittenbach, R. F., & Luce, M. F. (2011). The concept of voluntary consent. *The American Journal of Bioethics, 11*(8), 6–16. https://doi.org/10.1080/15265161.2011.583318

Pundi, K., Perino, A. C., Harrington, R. A., Krumholz, H. M., & Turakhia, M. P. (2020). Characteristics and strength of evidence of COVID-19 studies registered on ClinicalTrials.gov. *JAMA Internal Medicine, 180*(10), 1398–1400. https://doi.org/10.1001/jamainternmed.2020.2904

FURTHER READING

Adashi, E. Y., Walters, L. B., & Menikoff, J. A. (2018). The Belmont Report at 40: Reckoning with time. *American Journal of Public Health, 108*(10), 1345–1348.

Hawley, K. (2019). *How to be trustworthy*. Oxford University Press.

Israel, M., & Hay, I. (2006). *Research ethics for social scientists*. Sage Publications.

Parvizi, J., Tarity, T. D., Conner, K., & Smith, J. B. (2007). Institutional review board approval: Why it matters. *Journal of Bone and Joint Surgery. 89*(2), 418–426.

43

COVID-19-Related Community Sentiment Studies

Best Practices and Methodological Considerations

EVAN MURPHY AND BREANNA BOPPRE ■

The novel coronavirus COVID-19 shook communities across the globe. In the United States alone, there have been over 34 million COVID-19 infections and over 600,000 deaths at the time of this writing (June 2021; Centers for Diseases Control and Prevention, 2021). For those fortunate enough not to be infected with COVID-19 or to need to deal with infections of their family and friends, there were still dramatic changes to everyday life (see Chapter 2 for more on how the pandemic changed life). Daily routines of nearly all Americans were impacted through legal actions such as stay-at-home orders, mask mandates, school closures, and social distancing policies that were first enacted in March 2020 (see Chapter 3 for more on COVID-19 policies).

U.S. legal agencies were forced to adapt through significant shifts in daily processes. From courts to corrections, procedural changes were made across the legal system to address public health concerns, while maintaining the rule of law. For example, agencies have had to rely on remote methods for a variety of necessary commitments, such as court hearings, appointments, and treatment (see Chapter 5 for more on the legal system and COVID-19). These conditions not only created unprecedented challenges for the legal system but also opened distinct opportunities for policy reform (J. M. Miller & Blumstein, 2020).

Throughout the pandemic, community sentiment has impacted policy changes, including within the legal system. For example, community sentiment has shaped the prioritization of vaccinating incarcerated people. Following the guidance of the Centers for Disease Control and Prevention, several states have prioritized the vaccination of incarcerated people by placing them in the first wave of their

Evan Murphy and Breanna Boppre, *COVID-19-Related Community Sentiment Studies* In: *The Social Science of the COVID-19 Pandemic.* Edited by: Monica K. Miller, Oxford University Press. © Oxford University Press 2024.
DOI: 10.1093/oso/9780197615133.003.0043

vaccination plan.[1] However, some states have been forced to amend their vaccination plan due to community backlash. In Colorado, a Denver op-ed article argued that the state's vaccination plan would provide COVID-19 immunization to a "mass murderer" before the elderly and those with chronic health conditions.[2] A few weeks later after an uproar from his constituents, Colorado's governor revised the state's vaccination plan by removing incarcerated people from the plan entirely—presumably placing them last on the list for vaccinations despite higher risk of COVID-19 exposure than the general public. This example highlights the power that community sentiment can have on important policy decisions among different social groups in society.

The COVID-19 pandemic has created research needs and opportunities to understand community sentiment. In this chapter, we discuss community sentiment toward legal actions (i.e., laws, policies, or procedures) relevant to the COVID-19 pandemic. We begin by explaining what community sentiment is, describing how it is measured, and providing an overview of individual differences that can impact community sentiment. We then discuss methodological considerations for community sentiment research given the current constraints of the COVID-19 pandemic. We discuss the advantages of qualitative and mixed-methods community sentiment research and the opportunities that virtual platforms (e.g., Zoom) provide researchers who want to study hard-to-reach populations. Finally, we discuss the importance of disseminating quality research despite the pressure to publish research quickly.

COMMUNITY SENTIMENT

At a basic level, sentiment can be understood as a person's attitude toward or opinion about some attitude object. However, *community* sentiment is broader than just one person's attitude: It represents a collective attitude. Community sentiment can be defined as the collective attitudes or opinions of a given population about some attitude object (M. K. Miller & Chamberlain, 2015). People can have sentiment about anything, including policies, laws, and social issues; the list is endless. The present chapter focuses on sentiment toward legal actions (i.e., laws, policies, or procedures) relevant to the COVID-19 pandemic.

Measuring and understanding community sentiment about legal actions is important for several reasons. First, sentiment toward laws is a unique type of sentiment because laws affect everyone, can impact some social groups more than others, and can have significant consequences for society (M. K. Miller & Chamberlain, 2015). Second, sentiment can affect how the law is interpreted and enforced and how people who are affected by the law view the legal system generally (e.g., the legal system's perceived legitimacy; M. K. Miller & Chamberlain, 2015). Finally, understanding community sentiment is important because people are less likely to comply with legal actions or actors that they do not agree with or believe have legitimate authority over their behavior (Tyler, 2006).

Although considering community sentiment is important, there are a couple of reasons that policymakers should also be cautious. First, community sentiment can be measured improperly, and poorly conducted studies could produce erroneous results, which could lead lawmakers astray. Issues such as poorly conducted polls, poor sampling, vague questions, wording/order issues, and response options are some of the many issues that can affect the accuracy of community sentiment studies (M. K. Miller & Chamberlain, 2015). Second, even when a poll is conducted correctly, it still might not provide quality information about sentiment because of the characteristics of the respondents. Many people are ignorant about issues related to policy (Denno, 2000), are unable to tap into their own sentiment, or cannot communicate it properly (Blumenthal, 2003). Finally, community sentiment can also go against what is best for public health. For example, to slow the spread of COVID-19 and protect the public's health, lawmakers ignored antimasking community sentiment when implementing mask mandates.

The study of community sentiment is not limited to sentiment about existing laws, but also encompasses sentiment toward potential laws (e.g., COVID-19 vaccination passports). Measuring sentiment about potential laws provides context to understand whether people would vote for a law if it was on a ballot or whether they would comply with a law if it were to be enacted. Studies of community sentiment revealed what citizens believe the law "ought to be" (Finkel, 1995, p. 2). When lawmakers adopt laws that align with community sentiment, there are benefits for society more broadly, such as an increased sense of justice and government legitimacy among the public (M. K. Miller & Chamberlain, 2015).

Measuring Community Sentiment

When measuring community sentiment, there are two important decisions that need to be made: (1) What is the "community" that is being studied? and (2) What is the best method to measure their sentiment? Defining the community can be difficult and can depend on a variety of factors. The topic of study, the research question(s), and the legal application of a policy or law can all impact the community from which sentiment will be studied (M. K. Miller & Chamberlain, 2015). For example, a study that measured sentiment toward COVID-19 stay-at-home orders could vary dramatically if the community being studied were business owners, health professionals, or U.S. citizens. Similarly, we would expect different community sentiment between people in rural versus urban communities or red versus blue states.

In addition to defining the community, researchers also need to decide the best way to measure sentiment. Finkel (1995) suggested four ways of measuring community sentiment in the legal domain: legislative enactments, jury decisions, mock jury research, and public opinion polls. The first three can all be used as indirect measures of community sentiment (Finkel, 1995).

More direct approaches, such as public opinion polls, can provide a more pure and objective measure of a given community's sentiment. Polls can be conducted with representative samples and can provide a direct measure of sentiment within a given community. Public opinion polls are one of the most common methods to measure community sentiment; however, polls can be inaccurate if they measure sentiment that is specific to a time or place (i.e., transient sentiment), if they assess people who are not informed about a particular issue in question, or if they measure sentiment from people who are unable to accurately "tap" into their own sentiment (i.e., identify or communicate their sentiment; Blumenthal, 2003).

Determining the most appropriate method to measure community sentiment will largely depend on the researcher's goals and practical issues such as time and resources for a given project. Two particularly important methodological considerations for researchers are sampling and measurement error (Chamberlain & Shelton, 2015). Sampling error, or the difference between the sample and the population, is a consistent concern in community sentiment research. Often, community sentiment researchers extrapolate about the sentiment of an entire population (i.e., the community) by surveying a smaller subset of the population (i.e., the sample). The larger the difference between the sample and the population, the larger the sampling error. Probability sampling techniques help to reduce sampling error by allowing researchers to survey a representative random sample of a given population (Chamberlain & Shelton, 2015).

Measurement error is another issue to consider in community sentiment research. Measurement error refers to the differences between what a question is designed to measure and what it actually measures. Question wording, complexity, order, length, and response options are some of the many factors that can affect construct validity and measurement error (Tourangeau et al., 2000). The mode of response (e.g., in person, online, written, or oral) is another important measurement concern because it can impact how people respond (see Diamond, 2011; Tourangeau et al., 2000). For instance, people might be more willing to answer sensitive questions in an online survey compared to an in-person interview. In order to have an accurate measurement of community sentiment, researchers must be mindful of how their research methods could impact both sampling and measurement error.

Individual Differences in Community Sentiment

When conducting community sentiment research, there are several individual differences that researchers need to keep in mind. Individual differences in knowledge, personal relevance, emotion, and political orientation (or other personality variables) can all affect people's sentiment toward laws or policies. These are some of the factors that could be particularly important to consider when conducting research on community sentiment toward legal actions (i.e., laws, policies, or procedures) relevant to the COVID-19 pandemic.

KNOWLEDGE

The first individual difference to consider when conducting community sentiment research is the extent to which a person has knowledge about a particular law or policy. People with greater knowledge will likely have different community sentiment than those with less knowledge on a particular topic. Supreme Court Justice Thurgood Marshall captured this idea in his "ignorance hypothesis," which stated that people would have different attitudes toward the death penalty if they knew more about it (Finkel, 1995). Past research has shown the impacts of knowledge on community sentiment for topics such as the death penalty (Lambert et al., 2011), laws regulating pregnancy behaviors (Reichert & Miller, 2017), and affirmative consent policies (M. K. Miller, 2020).

When conducting community sentiment research toward legal actions and the COVID-19 pandemic, prior knowledge is a factor that should be taken into consideration. Those with greater knowledge about the symptoms, risks, and preventive behaviors associated with COVID-19 will likely be more supportive of legal actions that reduce the spread of the virus (e.g., mandating masks in correctional facilities). Indeed, more knowledge about COVID-19 is associated with support for protective behaviors such as avoiding crowds, wearing face masks, and following official guidelines (Ning et al., 2020).

Personal Relevance

In addition to individual differences in knowledge, community sentiment might differ because of the personal relevance that a particular topic has to a person. Personal relevance has been found to impact community sentiment for legal policies previously (M. K. Miller, 2020; M. K. Miller et al., 2018; Yelderman et al., 2018). In a study investigating community sentiment toward affirmative consent policies, women reported more positive sentiment than men. Although consent laws are equally important to both men and women, it was hypothesized that male participants perceived the policy as differentially personally relevant because men were more likely to worry about being accused of assault when compared to women (M. K. Miller, 2020).

When conducting community sentiment research toward legal actions and the COVID-19 pandemic, there are many personal relevance factors that could impact people's community sentiment. People who have previously been infected with COVID-19 will likely have very different levels of support for policies that look to slow the spread of the virus compared to people who have not been infected with the virus. Similarly, people who have family members who are incarcerated will likely be more supportive of early release policies, which look to reduce COVID-19 contagion in crowded correctional facilities by releasing those incarcerated for low-level offenses prior to their scheduled release date. Another personal relevance factor that could impact community sentiment is a person's health. People who are older or have underlying health conditions will likely be more supportive of COVID-19 policies that look to limit the spread of the virus due to the increased risks that the virus poses to them. For example, a cross-sectional survey conducted in the United States and Australia found that older people were significantly more supportive of stay-at-home orders than younger people (Czeisler et al., 2021).

Emotion

Emotions are another individual difference that can impact community sentiment. Often, our emotions are the first, and sometimes primary, source of information that is used as a basis of sentiment (M. K. Miller et al., 2015). When people are experiencing emotion, they can ignore logic and reason, instead focusing on gut instincts, first thoughts, and broad generalizations (i.e., the affect heuristic). For instance, Sicafuse and Miller (2014) found that many people based their sentiment toward human papilloma virus vaccination on emotions rather than logic. Other community sentiment studies have shown how emotions were associated with support for other legal policies (M. K. Miller et al., 2018; Yelderman et al., 2018).

Emotions similarly could affect community sentiment toward COVID-19 legal actions. The COVID-19 pandemic is undoubtedly an emotional experience for many. Fear, sadness, panic, and anxiety are some of the many emotions commonly felt throughout the pandemic (Adikari et al., 2021). The extent in which people feel these emotions could impact their attitude toward legal actions. Indeed, a recent study from Sweden found that both anger and fear were associated with support for more restrictive policies to limit the spread of the virus, while anxiety was associated with support for economic policies (e.g., increased sick leave; Renström & Bäck, 2021).

POLITICAL ORIENTATION

A final individual difference that could be particularly important to consider when conducting community sentiment research on COVID-19 legal actions is political orientation. Past research has found that community sentiment for legal policies can vary based on political orientation (e.g., Chomos & Miller, 2015; Sigillo et al., 2012). Indeed, throughout the COVID-19 pandemic there have been great differences between Republicans and Democrats in the perceived threat and need for government support in dealing with COVID-19.[3] Although there could be philosophical differences between Republicans and Democrats that are relevant to the COVID-19 pandemic (e.g., the role of the federal government), the politicization and polarization of COVID-19 news has also contributed to the polarization of U.S. COVID-19 attitudes (Hart et al., 2020; see Chapter 14 for more on the politics of COVID-19). A recent study has highlighted these political differences, finding that Republicans were less supportive of social distancing directives from governors' stay-at-home orders when compared to Democrats (Graham et al., 2020).

Although we have discussed individual differences in knowledge, personal relevance, emotion, and political orientation, this is far from an exhaustive list. These individual differences reflect only a few of the many factors that can impact community sentiment. There are numerous other individual differences, such as age, race, gender, and religiosity, that are not discussed in this chapter. Because individual differences are often related to legal attitudes, it is important for researchers to consider how these factors can impact community sentiment and how these relationships could differ based on the topic, timing, and sample of their study.

METHODOLOGICAL CONSIDERATIONS

When conducting community sentiment research during or about the COVID-19 pandemic, there are several methodological considerations to keep in mind (see

Chapter 42 for a discussion of the ethics of conducting COVID-19 research). This section will highlight the strengths of qualitative and mixed methods, the barriers and adaptations to data collection during the pandemic, and the importance of timely and accurate research dissemination.

Strengths in Qualitative and Mixed Methods

Given the distinct and new challenges faced by practitioners and community members, qualitative and mixed methodologies hold distinct advantages to studying sentiments about new issues related to the pandemic. Qualitative research typically uses an inductive approach in which the data and responses lead the research rather than predetermined theory or hypotheses (Creswell & Poth, 2018; Patton, 2015). Therefore, qualitative research, or the combination of qualitative and quantitative methods (mixed methods), can help build understandings of community sentiments without the constraints of solely predetermined measures, such as closed-ended survey questions or secondary data.

Barriers and Adaptations to Data Collection During the Pandemic

The COVID-19 pandemic has required a great deal of adaptations in daily routines and work—including work related to research. Conducting research amid the pandemic requires methodological adjustments while ensuring the quality of research is maintained. Scholars across the globe were faced with indirect barriers to conducting research, including adapting to remote teaching and increased caretaking responsibilities associated with remote schooling. With most children at home due to school and day care closures, increased child care responsibilities have disproportionately impacted women in academia (see Chapter 29 for more on women and families).[4] Ultimately, such conditions overshadow researchers' abilities to collect data as usual.

Researchers who traditionally used online or remote research methodologies, such as surveys or secondary data collection from official reports, faced fewer direct barriers in continuing such research during the pandemic. Surveys remain an effective way to measure community sentiment and hold the potential to capture large samples of community members. However, those conducting face-to-face research encountered distinct challenges during the pandemic to ensure the health and safety of both researchers and participants. Specifically, both researchers and participants were required to wear face masks at all times, pass COVID-19 screenings, and socially distance 6 feet apart in order to collect data. Such conditions were especially taxing in qualitative methodologies, as social distancing and masks can interfere with audio recording quality and the ability to build rapport during interviews and focus groups.

The pandemic caused researchers to rethink typical research strategies. Some scholars employed virtual methods in place of in-person primary data collection. Virtual platforms (e.g., Zoom) allowed researchers to engage with larger, representative samples across the United States or to connect with hard-to-reach populations directly impacted at the nexus of legal and COVID-19 policies. Even secondary data collection strategies evolved. For example, researchers in Australia qualitatively coded Twitter data to determine community sentiment toward COVID-19 government policies such as mask mandates, social distancing, and a wage subsidy program (Zhou et al., 2021).

Here, we provide an example of a mixed-methods study on sentiments toward correctional agencies' responses to the pandemic to illustrate research adaptations during the pandemic. Boppre and Novisky (2020) recruited over 300 people with incarcerated loved ones from across 40 states to participate in their online survey through social media and support groups across the nation. Using social media allowed for increased reach to potential participants, especially as social media and Internet usage increased during the pandemic.[5] Also, families impacted by incarceration would have been more difficult to reach in person due to stay-at-home orders and lockdowns within U.S. prisons.

Additionally, Boppre and Novisky (2020) used Zoom to conduct follow-up interviews remotely with a subset of their survey participants ($n = 35$). The virtual format allowed the researchers to connect with participants across various U.S. states versus one single location. Using Zoom also increased accessibility to participants who faced increased child care and varying work commitments. Thus, virtual recruitment and data collection methods held the potential to engage with more participants, particularly due to the constraints of the pandemic (i.e., stay-at-home orders).

Research Dissemination

Public criminology (e.g., Burgess-Proctor, 2018; Uggen & Inderbitzin, 2010) holds the potential to connect the public to criminological research, which is important especially due to the urgency of conditions during the pandemic related to legal policies and practices. Typical research dissemination can take considerable time to undergo peer review and publication, especially within the social sciences (Huisman & Smits, 2017). Researchers might consider other methods of dissemination to reach the public with more immediacy, such as social media (e.g., Twitter posters, animated abstracts, or GIFs; Morrison et al., 2020; Rivera, 2020) or op-eds (Rodriguez, 2018).

Nonetheless, researchers must be cautious when conducting and disseminating research quickly. For example, a recent study by Piquero and colleagues (2020b) examined the short-term effects of the pandemic's subsequent stay-at-home orders on domestic violence in Dallas, Texas. The study was published less than 3 months after the start of stay-at-home orders in Texas (March 24, 2020) and tracked domestic violence incidents from January 1 to April 27, 2020. Gonzalez and colleagues (2020) cautioned against the policy implications of such a short-term analysis with its methodological limitations related to the time frame and analytic approach. Gonzalez and colleagues (2020) noted that "inaccurate findings were disseminated to policymakers, other researchers and members of the public on social media (p. 1102)," which could lead to potential harmful policy shifts, such as the premature termination of stay-at-home orders.

While Piquero and colleagues (2020a) provided additional commentary addressing Gonzalez and colleagues' (2020) concerns, the study, subsequent commentaries, and media responses reflected the potential power and critiques over relatively quick research completion and dissemination. Researchers must utilize rigorous research methodologies and work collaboratively with media and policymakers to ensure accuracy in the interpretation of results. These precautions are important as the media holds potential to influence community sentiments as well (see Sigillo & Sicafuse, 2015, for a review).

CONCLUSION

Although the COVID-19 pandemic has created new obstacles for researchers, conducting community sentiment research remains crucial. With many new policies and procedures adopted during the COVID-19 pandemic, a plethora of unanswered questions remain. Community sentiment research, especially toward legal actions (i.e., policies, laws, and procedures), can provide lawmakers with an understanding of what the public wants and expects from the government. When lawmakers adopt laws or policies that align with community sentiment, there are direct benefits to society, such as a sense of justice and perceived government legitimacy.

NOTES

1. https://www.prisonpolicy.org/blog/2020/12/08/covid-vaccination-plans/
2. https://www.washingtonpost.com/health/2021/01/02/covid-vaccine-prisons/
3. https://www.pewresearch.org/politics/2020/06/25/republicans-democrats-move-even-further-apart-in-coronavirus-concerns/
4. https://www.insidehighered.com/news/2020/04/21/early-journal-submission-data-suggest-covid-19-tanking-womens-research-productivity; https://www.nature.com/articles/d41586-020-01135-9?error=cookies_not_supported&code=05ab5744-a88a-45a1-8fad-f87ff3eabaab
5. https://www.digitalcommerce360.com/2020/09/16/covid-19-is-changing-how-why-and-how-much-were-using-social-media/

REFERENCES

Adikari, A., Nawaratne, R., De Silva, D., Ranasinghe, S., Alahakoon, O., & Alahakoon, D. (2021). Emotions of COVID-19: Content analysis of self-reported information using artificial intelligence. *Journal of Medical Internet Research, 23*(4), 1–18. https://doi.org/10.2196/27341

Blumenthal, J. A. (2003). Who decides? Privileging public sentiment about justice and the substantive law. *University of Missouri-Kansas City Law Review, 72*, 1–21.

Boppre, B., & Novisky, M. (2020, November 18–21). *"I'm afraid he won't make it out alive": Perspectives on the COVID-19 Pandemic from Families of Incarcerated Persons* [Conference presentation]. CrimCon, virtual.

Burgess-Proctor, A. (2018). Doing public criminology in a politicized climate. *The Criminologist, 43*(6), 1–6.

Centers for Disease Control and Prevention. (2021). COVID data tracker [Data set]. https://covid.cdc.gov/covid-data-tracker/#datatracker-home

Chamberlain, J., & Shelton, D. E. (2015). Methods and measures used in gauging community sentiment. In M. K. Miller, J. A. Blumenthal, & J. Chamberlain (Eds.), *Handbook of community sentiment* (pp. 43–54). Springer.

Chomos, J. C., & Miller, M. K. (2015). Understanding how individual differences are related to community sentiment toward safe haven laws using a student sample. In M. K. Miller, J. A. Blumenthal, & J. Chamberlain (Eds.), *Handbook of community sentiment* (pp. 83–97). Springer.

Creswell, J. W., & Poth, C. N. (2018). *Qualitative inquiry and research design: Choosing among five approaches.* Sage Publications.

Czeisler, M. É., Howard, M. E., Robbins, R., Barger, L. K., Facer-Childs, E. R., Rajaratnam, S. M., & Czeisler, C. A. (2021). Early public adherence with and support for stay-at-home COVID-19 mitigation strategies despite adverse life impact: A transnational cross-sectional survey study in the United States and Australia. *BMC Public Health, 21*(1), 1–16. https://doi.org/10.1186/s12889-021-10410-x

Denno, D. W. (2000). The perils of public opinion. *Hofstra Law Review, 28*, 741–791.

Diamond, S. S. (2011). Reference guide on survey research. In *Reference manual on scientific evidence* (3rd ed., pp. 359–424). National Academies Press.

Finkel, N. J. (1995). *Commonsense justice: Jurors' notions of the law.* Harvard University Press.

Gonzalez, J. M. R., Molsberry, R., Maskaly, J., & Jetelina, K. K. (2020). Trends in family violence are not causally associated with COVID-19 stay-at-home orders: A commentary on Piquero et al. *American Journal of Criminal Justice, 45*(6), 1100–1110. https://dx.doi.org/10.1007%2Fs12103-020-09574-w

Graham, A., Cullen, F. T., Pickett, J. T., Jonson, C. L., Haner, M., & Sloan, M. M. (2020). Faith in Trump, moral foundations, and social distancing defiance during the coronavirus pandemic. *Socius: Sociological Research for a Dynamic World, 6*, 1–23. https://doi.org/10.1177/2378023120956815

Hart, P. S., Chinn, S., & Soroka, S. (2020). Politicization and polarization in COVID-19 news coverage. *Science Communication, 42*(5), 679–697. https://doi.org/10.1177/1075547020950735

Huisman, J., & Smits, J. (2017). Duration and quality of the peer review process: The author's perspective. *Scientometrics, 113*(1), 633–650. https://doi.org/10.1007/s11192-017-2310-5

Lambert, E. G., Camp, S. D., Clarke, A., & Jiang, S. (2011). The impact of information on death penalty support, revisited. *Crime & Delinquency, 57*(4), 572–599. https://doi.org/10.1177/0011128707312147

Miller, J. M., & Blumstein, A. (2020). Crime, justice & the COVID-19 pandemic: Toward a national research agenda. *American Journal of Criminal Justice*, *45*(4), 515–524. https://doi.org/10.1007/s12103-020-09555-z

Miller, M. K. (2020). Variations in community sentiment toward affirmative consent policies. *Criminal Justice Studies*, *34*(2), 173–183. https://doi.org/10.1080/14786 01X.2020.1824430

Miller, M. K., & Chamberlain, J. (2015). "There ought to be a law!" Understanding community sentiment. In M. K. Miller, J. A. Blumenthal, & J. Chamberlain (Eds.), *Handbook of community sentiment* (pp. 3–28). Springer.

Miller, M. K., Alvarez, M. J., & Weaver, J. (2018). Empirical evidence for AMBER alert as crime control theater: A comparison of student and community samples. *Psychology, Crime & Law*, *24*(2), 83–104. https://doi.org/10.1080/1068316X.2017.1390573

Morrison, M., Merlo, K., & Woessner, Z. (2020). How to boost the impact of scientific conferences. *Cell*, *182*(5), 1067–1071. https://doi.org/10.1016/j.cell.2020.07.029

Ning, L., Niu, J., Bi, X., Yang, C., Liu, Z., Wu, Q., Ning, N., Liang, L., Liu, A., Hao, Y., Gao, L., & Liu, C. (2020). The impacts of knowledge, risk perception, emotion and information on citizens' protective behaviors during the outbreak of COVID-19: A cross-sectional study in China. *BMC Public Health*, *20*(1), 1–12. https://doi.org/10.1186/s12889-020-09892-y

Patton, M. Q. (Ed.) (2015). *Qualitative research and evaluation methods: Integrating theory and practice* (4th ed.). Sage.

Piquero, A. R., Riddell, J. R., Bishopp, S. A., Narvey, C., Reid, J. A., & Piquero, N. L. (2020a). Reply to Gonzalez et al. *American Journal of Criminal Justice*, *45*(6), 1111–1118. https://dx.doi.org/10.1007%2Fs12103-020-09575-9

Piquero, A. R., Riddell, J. R., Bishopp, S. A., Narvey, C., Reid, J. A., & Piquero, N. L. (2020b). Staying home, staying safe? A short-term analysis of COVID-19 on Dallas domestic violence. *American Journal of Criminal Justice*, *45*(4), 601–635. https://dx.doi.org/10.1007%2Fs12103-020-09531-7

Reichert, J., & Miller, M. K. (2017). Social cognitive processes and attitudes toward legal actions: Does receiving information affect community sentiment? *Applied Psychology in Criminal Justice*, *13*(1), 70–95.

Renström, E. A., & Bäck, H. (2021). Emotions during the Covid-19 pandemic: Fear, anxiety, and anger as mediators between threats and policy support and political actions. *Journal of Applied Social Psychology*, *51*(8), 861–877. https://doi.org/10.1111/JASP.12806

Rivera, E. (2020). Create #AnimatedAbstracts and gifs in PowerPoint (+2 examples). Creative Research Communications. https://www.echorivera.com/blog/animatedab stracts

Rodriguez, N. (2018). Expanding the evidence base in criminology and criminal justice: Barriers and opportunities to bridging research and practice. *Justice Evaluation Journal*, *1*(1), 1–14. https://doi.org/10.1080/24751979.2018.1477525

Sicafuse, L. L., & Miller, M. K. (2014). An analysis of public commentary supporting and opposing mandatory HPV vaccination: Should lawmakers trust public sentiment? In M. K. Miller, J. Chamberlain, & T. Wingrove (Eds.), *Psychology, law, and the wellbeing of children* (pp. 234–254). Oxford University Press.

Sigillo, A. E., Miller, M. K., & Weiser, D. A. (2012). Attitudes toward nontraditional women using IVF: The importance of political affiliation and religious characteristics. *Psychology of Religion and Spirituality*, 4(4), 249–263. https://doi.org/10.1037/a0027940

Sigillo, A. E., & Sicafuse, L. L. (2015). The influence of media and community sentiment on policy decision-making. In M. K. Miller, J. A. Blumenthal, & J. Chamberlain (Eds.), *Handbook of community sentiment* (pp. 29–42). Springer.

Tourangeau, R., Rips, L. J., & Rasinski, K. (2000). *The psychology of survey response.* Cambridge University Press.

Tyler, T. R. (2006). Psychological perspectives on legitimacy and legitimation. *Annual Review of Psychology*, 57, 375–400. https://doi.org/10.1146/annurev.psych.57.102904.190038

Uggen, C., & Inderbitzin, M. (2010). Public criminologies. *Criminology & Public Policy*, 9(4), 725–749. https://doi.org/10.1111/j.1745-9133.2010.00666.x

Yelderman, L. A., Miller, M. K., Forsythe, S., & Sicafuse, L. (2018). Understanding crime control theater: Do sample type, gender, and emotions relate to support for crime control theater policies? *Criminal Justice Review*, 43(2), 147–173. https://doi.org/10.1177/0734016817710695

Zhou, J., Yang, S., Xiao, C., & Chen, F. (2021). Examination of community sentiment dynamics due to COVID-19 pandemic: A case study from a state in Australia. *SN Computer Science*, 2(3), 201–212. https://doi.org/10.1007/s42979-021-00596-7

FURTHER READING

Burstein, P. (2003). The impact of public opinion on public policy: A review and an agenda. *Political Research Quarterly*, 56(1), 29–40. https://doi.org/10.2307/3219881

Miller, M. K., Blumenthal, J. A., & Chamberlain, J. (Eds.). (2015). *Handbook of community sentiment.* Springer.

44

Strengthening Children and Youth Exposed to Multiple Community Stressors in Zagreb

Putting the Science Into Practice

GORDANA BULJAN FLANDER, IGOR MIKLOUŠIĆ,
TEA BREZINŠĆAK, ELLA SELAK BAGARIĆ,
AND VJEKOSLAV JELEČ ∎

EXPERIENCES OF THE ZAGREB COMMUNITY IN THE COVID-19 PANDEMIC

In the early Sunday morning of March 22, 2020, the people of Zagreb, Croatia, were roughly awakened by a strong earthquake. An earthquake of this intensity had not been recorded in Zagreb for the past 140 years. Within seconds, the earthquake caused widespread damage to the buildings, leaving a significant number of families homeless. The streets of the central, old part of the city became covered with pieces of facade and bricks, barely visible from the dust, making this part of the city unsafe for the days and months that followed. One young life was lost due to injuries sustained. Images emerged of mothers carrying their newborn babies on the street after a hospital evacuation in Zagreb as the snow started to fall, as well as footage and photos of the Zagreb football fan organization volunteers helping to transfer newborns in incubators to a safe location. The earthquake occurred in the first days of COVID-19 lockdown and strict stay-home orders. The tremors forced people to leave their homes and hindered their adherence to social distancing recommendations. For days, the authorities had encouraged people to stay home, but for many, home was now no longer a safe place or did not feel safe anymore. The earthquake was followed by a series of aftershocks,

Gordana Buljan Flander, Igor Mikloušić, Tea Brezinšćak, Ella Selak Bagarić, and Vjekoslav Jeleč, *Strengthening Children and Youth Exposed to Multiple Community Stressors in Zagreb* In: *The Social Science of the COVID-19 Pandemic*. Edited by: Monica K. Miller, Oxford University Press. © Oxford University Press 2024. DOI: 10.1093/oso/9780197615133.003.0044 culminating with strong earthquakes hitting the nearby cities of Petrinja and Sisak in late December 2020, causing distress and (re)traumatization. As in many other countries, the COVID-19 pandemic in Croatia was unquestionably marked by parallel crises and numerous individual challenges. All of this brought not only uncertainty, insecurity, and numerous losses—home, loved ones, health, but also a significant loss of quality of life, such as physical contact, warmth, and comfort.

A growing body of research points to mental health risks created by the COVID-19 pandemic for children and young people (Li et al., 2021; Ma et al., 2021; Racine et al., 2021), especially those who have experienced the effects of a pandemic on economic circumstances and daily life and delays in academic activities (Cao et al., 2020). In Zagreb, these risks have been exacerbated by a series of earthquakes, which is an event that poses a direct threat to the physical integrity and life of those affected, thus being a potentially traumatic event. The described circumstances posed a risk for toxic levels of stress that, depending on the developmental stage in which they occur, could lead to a number of negative long-term consequences for the development, physical, and mental health of children (Shonkoff & Garner, 2012).

For the community of mental health professionals in Croatia, this was by no means the first crisis they faced. Although the crisis response mechanisms were not particularly well established, the knowledge and experience gained during the Homeland war in the 1990s, and other crises since, served as a valuable guide. Once more, mental health professionals assumed responsibility and focused on protecting the rights and well-being of children, this time by ensuring the availability of mental health services for those who needed them, protecting children from side effects of crisis, such as the rise in family violence, and above all else enhancing their psychological resilience (see also Chapters 20 and 21 for more on resilience related to the pandemic).

This chapter presents the initiatives and strategies aimed at protecting mental health and well-being of children and youth in Zagreb. The chapter outlines the importance of psychological resilience and presents the steps taken by the newly founded Commission for the Protection of Mental Health of Children and Youth of the City of Zagreb to devise and implement a strategy to help and empower children, youth, and their families during the COVID-19 pandemic (see Chapter 29 for more on the impact of the pandemic on families). The strategy had four distinct segments; from empowering the community and mental health professionals alike, to engaging the media and conducting an extensive mental health screening in order to objectively assess the mental health status of the children and youth in Zagreb. Finally, opportunities for further research are also discussed. The chapter thus hopes to provide insights, as well as guidelines, for communities, mental health professionals, and governing bodies alike on how to use the available resources to mitigate the negative impact of the COVID-19 pandemic.

THE SCIENCE OF PSYCHOLOGICAL RESILIENCE

Psychological resilience describes a person's capacity for achieving positive adjustment when faced with trauma, adversity, or ongoing significant life stressors

(Luthar et al., 2000; Southwick et al., 2014; Zautra et al., 2010). With the onset of the COVID-19 pandemic, the issue of resilience was brought again to the forefront as we strive to understand the impact of the COVID-19 pandemic on mental health and plan policies to protect the children and youth from the stress brought on by the pandemic. This segment presents a systems view of resilience and examines ways in which resilience has been linked to various COVID-19 pandemic-related outcomes and guidelines.

The COVID-19 pandemic has proven to be a systemic problem that impacted not only the individual but also a broad range of systems on which a person relies and draws support from. For children, the effects of various restrictions and lockdowns span beyond the immediate effect of kindergarten, school, or college closures or the risk of infection. The limitations set forth to prevent the spread of the disease impacted their ability to physically socialize and play with their peers. Furthermore, many families experienced economic hardship, sudden loss of their closest family members to the disease, as well as heightened levels of stress for families whose members were in high-risk professions such as those in medical and other essential services. Finally, with the increased strain put on the medical system, children that suffered from chronic illnesses, or were in any way at risk, experienced stress related to the postponement of medical services. This cumulative negative experience of trauma on the well-being of children is well documented (Masten et al., 2015) and one of the reasons why the negative effects of the earthquake in Zagreb should be taken even more seriously.

In much the same way as the sources of stress can be seen as a cumulative system of negative influences on the mental health and well-being of individuals, resilience can also be seen as a capacity of a compound dynamic system to respond and adapt to these challenges (Masten, 2018). The psychological resilience system relies on not only the interpersonal traits of the children but also the quality of their relationships with their parents, peers, or caregivers. It also depends, for instance, on institutional resilience, preparedness of crisis response teams, availability of (mental) health services, and the ability of governments to maintain stability and offer economic relief.

The critical role of parents and families in protecting children from the adverse effects of the COVID-19 pandemic, as well the importance of providing support for children and their families alike, has already been documented (Masten, 2021). Some of the systemic approach guidelines for increasing psychological resilience of children and facilitating their adaptation to pandemic circumstances include acknowledging family-centered mental health services should constitute a public health mandate, implementing tailored monitoring and support systems for children and families, and improving access to mental health services through family-based and trauma-informed training for both mental health professionals and school base personnel (Stark et al., 2020). In line with this systems approach to human resilience (Masten & Motti-Stefanidi, 2020), efforts were undertaken to enhance the psychological resilience of children and youth by strengthening the psychological resources of children and families, as well as mental health and educational professionals whose support and protection they rely on.

THE PRACTICE OF COORDINATED COMMUNITY ACTION

Considering the disturbance at different levels of children's environment created by both earthquakes and the COVID-19 pandemic and limited resources, this endeavor called for coordinated actions and relying on existing resources and capacities of the city of Zagreb. Therefore, soon after the first earthquake in Zagreb, on April 29, 2020, the city of Zagreb established the Commission for the Protection of Mental Health of Children and Youth of the City of Zagreb (the commission), bringing together mental health experts working with children and youth, representatives of the city, and experts from the fields of education and culture. All members volunteered to contribute to the work of the commission. The commission aimed to promote psychological resilience by strengthening the capacity of their families, early childhood educators, teachers, and healthcare and social services experts in supporting and protecting them. In this way, the commission hoped to ameliorate the effects of multiple community stressors on the mental health of children and adolescents. The role of the commission was to use existing resources to promote intersectoral cooperation and cooperation between community, health, education, and social services in order to develop a well-coordinated, evidence-based approach. This section presents the four phases undertaken by the commission and targeted at promoting psychological resilience and mental health of children and youth:

1. *Strengthening the community*: Promoting psychological resilience of children and youth by providing trauma-informed services and materials for children and families
2. *Strengthening the healthcare and child protection system*: Increasing the capacity and quality of professional psychological support and the healthcare system
3. *Media engagement*: Raising the awareness on the importance of psychological resilience, mental health, and child abuse prevention through media appearances by experts and awareness-raising campaigns
4. *Identifying children at risk*: Conducting an extensive mental health screening

Strengthening the Community

The work of the commission began with identifying available resources targeted at promoting psychological resilience and mental health of children and youth. This step revealed an abundance of free resources aimed at children and youth, their families, and different professionals that were already available within the child and youth protection system in Zagreb. However, it also pointed to problems in making sure these resources reached those who needed them, inefficient allocation of human resources in their development, and gaps in creating a comprehensive approach, which was a result of an uncoordinated, crisis-based response. In order to cope with these issues, the commission created a web platform *Support on the Palm of Your Hand* (Podrška na dlanu; https://zagreb.hr/podrska-na-dlanu/158212), which included a selection of free e-resources categorized according to their target user (children, youth, parents, and experts), and a list of healthcare institutions that provided mental health services for children and youth. Using information and communication technologies enabled professionals to bypass social distancing measures and reach a large number of people.

The resources included different psychoeducation focused materials, articles with expert advice, e-books, booklets, and video materials. All of these aimed to

- provide information about common reactions to stressful or traumatic events and adaptive ways of coping
- promote social connectedness, play, and physical activity among children and youth
- promote positive parenting practices
- support parents in helping their children cope with school obligations
- support parents and other trusting adults in seeking mental health service for the child or young person when needed
- support families and professionals in protecting children from abuse and neglect
- maintain psychological well-being of parents and professionals
- develop a trauma-informed approach in delivering educational, healthcare, and social services

All of the resources were previously developed by professionals working in various health and social services institutions in Zagreb: psychologists, psychiatrists, pediatricians, social workers, and educators. The visibility of resources developed within various institutions also made it easier to focus the efforts of professionals on those areas that were lacking. Examples of shared e-resources for families, with titles translated from Croatian to English, include

- Booklet: *Children and Families Before, During and After the Earthquake*; provided information about common responses to trauma and ways of supporting children (Buljan Flander, Prijatelj, et al., 2020)
- Leaflets: *Small Kids, Big Worries: Stress in Early Childhood* (Brezinšćak & Selak Bagarić, 2020) and *Stressed Out Kids—Stress in Children and Adolescents* (Selak Bagarić & Brezinšćak, 2020) focused on common signs of stress in children and providing support
- Card game: *Cards for Rainy Days (and Social Distancing)* (Brezinšćak & Crnčević, 2020), containing 55 ideas for family activities to strengthen their relationship and build psychological resilience (also available in English, Greek, Romanian, Hungarian, and Macedonian)
- Workbook: *My Superhero and Me* (Buljan Flander, Raguž, et al., 2020), including activities focused on promoting emotion regulation skills and confidence

- *Illness in the family* (Knez Turčinović et al., 2020), a guide for families in coping with an illness of the child or other family member

One of the key resources in promoting the psychological well-being of parents and other adults caring for the well-being of children, helping them to guide children through challenging times, was a package of recommendations (Bagarić et al., 2020) developed by the Vrapče Psychiatric Clinic, the Reference Center of the Ministry of Health for psychosocial methods, the Croatian Society for Clinical Psychiatry of the Croatian Medical Association, the Mental Health and Addiction Prevention Service NZJZ "Dr. Andrija Štampar," and the Croatian Institute of Public Health. These resources aimed to help mental healthcare professionals provide psychosocial support, prevent burnout of healthcare workers, and serve as a guide for self-help of citizens in preventing the negative consequences of stress.

The information about the creation of the platform was shared with all preschools and schools in Zagreb, as well as social service centers and healthcare institutions under the governance of the city. Further, the commission developed e-resource packages for parents and professionals in the field of education. These were delivered to every preschool, primary school, and secondary school in Zagreb. The schools shared them with parents using available channels, ultimately reaching adults caring for over 12,000 children. Because no funding was available, the project was conducted relying exclusively on enthusiasm and readiness to collaborate.

With the support of the City Health Office and the City Office of Education, printed copies of some of the publications were delivered to families who lost their homes in Zagreb earthquakes and resided in temporary accommodation. The guidebook developed for parents of young children from birth to 3 years of age, *In Your Arms* (Selak Bagarić et al., 2020), also was given to families in printed form. Authored by psychologists, a psychiatrist, and a pediatric neurologist and inspired by the unsettling images of mothers of newborns on the day of the first Zagreb earthquake, the guidebook was also delivered to all maternity hospitals in Zagreb.

Strengthening the Healthcare and Child Protection System

In order to improve the availability and quality of psychological support provided to children and families affected by the COVID-19 pandemic and earthquakes, and to support those who support others, professionals from the commission joined forces with their colleagues in the Zagreb Child and Youth Protection Center and other professionals within the child protection system. The aims were to (1) strengthen skills and competencies of professionals working with children, youth, and their families in the areas of stress, trauma, and recovery; (2) provide support in nurturing a trauma-informed approach; and (3) facilitate keeping up with the growing body of research on the effects of COVID-19 pandemic on children and families. Throughout the year 2020, numerous webinars and conferences were organized, all free of charge for their participants.

Undoubtedly, the most important of them took place in late April 2020, when 180 psychologists, who would later continue to provide support via telephone lines during the COVID-19 pandemic, participated in a 3-day online training called *Psychological Support in Crisis Through Digital Platforms*. The training was organized by the city of Zagreb, Zagreb Child and Youth Protection Center, and Croatian Psychological Chamber and conducted by professionals of various backgrounds, including psychologists, psychiatrists, social workers, pediatricians, and law enforcement officers.

The collaboration would further inspire mental health, child protection, and education professionals and academics to embark on another shared journey. As a multidisciplinary approach response to providing support in and after the pandemic, a group of editors and authors created the e-book *Connected: Telephone and e-Counseling in the Face of the COVID-19 Pandemic* (Buljan Flander & Bogdan, 2021), which was once more made publicly available pro bono in Croatian and in English. The partners in the project were the city of Zagreb and the Croatian Psychological Chamber. The 200-page e-book, which brought together scientific research, recommendations, and the experiences of 16 experts from various fields, was described by reviewers as a "lasting trace of knowledge about the possibilities of telemedicine and psychological counseling in times of crisis, that will without a doubt ensure advantage even after the COVID-19 crisis" (Buljan-Flander & Bogdan, 2020). In addition to sections presenting available research on the impact of the COVID-19 pandemic on the mental health of children and adults, guidelines for providing psychological support and the importance of fostering resilience of clients as well as professionals, the authors also confronted the crises related to the rise in violence toward children.

Through collaboration with Zagreb Child and Youth Protection and the City Offices for Health and Education, a number of free webinars for professionals were organized, aiming to promote the quality of psychological support and encouraging timely response in protecting children from abuse and neglect in times of crises. Despite being aimed at professionals in Croatia, some were attended by a number of professionals in the region. The ones that sparked the most interest among the professional public were

- Webinar: *Pandemic COVID-19 and Mental Health of Children and Adolescents: Threat and Opportunity* (1,000 participants working in mental health, social services, and education)
- Webinar: *A Multidisciplinary Approach in the Diagnosis and Treatment of Childhood Trauma in a Family Environment* (1,000 participants working in the field of child protection)
- Online round table: *Stolen Childhood—A Dialogue of Experts and the Media in Protecting Children From Violence* (600 participants of various backgrounds)
- *Building Resilient Educational Systems in the Pandemic COVID-19: Support in Maintaining the Mental Health of Children and Their Families* (mental health and child development professionals working in primary and secondary schools of Zagreb)

Resource packages for empowering mental health professionals who work with children were delivered online to 60 preschools, 111 regular primary schools, 4 primary schools for students with disabilities, and 55 secondary schools; the health-care professionals in Zagreb; as well as the social protection system professionals. In addition to written resources we previously discussed, the packages included a selection of videos from previously mentioned professional training.

Media Engagement

Experience shows that media can be a valuable partner in promoting social change. In the era of social distancing, when people were encouraged to stay home, collaboration with the media also presented itself as a way of connecting professionals with the public in raising public awareness of mental health. Mental health professionals relied on media appearances to educate the public on common stress and trauma reactions, promote adaptive strategies of coping and psychological resilience, and support parents in guiding their children through COVID-19-related challenges, such as psychological distress, isolation, and online schooling. Further, professionals used the platform to warn the public, as well as decision makers, about the rise in violence against children, women, and other vulnerable groups. The most successful examples of collaboration between mental health professionals and media in 2020 included the following campaigns:

- Instagram campaign: *Share, Support, Withstand* was created and led pro bono by a team of digital marketing experts from the Degordian agency and psychologists from the Zagreb Child and Youth Protection Center during the lockdown in March 2020. Targeting young people, it aimed to encourage people to take care of their own mental and physical health, follow social distancing measures, empathize with at-risk groups, encourage positive communication through social media. The most popular influencers in Croatia joined the cause and shared the campaign templates on their profile along with hashtags #stayhome (#ostanidoma) and #hereforeachother (#tujednizadruge). The campaign spontaneously spread to the region through influencers (athletes, actors, singers, etc.), whose number of followers exceeded 2.5 million.
- Campaign: *More Courageous by the Day* not only focused on raising awareness on mental health of school-aged children, but also provided parents with tools that could support them in coping with COVID-19-related challenges. The campaign was inspired by the conclusions reached in the "mining" phase of the commission's work. As a part of the campaign, in September 2020 a workbook for children of the same name (Brezinšćak et al., 2020), authored by members of the commission and containing 60 pages of activities aimed to promote psychological resiliency of children, was distributed (26,000 copies) with the daily newspaper *Jutarnji list*. In October 2020, the commission delivered the

publication in printed form to Zagreb schools most damaged by the earthquake.

- In cooperation with the Zagreb Child and Youth Protection Center and the Degordian Agency, the Croatian Ministry of Interior launched a campaign named *Behind Closed Doors*, addressing a rise in violence against children and limited possibilities of seeking help and protection in social isolation. The campaign aimed to protect children from abuse by appealing to the civic courage and personal responsibility of individual people to prevent abuse by informing the system in a timely manner. The campaign was noticed by the Council of Europe (2021) and presented as an example of good practice. The short video depicted the life of a young girl named Mia, who remained closed with her abuser during the quarantine period by focusing on the doors of her home, thus reminding the viewer about children whose home was not a safe place. The name Mia was chosen because it was the most common name given to baby girls in Croatia in the past 3 years. The campaign was shared internationally by the European Crime Prevention Network (EUCPN, 2020).

Identifying Children at Risk

To allow early identification of psychological problems of children and youth, thus preventing the development of deeper negative consequences in their development and mental health, the Commission for the Protection of Mental Health of Children and Youth of the City of Zagreb conducted screening of school-aged children in Zagreb. The screening took place during February and March 2021, a year after the first major earthquake in Zagreb. Due to pandemic-related circumstances, many children took their classes online, some in periods of illness or self-isolation due to possible infection, and others continuously because they were at high risk of developing severe clinical manifestations of the illness. With this in mind, the commission decided to take a different approach. To take into account the experiences of all children equally, the screening was based on information provided by their parents. With the help of teachers, a link to the study was provided to all parents of children attending primary and secondary schools in Zagreb. The information was gathered using an online platform developed pro bono by an e-health company named Little Dot, safeguarding the confidentiality and anonymity of participants. The final sample included over 22,000 parents, thus gathering information about 1 in 4 children and adolescents in Zagreb (23% of primary school students and 24% of secondary schools students). Once more, the project was conducted with no funding.

A report on preliminary results (Buljan Flander et al., 2021) showed that most children (82%) had experienced earthquake-related and/or pandemic-related stressors. Most common stressors include self-isolation periods of the child (61%), a family member they live with (43%), or a close person outside their family (e.g., friends or teachers) (35%). Forty-three percent of children and adolescents had a close person outside their family who belonged to a high-risk group, while one in three lived with a family member at risk. The most severe stressors—hospitalization or loss of a family member or other close people—were the most infrequent. A significant proportion of children experienced changes in psychological functioning: About 1 in 10 children had significant anxiety and/or depressive symptoms, while about 1 in 7 faced a clinically significant level of symptoms of post-traumatic stress. Regarding the presence of these changes, no difference was found between children in primary and secondary schools, but it was shown that girls were at higher risk. Children who were more exposed to the effects of a pandemic, such as those whose family member or a close family member had COVID-19 or had experienced a loss, were also at increased risk.

To acquire a deeper insight into the experiences and well-being of parents, who are the main source of support and protection in the lives of their children, the Zagreb Child and Youth Protection Center conducted an online survey of almost 700 parents in Croatia during the COVID-19 health crisis, mostly of mothers (91%). These findings helped identify the needs of parents, thus informing the development of services focused on their needs and indirectly contributing to the well-being of their children. The main findings showed that the parental role was burdened by numerous concerns (80%), physical distancing measures (51%), emotional burdens (53%) and financial worries (55%). A significant number of parents (41.6%) felt an increased level of stress. One in five parents also reported increased levels of depression and one in four increased levels of anxiety (Buljan Flander et al., 2021).

FURTHER RESEARCH

The work of the commission shows an extensive effort made to put experience and theoretical knowledge of the mental health professionals in Zagreb into practice during one of the most severe (mental) health crises that have impacted the children in the city of Zagreb. The efforts of the commission included two extensive studies that were aimed at screening for mental health issues of children and assessing the well-being of their families. The studies provided the city of Zagreb, and its mental health professionals, invaluable information on the impact the two parallel crises had on children and youth in Zagreb. Ideally, studies in the future should consider a longitudinal framework where changes could be monitored over longer periods. Exposure to all of the distributed materials and perceived availability of mental health support should also be surveyed to identify room for improvement and other possible venues of dissemination of the educative materials. Finally, future research and policies should focus on new technologies and the promising prospects of telemedicine to provide even more sources of resilience, as is discussed in Chapter 20 of this volume.

CONCLUSION

The challenges that lie ahead are unknown. However, one thing is certain; the psychological resilience of children and adults stems from personal strength as well as from the support and resources offered by their environment. The safety and support that children have in their everyday life is the key to their recovery, and in order to provide it we need an extensive and informed collaboration between healthcare, education and social welfare experts, parents and families, institutions, and all other members and stakeholders in the community. The experiences of the Zagreb community provide guidelines, strategies, and materials that can be used to help direct professionals and communities alike when faced with some of the challenges the COVID-19 pandemic has brought to the world. The chapter highlighted four areas on which available resources were focused: strengthening the community, strengthening the healthcare and child protection system, media engagement, and identifying children at risk. A timely and extensive collaborative effort of local governing bodies, healthcare and educational institutions, and mental health experts, such as the one presented in this chapter, offers hope that a significant positive impact can be made in protecting the mental health and safety of children and youth, even with limited resources that are often a severe reality in the times of crises.

REFERENCES

Bagarić, Š., Bektić, J., Brečić, P., Bilić, V., Britvić, D., Buzina, N., Eterović, M., Ivandić, M., Jendričko, T., Koić, E., Kovač, M., Kušan Jukić, M., Marčinko, D., Martić-Biočina, S., Mihaljević-Peleš, A., Mužinić Marinić, L., Radić, K., Repovečki, S., Savić, A., . . . Vidović, D. (2020). Zaštita mentalnog zdravlja u krizi: stres, tjeskoba, strah - postupci označavanja i samopomoći postupak umirenja uznemirenih osoba. *Medix: specijalizirani medicinski dvomjesečnik, 141,* 6–50. https://zdravlje.gov.hr/UserDocsImages/2020%20Sanitarna/Preporuke%20za%20zastitu%20mentalnog%20zdravlja%20u%20krizi_Cjeloviti%20dokument.pdf

Brezinšćak, T., Buljan Flander, G., & Selak Bagarić, E. (2020). *Svakim danom sve hrabriji: Radna bilježnica koja osnažuje i gradi psihološku otpornost* [More courageous by the day: A workbook that strengthens and builds psychological resilience] [Brochure]. https://www.poliklinika-djeca.hr/publikacije/svakim-danom-sve-hrabriji-radna-biljeznica-koja-osnazuje-i-gradi-psiholosku-otpornost/

Brezinšćak, T., & Crnčević, N. (2020). Cards for rainy days (and social distancing) [Brochure]. https://childhub.org/ru/node/28091?language=sq

Brezinšćak, T., & Selak Bagarić, E. (2020). Mala djeca velike brige: Stres kod djece predškolske dobi [Small kids, big worries: Stress in early childhood] [Brochure]. https://www.poliklinika-djeca.hr/aktualno/novosti/letak-mala-djeca-velike-brige-stres-kod-djece-predskolske-dobi/

Buljan Flander, G., & Bogdan, A. (Eds.). (2020). *Connected: Telephone and online counselling in coping with the COVID-19 pandemic and its consequences.* Croatian Chamber of Psychology, the City of Zagreb, City Office for Health, Croatian

Chamber of Psychology and the Child and Youth Protection Centre of the City of Zagreb. https://www.poliklinika-djeca.hr/wp-content/uploads/2021/01/CONNEC TED-Telephone-and-Online-Counselling-in-Coping-with-the-COVID-19-Pande mic-and-Its-Consequences.pdf

Buljan Flander, G., Boričević Maršanić, V., Prijatelj, K., & Selak Bagarić, E. (2021). Roditeljstvo u pandemiji: Izazovi, rizici i prilike odrastanja. Izvjestaj istrazivanja o iskustvima roditelja u hrvatskoj tijekom Covid-19-zdravstvene krize [Parenting in the pandemic: Challenges, risks and opportunities] [Brochure]. https://www.poli klinika-djeca.hr/aktualno/novosti/roditeljstvo-u-pandemiji-izazovi-rizici-i-pril ike-odrastanja-izvjestaj-istrazivanja-o-iskustvima-roditelja-u-hrvatskoj-tijekom-covid-19-zdravstvene-krize

Buljan Flander, G., Mikloušić, I., Redžepi, G., Selak Bagarić, E., & Brezinšćak, T. (2021). Godinu dana poslije: Rezultati probira mentalnog zdravlja djece u Zagrebu [A year later: The results of child mental health screening in Zagreb]. Povjerenstvo za Zaštitu Djece i Mladih Grada Zagreba. https://www.poliklinika-djeca.hr/aktualno/ novosti/godinu-dana-poslije-rezultati-probira-mentalnog-zdravlja-djece-u-zagr ebu-kratki-izvjestaj

Buljan Flander, G., Prijatelj, K., & Roje Đapić, M. (2020). Djeca i obitelji prije, tijekom i nakon potresa [Children and families before, during and after the earthquake] [Brochure]. https://www.poliklinika-djeca.hr/aktualno/novosti/besplatna-publikac ija-djeca-i-obitelji-prije-tijekom-i-nakon-potresa/

Buljan Flander, G., Raguž, A., & Prijatelj, K. (2020). My superhero and me [Brochure]. https://www.poliklinika-djeca.hr/english/featured/workbook-for-children-my-superhero-and-me/

Cao, W., Fang, Z., Hou, G., Han, M., Xu, X., Dong, J., &Zheng, J. (2020). The psycho-logical impact of the COVID-19 epidemic on college students in China. *Psychiatry Research*, *287*, Article 112934. https://www.ncbi.nlm.nih.gov/pmc/articles/PMC 7102633/?fbclid=IwAR07Z9xB4k49ynqK1jhonKoBsEunkK-zZ7dhIXeIJD2v_Apn qftO4QIfFAU

Council of Europe. (2021). The COVID-19 pandemic and children: Challenges, responses and policy implications [Fact sheet]. https://rm.coe.int/covid-19-factsh eet-revised-eng/1680a188f2

European Crime Prevention Network (EUCPN). (2020). *Behind the door*. European Crime Prevention Network. https://eucpn.org/document/behind-the-door

Knez Turčinović, M., Kralj, D., Križan, V., & Škrlec, N. (2020). Illness in the family: A handbook for parents [Brochure]. https://www.poliklinika-djeca.hr/english/featu red/free-publication-disease-in-the-family-a-handbook-for-parents/

Li, Y., Wang, A., Wu, Y., Han, N., & Huang, H. (2021). Impact of the COVID-19 pan-demic on the mental health of college students: A systematic review and meta-analysis. *Frontiers in Psychology*, *12*, Article 669119, https://doi.org/10.3389/ fpsyg.2021.669119

Luthar, S. S., Cicchetti, D., & Becker, B. (2000). The construct of resilience: A critical evaluation and guidelines for future work. *Child Development*, *71*(3), 543–562. https://doi.org/10.1111/1467-8624.00164

Ma, L., Mazidi, M., Li, K., Li, Y., Chen, S., Kirwan, R., Zhou, H., Yan, N., Rahman, A., Weidong, W., & Wang, Y. (2021). Prevalence of mental health problems among chil-dren and adolescents during the COVID-19 pandemic: A systematic review and meta-analysis. *Journal of Affective Disorders*, *293*, 78–89. https://doi.org/10.1016/j.jad.2021.06.021

Masten, A. S. (2018). Resilience theory and research on children and families: Past, present, and promise. *Journal of Family Theory and Review*, *10*(1), 12–31. https://doi.org/10.1111/jftr.12255.

Masten, A. S. (2021). Family risk and resilience in the context of cascading COVID-19 challenges: Commentary on the special issue. *Developmental Psychology*, *57*(10), 1748.

Masten, A. S., & Motti-Stefanidi, F. (2020). Multisystem resilience for children and youth in disaster: Reflections in the context of COVID-19. *Adversity and Resilience Science*, *1*(2), 95–106. https://doi.org/10.1007/s42844-020-00010-w

Masten, A. S., Narayan, A. J., Silverman, W. K., & Osofsky, J. D. (2015). Children in war and disaster. In M. H. Bornstein, T. Leventhal, & R. M. Lerner (Eds.), *Handbook of child psychology and developmental science: Ecological settings and processes in developmental systems* (7th ed., pp. 704–745). John Wiley & Sons.

Racine, N., McArthur, B. A., Cooke, J. E., Eirich, R., Zhu, J., & Madigan, S. (2021). Global prevalence of depressive and anxiety symptoms in children and adolescents during COVID-19: A meta-analysis. *JAMA Pediatrics*, *175*(11), 1142–1150. https://doi.org/10.1001/jamapediatrics.2021.2482

Selak Bagarić, E., & Brezinšćak, T. (2020). Klinci pod stresom—Stres kod djece i adolescenata [Stressed out kids—stress in children and adolescents] [Brochure]. https://www.poliklinika-djeca.hr/aktualno/novosti/letak-klinci-pod-stresom-stres-kod-djece-i-adolescenata/

Selak Bagarić, E., Slijepčević Saftić, V., Prijatelj, K., & Boričević Maršanić, V. (2020). U tvom naručju: Vodic za roditelje kroz pustolovinu prve tri godine djetetova života [In your arms: A guide for parents through adventures of the first 3 years in a child's life] [Brochure]. https://www.poliklinika-djeca.hr/aktualno/novosti/besplatna-publikacija-u-tvom-narucju-vodic-za-roditelje-kroz-pustolovinu-prve-tri-godine-djetetova-zivota/

Shonkoff, J. P., & Garner, A. S. (2012). The lifelong effects of early childhood adversity and toxic stress. *Pediatrics*, *129*(1), 232–246. http://dx.doi.org/10.1542/peds.2011-2663

Southwick, S. M., Bonanno, G. A., Masten, A. S., Panter-Brick, C., & Yehuda, R. (2014). Resilience definitions, theory, and challenges: Interdisciplinary perspectives. *European Journal of Psychotraumatology*, *5*(1), Article 25338. https://doi.org/10.3402/ejpt.v5.25338

Stark, A. M., White, A. E., Rotter, N. S., & Basu, A. (2020). Shifting from survival to supporting resilience in children and families in the COVID-19 pandemic: Lessons for informing U.S. mental health priorities. *Psychological Trauma: Theory, Research, Practice, and Policy*, *12*(S1), S133–S135. https://doi.org/10.1037/tra0000781

Zautra, A. J., Hall, J. S., & Murray, K. E. (2010). Resilience: A new definition of health for people and communities. In J. W. Reich, A. J. Zautra, & J. S. Hall (Eds.), *Handbook of adult resilience* (pp. 3–29). The Guilford Press.

FURTHER READING

Buljan Flander, G., & Bogdan, A. (Eds.). (2020). *Connected: Telephone and online counselling in coping with the COVID-19 pandemic and its consequences.* Croatian Chamber of Psychology, the City of Zagreb, City Office for Health, Croatian Chamber of Psychology and the Child and Youth Protection Centre of the City of Zagreb. https://www.poliklinika-djeca.hr/wp-content/uploads/2021/01/CONNEC TED-Telephone-and-Online-Counselling-in-Coping-with-the-COVID-19-Pande mic-and-Its-Consequences.pdf

45

Researching Emotional Topics During Emotional Times

Reflecting on Best Practice for the Management and Negotiation of Emotional Labor in Qualitative Social Research

SAMANTHA HUGHES, SARAH LEMON, NATASHA STONEBRIDGE, AND SAM SCOTT ■

During the COVID-19 pandemic in 2020, three early career researchers (ECRs) from the United Kingdom found themselves carrying out in-depth interviews with front-line workers. In this chapter, the researchers share their experiences of this emotionally charged time and discuss the impact of performing emotional labor (EL) within this context. This chapter provides researchers with an understanding of EL, which will help with the recognition and management of their own emotions and, in doing so, help protect them from emotional harm while simultaneously enriching and enhancing their research (see also the chapters in Section Five of this volume for more on doing research during and about the pandemic more generally). Additionally, this chapter seeks to raise awareness of EL and highlight the importance of addressing the topic within the wider academic community.

EMOTION AND WORK IN THE COVID-19 PANDEMIC

On March 11, 2020, the World Health Organization (WHO) declared COVID-19 a global pandemic (WHO, 2020). To reduce mortality and morbidity rates, significant restrictive measures were implemented across the globe (see Chapter 3 of this volume). Many governments initiated lockdown measures, which included the closure of nonessential businesses; however, key workers, such as those in

Samantha Hughes, Sarah Lemon, Natasha Stonebridge, and Sam Scott, *Researching Emotional Topics During Emotional Times* In: *The Social Science of the COVID-19 Pandemic*. Edited by: Monica K. Miller, Oxford University Press.
© Oxford University Press 2024. DOI: 10.1093/oso/9780197615133.003.0045

health and social care roles, the community supply chain (e.g., supermarkets), or other emergency services were still required to work. The emotional toll of working in healthcare during the pandemic has been widely acknowledged in the media and academia (e.g., Kinsella et al., 2022; Liu et al., 2020; Sarabia-Cobo et al., 2021; Sumner & Kinsella, 2021). Healthcare workers believed it was their duty to keep working. However, fatigued from long working hours, distraught at their ever-increasing exposure to death, fearful for their own well-being and of spreading the virus to loved ones, the trauma they experienced was evident (see also Chapters 20 and 27 for more on trauma and the pandemic). One intensive care unit doctor[1] reported:

> I had a panic attack on the bus. . . . It was a baby's screams that set me off. . . . I was crying to myself, trying to blank out the distressing noise. It reminded me of the phone calls I've made to families bereaved by Covid . . . when you give them the worst news and hear their howls. It's piercing and sticks with you. (Anonymous, 2021)

Another relayed an experience shared by a colleague: "She has to get new clothes for her children because she can't bear the sound of zips anymore after having to zip up body bags" (Kinsella et al., 2022, p. 10). The last quotation was taken from an interview for the CV19 Heroes Project,[2] a study that we (Samantha, Natasha, and Sarah) were appointed to as research assistants and the catalyst for this chapter. The following section establishes the challenging nature of conducting social research during the COVID-19 pandemic and then focuses on the relevance of EL when carrying out such research.

Conducting Social Research in the Pandemic

The CV19 Heroes Project launched in March 2020 at the outset of the pandemic. It aims to track the well-being of front-line and key workers in the United Kingdom and Ireland during and in the aftermath of COVID-19. It is a multiphase, mixed-methods project comprising quantitative elements examining resilience, burnout, and well-being via electronic surveys (Sumner & Kinsella, 2021) and qualitative components via semistructured interviews (Kinsella et al., 2022). We were brought on board to conduct the interviews and support the project leads in the analysis of data.

Of the limited prior research investigating experiences of working during the pandemic, findings are bleak. Newcomb (2021), for example, reflected on suffering an emotional breakdown while struggling to balance the demands of work and being a mum and a researcher during an emotional time. Similarly, the media documented how remote working, research delays, economic fallout, and child care obligations had seen a rise in mental health concerns and burnout within the community.[3] As such, we became increasingly aware of our emotional vulnerabilities as researchers. From the outset of the CV19 Heroes Project, the project leads had communicated that the work would be emotionally demanding. Therefore, after engendering an open and safe environment, and before any data had been gathered, the project leads proposed peer support check-in with preplanned meetings throughout the interview period. Discussions ranged from offloading anxieties regarding difficult conversations, to asking questions about the project, and to discussing non-work-related stressors. We also set up a WhatsApp group in case we needed to engage outside of formal meetings, ensuring that personal and professional boundaries were acknowledged (i.e., we were there to offer a friendly ear, not to act as therapists). Alongside peer support, each interviewer engaged in a reflexive exercise postinterview, which could be referred to and shared with the group. Peer support and reflexivity have been previously noted as effective management strategies for researchers when studying emotional topics (Dickson-Swift et al., 2007; Newcomb, 2021; Waters et al., 2020); however, there is little guidance on effectively managing emotions in academia. This could, in part, be due to the historical understandings of emotions in research.

Historically, social scientists supported a positivist, scientific study of society that contended that research should be objective, context free, value free, bias free, and replicable. Within academia, positivism was considered the gold standard of research and scholars were trained to extract out their emotions, which were considered irrational, dangerous, and of lesser value than detached and objective positivistic inquiry. Subsequently, good researchers were those who could remain neutral and emotion free (Hubbard et al., 2001). However, the rise of interpretivism, which professed knowledge comprises multiple interpretations that are context dependent and value laden, placed subjective experience at the heart of social research (Lincoln & Guba, 1985), and, as such, the role of emotion became increasingly acknowledged within qualitative literature. There is now growing recognition that undertaking qualitative research can pose challenges for the researcher who adopts an active role in the process. Consequently, several studies have considered researchers' emotions, the impact these might have on their health and well-being and on the integrity of their work (e.g., Bundhoo & Lynch, 2021; Newcomb, 2021; Waters et al., 2020). However, studies are scarce and rarely involve the articulation of feelings or discuss how to systematically manage emotions (Bundhoo & Lynch, 2021; Dickson-Swift et al., 2009). This is of particular importance to understand since qualitative work requires researchers to perform *emotional labor*, which contributes additional pressure to an already challenging role.

Emotional Labor

Emotional labor is defined as the induction or suppression of private feelings, which are replaced with more socially acceptable emotions (Hochschild, 1983). The term was first introduced by Hochschild (1983) concerning flight attendants who were expected to be friendly despite how they were feeling and regardless of the stressfulness of the situation. Qualitative researchers have since been identified as persons that perform EL. For example, during interviews participants might talk about emotional experiences, and if these are particularly relatable to the researcher, these emotions could transfer to them. While the researcher might feel upset, they need to control their emotions, often through emotional suppression, to minimize harm and to maintain the integrity of their work. However, it can be difficult for researchers to comprehend which emotions to share to maintain the well-being of themselves and their participants while simultaneously trying to build rapport and gain the most insightful data possible (Hoffmann, 2007). Specific *feeling rules*, which are a shared set of guidelines that inform how people *should feel* within the associated discipline (Hochschild, 1983), help to dictate this decision. For example, the academic researcher is expected to present a competent and calm exterior during an interview, irrespective of the content or their personal views (Bundhoo & Lynch, 2021).

Practising EL is particularly challenging for ECRs and those working with sensitive or emotive topics (Waters et al., 2020). The flexible and open nature of feeling rules means that the level of emotion that the researcher *should* display is open for continual negotiation and debate. Some researchers believe it is important to be openly emotional as a way of connecting with participants, while others favor emotional suppression and, as such, consider emotional displays to be inappropriate and unprofessional (Dickson-Swift et al., 2009). This lack of clarity contributes a further stressor for ECRs, who are establishing their identities as academics while trying to learn the *right* way to perform (Seear & McLean, 2008).

Despite recommendations calling for training in EL, especially for ECRs and supervisory teams, for institutions to embrace a self-care ethos and for ethical proceedings to actively include the emotions of the researcher (Waters et al., 2020), we struggled to find practical applications. Therefore, we decided to reflect on our lived experiences as ECRs during the pandemic to initiate awareness and appreciation of EL within the academic community so that it might be more actively addressed.

PERSONAL REFLECTIONS

In exploring our experiences of researching during COVID-19, we tasked ourselves with writing a reflexive narrative in response to a series of questions, including (but not limited to) "Have you considered whether emotion should come into the research process and whether people acknowledge emotion enough in academia?" and "How did you feel during carrying out the project?" We analyzed our reflections using thematic analysis (Braun & Clarke, 2013), coding individually before coming together to discuss and refine our codes and candidate themes. In this section, three themes are presented: (1) acknowledgment; (2) responsibility; and (3) management. Subthemes are also discussed and represent the complex nature of EL. Figure 45.1 depicts a thematic map of our experiences.

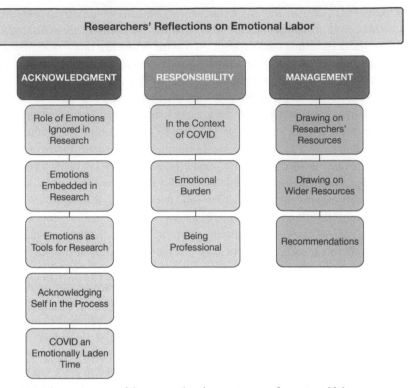

Figure 45.1 Thematic map of the researchers' experiences of emotional labor.

Acknowledgment

We felt that only after acknowledging EL within the research process can it begin to be managed. Paradoxically, however, we perceived that the "role of emotion is ignored in research" represented our first subtheme. Our reflections surmised this might be because the display of emotions in the context of academia is still largely stigmatized: "I think researchers feel less science-y if they reference an emotional reaction" (Natasha), putting pressure on researchers to remain objective, particularly ECRs still in search of their academic identity. We felt this could relate to positivist legacies and the failure of interpretivism to fully shift paradigms.

While we recognized increasing acknowledgment of emotions in qualitative research, we wondered if this was rather superficial: an obligation to abide by ethical standards as opposed to offering a more genuine and constructive consideration of the researchers' emotions. As Samantha stated: "Although reflexivity is a requirement in most qualitative research now, I feel like it remains an afterthought and is often only completed because it is obligatory to do so . . . with little regard for the researcher's thoughts and feelings themselves."

However underacknowledged emotions might be, our reflections overwhelmingly cited that "emotions are embedded in research"; they are both fundamental and inevitable within the research process. The following quotations highlight how particular stories evoked upsetting emotional reactions that stayed with us for some time after we collected and analyzed the data: "I had a very strong reaction to a participant who said [that] she wanted to tell others it was ok to walk away. This for some reason continues to stay with me" (Sarah) and

> a consultant working on a covid ward. They felt like a failure, surrounded by dying people they couldn't sit with and felt very upset at the fact that people were left to die without loved ones around them. They got very emotional, crying during the interview, which made me cry. (Natasha)

Having an emotional response during an interview is something we all struggled to negotiate. However, we acknowledged that we are all human beings, and, as such, emotions are inevitable, and we supported each other in the notion that it is OK to have an emotional response. Additionally, we recognized the importance of emotions in directing our research practices, concluding that the experiences and emotions we bring to our research inform our subjective positions. As such, we felt that it was important to disclose our emotions to a certain extent because "being transparent about [our] emotions [can] increase the integrity of research" (Samantha); audiences are able to navigate our decision-making processes and, in doing so, comprehend how and why we reached the conclusions that we did. This discussion helped with our confidence in viewing emotional disclosure as acceptable and of value, albeit the amount and intensity of emotional expressionism that is appropriate for us to show is something that we are all still learning. This links to another subtheme of acknowledgment: "emotions as tools for research," which presents the idea that acknowledging the influence of emotions can inform better practice.

Another key takeaway was the importance of "acknowledging self in the process." Practicing reflexivity covered this to a certain extent; however, as Sarah reflected: "The more involved the researcher is with their participants, the closer the contact, the more the subject is personal to them, then potentially the greater the cost of managing this whilst trying to remain objective for their research." Samantha gave an example of how the lockdown restrictions, enforced due to COVID-19, in which she had not seen family members in over a year, made her vulnerable to related interview content:

> As I continued to carry out interviews . . . I started to feel a little apprehensive. I thought it was perhaps talking about death. . . . But . . . [after] delving further into what was bothering me . . . it was times in which frontline workers spoke about loved ones not being able to be together in death, and the sense of hopelessness that that evoked for them. The fact that I am very close to my family made me able to envision myself in such situations and how I would feel not being able to see those close to me in their final hours . . . [that] was actually what got to me. (Samantha)

By acknowledging her emotions Samantha was able to implement management strategies, including learning to let go. This also alluded to the first step in managing EL: *to acknowledge it*.

Emotional labor was perceived to be ever present in our decision-making processes, for example in deciding which phenomena to explore in research: "As researchers, we get told to follow our passions, that's emotive" (Natasha). We further reflected that EL is present irrespective of whether our research is qualitative or quantitative:

> I do believe that there is a degree of EL in all research. . . . Researchers in the main choose to study areas that are important to them in some personal way, thereby any interaction with this data is likely to have some EL. (Sarah)

Finally, we noted that researching during the context of the pandemic added to the emotional burden of the work. The CV19 Heroes Project began during the first U.K. lockdown and at a time when people had been asked to stay in their homes for 3 months. Therefore, the strong subtheme of "COVID as an emotionally laden time" acknowledged that the backdrop to data gathering was an unusually emotional one: "We were experiencing a terrible time; I was hearing stories of people dying alone, empty supermarket shelves, people scared but going to work. It felt apocalyptic" (Natasha). This was also reflected in the data: "There was a sense for me that the participants needed to varying degrees to really 'get things off their chest'; it felt different to previous interviews I had carried out. . . . It was more an offloading by the participants" (Sarah).

Lockdown restrictions meant a change to work practices as researchers, working online and often in isolation. In addition, other outlets that we engaged in for our emotional well-being were curbed, such as volunteering:

> It's not essential and I couldn't live with the guilt of knowing that I had brought anyone to harm because of my decision to continue [volunteering] at that stage. . . . This conjured a lot of emotions within me, such as frustration but also admiration for the work frontline healthcare workers have to do. (Samantha)

Nevertheless, given the many restrictions, taking part in the project enabled us to reframe and redirect our emotional energy from hopelessness and distress to purpose and determination.

Responsibility

Another theme was "responsibility" and included the subtheme "in the context of COVID." First, we felt emotionally burdened by the responsibility of representing the voices of front-line workers and the importance of the work that they do: "It has made me more determined to get the voices of frontline workers out there so that people can understand more about what COVID is like for the people that come face to face with it every day" (Samantha). This enhanced our motivation to do the work regardless of personal feelings.

"Emotional burden" was strongly represented across the data and included within responsibility with the view that it was not only the burden shared by participants that was challenging but also the burden of doing a *good job* and of supporting each other as a team:

> There was a definite emotional impact on [us] in how [we] were addressing [our] personal feelings around the interviews and the topic of COVID. Although not perhaps verbally or formally acknowledged. (Sarah)

This hints at how, although we might not have been aware at the time, we were actively taking responsibility to manage our EL as a team, as Samantha and Sarah reflected: "I think that I would have felt more distressed by feeling like I had to hide my emotions and carry the responsibilities of what was disclosed in the interviews on my own" (Samantha); "I also felt a keen responsibility for my fellow researchers and the distress they sometimes expressed" (Sarah). Consideration about who takes on the burden was also discussed, and we struggled to understand where responsibility should lie:

> I do not feel like they [the project leads] should be put in a position where they feel the extra burden and responsibility for ensuring the emotional stability of those around them (i.e., they are not therapists!). . . . It is difficult to know where the boundary lies between responsibility, duty of care and professionalism. (Samantha)

Samantha highlighted how *feeling rules* or expected norms within academia could extenuate ECRs distress in feeling like they have a responsibility to carry the emotional burden on their own:

> I might not have shared my distress at the time due to expectations that dealing with emotional content is simply a part of the qualitative researcher's role as well as the fact that I was a very early career researcher and would not have had the confidence to confide in anyone. (Samantha)

This subtheme of "being professional" was repeated throughout in terms of maintaining healthy boundaries. Discussions centered on our ongoing struggle during interviews to balance expressions of empathy while maintaining emotional distance from our participants. While acknowledging that traditional scientific notions of professionalism are beginning to change, we also felt there is a long way to go before emotions are truly accepted and integrated as part of the research process: "For me researchers still remain reluctant to discuss their personal emotions and how these impacted the research, perhaps out of fear of the consequences (i.e., being perceived by others as 'unstable,' or not a 'proper' researcher)" (Samantha).

Not being professional, or being seen as a proper researcher due to an emotional element in the work was repeatedly cited, compounded by being an ECR: "As an ECR you're always questioning your ability, do you have the right tone and style of asking questions?" (Natasha).

There was also consideration of allocating time to support the group and a nod to power relations insomuch as we felt that significant support had been given to us, but we had concerns about how much aid was being offered to the project leads: "Perhaps given their responsibility towards us they felt they could not express [their true emotions]?" (Sarah).

Management

The final theme of management related to how EL had been managed throughout and the learnings gained. The first subthemes took a micro/macro approach: "drawing on researchers' resources" and "drawing on wider resources." Samantha reflected on how her past experiences (i.e., drawing on her wider resources) presented her with perspectives and skills that provided her with confidence in her ability (i.e., the researchers' resources) to manage challenging narratives:

> While I now feel confident in managing emotional content etc. and enjoy this responsibility as a qualitative researcher, before gaining my lived experiences I would not have been so confident in doing so, and as a result might have suffered elongated distress. (Samantha)

All of us drew on personal skills to manage EL, such as taught reflexivity or listening skills honed via counseling courses: "Learning about counseling skills has been an integral part of my learning to deal with emotional reactivity of myself and others in the research process" (Samantha). With regard to "drawing on wider resources," setting up and engaging in the peer support group also helped manage EL through learning new strategies from one another: "It was valuable to be aware of different responses by the different researchers allowing me to learn better ways to manage my EL" (Sarah). Defense mechanisms were also utilized, such as compartmentalization, which in this context delayed Natasha's emotional reaction:

> When you have two or three of those interviews a day or in a couple of days you have to put them in boxes and start afresh with the next one. I felt like I did do that. It was only talking about them with others that brought the emotion back. (Natasha)

Again, this highlighted the importance of acknowledging EL as researchers never know when it might affect them.

Acknowledging EL within research via permitting people to feel was also perceived as key to managing it. "I feel that I had a more than appropriate response to what I was hearing" highlighted a growing confidence for Natasha, accepting her emotional response to a particularly emotive interview.

Listening to one another and drawing on wider team resources also helped validate feelings: "Knowing that others were having similar thoughts to me [helped]" (Samantha). Hearing each other's experiences was also an opportunity to study one another's coping mechanisms (see also Chapters 20 and 21 for more on resilience and the pandemic). This went beyond the research, and there were times when the support group had a more social role, key when you consider the backdrop of the project: "Just seeing and talking with my peers, even if we did not discuss the research, helped to relieve some anxiety, particularly at the time when we were all pretty isolated due to a national lockdown" (Samantha).

Support groups and scheduling meetings irrespective of the need are repeated "recommendations" across the data. This final subtheme is explored further in terms of practical advice to consider at the design stage of any new study. Here it relates to the recommendations highlighted with a view to acknowledging and managing EL in the research process: "I think that considering this process and now being aware of the concept of 'emotional labour' will allow me to be a better researcher" (Sarah), and "regardless of our perceived want or need . . . it ensured that I confronted my experiences and emotions even when I was unaware that I needed to" (Samantha).

One recommendation is for EL to be explicitly referenced at ethical review: "From the outset when doing research and as part of the ethics process, the concept of EL should be considered alongside acknowledging subjectivity" (Sarah), and that guidance should be developed enabling researchers to consider the EL of themselves and others within the research process. As previously noted, the creation and use of a support group was also recommended. Limitations were observed in that we "are not therapists," and therefore we felt that consideration should be given to having a dedicated therapeutic supervisor, especially when "dealing with a particularly emotional subject or area where there is an element of lived experience" (Natasha).

LESSONS LEARNED AND RECOMMENDATIONS

The following learnings and recommendations are drawn from our reflections and informed by the limited literature. It is hoped these prove helpful for all researchers in managing EL.

Emotional Labor Is Central But Neglected in Social Research

Researchers are emotional beings and, as such, there will always be an element of EL within research. Although a formal statement of a researchers' subject position is used within qualitative work, this tends to have an intellectual analytical focus rather than an emotional one. Actively engaging with emotions through subject reflection at the outset will help researchers to acknowledge how the topic might arouse certain emotions and why. This will allow for better management of EL and the impact of this on researchers' decisions, data collection, analysis, and well-being.

Emotional Labor Varies According to Research Context

The impact of EL might depend on the type of research and the context. Quantitative research by design, it could be argued, generally requires less EL with participants. However, the motives that drive researchers, the data gathered, and interactions with supervisors and research bodies all require some management of EL. Qualitative work, in contrast, often requires EL, especially when engaging with participants, but the degree might depend on the type of research. Inquiry in which the researcher shares a lived experience with the participants or engages with participants who have suffered difficult or traumatic experiences could require higher levels of EL; this supports previous research findings (e.g., Bundhoo & Lynch, 2021; Waters et al., 2020).

Considerations for Managing Emotional Labor in Research

In the discussion that follows, we suggest how the management of EL could be incorporated into and facilitated by *everyone* within the research process, irrespective of level, thereby allowing the academic community and research to thrive. We summarize the points in Table 45.1.

Organization Level

We were privileged to have project leads who acknowledged the potential for EL from the outset and provided good support. However, we felt it difficult to comprehend who had, or should have, the ultimate responsibility for ensuring ECRs emotional stability during the research process.

Ethics procedures across academia dictate that physical and emotional well-being is paramount, and that harmful research must be avoided (see Chapter 42 for more on the ethics of pandemic-related research). However, we and others (e.g., Dickson-Swift et al., 2007, 2009) argue that more detailed consideration of EL is also needed. To facilitate awareness of EL, we recommend the topic should be incorporated within student research modules. In addition, reflection on EL should be part of ethics reviews, and, for highly emotional topics or where supervisors and researchers do not feel it appropriate to have open discussions, counseling services should be available (e.g., via employee assistance programs or similar). We were lucky in our own ECR context to have supporting individual people and institutions, but engagement with and reflections around EL should not be left to chance.

Table 45.1 Considerations for Managing Emotional Labor in Research

Level	Goal	Recommendations
Organizational	Foster a culture where EL is recognized, acknowledged, and valued as integral to the research process.	• EL is considered more explicitly within an institution's ethical framework. • Actively provide strategies that help academics manage EL during research. • Provide access to counseling services where appropriate and/or employee assistance support. • Include EL within undergraduate and postgraduate research design modules.
Group/project	Researcher well-being is incorporated within research design. Group communication is open and supportive.	• Ensure researchers can access supportive supervision. • Regular debriefing is set up as standard; include a postresearch debrief and self-care skills analysis. • Informal support should be set up (this could include supervisors, the research team, or a research buddy).
Individual	Researchers understand the potential impact of EL on their well-being and research and actively develop strategies to manage this.	• Attend training or complete assignments on EL and self-reflection. • Practice regular self-reflection. • Know and develop adaptive coping strategies. • Increase self-awareness and skills through basic counseling training. • Know where to access support.

GROUP/PROJECT LEVEL

Debrief meetings should be scheduled *before* data collection to ensure priority is given and include postproject sessions as both our reflections and others (e.g., Newcomb, 2021; Waters et al., 2020) indicate EL does not have an expiry date. Sessions should be an opportunity to discuss emotional experiences as appropriate utilizing reflective journals to provide a focus and aid discussion. Analyzing reflective notes through discussion allows for the processing of emotions and can provide detachment. Our reflections emphasized this as an invaluable learning experience and the opportunity to seek advice from peers.

Informal communication is also important, and to that end we recommend the use of instant messaging groups. One might include supervisors, fellow team researchers, or a buddy system with other students. We also acknowledged that we felt safe and supported within our team; however, this is not always the case. Team relationships, specifically power relations, are therefore an area for further exploration when considering best practice for managing EL.

INDIVIDUAL LEVEL

Basic counseling skills, active listening skills, and keeping personal reflective journals are highly recommended for building self-awareness; they all help manage EL both in the moment and thereafter. Researchers should reflect on and analyze their own skills and coping mechanisms regularly to develop their own resources and also identify gaps where they could need further support or training.

In line with previous research (e.g., Bundhoo & Lynch, 2021), our reflections indicated that keeping a research diary is a valuable tool in which reflections on EL can be easily included; practicing emotional reflexivity builds self-awareness and skills for future research. Furthermore, integrating your reflexive journal into research accounts can add depth and transparency to your decision-making processes, thereby enhancing the integrity of the work. Being reflexive is not an easy task, however, so there is an opportunity here for institutions to provide relevant training.

CONCLUSION

Given interpretivism is now a widely accepted research paradigm, it is surprising how few scholars have reflected methodologically on the role of emotion and EL in social research. This chapter has addressed this gap within the context of ECRs engaged in qualitative enquiry into front-line workers during the COVID-19 pandemic. While the scale and nature of EL will vary according to the research context, some form of EL is likely in all social research. This chapter has underlined the importance of managing emotion to ensure the research is able to succeed, and that researchers can flourish in often difficult circumstances.

NOTES

1. https://www.telegraph.co.uk/health-fitness/mind/life-icu-doctor-have-panic-atta cks-bus-way-hospital/?fbclid=IwAR2VXo8Is08v6cpM2Ke0Pc_m48r0iI7Na7Ca qs_j17NlytgoEbk4BvwL6vY
2. https://cv19heroes.wordpress.com
3. https://www.nature.com/articles/d41586-021-00663-2

REFERENCES

Anonymous. (2021, January 15). The life of an ICU doctor: "I have panic attacks on the bus on the way to the hospital." *The Telegraph.* https://www.telegraph.co.uk/ health-fitness/mind/life-icu-doctor-have-panic-attacks-bus-way-hospital/?fbclid= IwAR2VXo8Is08v6cpM2Ke0Pc_m48r0iI7Na7Caqs_j17NlytgoEbk4BvwL6vY

Braun, V., & Clarke, V. (2013). *Successful qualitative research: A practical guide for beginners.* Sage.

Bundhoo, D., & Lynch, K. (2021). Pacing emotional labour of qualitative research in an intractable conflict environment. *Area, 53*(1), 47–55. http://dx.doi.org/10.1111/ area.12640

Dickson-Swift, V., James, E. L., Kippen, S., & Liamputtong, P. (2007). Doing sensitive research: What challenges do qualitative researchers face? *Qualitative Research, 7*(3), 327–353. https://doi.org/10.1177%2F1468794107078515

Dickson-Swift, V., James, E. L., Kippen, S., & Liamputtong, P. (2009). Researching sensitive topics: Qualitative research as emotion work. *Qualitative Research, 9*(1), 61–79. https://doi.org/10.1177%2F1468794108098031

Hochschild, A. R. (1983). *The managed heart: Commercialization of human feeling.* University of California Press.

Hoffmann, E. A. (2007). Open-ended interviews, power, and emotional labor. *Journal of Contemporary Ethnography, 36*(3), 318–346. https://doi.org/10.1177%2F089124160 6293134

Hubbard, G., Backett-Milburn, K., & Kemmer, D. (2001). Working with emotion: Issues for the researcher in fieldwork and teamwork. *International Journal of Social Research Methodology, 4*(2), 119–137. http://dx.doi.org/10.1080/13645570116992

Kinsella, E. L., Hughes, S., Lemon, S., Stonebridge, N., & Sumner, R. C. (2022). "We shouldn't waste a good crisis": The lived experience of working on the frontline through the first surge (and beyond) of COVID-19 in the U.K. and Ireland. *Psychology and Health, 37*(2), 151–177. https://doi.org/10.1080/08870446.2021.1928668

Lincoln, Y. S., & Guba, E. G. (1985). *Naturalistic inquiry.* Sage.

Liu, Q., Luo, D., Haase, J. E., Guo, Q., Wang, X. Q., Liu, S., Xia, L., Liu, Z., Yang, J., & Yang, B. X. (2020). The experiences of health-care providers during the COVID-19 crisis in China: A qualitative study. *The Lancet Global Health, 8*(6), 790–798. https:// doi.org/10.1016/S2214-109X(20)30204-7

Newcomb, M. (2021). The emotional labour of academia in the time of a pandemic: A feminist reflection. *Health Promotion Practice, 20*(2), 247–255. https://doi. org/10.1177%2F1473325020981089

Sarabia-Cobo, C., Pérez, V., de Lorena, P., Hermosilla-Grijalbo, C., Sáenz-Jalón, M., Fernández-Rodríguez, A., & Alconero-Camarero, A. R. (2021). Experiences of geriatric nurses in nursing home settings across four countries in the face of the COVID-19 pandemic. *Journal of Advanced Nursing, 77*(2), 869–878. https://doi.org/10.1111/jan.14626

Seear, K. L., & McLean, K. E. (2008). Breaking the silence: The role of emotional labour in qualitative research. In T. Majoribanks, J. Barraket, J. S. Chang, A. Dawson, M. Guillemin, M. Henry-Waring, A. Kenyon, R. Kokanovic, J. Lewis, D. Lusher, D. Nolan, P. Pyett, R. Robins, D. Warr, & J. Wyn (Eds.), *The annual conference of the Australian Sociological Association 2008. Re-imagining sociology: Conference publication proceedings* (pp. 1–16). The Australian Sociological Association (TASA).

Sumner, R. C., & Kinsella, E. L. (2021). Grace under pressure: Resilience, burnout, and wellbeing in frontline workers in the U.K. and Republic of Ireland during the SARS-CoV-2 pandemic. *Frontiers in Psychology, 11*, 576229. https://doi.org/10.3389/fpsyg.2020.576229

Waters, J., Westaby, C., Fowler A., & Phillips J. (2020). The emotional labour of doctoral criminological researchers. *Methodological Innovations, 13*(2), 1–12. https://doi.org/10.1177%2F2059799120925671

World Health Organization (WHO). (2020). WHO director-general's opening remarks at the media briefing on COVID-19 11 March 2020. https://www.who.int/director-general/speeches/detail/who-director-general-s-opening-remarks-at-the-media-briefing-on-covid-19---11-march-2020

FURTHER READING

Loughran, T., & Mannay, D. (2018). *Emotion and the researcher: Sites, subjectivities, and relationships* (Studies in qualitative methodology, Vol. 16). Emerald Publishing Limited. https://doi.org/10.1108/S1042-319220180000016001

Pascoe Leahy, C. (2021). The afterlife of interviews: Explicit ethics and subtle ethics in sensitive or distressing qualitative research. *Qualitative Research, 22*(5), 777–794. https://doi.org/10.1177/14687941211012924

Selecting Personality and Individual Difference Theories to Predict COVID-19 Sentiment and Behaviors

PAUL G. DEVEREUX ■

In doing research that is helpful in understanding the response to the COVID-19 pandemic, researchers must determine which theories are best suited to explain the phenomenon.

In this chapter, I use Bendassolli's (2014) definition of theory as "webs of interlocking concepts that facilitate the organization of empirical material by providing explicit interpretive frameworks that researchers use to make their data intelligible and justify their choices and methodological decisions" (p. 166). Stated more simply, theories are an explanation of the way things work (Collins & Stockton, 2018). Theories are not statements of certainty; they are tentative explanations of how phenomena operate. For example, theories might provide ideas about what influences sentiments or behavior and the potential outcomes or consequences of having those sentiments or performing that behavior. In other words, theory provides ideas about why something occurs, for example, why don't people wear masks? In this chapter, I provide an overview of how theories can be used to explain sentiment and behaviors by using three theories as case studies for this current public health situation. The goal is not to present an extensive overview of each theory as that is done elsewhere; rather, the point is to highlight theories that might be applicable to the pandemic illustrating how the theory can be applied and used to derive research questions and testable hypotheses.

Theory is key to the research process in a number of important ways. Theory helps researchers explain the data and study results by providing a framework for

Paul G. Devereux, *Selecting Personality and Individual Difference Theories to Predict COVID-19 Sentiment and Behaviors*
In: *The Social Science of the COVID-19 Pandemic*. Edited by: Monica K. Miller, Oxford University Press.
© Oxford University Press 2024. DOI: 10.1093/oso/9780197615133.003.0046

their findings. Theories also guide researchers where to look (and also where not to look) for what is relevant or not relevant for a study of a given topic. Theories provide guidance on how variables are supposed to act (e.g., increasing or decreasing another factor; operating together or in isolation) either as causal influences on other variables or, more simply, how they are associated with each other. Theories are also written at a general enough level that they can apply to other contexts, persons, or events. These general explanations then allow researchers to make specific predictions about a certain issue. In these ways, theory helps develop research questions and testable hypotheses.

Furthermore, they help to answer questions such as which variables should be measured in a study and the appropriate sample(s) to be researched. Guiding the study's design, theory helps with standardizing measurement using common metrics articulated by the theory. This standardization helps researchers to consistently measure the same things in the same ways, which allows for building a common literature base for the research topic. Findings from a study inform the chosen theory by either extending its propositions to other situations or limiting its scope when the data do not support either it or its components. Beyond one study, theory also connects a study to the literature and allows for research to build in a systematic way as theoretical concepts and ideas are either supported or refuted. In these ways, theories are open to being disproved via the scientific method.

As one consideration, a good theory should be practical and be applicable to real-world contexts. Kurt Lewin famously said: "Nothing is as practical as a good theory" (Lewin, 1943). However, work continues to be needed to translate theory into actions like public health interventions. In this chapter, I present guidance on how to select theories as they relate to the COVID-19 pandemic.

SELECTING SOCIAL SCIENCE THEORIES THAT INFORM SENTIMENT AND BEHAVIORS

Social science and the field of social psychology in particular aim to understand how humans make sense of and respond to their social environment. COVID-19 containment measures require changes to behavior. Changes to behavior typically arise from a person's attitudes and perceptions about the behavior and their evaluations of the outcomes of performing that behavior (see Chapter 17 for more on how attitudes shape COVID-19 behavior). A person might consider whether there will be a positive or negative outcome if they engage in that behavior. How they answer that question will influence their likelihood of performing that behavior. Many of the topics studied in social psychology, such as personality and individual differences in prosociality (see Chapter 13 for more on prosocial behavior and pandemic behavior), empathy (Pfattheicher et al., 2020), narcissism (Nowak et al., 2020), self-efficacy (Chong et al., 2020), and political affiliation (see Chapter 3 for more on the political aspects of COVID-19) should be expected to affect both how one thinks about and experiences the pandemic and how one responds to it. There are many social science theories to choose from that address these topics.

As a new researcher, the initial step in selecting theories is becoming familiar with relevant theories by reading the scientific literature. Researchers must be aware of the conversation that is happening among researchers about the topics of interest and, specific to theory, how they attempt to explain that phenomenon using theory.

The next question is how to choose among the available theories for a research question. For example, if researchers are focused on what explains behavior in a given situation or context, an important next step is to define the parameters of the situation. A good understanding of the situation requires demarcating its features, boundaries, and specific components. The current pandemic, a situation concerning a communicable disease, has many components: heightened emotions of fear; potentially deadly outcomes; differential impact (i.e., some people might be more at risk than others); changes to public behavior; restrictions on behaviors; government mandates (see Chapter 3 for more on COVID-19 policies); the necessity for collective behavior (see Chapter 16); and concern about others. It might not be possible to examine the entirety of the situation, so the researcher must decide which components are most important for their interests. For example, it might be one's focus to examine in particular humans' fear of disease and the behaviors that are associated with this fear, such as victim blaming and prejudice toward groups who are believed to be responsible for spreading disease (see Chapter 23 for more on prejudice related to COVID-19). Regardless of the particular context being studied, in deciding on a theory, researchers need to educate themselves on not only the topic at hand but also theories that might apply to the topic.

The next step after possible theories have been identified is to evaluate their fit to the situation of interest. Questions to guide one through this process include, Was the theory developed for this specific topic? Or, was it developed for related topics? That is, has the theory been used and studied with similar topics before? If so, how much evidence is supported by the theory? How many of its constructs are applicable to the current situation? For example, some components of the health belief model (HBM), such as the perceived benefits of social distancing might better explain reactions to the virus than other components, like perceived severity of the disease outcome, which might not be as motivating if people do not feel at risk (Skinner et al., 2015). Ideally, previous research would provide guidance on which concepts of a theory hold up to empirical testing in the chosen topic area.

If researchers find that multiple theories could be appropriate, which should they choose? They could make decisions based on conceptual or empirical fit. Regarding the concepts of the theory, is one theory more parsimonious than another (Pedhazur & Schmelkin, 1991)? In other words, does it involve fewer assumptions and is stated more simply than the other one? Perhaps that one is a stronger theory than one that is perhaps unnecessarily complicated in its explanations. A researcher might choose the theory with stronger evidence and research findings to support it. Does one make more accurate predictions supported by research about the topic than another? Does one theory cover a broader range of the phenomenon than another (Singleton & Straits, 2018)? Does the theory accurately predict or explain new facts or circumstances? Alternatively, maybe the researcher should choose a theory that appears relevant but hasn't been applied to the topic yet?

A researcher might decide to incorporate more than one theory in the study and compare the theories to see which ones result in better evidence and provide better explanations for the research issues. More than one theory might be needed, as in a case in which a researcher uses a second theory to fill in gaps of the first theory. For example, the HBM does not speak to the readiness of someone to perform a behavior like behavior stage theories do. These theories, such as the transtheoretical model (Prochaska et al., 2015), describe stages of change that identify which readiness phase a participant is in (e.g., not considering a behavior change vs. being ready and motivated to make a change). The researcher in this case could decide to include elements of both theories. That is, the HBM could be used to measure a person's perceived disease susceptibility, and then that information could be compared with their stage of readiness for behavior change. Next, I provide a case study of three theories that could be applied to the pandemic. I demonstrate how exploring the theory's constructs can help to make predictions and when a researcher might need to develop their own theory.

Belief in a Just World

The belief in a just world theory aims to explain people's attributions about threatening events and describe cognitive differences among people. The theory is centered on the idea that humans prefer to see the world as orderly, fair, and just (Lerner & Miller, 1978). Seeing the world in this way makes life more tolerable and less threatening to humans because if the world is just, people get what they deserve and deserve what they get. This belief serves a functional purpose, allowing people to hope that good deeds and hard work will lead to positive outcomes. There is a very strong cultural component to this belief, which is taught and reinforced in many ways, such as through religions (good people go to heaven; sinners go to hell), movies in which the good guy wins and the bad guys are punished, the ethos of Santa Claus keeping his naughty and nice lists, the idea of karma, and the belief is reflected in statements like "what goes around comes around."

Just world beliefs (JWBs) have been associated with authoritarianism, work ethic, locus of control (LOC; Rubin & Peplau, 1975), and religiosity (Furnham & Reilly, 1991). As mentioned, these are individual differences, with some people having more of a need for this belief than others. There are benefits to having JWBs also as they are associated with better coping and reduced stress (for a review, see Furnham, 2003). However, there is a downside to believing that if good things happen to people then it is because they deserved them. These beliefs lead to strategies to maintain a belief that the world is fair and just, and one of these strategies identified is victim blaming. Blaming the victim can be a consequence of believing that if something bad happens to someone they somehow deserved it as well. The support of rape myths, which are false beliefs that people who are raped did something to deserve it (e.g., wore certain clothes or acted in a certain way) has been linked to beliefs in a just world (Vonderhaar & Carmody, 2014).

With its potential to bring sickness and death, the COVID pandemic can be a source of threat to people. People naturally try to avoid bad outcomes, like contracting disease, and do not want to believe they are susceptible to bad outcomes, so they will do what they need to do to keep the danger away from them, including using the cognitive reframing associated with JWBs. For example, to maintain their belief that the world is just, a person might wear a mask and then if it helps prevent them from getting sick, that helps reinforce the belief that the world is fair because they did what was asked of them and were treated (rewarded) accordingly.

Belief in a just world theory allows researchers to make predictions about attributions during a threatening time. Because the theory is explicitly concerned with how humans make strong links between behaviors and outcomes, it can be used to predict why someone would engage in containment behaviors. People who hold high levels of this belief would be expected to engage in ways that maintain their belief that the world is orderly and stable because of the strong link in their minds between behaviors and outcomes. Similar to the acceptance of rape myths, it might also explain why some argue those who got COVID somehow deserved it, whether it be their unwillingness to protect themselves or due to other reasons. It can also explain people's lack of willingness to support help for those with the disease—because of the belief that it is due to their own fault. Alternatively, if people with JWBs are made to feel that a victim is innocent and can help the victim, they will (Lerner & Simmons, 1966).

There is support for the theory as it applies to the pandemic. In a study examining beliefs in a just world during the coronavirus pandemic, people higher in JWB reported more positive emotions and seeing that others got negative outcomes was reassuring in affirming the sense that the world is indeed fair (Wang et al., 2020). Other studies could examine how high JWBs make people feel less vulnerable to the disease, which is predicted by the theory. How JWBs lead to more or less adherence to containment measures is an empirical question to be studied.

Locus of Control

The idea of an LOC arose during the time when an inner-outer self metaphor in personality psychology became popular in the mid-20th century. These are typically distinctions made between the "true" inner self and what was presented to the "outer" world. An LOC refers to a belief that either one is in control of the events in their life (inner LOC) or external forces are largely responsible for the outcomes in life (Rotter, 1954). A person who believes that chance or fate determines life circumstances would have a higher external LOC. Since its development, there has been an extensive record of studies examining this construct, with differences in well-being related to one's LOC. In general, an external LOC is related to higher reports of stressful experiences and psychological and physical problems (Sharif, 2017).

Believing one is in control of a life event can lead a person to take steps to control illness. For instance, youth with chronic health conditions who had a higher internal LOC were more likely to adhere to their injectable medications (Nazareth et al., 2016). In contrast, youth with a higher "chance" external LOC had more emergency department visits, and those with "other" external LOC spent more nights at the hospital. This also relates to other outcomes as well; patients with epilepsy who had higher internal LOC scores had better controlled seizures (Asadi-Pooya et al., 2007), and patients with HIV and higher internal LOC had better physical quality of life (Préau et al., 2005). In a study of low-income, young adult Latinas in the United States, having an internal LOC was associated with more Internet searching for health-related information (Roncancio et al., 2012).

Using the LOC to make predictions during the COVID-19 pandemic, it could be argued that those who have higher internal LOC would be more likely to follow public health guidelines as they would see outcomes as more "in their own hands," whereas people who have an external LOC would be less likely to comply as they might think it is fate or God's plan that determines whether they get sick. Researchers could examine the pandemic's impact on people with different levels of control beliefs. A related study examined adults in the United States and Europe during the COVID-19 pandemic and found that having a higher external LOC was associated with mental health symptoms of depression, stress, and anxiety (Sigurvinsdottir et al., 2020). Measuring people's LOC could be used also to test the effectiveness of pandemic-related messages. For example, if someone has a high internal LOC, they might be more responsive to messages about what they can do to prevent contracting COVID-19 than someone with high external LOC. A person with high external LOC might be more motivated by messages, either positive or negative, about the vaccines.

Moral Disengagement

Moral disengagement (MD) is an apt theory to apply to the COVID pandemic because it concerns itself with reasons why people do not feel the rules apply to them (Bandura, 2002). Similar to other chapters in this volume that explain how reactance theory (Brehm, 1972; see Chapter 8) or political attitudes[1] (see Chapter 33) can influence containment behaviors, a major concern has been to understand the people who do not follow the social distancing or mask-wearing guidelines.

According to Bandura, who developed the theory, there are different mechanisms that people use to justify why a moral action is not needed, such as displacement of responsibility, which places responsibility for the immoral action on those in authority, and minimization of consequences, which refers to downplaying the severity or existence of harm (Bandura, 2002). MD also allows for an examination of individual differences in response to the pandemic as not everyone engages in this process and not for all situations.

Moral disengagement has been associated with social distancing guidelines (Alessandri et al., 2020) in Italy. In a study the authors conducted examining influences on COVID containment behaviors, we examined MD, JWBs, LOC, and beliefs about the pandemic (e.g., it was planned by people in power or that the response has been extreme) in a sample of adults throughout the United States (Devereux et al., 2021). Compared to the other measures, MD was the biggest influence on whether people supported the public health guidelines, with those with higher scores on MD less likely to support the protocols. Our study supports that MD provides justification for why people do not need to follow the rules during the pandemic and place their interests as more important than society's (Shu et al., 2011). Although MD was the strongest predictor, JWBs and having an internal LOC were also associated with adherence. Our findings specific to the pandemic are consistent with previous evidence that LOC was associated with actions that promote and protect health (Weiss & Larsen, 1990). Similarly, the more a person believes the world is fair and that people get what they deserve, the more likely they were to follow the public health guidelines, which supports previous research demonstrating that for events that are controllable, people with high JWBs will take action to reaffirm their belief in a fair world in which there are consequences for actions (Furnham, 2003).

Moral disengagement is relevant for COVID because it provides a framework in which to understand people's explanations for not following public health guidelines designed to keep themselves and others safe. Examining which of the MD mechanisms (e.g., displacement of responsibility or minimization of consequences) also helps to inform how messages should be framed to target the rationale for not adhering to the guidelines. Similar to the other theories, it can be used to tailor messages to people who are more likely to engage in MD.

These examples of theories were selected to show how theory can be relevant and applied to the COVID-19 pandemic and used to develop research questions. Knowing the literature, knowing the features of the situation the researchers want to apply theory to, and then brainstorming questions derived from the theory that might be worth pursuing are the initial steps in applying theory to a research topic. Obtaining feedback and input on research ideas for the study questions is an important next step in refining one's ideas and coming up with an interesting and worthwhile research question.

WHEN TO CREATE A NEW THEORY

If theories are incomplete, researchers might need to incorporate ideas from other theories to add to the identified theory or add their own ideas for the theory. Theories can be incomplete for a number of reasons. For example, aspects of the theory might not readily apply to the situation. Or, it might be an intriguing idea but not well supported by other studies. Or, there might be only limited support for the theory, with all the evidence coming from the same few researchers. A well-supported theory would contain evidence from multiple studies across multiple settings conducted by many different researchers.

Related here also is considering the methods that comprise the evidence base for the theory. Do the findings all result from the same methodology (e.g., only self-report)? In this case, there might be a concern about what is called a monomethod bias (Pedhazur & Schmelkin, 1991), and it would be important therefore to extend the testing of the theoretical constructs using multiple methods, such as observation or direct assessment of behavior. Similarly, is all the evidence from a theory from the same population, such as White college students? A stronger theory would have been tested in a variety of samples of people of different demographic groups, including gender, age, culture, and race/ethnicity. Researchers would also want to see how the theory holds up in other settings, although researchers recognize that a theory might predict what happens in one setting but not another. For example, the LOC theory might explain COVID containment behaviors in the United States, which is a more individualistic society than in a collectivistic society such as Japan (see Chapters 16 and 35 for more on culture and the pandemic). Finally, researchers should question theory if the studies on it have only been applied to a limited number of topics. In these cases, in which existing theory is lacking, researchers might be in a position to consider their own explanations for the phenomenon and thus contribute to the creation of theory.

CONCLUSION

There are many strongly supported and well-developed theories to choose from in the social sciences. The task of the researcher is to identify the right theory for their research question. As was evident with the case of the COVID-19 pandemic, theories can explain the public's response to this deadly virus. Theories provide researchers "a way of seeing," a particular point of view of how factors come together and interact to influence behaviors. But theories are also a way of "not seeing" (Pedhazur & Schmelkin, 1991). Theories allow researchers to focus on specific variables but at the exclusion of others. As important as they are in advancing science, it is also important to remember they provide one lens for us but not the entire picture.

NOTE

1. Igielnik, R. (June 23, 2020). *Most Americans say they regularly wore a mask in stores in the past month; fewer see others doing it.* Pew Research Center. Retrieved from https://www.pewresearch.org/short-reads/2020/06/23/most-americans-say-they-regularly-wore-a-mask-in-stores-in-the-past-month-fewer-see-others-doing-it/

REFERENCES

Alessandri, G., Lorenzo, F., Tisak, M. S., Crocetti, E., Crea, G., & Avanzi, L. (2020). Moral disengagement and generalized social trust as mediators and moderators of rule-respecting behaviors during the COVID-19 outbreak. *Frontiers in Psychology, 11,* 2102. https://doi.org/10.3389/fpsyg.2020.02102

Asadi-Pooya, A. A., Schilling, C. A., Glosser, D., Tracy, J. I., & Sperling, M. R. (2007). Health locus of control in patients with epilepsy and its relationship to anxiety, depression, and seizure control. *Epilepsy & Behavior, 11*(3), 347–350. https://doi.org/10.1016/j.yebeh.2007.06.008

Bandura, A. (2002). Selective moral disengagement in the exercise of moral agency. *Journal of Moral Education, 31*(2), 101–119. https://doi.org/10.1080/0305724022014322

Bendassolli, P. F. (2014). Reconsidering theoretical naïveté in psychological qualitative research. *Social Science Information, 53,* 163. https://doi.org/10.1177/0539018413517181

Brehm, J. W. (1972). *Responses to loss of freedom: A theory of psychological reactance.* General Learning Corporation.

Chong, Y. Y., Chien, W. T., Cheng, H. Y., Chow, K. M., Kassianos, A. P., Karekla, M., & Gloster, A. (2020). The role of illness perceptions, coping, and self-efficacy on adherence to precautionary measures for COVID-19. *International Journal of Environmental Research and Public Health, 17*(18), 6540. https://doi.org/10.3390/ijerph17186540

Collins, C. S., & Stockton, C. M. (2018). The central role of theory in qualitative research. *International Journal of Qualitative Methods, 17*(1), 1–10. https://doi.org/10.1177/1609406918797475

Devereux, P. G., Miller, M. K., & Kirshenbaum, J. (2021). Moral disengagement, locus of control, and belief in a just world: Individual differences relate to adherence to COVID-19 guidelines. *Personality and Individual Differences, 182,* 111069. https://doi.org/10.1016/j.paid.2021.111069

Furnham, A. (2003). Belief in a just world: Research progress over the past decade. *Personality and Individual Differences, 34*(5), 795–817. https://doi.org/10.1016/S0191-8869(02)00072-7

Furnham, A., & Reilly, M. (1991). A cross-cultural comparison of British and Japanese Protestant work ethic and just world beliefs. *Psychologia: An International Journal of Psychology in the Orient, 34*(1), 1–14.

Lerner, M. J., & Miller, D. (1978). Just world research and the attribution process. *Psychological Bulletin, 85,* 1030–1051.

Lerner, M. J., & Simmons, C. H. (1966). Observer's reaction to the "innocent victim": Compassion or rejection? *Journal of Personality and Social Psychology, 4,* 203–210.

Lewin, K. (1943). Psychology and the process of group living. *Journal of Social Psychology, 17,* 113–131.

Nazareth, M., Richards, J., Javalkar, K., Haberman, C., Zhong, Y., & Rak, E. (2016). Relating health locus of control to health care use, adherence, and transition readiness among youths with chronic conditions, North Carolina, 2015. *Preventing Chronic Disease, 13,* 160046. https://dx.doi.org/10.5888/pcd13.160046

Nowak, B., Brzóska, P., Piotrowski, J., Sedikides, C., Żemojtel-Piotrowska, M., & Jonason, P. K. (2020). Adaptive and maladaptive behavior during the COVID-19 pandemic: The roles of Dark Triad traits, collective narcissism, and health beliefs. *Personality and Individual Differences*, *167*(1), 110232. https://doi.org/10.1016/j.paid.2020.110232

Pedhazur, E. J., & Schmelkin, L. P. (1991). *Measurement, design, and analysis: An integrated approach*. Lawrence Erlbaum Associates.

Pfattheicher, S., Nockur, L., Böhm, R., Sassenrath, C., & Petersen, M. B. (2020). The emotional path to action: Empathy promotes physical distancing and wearing of face masks during the COVID-19 pandemic. *Psychological Science*, *31*(11), 1363–1373. https://doi.org/10.1177/0956797620964422

Préau, M., Vincent, E., Spire, B., Reliquet, V., Fournier, I., Michelet, C., Leport, C., & Morin, M. (2005). Health-related quality of life and health locus of control beliefs among HIV-infected treated patients. *Journal of Psychosomatic Research*, *59*(6), 407–413. https://doi.org/10.1016/j.jpsychores.2005.06.005

Prochaska, J. O., Redding, C. A., & Evers, K. E. (2015). The transtheoretical model and stages of change. In K. Glanz, B. K. Rimer, & K. Viswanath (Eds.), *Health behavior: Theory, research, and practice* (5th ed., pp. 125–148). Jossey-Bass.

Roncancio, A. M., Berenson, A. B., & Rahman, M. (2012). Health locus of control, acculturation, and health-related Internet use among Latinas. *Journal of Health Communication*, *17*(6), 631–640. https://doi.org/10.1080/10810730.2011.635767

Rotter, J. B. (1954). *Social learning and clinical psychology*. Prentice-Hall.

Rubin, Z., & Peplau, L. A. (1975). Who believes in a just world? *Journal of Social Issues*, *31*, 65–90.

Sharif, S. P. (2017). Locus of control, quality of life, anxiety, and depression among Malaysian breast cancer patients: The mediating role of uncertainty. *European Journal of Oncology Nursing*, *27*, 28–35. https://doi.org/10.1016/j.ejon.2017.01.005

Shu, L. L., Gino, F., & Bazerman, M. H. (2011). Dishonest deed, clear conscience: When cheating leads to moral disengagement and motivated forgetting. *Personality and Social Psychology Bulletin*, *37*(3), 330–349. https://doi.org/10.1177/0146167211398138

Sigurvinsdottir, R., Thorisdottir, I. E., & Gylfason, H. F. (2020). The impact of COVID-19 on mental health: The role of locus on control and internet use. *International Journal of Environmental Research and Public Health*, *17*(19) 6985. https://doi.org/10.3390/ijerph17196985

Singleton, R. A., & Straits, B. C. (2018). *Approaches to social research*. Oxford University Press.

Skinner, C. S., Tiro, J., & Champion, V. L. (2015). The health belief model. In K. Glanz, B. K. Rimer, & K. Viswanath (Eds.), *Health behavior: Theory, research, and practice* (5th ed.) (p. 75–94). Jossey-Bass.

Vonderhaar, R. L., & Carmody, D. C. (2014). There are no "innocent victims": The influence of just world beliefs and prior victimization on rape myth acceptance. *Journal of Interpersonal Violence*, *30*(10), 1615–1632. https://doi.org/10.1177/0886260514549196

Wang, J., Wang, Z., Liu, X., Yang, X., Zheng, M., & Bai, X. (2020). The impacts of a COVID-19 epidemic focus and general belief in a just world on individual emotions.

Personality and Individual Differences, 168, 110349. https://doi.org/10.1016/j.paid.2020.110349

Weiss, G. L., & Larsen, D. L. (1990). Health value, health locus of control, and the prediction of health protective behaviors. *Social Behavior and Personality: An International Journal, 18*(1), 121–135. https://doi.org/10.2224/sbp.1990.18.1.121

FURTHER READING

Bandura, A. (2016). *Moral disengagement: How people do harm and live with themselves.* Worth Publishers.

Hafer, C. L., & Bégue, L. (2005). Experimental research on just-world theory: Problems, developments, and future challenges. *Psychological Bulletin, 131*(1), 128–167. https://doi.org/10.1037/0033-2909.131.1.128

Joas, H., & Knöbl, W. (2014). *Social theory: Twenty introductory lectures.* Cambridge University Press.

Wallston, B. S., & Wallston, K. A. (2020). Social psychological models of health behavior: An examination and integration. In A. Baum, S. E. Taylor, & J. E. Singer (Eds.), *Handbook of psychology and health* (Vol. 4, pp. 23–54). Routledge. https://doi.org/10.4324/9781003044307

47

From Threats to Defenses

Theoretical and Statistical Suggestions to Investigate and Explain the Psychological Phenomena of COVID-19

ROBIN WILLARDT, CHIARA A. JUTZI,
PETRA C. SCHMID, AND EVA JONAS ∎

All around the world, the COVID-19 pandemic caused an unprecedented interruption of daily life: Lockdown measures left people restricted in their personal freedom, choices, and possibilities (see Chapters 1 and 3 for more on pandemic policies, and Chapter 8 for more on behavior related to restricted freedom) and an unsettling state of uncertainty caused by a lack of knowledge about the virus persists to this day. Furthermore, the virus poses a physical (and potentially deadly) danger to one's own health.

At the same time, an increase in conspicuous psychological phenomena such as heightened states of negative emotions (Burke et al., 2020), a disproportionate amount of toilet paper bulk buying,[1] the belief that the virus was artificially created by Bill Gates (Goodman & Carmichael, 2020; see Chapters 13 and 38 for more on misinformation), or resentment against people of Asian descent[2] could be observed. As the pandemic progressed, new phenomena, such as vaccine distrust (Peretti-Watel et al., 2020) or noncompliance with government-directed anti-COVID measures (Neumann-Böhme et al., 2020), have occurred. While some of these phenomena are partially overlapping and related to each other, as in the case of people's conspiracy beliefs and their hesitation to get vaccinated (Bertin et al., 2020; Salali & Uysal, 2020), others appear to be unrelated or even contradictory to each other. This is, for example, the case when considering the acts of solidarity (see Chapters 21 and 41 for more on collective responses to the pandemic) on the one hand and the incidents of racial bias and prejudice during the pandemic (see Chapter 23 for more on pandemic-related discrimination) on the other hand.

The purpose of this chapter is to offer guidance on how to investigate these diverse, partly contradictory, and potentially COVID-19-related phenomena.

Robin Willardt, Chiara A. Jutzi, Petra C. Schmid, and Eva Jonas, *From Threats to Defenses* In: *The Social Science of the COVID-19 Pandemic.* Edited by: Monica K. Miller, Oxford University Press. © Oxford University Press 2024.
DOI: 10.1093/oso/9780197615133.003.0047

We first note that the COVID-induced interruptions in the form of uncertainty, lack of control, and mortality salience (among others) represent psychological threats that have been investigated in separate lines of research since before the pandemic (e.g., Hogg, 2007; Kay & Eibach, 2013; Pyszczynski et al., 1999). Each of these streams of research uses its own, largely isolated, theoretical framework to explain the emotional, cognitive, and behavioral effects of a given psychological threat. Interestingly, these threats induce effects that closely resemble the psychological phenomena that could be observed during the pandemic, such as conspiracy beliefs or intergroup bias (Jutzi et al., 2020; Reiss et al., 2020). As pandemic-induced interruption of daily life fostered multiple threats at the same time, though (Bland, 2020; Kachanoff et al., 2020), a singular stream of threat research might not fully capture the multidimensional threat nature of COVID-19.

We thus propose taking an integral approach with the general process model of threat and defense (GPMTD; Jonas et al., 2014) serving as a theoretical foundation. Based on the behavioral activation system (BAS) and behavioral inhibition system (BIS; Gray & McNaugthon, 2000), the model describes a singular mechanism through which threats induce anxiety and behavioral inhibition. Consequently, they lead to distal defense reactions that lower anxiety and reestablish a behavioral approach. These reactions are thought to be mirrored in the psychological phenomena associated with the pandemic (Reiss et al., 2020). Assuming that the threatening nature of COVID-19 triggers the mechanism outlined by the GPMTD and is therefore responsible for a given phenomenon, a researcher might nevertheless be interested in investigating threats separately and their potential individual as well as interacting effects on phenomena associated with COVID-19. The reason for this is that a given psychological phenomenon of COVID-19 might be affected by only certain threats implicated in COVID-19 (Shepherd et al., 2011). Furthermore, the magnitude of the effect of a given threat might vary depending on interindividual differences (e.g., Agroskin et al., 2016) as well as currently salient goals and norms (e.g., McGregor et al., 2013). We therefore recommend and discuss the use of structural equation modeling (SEM). As will be discussed in this chapter, this statistical analysis technique is well suited to investigate hypotheses regarding (1) global effects of the threatening nature of COVID-19 as suggested by the GPMTD as well as (2) individual and interacting effects of specific threats and their motivational-affective underpinnings on psychological phenomena associated with the current pandemic. The goal of this chapter is therefore to provide researchers with theoretical and methodological recommendations to effectively investigate threat-induced effects on COVID-19-related phenomena.

THE PSYCHOLOGICAL IMPACT OF COVID-19: A VARIETY OF POSSIBLE OUTCOMES AND MECHANISMS

As described above, the COVID-19 pandemic has been associated with a long list of consequential psychological phenomena, such as conspiratorial ideation (e.g., Bill Gates implanting microchips through vaccinations); conspicuous behavior (e.g., bulk buying toilet paper); or intergroup biases (e.g., resenting people of Asian descent). When investigating their origins, it is noteworthy that in past research, many of these phenomena have been found to be induced by psychological threats such as uncertainty, a lack of personal control, or the salience of death (e.g., Arndt et al., 2004; Hogg & Adelman, 2013; Newheiser et al., 2011). Importantly, these threats are also implicated in the current pandemic: First, COVID-19 has restricted one's freedom to travel, to meet friends, as well as to work, and therefore has decreased one's level of personal control (United Nations World Tourism Organization, 2020). Furthermore, the lack of knowledge about the virus itself, its spread, its contagiousness, and the way people might react to the prolonged presence of the virus in their everyday life has caused uncertainty.[3] Last, news about rising death tolls around the globe caused death awareness and represented a continuous reminder of one's own mortality (Pyszczynski et al., 2020; see Chapter 35 for more on pandemic related mortality salience). That is why the pandemic has been considered a "superthreat" (Jutzi et al., 2020), meaning that it unearths several psychological threats known to lead to consequential emotional, cognitive, and behavioral phenomena.

Hence, a prominent idea in past research on COVID-19 has been that the psychological phenomena that co-occurred with the spread of COVID-19 could be due to the threats that the pandemic entails (Bland, 2020; Kachanoff et al., 2020). This idea leaves researchers with different paths to take since a given COVID-19-related phenomenon can theoretically be explained by several different threats at the same time. For instance, both mortality salience and a lack of personal control are both well-researched psychological threat variables that have been associated with increased levels of ingroup bias (Agroskin et al., 2016; Agroskin & Jonas, 2013; Fritsche et al., 2008). Assuming that COVID-19 increases the salience of one's own death and one's lack of control, both threats could potentially be responsible for an increased level of ingroup bias during the pandemic. The GPMTD (Jonas et al., 2014) outlines a theoretical foundation to assess globally whether psychological phenomena associated with COVID-19 are caused by its threatening nature. As such, this model is able to provide a theoretical foundation to explain multiple observed phenomena around COVID-19 without having to choose between individual threats.

THE GENERAL PROCESS MODEL OF THREAT AND DEFENSE

Past threat research has relied on isolated theoretical frameworks and mechanisms to explain the effects of specific threats on behavior, cognition, and emotion. Despite their differences, the individual threats often resulted in quite similar, if not identical, reactions, as illustrated by the example of ingroup bias. Pointing out this overlap between the reactions toward different investigated threats in past literature, the purpose of the GPMTD was to unite the fragmented literature on threats and their consequences. It did so by suggesting an integrative process through which the various, yet similar, reactions toward different threats can be explained.

The GPMTD proposes that, even though the various lines of research differed regarding the investigated threats and the proposed mechanisms that explained the consequences of threats, they all shared the idea that "threats result from some experience of discrepancy between an expectation or desire and the current circumstances" (Jonas et al., 2014, p. 229). Different types of threat are all characterized by these discrepancies: Threats to personal control, for instance, highlight the divergence between freedom and restriction, such as restrictions imposed due to the COVID-19 pandemic. Threats to people's own lives as caused by the severe acute respiratory syndrome coronavirus 2 (SARS-CoV-2) remind them of the discrepancy between their wish for an endless life and their own finiteness. This threat-induced discrepancy then triggers proximal defense reactions by activating the BIS. These reactions consist of hypervigilance, anxious arousal, avoidance motivation, and inhibition of all ongoing behaviors (Gray & McNaughton, 2000; Jonas et al., 2014).

A continuously activated BIS is unpleasant and can hinder goal pursuit. Hence, people are motivated to downregulate BIS through distal defenses. These distal defenses mute the BIS while reactivating the BAS. Some of these distal defenses are directed at the cause of the threat, hence offering direct resolution, such as adherence to hygiene rules or self-imposed restriction of social contacts to prevent further spread of COVID-19. Other defenses are of purely palliative nature. An example already used in Chapter 6 of this book is the belief in corona-related conspiracies: Following the belief that the virus was artificially developed by the Chinese government or by Bill Gates does not tackle the threat itself. According to the GPMTD, this palliative defense nevertheless fulfills a purpose by lowering the threat-induced behavioral inhibition and anxiety while reinstating behavioral activation.

To summarize, the GPMTD explains the abundant and at times seemingly irrational reactions to psychological threats through a common process. Its theoretical contribution lies in the bridging of fragmented lines of research on psychological threats and their potential consequences. Considering the COVID-19 pandemic, though, we propose that the GPMTD also yields applied value. As described in this chapter, several reasons emerge why the GPMTD is well suited to serve as a theoretical foundation for conducting research on the psychological phenomena associated with COVID-19.

APPLYING THE GENERAL PROCESS MODEL OF THREAT AND DEFENSE TO PSYCHOLOGICAL RESEARCH ON COVID-19

First, and as outlined in this chapter, the GPMTD proposes an affect-driven motivational process to explain how the occurrence of threats lead to the emergence of defense reactions (i.e., COVID-19-related psychological phenomena). Unlike other models arguing for an affect-free mechanism (see Lambert et al., 2014, for a criticism on these models), this process fits the emotional characteristic of the current pandemic (Burke et al., 2020; Lwin et al., 2020). The model also gives a potential explanation for seemingly irrational behaviors associated with the pandemic, such as pandemic bulk buying: According to the GPMTD, these behaviors are palliative defenses that might not lower the threat(s) at hand but nevertheless provide relief from threat-induced anxiety. Moreover, past research has validated the model's proposed mechanism as well as its capacity to predict the affective, cognitive, and behavioral consequences of a diverse range of threats (e.g., Jutzi et al., 2020; Reiss et al., 2020). Several of the threats included in the model, such as uncertainty, lack of personal control, and mortality salience, are also part of the COVID-19 superthreat (Jutzi et al., 2020). Furthermore, the model has already been successfully applied to the current pandemic: As outlined in the beginning of this chapter, the psychological investigation of COVID-19 and its consequences poses the problem of a multitude of potential threats to examine. To solve this problem and in line with the integrative approach of the GPMTD, recent studies by Jutzi and colleagues (2020) and Reiss and colleagues (2020) used a discrepancy scale (see Box 47.1) specifically tailored to capture the main threats implicated in COVID-19. The development of this scale was based on the GPMTD's assumption that all threats, regardless of their nature, lead to a state of discrepancy. Hence, the items of the scale assess the magnitude of discrepancy induced by the individual threats implicated in COVID-19.

With the help of this scale, Reiss and colleagues (2020) reported a positive correlational relationship between threat-induced COVID-19 discrepancy and behavioral inhibition as well as a negative correlation between threat-induced COVID-19 discrepancy and behavioral activation. This means the discrepant experience unearthed by the threats of the pandemic was indeed associated with higher BIS activation, as supposed by the GPMTD. In line with these findings, Jutzi and colleagues (2020) measured and manipulated people's threat-induced COVID-19 discrepancy and found positive relationships between heightened discrepancy and ingroup entitativity, control restoration motivation, system justification, conspiratorial beliefs, and passive party support via increased BIS activation.

The use of this scale assessing an overall COVID-19 threat-level score shows how the GPMTD can help to solve the question of what variables to investigate regarding the potential psychological consequences of COVID-19 caused by its threatening nature: By assuming a common underlying mechanism through which the threats entailed in COVID-19 affect humans, the model allows researchers to globally test whether the threats implicated in the pandemic might be responsible for COVID-19-related phenomena, such as conspiracy beliefs or ingroup bias, which, according to the GPMTD, represent distal defenses aimed at lowering anxious arousal and behavioral inhibition. This approach is especially useful if a researcher wants to know whether the threatening nature of COVID-19 in general is responsible for a given psychological phenomenon associated with the pandemic.

Box 47.1

Item List of the Discrepancy Scale Used by Jutzi and Colleagues (2020) and Reiss and Colleagues (2020)

Despite the Coronavirus, I can do just about anything I really set my mind to. *(R)*

The Coronavirus determines most of what I can and cannot do.

Because of the Coronavirus, what happens in my life is currently beyond my control.

The Coronavirus interferes with the things I want to do.

The unpredictability of the Coronavirus outbreak does not bother me. *(R)*

During the Corona pandemic, not having all the information I need is frustrating.

I can't stand that the Coronavirus outbreak took me by surprise.

The uncertainty surrounding the Coronavirus keeps me from living a fulfilled life.

I doubt that I can deal efficiently with unexpected consequences of the Coronavirus.

Even if I invest the necessary effort, I cannot solve the problems that arise with the Coronavirus.

I can remain calm during the Corona pandemic because I can rely on my coping abilities. *(R)*

If the Coronavirus causes problems for me, I am sure I will find a solution for them. *(R)*

The Corona pandemic surprised me.

I expected the Corona outbreak. *(R)*

The current Corona situation was predictable. *(R)*

Note. Items marked with "R" are reverse coded. From "Between Conspiracy Beliefs, Ingroup Bias, and System Justification: How People Use Defense Strategies to Cope With the Threat of COVID-19," by C. A. Jutzi, R. Willardt, P. C. Schmid, and E. Jonas, 2020, *Frontiers in Psychology*, *11*, 578586, 1–16. https://doi.org/10.3389/fpsyg.2020.578586. Reproduced under a CC BY 4.0 license.

As discussed in the next section of this chapter, there are nevertheless several reasons for also investigating each of the threats implicated in COVID-19 separately.

INDIVIDUAL THREATS AND THEIR RELEVANCE FOR COVID-19 RESEARCH

Past research has shown that the effects of individual threats on a given defense reaction can interact with each other. In a study by Fritsche and colleagues (2013), for instance, outgroup derogation increased when the perceived homogeneity of one's group was threatened, but only when this homogeneity threat co-occurred with low levels of personal control. Hence, certain psychological phenomena of COVID-19 might occur only when two specific threats are present simultaneously. Moreover, not all defense reactions are equally affected by all threats (Shepherd et al., 2011), and whether individual threats lead to specific defense reactions can depend on personality traits (Agroskin et al., 2016; McGregor et al., 2005; Poppelaars et al., 2018) and the salience of specific goals and norms (Fritsche et al., 2010; McGregor et al., 2013). This means that researchers might find a specific threat associated with COVID-19 to lead to a defense reaction for a specific participant pool (e.g., elderly people; see Chapter 48 for more on individual differences) or situation (e.g., right before a new lockdown) but might not find the same effect for a different population or situation. They might also find a specific COVID-related defense reaction to occur for one threat implicated in COVID-19 but not for another one.

Individual threats can also differ from each other regarding their physiological and self-rated properties. For instance, Reiss et al. (2021) recently compared different threats in body heat maps and found different arousal locations for distinct threat types. Asking participants where they felt "aroused" in their body helped to create maps of (de)activation that show different patterns for distinct threat types. The authors also clustered threat types and their properties and found three distinct threat patterns that differed significantly from a control condition cluster. Mortality salience formed a distinct cluster standing on its own, while freedom and meaning threats were grouped together in one cluster. The third threat cluster was a larger one consisting of uncontrollability, insecurity, and isolation.

Given this past research, it can be informative to test how specific threats contribute to and interact on a psychological phenomenon associated with COVID-19. Identifying the individual threats responsible for a given psychological phenomenon associated with COVID-19 is also relevant for the successful development of interventions: Assuming that, by applying the GPMTD, researchers find indication for a link between the threat-induced COVID-19 discrepancy and intergroup bias, they might want to explore ways to lower the intergroup bias caused by the pandemic. Doing so requires researchers to establish what threat(s) implicated in COVID-19 is/are driving heightened intergroup bias because different threats require different intervention strategies. For example, whereas the lack of control imposed by the pandemic might be lowered by communication strategies that increase perceived personal freedom, experienced mortality salience calls for communication strategies that prevent the audience from being directly and frequently confronted with the possibility of dying due to the virus. In order to test, recommend, and implement such threat-lowering strategies, one has to know what threat(s) within COVID-19 must be targeted to successfully and significantly lower an unwanted psychological phenomenon associated with the pandemic.

So far, the chapter first showed the advantages of using the GPMTD to test the overall threat-induced effects of COVID-19 on psychological phenomena.

Thereafter, reasons for the investigation of individual threats in order to assess their unique and possibly interacting effects were outlined. To investigate (1) whether a given psychological phenomenon associated with COVID-19 is generally caused by the threats it entails and (2) which individual threats cause specific COVID-19-related phenomena, the last section of this chapter now describes the advantages of using SEM as an analysis technique when planning and analyzing one's next COVID-19 study.

STRUCTURAL EQUATION MODELING AS THE STATISTICAL TOOL OF CHOICE

Structural equation modeling allows the testing of complex structural constellations between a given set of variables (Bollen, 1989; Brown, 2015). It does so by comparing an observed covariance matrix (or sometimes correlation matrix) where all variables are allowed to covary freely with the matrix resulting from a proposed model in which covariations between variables are restricted (e.g., by only allowing Variable A to covary with Variable C via a mediator Variable B). If the model-implied covariance matrix can closely reproduce the observed (i.e., empirical) covariance matrix of the data, good model fit is achieved, and one can thus conclude that the proposed model explains the observed data well. Among other advantages, SEM allows the testing of different relationships between a multitude of predictors, mediators, moderators, and outcome variables. Models are therefore able to test whether the simultaneous effect of multiple predictor or independent variables on outcome or dependent variables run via mediator and moderator variables. Furthermore, models can include several outcome variables or, in an experimental setup, dependent variables. This creates (almost) complete freedom in specifying theory-driven models and renders repetitive and separate analyses for each outcome or dependent variable one wants to test obsolete.

The properties of SEM make it a useful statistical tool for research on the psychological phenomena associated with COVID-19 based on the GPMTD (Reiss et al., 2020): For instance, a researcher can assess participants' overall COVID-19 threat level (e.g., with the discrepancy scale mentioned previously), their level of activated BIS (indicated, i.e., via state anxiety), and their engagement with a psychological phenomenon hypothesized to be caused by COVID-19 (e.g., Kachanoff et al., 2020; Reiss et al., 2020). SEM can now test whether participants' overall COVID-19 threat level affects the psychological phenomenon via increased BIS activation as would be predicted by the GPMTD. Since SEM allows the inclusion of more than one outcome variable in a given model, the proposed mediated relationship between participants' overall COVID-19-threat level and several psychological phenomena can be tested at the same time. SEM is also well suited to investigate individual threats and their unique as well as interacting effects on COVID-19 phenomena. For instance, a researcher can assess uncertainty, lack of control, and mortality salience as individual variables and test a model in which all three threats are allowed to covary with the level of activated BIS, which in turn is allowed to covary with one or several COVID-19 phenomena. In this model, it is possible to investigate how strongly the individual threats differ in magnitude regarding their indirect effects on COVID-19-related phenomena (Reiss et al., 2020). Similarly, a model in which two or more threats are hypothesized to interact with each other can be tested.

CONCLUSION

Many of the COVID-related psychological phenomena mentioned in this chapter can have detrimental consequences such as verbal and physical abuse against individuals of Asian descent due to COVID-related outgroup derogation (Lee, 2020) or the resurgence of incidence rates due to a lack of adherence to anti-COVID measures (Lange & Monscheuer, 2021). This shows the importance of answering the question of whether and how COVID-19 causes the aforementioned phenomena. Because the outbreak of the pandemic induced many threats potentially responsible for the psychological phenomena associated with COVID-19, investigating and potentially identifying those threats can seem daunting and somewhat overwhelming from a researcher's perspective.

As one possible approach to solve this problem, research during the pandemic has frequently referred to individual threats and their respective theoretical frameworks to explain psychological phenomena possibly associated with COVID-19. Often, though, these consequences can be explained by several threat-related concepts at the same time. Who is to say, for example, whether noncompliance with governmental measures to restrict the spread of the virus is due to cognitive dissonance (see Chapter 6), perceived uncertainty (see Chapter 10), safety anxiety (see Chapter 11), or a combination of those?

Hence, the purpose of this chapter was to suggest one possible pathway to systematically investigate the potential causes of COVID-related phenomena. As suggested by the GPMTD, the different threats entailed in COVID-19 might cause COVID-related phenomena through the same underlying mechanism: These different threats activate the BIS, triggering inhibition of all ongoing behaviors as well as hypervigilance, anxious arousal, and avoidance motivation. At the same time, distal defense reactions in the form of COVID-related phenomena such as conspiracy beliefs or intergroup bias are elicited in order to mute the BIS, lower anxiety, and reactivate BAS. Through this proposed mechanism, researchers do not have to justify the selection of one specific threat implicated in the current pandemic. Rather, they can use SEM as a statistical tool to globally investigate the relationship between COVID-19-related threats and the phenomena they potentially cause. At the same time, a researcher can use the GPMTD as a theoretical foundation to hypothesize and test the individual as well as interacting effects of threats implicated in COVID-19.

On a final note, it should be mentioned that COVID-19 is not the only consequential challenge that incorporates different threat facets. Other superthreats, such as migrant crises or climate change (Salas et al., 2020), also consist of several psychological threats, pose challenges, and possibly trigger psychological threat reactions. Thus, this chapter's proposed approach for investigating the psychological phenomena associated with COVID-19 is meant not only to be applied to the current pandemic, but also can help to investigate present and future superthreats of various kinds.

NOTES

1. https://www.theguardian.com/uk-news/2020/mar/15/panic-buying-sweeps-sto res-despite-appeal-for-responsible-shopping
2. https://www.nytimes.com/2020/03/23/us/chinese-coronavirus-racist-attacks.html
3. https://theconversation.com/learning-to-cope-with-uncertainty-during-covid-19- 151420

REFERENCES

Agroskin, D., & Jonas, E. (2013). Controlling death by defending ingroups—Mediational insights into terror management and control restoration. *Journal of Experimental Social Psychology, 49*(6), 1144–1158. https://doi.org/10.1016/j.jesp.2013.05.014

Agroskin, D., Jonas E., Klackl J., & Prentice, M. (2016). Inhibition underlies the effect of high need for closure on cultural closed-mindedness under mortality salience. *Frontiers in Psychology, 7,* 1583, 1–16. https://doi.org/10.3389/fpsyg.2016.01583

Arndt, J., Solomon, S., Kasser, T., & Sheldon, K. M. (2004). The urge to splurge: A terror management account of materialism and consumer behavior. *Journal of Consumer Psychology, 14*(3), 198–212. https://doi.org/10.1207/s15327663jcp1403_2

Bertin, P., Nera, K., & Delouvée, S. (2020). Conspiracy beliefs, rejection of vaccination, and support for hydroxychloroquine: A conceptual replication-extension in the COVID-19 pandemic context. *Frontiers in Psychology, 11,* 565128, 977–982. https:// doi.org/10.3389/fpsyg.2020.565128

Bland, A. M. (2020). Existential givens in the COVID-19 crisis. *Journal of Humanistic Psychology, 60*(5), 710–724. https://doi.org/10.1177/0022167820940186

Bollen, K. A. (1989). *Structural equation modeling with latent variables.* Wiley.

Brown, T. A. (2015). *Confirmatory factor analysis in applied research* (2nd ed.). Guilford Press.

Burke, T., Berry, A., Taylor, L. K., Stafford, O., Murphy, E., Shevlin, M., McHugh, L., & Carr, A. (2020). Increased psychological distress during COVID-19 and quarantine in Ireland: A national survey. *Journal of Clinical Medicine, 9*(11), 3481. https://doi. org/10.3390/jcm9113481

Fritsche, I., Jonas, E., Ablasser, C., Beyer, M., Kuban, J., Manger, A. M., & Schultz, M. (2013). The power of we: Evidence for group-based control. *Journal of Experimental Social Psychology, 49*(1), 19–32. https://doi.org/10.1016/j.jesp.2012.07.014

Fritsche, I., Jonas, E., & Fankhänel, T. (2008). The role of control motivation in mortality salience effects on ingroup support and defense. *Journal of Personality and Social Psychology, 95*(3), 524. https://doi.org/10.1037/a0012666

Fritsche, I., Jonas, E., Kayser, D. N., & Koranyi, N. (2010). Existential threat and compliance with pro-environmental norms. *Journal of Environmental Psychology, 30*(1), 67–79. https://doi.org/10.1016/j.jenvp.2009.08.007

Goodman, J., & Carmichael, F. (2020, May 30). *Coronavirus: Bill Gates "microchip" conspiracy theory and other vaccine claims fact-checked*. British Broadcasting Corporation (BBC). https://www.bbc.com/news/52847648

Gray, J. A., & McNaughton, N. (2000). *The neuropsychology of anxiety: An enquiry into the function of the septo-hippocampal system*. Oxford University Press. https://doi.org/10.1093/acprof:oso/9780198522713.001.0001

Hogg, M. A. (2007). Uncertainty–identity theory. *Advances in Experimental Social Psychology, 39*, 69–126. https://doi.org/10.1016/S0065-2601(06)39002-8

Hogg, M. A., & Adelman, J. (2013). Uncertainty-identity theory: Extreme groups, radical behavior, and authoritarian leadership. *Journal of Social Issues, 69*(3), 436–454. https://doi.org/10.1111/josi.12023

Jonas, E., McGregor, I., Klackl, J., Agroskin, D., Fritsche, I., Holbrook, C., Nash, K., Proulx, T., & Quirin, M. (2014). Threat and defense: From anxiety to approach. In J. M. Olson & M. P. Zanna (Eds.), *Advances in experimental social psychology* (Vol. 49, pp. 219–286). Academic Press. https://doi.org/10.1016/B978-0-12-800052-6.00004-4

Jutzi, C. A., Willardt, R., Schmid, P. C., & Jonas, E. (2020). Between conspiracy beliefs, ingroup bias, and system justification: How people use defense strategies to cope with the threat of COVID-19. *Frontiers in Psychology, 11*, 578586, 1–16. https://doi.org/10.3389/fpsyg.2020.578586

Kachanoff, F. J., Bigman, Y. E., Kapsaskis, K., & Gray, K. (2020). Measuring realistic and symbolic threats of COVID-19 and their unique impacts on well-being and adherence to public health behaviors. *Social Psychological and Personality Science, 12*(5), 603–616. https://doi.org/10.1177/1948550620982198

Kay, A. C., & Eibach, R. P. (2013). Compensatory control and its implications for ideological extremism. *Journal of Social Issues, 69*(3), 564–585. https://doi.org/10.1111/josi.12029

Lambert, A. J., Eadeh, F. R., Peak, S. A., Scherer, L. D., Schott, J. P., & Slochower, J. M. (2014). Toward a greater understanding of the emotional dynamics of the mortality salience manipulation: Revisiting the "affect-free" claim of terror management research. *Journal of Personality and Social Psychology, 106*(5), 655–678. https://doi.org/10.1037/a0036353

Lange, M., & Monscheuer, O. (2021). Spreading the disease: Protest in times of pandemics. ZEW-Centre for European Economic Research Discussion Paper *No. 21-009*. SSRN. https://dx.doi.org/10.2139/ssrn.3787921

Lee, B. Y. (2020, February 18). How COVID-19 coronavirus is uncovering anti-Asian racism. *Forbes*. https://www.forbes.com/sites/brucelee/2020/02/18/how-covid-19-coronavirus-is-uncovering-anti-asian-racism/#437a2e9729a6

Lwin, M. O., Lu, J., Sheldenkar, A., Schulz, P. J., Shin, W., Gupta, R., & Yang, Y. (2020). Global sentiments surrounding the COVID-19 pandemic on Twitter: Analysis of Twitter trends. *JMIR Public Health and Surveillance, 6*(2). e19447. https://doi.org/10.2196/19447

McGregor, I., Nail, P. R., Marigold, D. C., & Kang, S. J. (2005). Defensive pride and consensus: Strength in imaginary numbers. *Journal of Personality and Social Psychology, 89*(6), 978–996. https://doi.org/10.1037/0022-3514.89.6.978

McGregor, I., Prentice, M., & Nash, K. (2013). Anxious uncertainty and reactive approach motivation (RAM) for religious, idealistic, and lifestyle extremes. *Journal of Social Issues, 69*(3), 537–563. https://doi.org/10.1111/josi.12028

Neumann-Böhme, S., Varghese, N. E., & Sabat, I. (2020). Once we have it, will we use it? A European survey on willingness to be vaccinated against COVID-19. *European Journal Health Economics.* 21, 977–982. https://doi.org/10.1007/s10198-020-01208-6

Newheiser, A. K., Farias, M., & Tausch, N. (2011). The functional nature of conspiracy beliefs: Examining the underpinnings of belief in the Da Vinci Code conspiracy. *Personality and Individual Differences, 51*(8), 1007–1011. https://doi.org/10.1016/j.paid.2011.08.011

Peretti-Watel, P., Seror, V., Cortaredona, S., Launay, O., Raude, J., Verger, P., Fressard, L., Beck, F., Legleye, S., L'Haridon, O., Léger, D., & Ward, J. K. (2020). A future vaccination campaign against COVID-19 at risk of vaccine hesitancy and politicisation. *The Lancet Infectious Diseases, 20*(7), 769–770. https://doi.org/10.1016/S1473-3099(20)30426-6

Poppelaars, E. S., Harrewijn, A., Westenberg, P. M., & van der Molen, M. J. W. (2018). Frontal delta-beta cross-frequency coupling in high and low social anxiety: An index of stress regulation? *Cognitive, Affective, & Behavioral Neuroscience, 18*(4), 764–777. https://doi.org/10.3758/s13415-018-0603-7

Pyszczynski, T., Greenberg, J., & Solomon, S. (1999). A dual-process model of defence against conscious and unconscious death-related thoughts: An extension of terror management theory. *Psychological Review, 106*(4), 835–845. https://doi.org/10.1037/0033-295X.106.4.835

Pyszczynski, T., Lockett, M., Greenberg, J., & Solomon, S. (2020). Terror management theory and the COVID-19 pandemic. *Journal of Humanistic Psychology, 61*(2), 173–189. https://doi.org/10.1177/0022167820959488

Reiss, S., Franchina, V., Jutzi, C., Willardt, R., & Jonas, E. (2020). From anxiety to action—Experience of threat, emotional states, reactance, and action preferences in the early days of COVID-19 self-isolation in Germany and Austria. *PLoS One, 15*(12), e0243193. https://doi.org/10.1371/journal.pone.0243193

Reiss, S., Leen-Thomele, E., Klackl, J., & Jonas, E. (2021). Exploring the landscape of psychological threat: A cartography of threats and threat responses. *Social and Personality Psychology Compass, 15*(4), e12588. https://doi.org/10.1111/spc3.12588

Salali, G. D., & Uysal, M. S. (2020). COVID-19 vaccine hesitancy is associated with beliefs on the origin of the novel coronavirus in the U.K. and Turkey. *Psychological Medicine, 52*(15), 3750–3752. https://doi.org/10.1017/S0033291720004067

Salas, R. N., Shultz, J. M., & Solomon, C. G. (2020). The climate crisis and Covid-19—A major threat to the pandemic response. *New England Journal of Medicine, 383*(11), e70. https://doi.org/10.1056/NEJMp2022011

Shepherd, S., Kay, A. C., Landau, M. J., & Keefer, L. A. (2011). Evidence for the specificity of control motivations in worldview defense: Distinguishing compensatory control from uncertainty management and terror management processes. *Journal of Experimental Social Psychology, 47*(5), 949–958. https://doi.org/10.1016/j.jesp.2011.03.026

United Nations World Tourism Organization. (2020, April 17). COVID-19 related travel restrictions. UNWTO. https://www.unwto.org/covid-19-travel-restrictions

FURTHER READING

Jonas, E., McGregor, I., Klackl, J., Agroskin, D., Fritsche, I., Holbrook, C., Nash, K., Proulx, T., & Quirin, M. (2014). Threat and defense: From anxiety to approach. In J. M. Olson & M. P. Zanna (Eds.), *Advances in experimental social psychology (Vol. 49,* pp. 219–286). Academic Press. https://doi.org/10.1016/B978-0-12-800052-6.00004-4. The chapter entails a comprehensive overview of the GPMTD, distinguishes it from other theories, and is therefore a must-read for anyone who wants to delve further into threat and defense research.

Jutzi, C. A., Willardt, R., Schmid, P. C., & Jonas, E. (2020). Between conspiracy beliefs, ingroup bias, and system justification: How people use defense strategies to cope with the threat of COVID-19. *Frontiers in Psychology, 11,* 578586. https://doi.org/10.3389/fpsyg.2020.578586. This recent article applies the GPMTD to the current pandemic and investigates how the effect of COVID-19 threat on worldview defenses is mediated by BIS activation.

48

Moving Past the Pandemic

Lessons Learned From Social Science

MONICA K. MILLER ■

INTRODUCTION

Without a doubt, the COVID-19 pandemic changed the world in countless ways. Many of these changes were cataloged in this book, especially in the four chapters in Section one. Spires and Miller opened the book with a summary of the many ways the world changed—from education and employment to social events and protesting. Everett's chapter focused on the laws and court rulings that were developed during the COVID-19 pandemic, while Lanterman conducted an ethical analysis of many of the unique and evolving dilemmas that arose during the pandemic. Bornstein and Miller discussed many of the public health policies that were adopted in response to the pandemic. These chapters illustrate the many ways the world changed as a result of the pandemic—and suggest how the future will forever be marked by the pandemic.

Although it would be possible to write numerous books on how the pandemic changed the world, this book focused on one specific area: social science. Specifically, this book's aim was to offer a variety of ways in which social science played a part in the pandemic. In doing so, several themes emerged. First, the theme of "well-being" emerged in many ways, ranging from the well-being of individual people, small groups (including relationships), and societies. Second, the themes of resilience and positivity arose in many chapters. Some authors focused on both individual and group resilience, while others focused on the positive changes that arose due to the pandemic. A third theme was that of trust in authorities: how leaders encouraged trust and how trust was dependent on psychological processes and personal experiences.

Finally, the fourth theme was that of future directions for research. As editor, I hope that this theme represents the biggest contribution of the book. Authors

Monica K. Miller, *Moving Past the Pandemic* In: *The Social Science of the COVID-19 Pandemic.* Edited by: Monica K. Miller, Oxford University Press. © Oxford University Press 2024. DOI: 10.1093/oso/9780197615133.003.0048 highlighted the lessons learned from the pandemic and suggested ways that social science can help repair the initial harms caused by the pandemic, address the ongoing effects of the pandemic, and prepare for future crises by focusing on both the negative and positive outcomes of the pandemic. Not only can social science researchers use the ideas included here as a foundation for future research, but also I hope that it will promote well-being of people and society.

WELL-BEING

The first theme that emerged across many chapters in this volume is that of well-being. Well-being is the physical or mental health of a person, a small group (e.g., family), or society. Most obviously, the pandemic affected the physical well-being of those who contracted the virus. But, it also affected families who struggled with quarantining and working from home. It also affected societies as economies struggled and unrest emerged in the form of protests and refusal to obey health mandates. These are but a few examples of how the pandemic affected well-being.

Personal Well-Being

Many of the chapters in this book focused on well-being at the person level. This includes psychological processes that could affect either physical or mental well-being. Factors related to a person's gender or race could affect their well-being during the pandemic. For instance, gender norms can affect well-being if they put a person at higher risk of infection. Uysal and colleagues noted that men who subscribe to masculine and patriarchal norms are less risk avoidant, putting them at greater risk of contracting COVID. Race also plays a role in a person's well-being. Willis-Esqueda and Estrada-Reynolds discussed how structural and systemic disadvantages have made Native Americans, Latinos, and Blacks more vulnerable to well-being threats related to employment, education, and income. For instance, minorities are less likely to have occupations that allow them to work from home. Instead, they face risks in face-to-face occupations that leave them at heightened risk for infection.

In addition to social level risk factors (gender and racial factors), several social cognitive judgment errors put people at risk for infection harming physical well-being. First, Miller and Cabell noted how people intentionally seek information and sources (e.g., friends, news) that support their preexisting opinions and avoid information and sources that discredit their opinions. This can prevent changes in opinions (e.g., that vaccines are ineffective) that could promote well-being. A second judgment error was discussed by Nese and colleagues, who described how people often choose the certain and immediate benefits (e.g., going out with friends) over long-term and less certain benefits (e.g., preventing a possible infection). Third, Zell and Sedikides suggested that self-enhancement could lead people to believe that their COVID-19-related behaviors (e.g., their knowledge, health, likelihood of infection, and recovery time) would be more favorable than that of others. This bias could lead to risky behavior. Finally, Kim and colleagues discussed how reactance theory would predict that prevention measures (e.g., stay-home orders) likely made some people feel that their personal freedom was threatened. As such, these people reacted by engaging in these forbidden activities anyway—violating government-issued orders and even sometimes resorting to protesting and violence. As a result of these judgment errors, the individual person's own *physical* well-being is threatened (e.g., they might contract the virus or experience negative outcomes related to their reactions).

Other chapters focused more on *mental* well-being. For instance, Wildschut and Sedikides highlighted how boredom and loneliness can negatively affect psychological adjustment during the pandemic. Garfin and Estes discussed the public mental health crisis that arose from the pandemic. Contributing factors include personal losses (e.g., loss of health or loved ones), secondary stressors (e.g., job loss), and policies designed to mitigate viral spread (e.g., social distancing). A variety of losses and life changes harmed the mental well-being of many people.

Researchers are not immune to mental health effects—and could even be at heightened risk if they are conducting research with people who have suffered greatly due to the pandemic. Hughes et al. used the theoretical framework of "emotional labor" to describe some of the emotional aspects of conducting such research. All of these examples illustrate how the pandemic affected personal well-being.

Group Well-Being

Some chapters focused on well-being at the small-group level. These groups could be dyads such as romantic relationships or doctor-patient relationships. They could also be friend groups, families, or organizations. For instance, Capraro et al. discussed science-based messaging that could encourage prosocial and cooperative responses to the COVID-19 pandemic (e.g., distancing and mask wearing), prevent spreading the virus, and protect the well-being of one's social and familial groups. Such interventions would only work, however, if the group perceived the virus as a threat. Kityama noted that many people might have suspected that COVID-19 was a threat; however, they failed to act if most people in their social group were not taking actions to mitigate the spread of the virus. In these groups, a collective failure to act results when every person in the group underestimates other group members' anxiety related to the threat—an effect called pluralistic ignorance. As a result, the entire social group could face threats to their well-being if they fail to act because they are all making the same judgment error—that no one else is concerned—ultimately increasing risk of infection in that group.

In addition to the threats to group-level physical well-being posed by infection, the pandemic posed threats to the well-being of social *relationships*. Bayer and colleagues used the transformational framework to examine how social media hindered or encouraged efforts to maintain relationships with other people during the pandemic. As such, the health of these relationships could be enhanced or harmed by restrictions on gatherings and other policies leading to isolation.

Some family groups were especially vulnerable to the well-being threats during the pandemic. For instance, Mortensen et al. focused on mothers' mental health and parenting ability. They noted that mothers were disproportionally affected during the pandemic as they dealt with changing child care and schooling situations—while also trying to manage a career. The resulting instability produced threats to the family system and functioning, which the authors studied using a family systems approach.

More broadly, the well-being of relationships of all types was threatened. Pietromonaco and Overall discussed the challenges couples faced, including new financial burdens, changes to children's routines, and loss of normalcy. Such challenges, coupled with preexisting stressors, could affect a couple's ability to be supportive and their overall relationship quality. In extreme instances, the pandemic increased the risk of family abuse. Peoples and Furlano noted how the pandemic led to constrained networks and remote interactions (e.g., online school and employment, stay-home orders). These limitations on social support can increase the risk for family abuse (mental and physical) and deterioration of the family unit. All of these examples highlight the pandemic's effects on small groups.

Societal Well-Being

Some of the book's chapters focused on well-being at the societal level. For instance, the pandemic heightened social inequality, created social disruption and prompted widespread moral panic. Although the virus created a global threat, each individual person played an important role as they chose whether to get vaccinated or wear a mask. Such compliance varied by characteristics of the society (e.g., individualistic culture). In this way, each individual person's acts affect the well-being of society.

The interaction between the individual person and greater society was critical to pandemic outcomes in many aspects. For instance, Devereux and colleagues suggested that science-based public health messages can encourage people to promote global physical well-being by receiving a vaccine, noting that millions worldwide will need to be vaccinated to effectively end the pandemic. This means every person can act to promote societal well-being, but this does not always happen. Kityama applied the principles of "tragedy of the commons" to the pandemic. This concept refers to harm individual people cause to the public good (e.g., a virus-free environment) when they focus instead on their selfish personal interests (e.g., not wearing a mask). Individualist societies that value each person's autonomy and freedom over the collective good might experience this phenomenon more than collectivist societies.

Acting in selfish ways that harm the greater societal well-being was but one negative aspect of the pandemic. Gjonska noted that the pandemic caused an increased sense of alarm, fear, anxiety, and depression globally. This resulted in moral panic, a social phenomenon characterized by overreactions toward people, groups, behaviors, and events that were perceived as threats. The chapter by Kityama and the chapter by Estrada-Reynolds and Willis-Esqueda both expanded on this concept by focusing on xenophobia, prejudice, and stigma associated with the pandemic. Crimes against Asian Americans highlight how fear and stress of the pandemic exaggerated the tendency to dislike members of one's outgroup, especially if they are blamed for the pandemic. In this way, the pandemic harmed society by creating unrest, violence, and inequality (see generally Bresnahan et al., 2023, for a review of 50 articles about pandemic-related anti-Asian stigma).

Furthering this notion, Berthelot and Bornstein noted how the COVID-19 pandemic exacerbated the structural inequality in health and healthcare. Specifically, they used theory to explain how people of color, older adults, and those of low socioeconomic status had more negative health outcomes than other groups in society. Similarly, Bilewicz and Babińska concluded that countries and minority groups that have experienced historical and personal victimization could develop maladaptive responses to COVID-19 (e.g., failure to comply). These phenomena can shape society, amplifying social disparities that negatively affect well-being.

While some threats to social well-being affect the entire society, some target one type of culture or subgroup more than others. For instance, Gelfand and colleagues noted: "Cultures that are 'tight' tend to have strict social norms and strict penalties for deviance (e.g., China, Japan) compared to 'loose' (e.g., United States, Brazil) cultures with permissive behavior and weak social norms"; this highlights how looseness can be detrimental to some societies during the pandemic. Specifically, loose cultures might be more prone to longer term, more extreme negative outcomes (e.g., more deaths) than tight cultures.

Similarly, countries that have had traumatic lived experiences were exposed to more extreme effects on social well-being. Jeftić and Sasao examined how some containment measures (e.g., curfew and lockdown) might affect the mental well-being of some societies more than others. Specifically, they found that these measures acted as trauma reminders for people who survived the 1992–1995 war in Bosnia. They concluded that societies previously affected by war can experience more extreme PTSD symptoms and higher levels of perceived stress.

Lin and Druckman noted how the existential threat caused by the pandemic resulted in political polarization, which divided many countries, including the United States. Horner et al. noted that "people strived to uphold and affirm their worldviews as well as maintain a sense of value and meaning" and that this "intensified concerns with other social issues and increased the motivation for things such as protests in support of the Black Lives Matter movement among many liberals and claims of fraud in results of the 2020 presidential election among many conservatives." Such polarization negatively affects society well-being when parties' beliefs become so dissimilar that the parties cannot cooperate or tolerate differences.

Horner et al. noted how "death awareness" prompted more favorable attitudes toward products made domestically compared to products made in other countries. This chapter, along with the chapter authored by Estrada-Reynolds and

Willis-Esqueda, also noted how the pandemic increased xenophobia, racism, and stereotyping. These chapters gave examples such as calling the virus the "China virus," avoiding Chinese restaurants, and committing hate crimes against Asians. Additionally, West and Yelderman relied on theory to describe how societies might become more conservative in their moral beliefs and behaviors. This has implications for intergroup relations and society as a whole. For instance, ingroup favoritism and outgroup bias could increase—leading to disproportionately harsh punishment for minority groups.

Finally, Tyrala noted that there could be global repercussions of the pandemic. This chapter described how a capitalist economy produces dangerous asymmetrical power between countries. This increases social divides and inequality among countries, making it difficult to have a global response to crises such as a pandemic. All of these examples illustrate how the pandemic had negative effects on societal well-being.

RESILIENCE AND POSITIVE OUTCOMES OF THE PANDEMIC

A second theme that emerged from the chapters was that of resilience and positivity associated with the pandemic. These chapters indicated how social science can explain instances of individual and group-level resilience that occurred during the pandemic. Others highlighted the positive outcomes that also arose from the pandemic. People helped their neighbors and got vaccinated to promote the greater good. Kinsella and Sumner encouraged researchers to study both the trauma and the positive outcomes associated with the pandemic. They shared their experiences conducting research related to the pandemic—focusing on both negatives (e.g., anxiety) and positives (e.g., post-traumatic growth) of the frontline workers they studied.

More broadly, the authors in this book highlighted both individual-level and group-level resilience. Garfin and Estes highlighted how "individual factors and emerging resources (e.g., telehealth online self-care apps) have the potential to increase resilience and recovery for individuals grappling with the psychological effects of COVID-19-related distress."

As for group-level resilience, Cocking et al. noted how groups acted (typically in an orderly fashion) in solidarity and cooperation. They explained this solidarity using the social identity model of collective psychosocial resilience. This model suggests that people develop a shared social identity in response to experiencing a common crisis. This shared identity results in cooperation and social support seen widely during the pandemic. Flander et al. described such helping behavior that arose in Croatia to promote mental health and psychological resilience of children and families. Similarly, Horner and colleagues noted that the pandemic prompted some people to keep death-related anxiety at bay by reaffirming their values and meaning in life. They offered suggestions for how these motivations could be encouraged post-pandemic to encourage prosocial and benevolent values.

In addition to resilience, there were many other positive things that emerged during the pandemic. Horner and colleagues noted that many people sought meaning and self-worth by pursuing new goals, hobbies, and creative social events (e.g., Zoom get-togethers). Further, coping mechanisms based in psychology also brought about positive outcomes for some people, as noted by Wildschut and Sedikides. They illustrated how nostalgia can promote social connectedness and strengthen a person's meaning in life. Nostalgia reduces the negative impacts of the pandemic by reducing boredom and distress and promoting homeostasis. Such concepts could be used to create preventions or treatments to promote health.

Multiple chapters discussed how the pandemic can be used to create a more positive future. Van der Linden noted how the pandemic furthered an existing movement to study how to prevent misinformation. Tools such as their browser game *Go Viral!* could help people build psychological resistance against fake news in order to prevent misinformation from spreading. As such, the pandemic has helped develop a tool for prevention of the spread of both current and future misinformation regarding many topics. Also looking to the future, Wojcik suggested how the pandemic could be used as a springboard to encourage societies to restart their economies in more environmentally friendly ways. They suggested several ways that behaviors and beliefs could be transformed in order to support a more sustainable future.

TRUST IN AUTHORITIES

Another theme found in multiple chapters is that of trust of authorities— specifically healthcare providers and government leaders. For instance, Stedham and Mueller noted how some leaders were much more effective than others during the pandemic. Transformational leaders are more trustworthy because they behave in particular ways, including "individualized consideration, intellectual stimulation, inspirational motivation, and idealized influence." These behaviors create a shared sense of togetherness rather than a sense of "everyone for themselves." As such, authorities' decisions and behaviors played a role in the development of trust with those they lead.

The behavior of individual people also affected trust. For instance, Blank noted how individual psychological processes affect how much a person trusts authorities. He described the process of hindsight bias (in which a person sees an outcome as foreseeable) and outcome bias (in which a person evaluates another person's behavior based on the outcome). In both of these processes, a person is blamed for a bad outcome, even if the outcome was uncertain—as many things were with the pandemic. When someone engages in these biased processes, it can negatively affect their trust in the person who is blamed for behaving in a way that had a negative outcome, even though the outcome was not foreseeable based on knowledge available at the time of the behavior.

Trust is particularly relevant to some groups who have historically weak relationships with authorities. As noted, the chapter by Berthelot and Bornstein noted that many structural inequalities were exacerbated by COVID-19. For instance, people of a minority race were less likely to live near a vaccination site or have transportation to travel to a site. More broadly, they were more likely to have face-to-face jobs and were less likely to have the resources (Internet and technology) to do school from home, as discussed by Willis-Esqueda and Estrada-Reynolds. The authors of these two chapters, as well as the chapter by Bilewicz and Babińska, discussed issues related to both historical and contemporary (mis)trust of those who are of a minority group.

There are a number of negative consequences that result from mistrust in authorities. Bornstein and Emler noted that people's trust in their healthcare providers and healthcare systems plays an important part in protecting people's physical health—while noting that such relationships are uniquely strained by the COVID-19 pandemic. Theory on trust in such relationships provides important insight as to how COVID-19 affects well-being. Gjoneska's chapter expanded on this issue of trust by noting that a lack of scientific consensus and distrust in public authorities resulted in moral grandstanding and disengagement for some, who then refused to comply with measures (e.g., vaccines) that could protect physical health. More broadly, Tyrala noted that the pandemic has created mistrust among societies, which can hinder public health measures and cooperation.

FUTURE DIRECTIONS

Most of the chapters in this book offered directions for future research and policy. Some of these future directions are psychological in nature; for instance, Siev and colleagues discussed how characteristics of an attitude (e.g., attitude strength) and message (e.g., one or two sided) can affect someone's willingness to attend to that message designed to persuade them to comply with pandemic guidelines. Similarly, Landy and Perry offered theory-based recommendations for improving messages, which could improve pandemic outcomes. A related future direction is to test group differences and individual differences. For instance, Prusaczyk and colleagues suggested that sexual objectification might lead men and women to respond differently to a threat such as the COVID-19 pandemic. Thus, future research could further study gender differences to determine whether some strategies would be differentially effective in encouraging compliance with protective measures. Similarly, Devereaux discussed various individual differences, such as just world beliefs, moral disengagement, and locus of control. Each of these personal traits involve judgments about the world, and these judgments in turn affect a person's behavior. Thus, by understanding *who* is most likely to comply— or not—it is possible to design more effective messages to promote compliance.

Finally, some future directions concern how to do research. Murphy and Boppre offered advice on how to conduct community sentiment research related to the pandemic, while Schoenegger and Pummer offered suggestions to address ethical issues in future research. Tuominen and Valli suggested that future researchers use a systematic approach to studying the effects of the pandemic and other crises, using dream reports as an example. Finally, Willardt et al. offered suggestions for choosing theory and statistics when studying complex topics like the pandemic.

CONCLUSION

The pandemic had an undeniable effect on nearly every aspect of life as we know it. As with many social events, social scientists jumped to action to study relevant behaviors, beliefs, and events. They explained what happened and predicted what will happen. They relied on "lessons learned" to offer suggestions for the future. At the core of all of this is theory. Social psychological theories have provided a helpful foundation for such study and analysis. The contributing authors have offered their valuable insights about how the pandemic interacted with social science. It is hoped that the theories and research offered here will prompt more such research, as indicated by the subtitle "A Call to Action."

As editor of this volume, I hope that the ideas put forth by these scholars will be useful in shaping future research, policy, and behavior. The lessons learned thus far, coupled with yet-to-be-tested theories, suggest numerous avenues for future research. Not only can this research help individual people and societies heal from the pandemic, but also it can help us prepare for future crises that are sure to arise. As researchers look to the future, we hope that the research and theory contained within can help promote a healthier tomorrow.

REFERENCE

Bresnahan, M., Zhu, Y., Hooper, A., Hipple, S., & Savoie, L. (2023). The negative health effects of anti-Asian stigma in the U.S. during COVID-19. *Stigma and Health, 8*(1), 115–123. https://doi.org/10.1037/sah0000375

INDEX

For the benefit of digital users, indexed terms that span two pages (e.g., 52–53) may, on occasion, appear on only one of those pages.

Tables, figures, and boxes are indicated by *t*, *f*, and *b* following the page number